Medical Terminology

Simplified

Fourth Edition

A Programmed Learning Approach by Body System

Medical Terminology

Simplified
Fourth Edition

A Programmed Learning Approach by Body System

Barbara A. Gylys (GĬL-ĭs), BS, MEd, CMA-A

Professor Emerita
College of Health and Human Services
University of Toledo
Toledo, Ohio

Regina M. Masters, BSN, MEd, RN, CMA

Medical Assisting Adjunct Faculty
Herzing University
Toledo, Ohio

F.A. Davis Company • Philadelphia

F. A. Davis Company
1915 Arch Street
Philadelphia, PA 19103
www.fadavis.com

Printed in the United States of America

Last digit indicates print number: 10 9 8 7 6 5 4

Senior Acquisitions Editor: Andy McPhee
Manager of Content Development: George W. Lang
Developmental Editor: Brenna H. Mayer
Art and Design Manager: Carolyn O'Brien

As new scientific information becomes available through basic and clinical research, recommended treatments and drug therapies undergo changes. The author(s) and publisher have done everything possible to make this book accurate, up to date, and in accord with accepted standards at the time of publication. The author(s), editors, and publisher are not responsible for errors or omissions or for consequences from application of the book, and make no warranty, expressed or implied, in regard to the contents of the book. Any practice described in this book should be applied by the reader in accordance with professional standards of care used in regard to the unique circumstances that may apply in each situation. The reader is advised always to check product information (package inserts) for changes and new information regarding dose and contraindications before administering any drug. Caution is especially urged when using new or infrequently ordered drugs.

Library of Congress Cataloging-in-Publication Data

Gylys, Barbara A.
    Medical terminology simplified: a programmed learning approach by body system/Barbara A. Gylys, Regina M. Masters.
    —4th ed.
      p.; cm.
    Includes index.
    ISBN 978-0-8036-2091-9
    1. Medicine—Terminology—Programmed instruction. I. Masters, Regina M., 1959- II. Title.
    [DNLM: 1. Terminology as Topic—Programmed Instruction. W 15 G997md 2010]
    R123.G935 2010
    610.1'4—dc22   2009041811

What's INSIDE...▶

Empower yourself with programmed learning and word building the *SIMPLIFIED WAY!*

MEDICAL TERMINOLOGY SIMPLIFIED
A Programmed Learning Approach by Body System, 4th Edition

HOW IT WORKS?

- Frame-based technique reinforces learning, not memorization.
- BONUS bookmark lets you quiz yourself by covering the answers.
- Content organized into small, easy-to-grasp sections, perfect for self-paced learning.
- Word-building concepts develop your knowledge step-by-step.
- Bonus interactive resources: Audio CD, Term*Plus* 3.0, and Davis*Plus* make learning an interactive, multimedia experience.

CHAPTER OBJECTIVES AND OUTLINES
provide guidance for the content to come.

chapter 1 Introduction to Programmed Learning and Medical Word Building

PROGRAMMED LEARNING
builds your medical vocabulary frame by frame and actively involves you in the process.

COMMONLY USED
prefixes, suffixes, and combining forms appear throughout.

Bonus Bookmark Study Tool!

Barbara A. Gylys
Regina M. Masters

MEDICAL RECORD ACTIVITIES

provide real-world case studies and critical-thinking exercises, including patient diagnosis and evaluation.

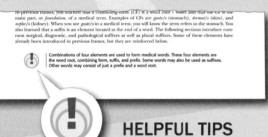

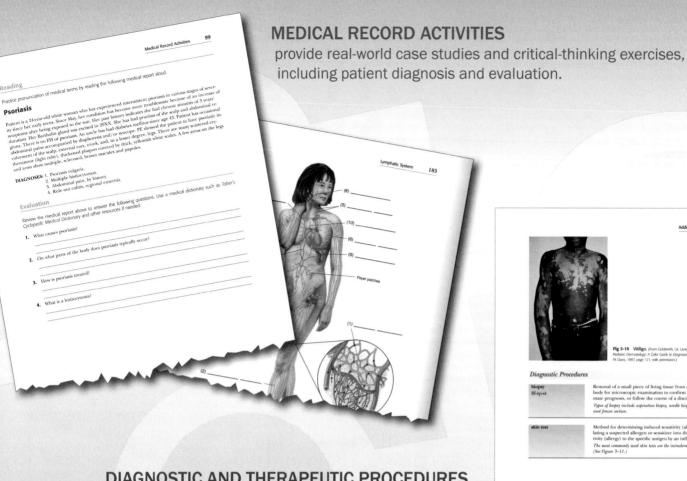

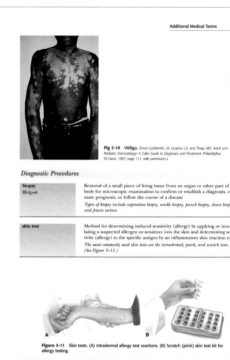

DIAGNOSTIC AND THERAPEUTIC PROCEDURES

clearly show how diseases and disorders are diagnosed and treated.

HELPFUL TIPS

appear throughout with an easy-to-locate **"!"** icon.

BULL'S-EYE ICONS

identify corresponding material online at Davis*Plus*.

EXERCISE AND ACTIVITY WORKSHEETS

in each chapter help you track your progress and prepare for quizzes and tests.

BRILLIANT FULL-COLOR ILLUSTRATIONS
leap from the page and enhance your understanding.

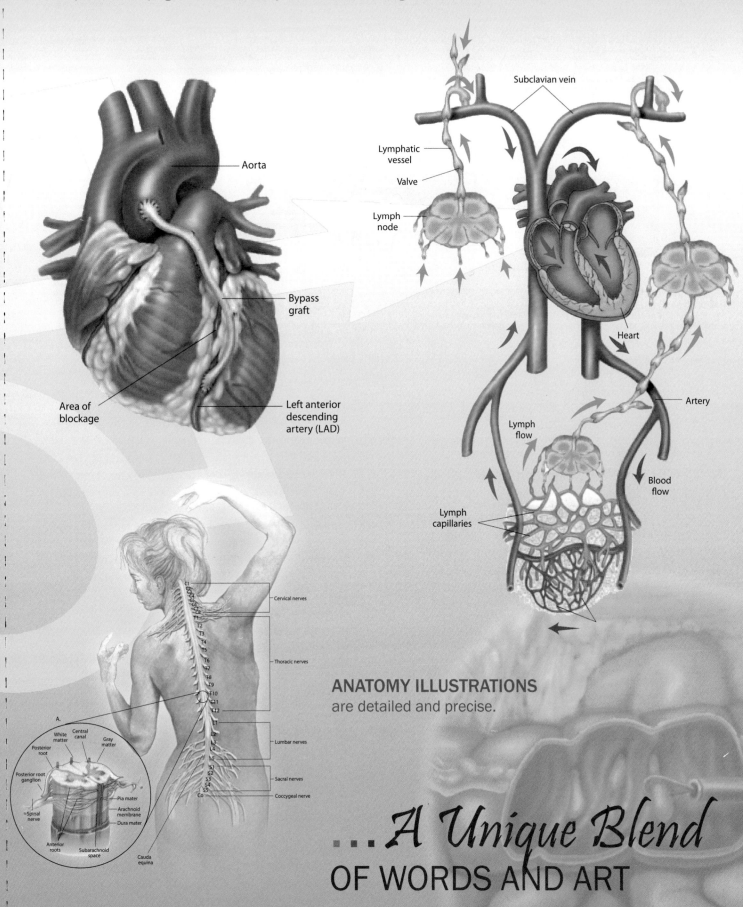

Aorta

Bypass graft

Area of blockage

Left anterior descending artery (LAD)

Subclavian vein

Lymphatic vessel

Valve

Lymph node

Heart

Lymph flow

Artery

Blood flow

Lymph capillaries

Cervical nerves

Thoracic nerves

Lumbar nerves

Sacral nerves

Coccygeal nerve

A.

White matter

Central canal

Gray matter

Posterior root

Posterior root ganglion

Spinal nerve

Anterior roots

Subarachnoid space

Pia mater

Arachnoid membrane

Dura mater

Cauda equina

ANATOMY ILLUSTRATIONS
are detailed and precise.

...A Unique Blend
OF WORDS AND ART

A COMPLETE LEARNING & TEACHING EXPERIENCE!

The full **Medical Terminology Simplified** package features the text, Term*Plus* 3.0*, Audio CD, and resources online at Davis*Plus*.

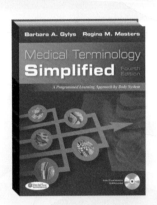

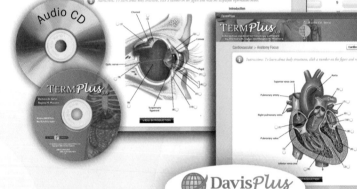

- **Audio CD**
  - Listen-and-Learn activities for more than 300 terms.

- **Term*Plus* 3.0***
  - Competency-based, self-paced.
  - Mac and PC compatible.
  - Interactive exercises, including anatomy labeling, crossword puzzles, word drag-and-drop, and word scrambles.

- **Student Resources Online at Davis*Plus***
  (No fee. No password. No registration.)
  - Audio pronunciations—downloadable to an iPod or MP3 player for study on the go.
  - Flash Card and Medical Record activities.
  - Word Search activities.
  - Animations—almost 20 in all.

  * Term*Plus* 3.0 available with full package only.

INSTRUCTOR RESOURCES
Available Upon Adoption
Online at Davis*Plus* and on CD-ROM

- **Activity Pack**—Instructor's Guide containing course outlines, bonus medical record activities, crossword puzzles, and more.
- **Interactive Teaching Tool**—51 body system activities.
- **Electronic Test Bank**—Customizable Wimba Test Bank with more than 850 questions.
- **Image Ancillary**—Nearly 200 images from the book.
- **PowerPoint Presentations**—4 PowerPoint presentations: Lecture Notes, MedTerm Tester (compatible with clicker technology,) MedTerm Workout, and Name that Part. ("READ ME" files provide tips for use.)
- **Additional Resources**—Supplemental medical record activities, pronunciations, flash cards, animations, and more, online at Davis*Plus*.

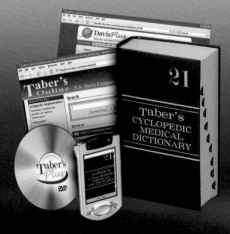

TABER'S CYCLOPEDIC MEDICAL DICTIONARY, 21ST EDITION

Edited by Donald Venes, MD, MSJ

Taber's brings meanings to life! To thrive in the ever-changing world of health care, you need a respected, trusted, and cutting-edge cyclopedic resource. In hand, online, or on your mobile device—anywhere and everywhere—turn to Taber's 21 and the Taber's*Plus* DVD.

WWW.FADAVIS.COM

This Book is Dedicated with Love

to my best friend, colleague, and husband, Julius A. Gylys
and
to my children, Regina Maria and Julius A., II
and
to Andrew Masters, Julia Masters,
Caitlin Masters, Anthony Mychal Bishop-Gylys,
and Matthew James Bishop-Gylys

—BARBARA GYLYS

to my mother, best friend, mentor, and co-author, Barbara A. Gylys
and
to my father, Julius A. Gylys
and
to my husband, Bruce Masters, and my children Andrew, Julia, and Caitlin,
all of whom have given me continuous encouragement and support

—REGINA MASTERS

Preface

The fourth edition of *Medical Terminology Simplified: A Programmed Learning Approach by Body System* continues to reflect current trends and new approaches to teaching medical terminology. This edition includes a variety of special features to make studying medical terminology a more rewarding experience. The new features have been developed based on feedback from instructors and students. A review of the "What's Inside" section provides explanations and illustrations about all of the text's distinctive features. The design and flexibility of *Simplified*, 4th edition, enables its use as a self-instructional book or in traditional lecture and classroom environments. The organization and pedagogical devices are designed to help instructors teach and students learn medical terminology easily and quickly. When students use the available learning tools, they will find the language of medicine stays with them and they can quickly apply the terminology in the clinical field.

This edition also continues to present eponyms without showing the possessive form, such as Alzheimer disease, Down syndrome, and Parkinson disease. Medical dictionaries as well as the American Association for Medical Transcription and the American Medical Association support these changes. New to this edition is a summary of common symbols as well as an updated list of "do-not-use" abbreviations found in Appendix E, Abbreviations and Symbols. In addition, all outdated medical terms in the textbook have been replaced with the most recent, state-of-the-art terms.

Helping Learners of All Styles

All enhancements and new material in the fourth edition are constructed to improve retention and make the study of medical terminology more enjoyable and engaging. One of the top priorities of this edition, as more and more students identify themselves as visual learners, is to ensure that the illustrations in the text and ancillary products are as helpful to students as possible. Many of the figures depicting the toughest topics for students to grasp have been newly developed; others from the previous edition have been enhanced for more clarity and ease of understanding. Thus, one of the most extraordinary features of this edition is the collection of all-new, visually outstanding, full-color illustrations. They are extremely useful as your students learn the association of medical terms to anatomy, physiology, pathology, and medical treatments of the human body. All of the artwork presents precise depictions of medical terms in action. Full-color figures enable you to see a true representation of the body system, pathological condition, or operative procedure.

It is clear among educators that the most effective method of learning medical terminology is to associate the terms in their appropriate relationship to the human body. This method includes acquiring an understanding of anatomy and physiology, the types of treatments used to cure various disorders, and the disease processes of the human body—all of which are covered in *Simplified*, 4th edition.

Programmed Learning Approach

The programmed learning approach of this book presents a word-building method for developing a medical vocabulary in an effective and interesting manner. A student can use it in a traditional classroom setting or with guidance from an instructor for independent study. The workbook text format is designed to guide the student through exercises that teach and reinforce medical terminology.

The programmed-learning technique makes use of *frames*, isolated pieces of information that, together, give the student the building blocks of medical terminology. The frames, each numbered with the chapter number and then the frame number within that chapter, allow students to learn at their own pace and in their own way. Each frame contains not only information about terminology but also fill-in lines students can use to reinforce understanding of the information. The student can find the answer to each fill-in line in the frame's answer box, located at the left of the page.

The key to using frames wisely is the bookmark included with every book. Students should use it to cover the answer column to verify their understanding of the content provided in the frame. Pronunciation keys for all medical words are also included in the frame answer boxes. Newly designed pronunciation guides in each chapter help students pronounce medical terms correctly.

New Features

To continue developing a contemporary teaching and learning package, we have implemented a number of insightful suggestions from numerous educators and students and updated each body system chapter, including:

- *Newly designed medical specialty section at the beginning of each body system chapter* shows students the connection between the body system and its respective medical specialty. This enhancement provides students with an understanding of the responsibilities of health care professionals in various branches of medicine.
- *New summaries of common suffixes and prefixes are presented in Chapter 1.* The tables also include an interactive activity to reinforce the student's knowledge of presented medical terms.
- *Enhanced objectives at the beginning of each chapter* continue to help students understand what is essential in the chapter. The reviews and activities are linked directly to these objectives, so both instructors and students can better evaluate competency in each area of study. If the student has not mastered a certain area, they can apply the objectives as a study instrument to help their understanding of the chapter.
- *New pronunciation guides* help students pronounce medical terms correctly.
- *Newly designed Additional Medical Terms section* helps students understand the connection between common signs, symptoms, and diseases and their diagnoses as well as the rationale behind methods of medical and surgical treatments selected for a particular disorder.
- *New flash-card activities* are now available by visiting *http://davisplus.fadavis.com/gylys/simplified* and downloading each chapter's *Listen-and-Learn* exercises. A special icon with instructions directs students to the site so they can preview, practice, and reinforce word elements presented in the chapter.
- *New Symbols section* in the Abbreviations appendix lists common symbols used in charting and other areas of health care.
- *Enhanced translations appendix* makes it easier for health-care providers who do not speak Spanish to communicate with their Spanish-speaking patients.

The popular and effective features found in the previous edition have been expanded and enhanced. Here's a breakdown of those features:

- *Chapter 1* introduces the programmed learning and the medical word-building approach. It also includes a summary of common suffixes and prefixes used in medical word building.
- *Chapter 2* discusses the structural organization of the human body.
- *Chapters 3 to 11* are organized according to specific body systems and may be taught in any sequence. These chapters include key anatomical and physiological terms; anatomy and physiology; combining forms, suffixes, and prefixes; terms related to signs, symptoms, and diseases as well as diagnostic, surgical and medical procedures; and abbreviations. Included are section reviews and medical record activities. All activities allow self-assessment and evaluation of competency.

Appendices

The textbook's appendices also offer learning tools to help reinforce the information presented in the chapters. Your students will also find the appendices useful for study, review, and reference as they begin their careers in the allied heath field:

- *Appendix A: Glossary of Medical Word Elements* contains alphabetical lists of medical word elements with corresponding meanings.
- *Appendix B: Answer Key* provides answers to anatomical labeling and section and chapter reviews as well as the medical records activities.
- *Appendix C: Index of Diagnostic, Medical, and Surgical Procedures* summarizes procedures covered in the textbook that establish a diagnosis as well as various methods of treatment.
- *Appendix D: Drug Classifications* provides information on prescription and nonprescription drugs used for the treatment of various medical conditions.

- *Appendix E: Abbreviations and Symbols* summarizes commonly used medical abbreviations and symbols, including their meanings.
- *Appendix F: Medical Specialties* provides a summary and description of medical specialties.
- *Appendix G: Spanish Translations* is a newly enhanced appendix of English-to-Spanish vocabulary and phrases relevant to various medical specialties. It is intended to help health-care providers who do not speak Spanish but who encounter Spanish-speaking patients in the medical environment.

Teaching and Learning Package

Numerous teaching aids are available free of charge to instructors who adopt the fourth edition of *Medical Terminology Simplified: A Programmed Learning Approach by Body System*. These supplemental teaching aids contain an abundance of information and activities to help students retain what they have learned in a given chapter. The various types of ancillary tools are designed to enhance course content that ensures students a program of excellence in a medical terminology curriculum. The ancillary products will also help you plan course work and provides you with various types of presentations to reinforce the learning process. These teaching aids include the Instructor's Resource Disk and DavisPlus, a web-based resource.

Instructor's Resource Disk

The Instructor's Resource Disk (IRD) contains an abundance of supplemental teaching aids designed to help students learn medical terminology and help instructors plan course work and enhance presentations. You can use these teaching tools in various educational settings, including the traditional classroom, distance learning, or independent studies. When you integrate them into course content, they will provide a sound foundation for developing an extensive medical vocabulary and guarantee a full program of medical terminology excellence for all of your students. The IRD includes:

- Activity Pack
- PowerPoint presentations, including Lecture Notes, MedTERM Workout, Name that Part, and MedTerm Tester
- Interactive Teaching Tool (ITT)
- Image bank with easily retrievable images
- Wimba computerized test bank, a powerful, user-friendly test-generation program

Activity Pack: Your Instructional Resource Kit

The Activity Pack is a resource full of instructional support for using the textbook and ancillary products. It is available in PDF format on the IRD. A bound copy of the entire Activity Pack is also available upon request. In addition, instructors who wish to custom tailor the material can request the Activity Pack in a Microsoft Word document. The fourth edition of the Activity Pack includes:

- *Course Outlines.* Suggested course outlines help you determine a comfortable pace and plan the best method of covering the material presented in the textbook.
- *Clinical Connection Activities.* These activities integrate clinical scenarios in each chapter as a solid reinforcement of content. Feel free to select activities you deem suitable for your course and decide whether the students should complete the activity independently, with peers, or as a group project.
- *Student and Instructor-Directed Activities* are updated teaching aids with new ones added for this edition. They offer a variety of activities for each body system chapter. Activities can serve as course requirements or supplemental material. In addition, you can assign them as individual or collaborative projects. For group projects, Peer Evaluation Forms are provided.
- *Oral and Written Research Projects.* The research projects provide an opportunity for your students to hone their research skills. The *Community and Internet Resources* section offers an updated list of technical journals, community organizations, and Internet sources that students can use to complete the oral and written projects. This section also includes an evaluation template for the oral and written research projects. These projects will add variety and interest to your course while reinforcing the learning process.

- *Anatomy Test Questions.* You can use the anatomy test questions for anatomy review or as a testing device. These questions also include an illustration for each body system chapter. An answer key is also provided.
- *Supplemental Medical Record Activities.* We have updated the supplemental medical record activities and added new activities to this edition. As in the textbook, these medical record activities use common clinical scenarios to show how the student would use medical terminology in the clinical area to document patient care. Each medical record includes activities for terminology, pronunciation, and medical record analysis. In addition, each medical record focuses on a specific medical specialty. You can use these records for group activities, oral reports, medical coding activities, or individual assignments. The medical records are designed to reinforce and enhance terminology presented in the textbook. An answer key is also provided.
- *Crossword Puzzles.* These fun, educational activities reinforce material covered in each body system chapter. You can use them for an individual or group activity, an extra credit opportunity, or "just for fun." An answer key is included for each puzzle.
- *Anatomy Coloring Activities.* Anatomy coloring activities, included for each body-system chapter, help reinforce the positions of the main organs that compose a particular body system.
- *Terminology Answer Keys.* In response to requests we have received from instructors like you, this section summarizes the answers to the *Terminology* tables in the medical records sections of the textbook. This added feature provides instructional support in using the textbook and assists you in correcting terminology assignments.
- *Master Transparencies.* The transparency pages offer large, clear, black-and-white medical illustrations from selected figures in the text. We have chosen each for its value in reinforcing lecture information. These master transparencies, provided for each body system, are perfect for making overhead transparencies or teaching with a document camera.

PowerPoint Presentations

This latest edition of *Simplified's* Activity Pack contains four *PowerPoint* presentations for your use:

- *Lecture Notes* provides an outline-based presentation for each body system chapter. It contains a chapter overview, the main functions of the body system, and selected pathology, vocabulary, and procedures for each. Full-color illustrations from the textbook are also included.
- *MedTERM Workout* is an interactive presentation in which key terms from a chapter swoop into view each time the presenter clicks the mouse. You can ask students to say the term aloud; define the term; identify the suffix, prefix, combining form, or combining element in each term; or provide other feedback before advancing to the next term.
- *Name that Part* is a unique interactive PowerPoint presentation that allows you to guide students in identifying specific parts of a body system.
- *MedTerm Tester* is an interactive clicker technology classroom activity that you can use for pathology review, short quizzes, or reinforcing course content.

Interactive Teaching Tool

The Interactive Teaching Tool (ITT) is a brand-new instructional aid for use in the classroom. The tool is an Adobe Flash application of images from the book, followed by questions and answers relevant to the illustration. You can zoom in to enlarge images and test students' knowledge as you lead discussion of the content.

Image Bank

New to this edition is an Adobe Flash–based image bank that contains all illustrations from the textbook. It is fully searchable and allows users to zoom in and out and display a JPG image of an illustration that can be copied into a Microsoft Word document or PowerPoint presentation.

Wimba Electronic Test Bank

This edition offers a powerful test-generating program called *Wimba.* It enables you to create custom-made or randomly generated tests in a printable format from a test bank of more than 850 test items, with 150 new test items for this edition. The test bank includes multiple-choice, true-false, and matching questions.

Because of the flexibility of the Wimba test-generating program, you can edit questions in the test bank to meet your specific educational needs. Therefore, if you wish to restate, embellish, or streamline questions or change distractors, you can do so with little effort. You can also add questions to the test bank. The Wimba program is available for Macintosh on request.

DavisPlusTeaching Tools

The DavisPlus web site, found at *http://davisplus.fadavis.com/gylys/simplified* is a study companion web site for *Simplified*, 4th edition. It provides activities to accelerate learning and reinforce information presented in each chapter. Special icons found within the chapters tells students when it is most advantageous to integrate the activities on the DavisPlus web site into their studies. All online exercises provide instructions for completing the various activities. The multimedia activities available on DavisPlus include:

- pronunciations of newly introduced medical terms from the word elements tables (chapters 2 through 11) to improve retention
- flash-card activities for preview and practice to reinforce word elements presented in the chapter
- medical record exercises (Chapters 3 through 11) that allow students to click highlighted terms in the medical record and hear their pronunciations and meanings to strengthen understanding of terms
- animations, such as exploration of the pathology of gastroesophageal reflux disease (GERD) or the various stages of pregnancy and delivery, to help students better understand complex processes and procedures
- word search games that present a variety of medical terms to reinforce word recognition and spelling in a fun activity

Audio CD

One audio CD is included free of charge in each textbook. The audio CD contains *Listen-and-Learn* exercises designed to strengthen spelling, pronounciation, and meanings of selected medical terms. They include pronunciation and spelling exercises for Chapters 2 through 11. The exercises provide continuous reinforcement of correct pronunciation, spelling, and usage of selected medical terms.

Medical secretarial and medical transcription students can also use the CD to learn beginning transcription skills by typing each word as it is pronounced. After typing the words, they can correct spelling by referring to the textbook or a medical dictionary. Finally, to evaluate student competency, a *Pronunciation, Spelling, and Transcription Activity Template* is provided in the Activity Pack.

TermPlus

Term*Plus* v3.0 is a powerful, interactive CD-ROM program offered with some texts, depending on which version has been selected. Term*Plus* is a competency-based, self-paced, multimedia program that includes graphics, audio, and a dictionary culled from *Taber's Cyclopedic Medical Dictionary*, 20th edition. Help menus provide navigational support. The software comes with numerous interactive learning activities, including:

- Anatomy Focus
- Tag the Elements-and-Drop)
- Spotlight the Elements
- Concentration
- Build Medical Words
- Programmed Learning
- Medical Vocabulary
- Chart Notes
- Spelling
- Crossword Puzzles
- Word Scramble
- Terminology Teaser

All activities can be graded and the results printed or e-mailed to an instructor. This feature makes the CD-ROM especially valuable as a distance-learning tool because it provides evidence of student drill and practice in various learning activities.

How to Use This Book

This self-instructional book is designed to provide the student with skills to learn medical terminology easily and quickly. A review of the "What's Inside" section provides insight, both visually and in narrative, into all of the text's distinctive features. The book's design and flexibility enables its use as a self-instructional book or one that can be used in traditional lecture and classroom environments. The following distinctive features are included in this learning package:

- The programmed learning approach presents a word-building method for developing a medical vocabulary in an effective and interesting manner. It is designed for use in a traditional classroom setting or for independent study with an instructor.
- The workbook-text format is designed to guide you through exercises that teach and reinforce medical terminology.
- Numerous activities in each unit are designed to enable the student to be mentally and physically involved in the learning process. With this method the student will not only understand but also remember the significant concepts of medical word building.
- Students learn by active participation. In this book, students write answers in response to blocks of information, complete section review exercises, and analyze medical reports. If a student is not satisfied with her level of comprehension after the review exercises, reinforcement frames direct the student to go back and rework the corresponding informational frames.
- New to this edition is a special icon in each chapter that directs the student to visit the *DavisPlus* web site at *http://davisplus.fadavis.com/gylys/simplified* for a flash-card review of word elements covered in the chapter.
- The *Listen-and-Learn* exercises provide reinforcement of pronunciation, definitions, and spelling practice of medical terms. The terms and pronunciations are now available by visiting the *DavisPlus* web site at *http://davisplus.fadavis.com/gylys/simplified.*
- Pronunciation keys for all medical words are included in the frame answer boxes and help the student pronounce each term correctly. Newly designed pronunciation guides in each chapter help students understand the pronunciation key for more accurate understanding of pronunciations.
- The appendices include many tools students can use as references when they begin working in the clinical field

We hope the pedagogical and visual features of *Medical Terminology Simplified: A Programmed Learning Approach by Body System,* 4th edition, make learning the language of medicine an exciting and rewarding process. We invite you to continue the tradition of sending your suggestions to the F.A. Davis Company so that we can consider them for the next edition.

BARBARA A. GYLYS
REGINA M. MASTERS

Reviewers

The authors extend a special thanks to the clinical reviewers and students who read and edited the manuscript and provided detailed evaluations and ideas for improving the textbook package.

We thank **Collette Bishop Hendler, RN, BS, CCRN,** ICU Clinical Leader at Abington (Pennsylvania) Memorial Hospital, for her thorough reviews and thoughtful feedback that helped improve the excellence of the final text and Activity Pack.

We are also grateful to **Sandra Andreev, BA,** George Washington University, for her meticulous review of the textbook, electronic testbank, and Activity Pack. Her forthright criticisms and helpful suggestions added immeasurably to the quality of the final text.

We extend our appreciation to **Laurie A. Pusczewicz,** Lecturer in the Department of Foreign Languages at the University of Toledo, for editing the Glossary of English-to-Spanish Translations and **Ticiano Alegre, MD**, Professor of Anatomy and Physiology at North Lake College, Arlington, Texas, for reviewing it.

Lastly, we extend our deepest gratitude to the following students:

- **Caitlin Masters,** a student at Indiana University in Indiana, who worked through the entire final copy of the textbook, evaluated the question bank, assisted in the audio recording template, and provided detailed suggestions for improving the textbook and Activity Pack.
- **Julia M. Masters, BS,** a fourth-year medical student at West Virginia School of Osteopathic Medicine in Lewisburg, who critiqued various sections of the manuscript.

F. A. Davis Medical Assistant Advisory Board

Pat Moeck, PhD, MBA, CMA (AAMA)
Director
Medical Assisting Program
El Centro College
Dallas, TX

Sharon Eagle, RN, MSN
Faculty
Nursing Program
Wenatchee Valley Community College
Wenatchee, WA

Marcie Jones, BS, CMA (AAMA)
Program Chair
Medical Assisting Program
Gwinnett Technical College
Lawrenceville, GA

Joanne Leming
Director
Allied Health Programs
Nevada Career Institute
Las Vegas, NV

Marti Lewis, EdD, RN, CMA-AC (AAMA)
Former Dean (retired)
Mathematics, Engineering, Science, and Health
Olympic College
Bremerton, WA

Lorraine Fleming McPhillips, MS, MT (ASCP), CMA (AAMA)
Allied Health Education Specialist
Branford, CT

Susan Perreira, MS, CMA (AAMA), RMA
Associate Professor and Coordinator
Medical Assisting Program
Capital Community College
Hartford, CT

Marilyn Reeder, MS, CMA (AAMA), CNA, CHUC
Instructor
Health Sciences and Medicine
GASC Technology Center
Flint, MI

Amy Semenchuk, RN, BSN
Department Chair
Health Occupations
Rockford Business College
Rockford, IL

Carol Tamparo, PhD, CMA (AAMA)
Former Dean of Health Sciences & Business (retired)
Lake Washington Technical College
Tacoma, WA

Claire Travis, BA, MA (Educ), MBA, CPHQ
Director
Allied Health
Salter School
Worcester, MS

LaTanya Young, RMA, PA-C, MMSc, MPH
Assistant Professor and Coordinator
Medical Assisting Program
Clayton State University
Morrow, GA

Acknowledgments

The fourth edition of *Medical Terminology Simplified: A Programmed Learning Approach by Body System* was greatly improved by comments that the authors received from the many users of previous editions—both educators and students. Although there are too many people to acknowledge individually, we are deeply grateful to each one. As in the past, the editorial and production staffs at F. A. Davis have inspired, guided, and shaped this project. The authors would like to acknowledge the valuable contributions of F .A. Davis's editorial and production team who were responsible for this project:

- Andy McPhee, Senior Acquisitions Editor, provided the overall design and layout for the fourth edition. He was instrumental in assisting the authors in designing a wide variety of state-of-the-art pedagogical products within the text to aid students in their learning activities and to help instructors plan course work and presentations. These teaching aids are described in the "Teaching and Learning Package" section of the Preface.
- George W. Lang, Manager of Content of Development, expertly guided the manuscript through the developmental and production phases of the process.
- Brenna H. Mayer, Developmental Editor, systematically and meticulously read the manuscript, helping it along at every stage. Her patience, creativity, and untiring assistance and support during this project were greatly appreciated, and the authors are grateful for all of her help.
- Margaret Biblis, Publisher, once again provided her support and efforts for the quality of the finished product.

We also acknowledge and thank our exceptionally dedicated publishing partners who helped guide and shape this large project:

Stephanie A. Casey, *Administrative Assistant*
Robert Butler, *Production Manager*
Yvonne N. Gillam, *Developmental Editor*
Kate Margeson, *Illustrations Coordinator*
Frank Musick, *Developmental Editor, Electronic Publishing*
Carolyn O'Brien, *Art and Design Manager*
David Orzechowski, *Managing Editor*
Kirk Pedrick, *Electronic Product Development Manager, Electronic Publishing*
Elizabeth Y. Stepchin, *Developmental Associate*

We also we extend our sincerest gratitude to Neil Kelly, Director of Sales, and his staff of sales representatives, whose continued efforts have undoubtedly contributed to the success of this textbook.

Contents at a Glance

APPENDICES

Contents

Chapter **4**

Respiratory System

Chapter **5**

Cardiovascular and Lymphatic Systems

Chapter **7**

Urinary System   271

Chapter **8**

Reproductive Systems

Chapter **9**

Endocrine and Nervous Systems

Appendices

1 Introduction to Programmed Learning and Medical Word Building

OBJECTIVES

Upon completion of this chapter, you will be able to:

- Learn medical terminology by using the programmed learning technique.
- Identify and define four elements used to build medical words.
- Analyze and define the various parts of a medical term.
- Apply the rules learned in this chapter to pronounce medical words correctly.
- Define and provide examples of surgical, diagnostic, pathological, and related suffixes.
- Apply the rules learned in this chapter to write singular and plural forms of medical words.
- Locate and apply guidelines for pluralizing terms.
- Practice pronouncing the medical terms presented in this chapter.
- Demonstrate your knowledge of this chapter by successfully completing the activities.

Instructions

In the first few pages, you will learn the most efficient use of this self-instructional programmed learning approach.

First remove the sliding card and cover the left-hand answer column with it.

1-1 This text is designed to help you learn medical terminology effectively. The principal technique used throughout the book is known as *programmed learning,* which consists of a series of teaching units called *frames.*

Each frame presents information and calls for an answer on your part. When you complete a sentence by writing an answer on the blank line, you are learning information by using the programmed learning technique. A frame consists of a block of information and a blank line. The purpose

answer

of the blank line is to write an _____.

1-2 Slide the card down in the left column to see the correct answer. After you correct the answer, read the next frame.

---

answer

1-3 It is important to keep the left-hand answer column covered until you write your _____.

---

learning

1-4 Several methods are employed in this book to help you master medical terminology, but the main technique used is called programmed _____.

---

answer(s)

1-5 After you write your answer, it is important to verify that it is correct. To do so, compare your answer with the one listed in the left-hand answer column.
To obtain immediate feedback on your responses, you must verify your _____.

 Study frames in sequence, because each frame builds on the previous one. Words are reviewed and repeated throughout the book to reinforce your learning. Consequently, you do not need to memorize every word that is presented.

---

one

1-6 The number of blank lines in a frame determines the number of words you write for your answer. Review the number of blank lines in Frame 1–5. It has _____ blank line(s). Therefore, the answer requires one word.

---

two, lines

1-7 A frame that requires two answers will have _____ blank _____.

1-8 In some frames, you will be asked to write the answer in your own words. In these instances, there will be one or more blank lines across the entire frame.
List at least two reasons why you want to learn medical terminology. Keep these objectives in mind as you work through the book.

_____

_____

Do not look at the answer column before you write your response and do not move ahead in a chapter. Progress in developing a medical vocabulary depends on your ability to learn the material presented in each frame.

frame	**1-9** Completing one frame at a time is the most effective method of learning. To achieve your goal of learning medical terminology, complete one _____ at a time.
back	**1-10** Whenever you make an error, it is important to go back and review the previous frame(s). You need to determine why you wrote the wrong answer before proceeding to the next frame. You may always go _____ and review information you have forgotten. Just remember, do not look ahead.
correct, check, *or* verify	**1-11** Do not be afraid to make a mistake. In programmed learning, you will learn and profit by your mistakes if you correct them immediately. Always _____ your answer immediately after you write it.
answer	**1-12** Because accurate spelling is essential in medicine, correct all misspelled words immediately. Do so by comparing your answer with the one in the left-hand _____ column.
correctly *or* accurately	**1-13** In medicine, it is important to spell correctly. Correct spelling can be a crucial component in determining the validity of evidence presented in a malpractice lawsuit. A physician can lose a lawsuit because of misspelled words that result in a misinterpreted medical record. To provide correct information, medical words must be spelled _____ in a medical record.

Word Elements

A medical word consists of some or all of the following elements:

- Word root
- Combining form
- Suffix
- Prefix.

How you combine these elements and whether all or some of them are present in a medical word determine the meaning of a word. The purpose of this chapter is to help you learn to identify these elements and use them to form medical terms.

suffix, prefix	**1-14** The four elements that are used to build a medical word are the word root, combining form, _____, and _____.
elements *or* parts	**1-15** Medical terminology is not difficult to learn when you understand how the *elements* are combined to form a word. To develop a medical vocabulary, you must understand the _____ that form medical words.

Word Roots

A *word root* is the main part or foundation of a word; all medical words have at least one word root.

teach	**1-16** In the words *teacher, teaches, teaching,* the word root is _____.

speak	**1-17** In the words *speaker, speaks, speaking,* the word root is _____.

1-18 Identify the roots in the following words:

Word	Root
reader	_____
spending	_____
playful	_____

read
spend
play

 A word root may be used alone or combined with other elements to form another word with a different meaning.

1-19 Review the following examples to see how roots are used alone or with other elements to form words. The meaning of each term in the right-hand column is also provided.

Root as a Complete Word	Root as a Part of a Word
alcohol	**alcohol**ism (condition marked by impaired control over alcohol use)
sperm	**sperm**icide (agent that kills sperm)
thyroid	**thyroid**ectomy (excision of the thyroid gland)

1-20 Throughout the book, a slash is used to separate word elements, as shown in the following examples. Write the word roots in the right-hand column for each of these terms:

alcohol	alcohol/ic _____
dent	dent/ist _____
lump	lump/ectomy _____
insulin	insulin/ism _____
gastr	gastr/itis _____

1-21 In medical words, the root usually indicates a body part (anatomical structure). For example, the root in *cardi/al, cardi/ac,* and *cardi/o/gram* is _____ and it means heart.

cardi

1-22 You will find that the roots in medical words are usually derived from Greek or Latin words. Some examples include *dent* in the word *dent/ist*, *pancreat* in the word *pancreat/itis*, and *dermat* in the word *dermat/o/logist*.

Underline the roots in the following words:

<u>dent</u>/al
DĔN-tăl

dent/al

<u>pancreat</u>/itis
păn-krē-ă-TĬ-tĭs

pancreat/itis

<u>dermat</u>/o/logist
dĕr-mă-TŎL-ō-jĭst

dermat/o/logist

---

part

1-23 In Frame 1–22, the root *dent* means *tooth,* *pancreat* means *pancreas,* and *dermat* means *skin.* All three roots indicate a body _____.

Combining Forms

A *combining form* (CF) is created when a word root is combined with a vowel. This vowel is usually an **o**. The vowel has no meaning of its own, but enables two word elements to be linked.

1-24 Like the word root, the CF is the basic foundation on which other elements are added to build a complete word. In this text, a combining form will be listed as word root/vowel, such as *dent/o* and *gastr/o.*
A word root + a vowel (usually an **o**) forms a new element known as

combining form

a _____ _____.

---

therm/o

gastr/o

1-25 The CF in *therm/o/meter* is _____ / _____.
The CF in *gastr/o/scope* is _____ / _____.

1-26 *Gastr/o* is an example of the word element called a

combining form

gastr, o

_____ _____.

Root in *gastr/o* is _____; the combining vowel is _____.

1-27 List the combining vowel in each of the following elements:

o

arthr/o _____

o

phleb/o _____

o

lith/o _____

<u>therm</u>/o
<u>abdomin</u>/o
<u>nephr</u>/o

1-28 Underline the word root in the following combining forms:
therm/o
abdomin/o
nephr/o

1-29 Use the combining vowel *o* to change the following roots to combining forms, and separate the elements with a slash.

Root	Combining Form (Root + Vowel)
cyst	_____
arthr	_____
leuk	_____
gastr	_____

cyst/o

arthr/o

leuk/o

gastr/o

1-30 Usually, the combining vowel is an *o*, although other vowels may be encountered occasionally.

The combining vowel is usually an _____.

o

1-31 Instead of joining the two elements *chem* and *-therapy* directly, the combining vowel *o* is attached to the root to form the word *chem/o/therapy*. The vowel has no meaning of its own, but enables two elements to be connected to each other.

Use the combining vowel to build medical terms below. *Chem/o/therapy* is given as an example.

Word Root	Suffix		Medical Term
chem	-therapy	*becomes*	*chem/o/therapy*
dermat	-logy	*becomes*	_____ / ___ / _____
encephal	-graphy	*becomes*	_____ / ___ / _____
neur	-logy	*becomes*	_____ / ___ / _____
therm	-meter	*becomes*	_____ / ___ / _____

chem/o/therapy
kē-mō-THĔR-ă-pē

dermat/o/logy
dĕr-mă-TŎL-ō-jē

encephal/o/graphy
ĕn-sĕf-ă-LŎG-ră-fē

neur/o/logy
nū-RŎL-ō-jē

therm/o/meter
thĕr-MŎM-ĕ-tĕr

1-32 The words in Frame 1–31 are easier to pronounce because the word roots are linked with the combining vowel *o*.

To make a word easier to pronounce, attach a combining _____ to the word root.

vowel

1-33 Although you may not know the meaning of all the words in this unit, you have already started to learn the word-building system by identifying the basic _____ of a medical word.

elements *or* parts

1-34 Understanding the word-building system will help you decipher the meanings of medical terms.

Using the word-building system to identify basic elements of a medical word will help you learn _____ terminology.

medical

dermat **dermat/o**	**1–35** In the word *dermat/o/logy,* the root is _____ ; the combining form is _____ / _____.

 A combining vowel is used to link a root to another root to form a compound word. This holds true even if the next root begins with a vowel, as in *gastr/o/enter/itis.*

o	**1–36** In the word *gastr/o/enter/itis,* the roots **gastr** (*stomach*) and **enter** (*intestine*) are linked together with the combining vowel _____.
leuk, cyt **-penia**	**1–37** The roots in *leuk/o/cyt/o/penia* are _____ and _____. The suffix is _____.
leuk/o, cyt/o	**1–38** Identify the CFs in *leuk/o/cyt/o/penia:* _____ / _____ and _____ / _____.
electr/o, cardi/o	**1–39** List the CFs in *electr/o/cardi/o/gram:* _____ / _____ and _____ / _____.
back	**1–40** You are now using the programmed learning method. If you are experiencing difficulty writing the correct answers, go back to Frame 1–1 and rework the frames. To master material that has been covered, you can always go _____ to review the frames.

 Throughout the subsequent frames, all word roots and combining forms that stand alone are set in boldface.

Suffixes

A *suffix* is a word element located at the end of a word. Substituting one suffix for another suffix changes the meaning of the word. In medical terminology, a suffix usually indicates a procedure, condition, disease, or part of speech. In this text, a suffix that stands alone is preceded by a hyphen.

suffix	**1–41** The element at the end of a word is called the _____.
play/er **read/er** **speak/er**	**1–42** *Play, read,* and *speak* are complete words and also roots. Add the suffix *-er* (meaning *one who*) to each root to modify its meaning. **Play** becomes _____ / _____. **Read** becomes _____ / _____. **Speak** becomes _____ / _____.

one who	**1–43** By attaching the suffix -er (one who) to **play, read,** and **speak,** we create nouns that mean:
one who	*Play*/er means _____ _____ *plays.*
one who	*Read*/er means _____ _____ *reads.*
	Speak/er means _____ _____ *speaks.*

ⓘ | A word root links a suffix that begins with a vowel.

1–44 Link the following roots with suffixes, each of which begins with a vowel. Then practice pronouncing the terms aloud by referring to the pronunciations in the left-hand answer column.

Word Root	Suffix		Medical Term
tonsill	-itis	*becomes*	_____ / _____
gastr	-ectomy	*becomes*	_____ / _____
arthr	-itis	*becomes*	_____ / _____

Left answer column:
tonsill/itis
tŏn-sĭl-Ī-tĭs
gastr/ectomy
găs-TRĔK-tō-mē
arthr/itis
ăr-THRĪ-tĭs

1–45 Changing the suffix modifies the meaning of the word. In the word *dent/al,* **dent** is the word _____ and -al is the _____.

root, suffix

1–46 A *dent/ist* is a specialist in teeth. *Dent/al* means *pertaining to teeth.* Simply changing the suffix gives the word a new meaning.

The suffix in *dent/ist* is _____. It means *specialist.*

-ist

The suffix in *dent/al* is _____. It means *pertaining to.*

-al

ⓘ | A combining form (root + o) links a suffix that begins with a consonant.

1–47 Change the following roots to combining forms and link them with suffixes that begin with a consonant. Then practice pronouncing the terms aloud by referring to the pronunciations in the left-hand answer column.

Word Root	Suffix		Medical Term
scler	-derma	*becomes*	_____ / ____ / _____
mast	-dynia	*becomes*	_____ / ____ / _____
arthr	-plasty	*becomes*	_____ / ____ / _____

Left answer column:
scler/o/derma
sklĕr-ō-DĔR-mă
mast/o/dynia
măst-ō-DĬN-ē-ă
arthr/o/plasty
ĂR-thrō-plăs-tē

1-48 Throughout the book, whenever a suffix stands alone, it will be preceded by a hyphen, as in *-oma (tumor)*. The hyphen indicates another element is needed to transform the suffix into a complete word.

hyphen

A suffix that stands alone will be preceded by a _____.

 Pronouncing medical words correctly is crucial because mispronunciations can result in incorrect medical interpretations and treatments. In addition, misspelled terms in a medical report may become a legal issue. Learning how to pronounce and spell medical terms is a matter of practice. To familiarize yourself with medical words, make it a habit to pronounce a word aloud each time you see the pronunciation listed in the answer column.

1-49 Underline the suffixes in the following words:

dent/ist
DĔN-tĭst

dent/ist

arthr/o/centesis
ăr-thrō-sĕn-TĒ-sĭs

arthr/o/centesis

neur/algia
nū-RĂL-jē-ă

neur/algia

angi/oma
ăn-jē-Ō-mă

angi/oma

gastr/ic
GĂS-trĭk

gastr/ic

nephr/itis
nĕf-RĪ-tĭs

nephr/itis

scler/o/derma
sklĕr-ō-DĔR-mă

scler/o/derma

1-50 Elements preceding a suffix can be a root or a combining form. Review Frame 1–49 and list the

arthr/o, scler/o

combining forms preceding suffixes: _____ / _____ *and*
_____ / _____

roots preceding suffixes:

dent, neur, angi, gastr, nephr

_____, _____, _____, _____, *and* _____.

Find answers to this frame in Appendix B, Answer Key, page 548.

1-51 Analyze the following medical terms by identifying their elements. The first is completed as an example. The vowel has no meaning of its own, but enables two elements to be connected.

Medical Term	Combining Form (root + o)		Word Root	Suffix
arthr/o/scop/ic ăr-thrōs-KŎP-ĭk	_arthr_	/ _o_	_scop_	_-ic_
erythr/o/cyt/osis ĕ-rĭth-rō-sī-TŌ-sĭs	_____	/ ____	_____	_____
append/ix ă-PĔN-dĭks	_____	/ ____	_____	_____
dermat/itis dĕr-mă-TĪ-tĭs	_____	/ ____	_____	_____
gastr/o/enter/itis găs-trō-ĕn-tĕr-Ī-tĭs	_____	/ ____	_____	_____
orth/o/ped/ic or-thō-PĒ-dĭk	_____	/ ____	_____	_____
oste/o/arthr/itis ŏs-tē-ō-ăr-THRĪ-tĭs	_____	/ ____	_____	_____
vagin/itis văj-ĭn-Ī-tĭs	_____	/ ____	_____	_____

1-52 The examples in Frame 1–51 show how medical words can be formed by various combinations of combining forms, roots, and

suffixes

_____.

Three Rules of Word Building

There are three important rules of word building:

- **Rule 1:** A word root links a suffix that begins with a vowel.
- **Rule 2:** A combining form (root + *o*) links a suffix that begins with a consonant.
- **Rule 3:** A combining form (root + *o*) links a root to another root to form a compound word. (This rule holds true even if the next root begins with a vowel.)

1-53 **Rule 1:** In the following examples, use a word root to link suffixes that begin with a vowel.

Word Root	Suffix		Medical Word
leuk	-emia	*becomes*	_____ / _____
cephal	-algia	*becomes*	_____ / _____
gastr	-itis	*becomes*	_____ / _____
append	-ectomy	*becomes*	_____ / _____

leuk/emia
loo-KĒ-mē-ă
cephal/algia
sĕf-ă-LĂL-jē-ă
gastr/itis
găs-TRĪ-tĭs
append/ectomy
ăp-ĕn-DĔK-tō-mē

1-54 **Rule 2:** In the following examples, use a combining form (root + *o*) to link the suffixes that begin with a consonant.

Word Root	Suffix		Medical Term
gastr	-scope	*becomes*	_____ / _____ / _____
men	-rrhea	*becomes*	_____ / _____ / _____
angi	-rrhexis	*becomes*	_____ / _____ / _____
ureter	-lith	*becomes*	_____ / _____ / _____

gastr/o/scope
GĂS-trō-skōp
men/o/rrhea
mĕn-ō-RĒ-ă
angi/o/rrhexis
ăn-jē-ō-RĔK-sĭs
ureter/o/lith
ū-RĒ-tĕr-ō-lĭth

1-55 **Rule 3:** In the following four examples, apply the rule, "Use a combining form (root + *o*) to link a root to another root to form a compound word." (This rule holds true even if the next root begins with a vowel.)

oste/o/chondr/itis
ŏs-tē-ō-kŏn-DRĪ-tĭs
oste/o/chondr/oma
ŏs-tē-ō-kŏn-DRŌ-mă
oste/o/arthr/itis
ŏs-tē-ō-ăr-THRĪ-tĭs
gastr/o/enter/itis
găs-trō-ĕn-tĕr-Ī-tĭs

oste + *chondr* + *-itis* becomes _____ / _____ / _____ / _____.

oste + *chondr* + *-oma* becomes _____ / _____ / _____ / _____.

oste + *arthr* + *-itis* becomes _____ / _____ / _____ / _____.

gastr + *enter* + *-itis* becomes _____ / _____ / _____ / _____.

1-56 Would you use a *word root* or a *combining form* as a link to the suffixes *-algia, -edema,* and *-uria?* _____ _____

word root

cardi/o/gram
KĂR-dē-ō-grăm

Rule 2: A combining form (root + *o*) links a suffix that begins with a consonant.

1–57 Refer to the three rules of word building on page 10 to complete frames 1–57 to 1–62.

Form a word with **cardi** and *-gram:* _____ / _____ / _____
(root)   (suffix)

Summarize the rule that applies in this frame.

Rule 2: _____

_____

---

carcin/oma
kăr-sĭ-NŌ-mă

Rule 1: A word root links a suffix that begins with a vowel.

1–58 Form a word with **carcin** and *-oma:* _____ / _____
(root)   (suffix)

Summarize the rule that applies in this frame.

Rule 1: _____

_____

---

enter/o/cyst/o/plasty
ĕn-tĕr-ō-SĬS-tō-plăs-tē

Rule 3: A CF links a root to another root to form a compound word.

Rule 2: A CF links a suffix that begins with a consonant.

1–59 Complete the following frames to reinforce the three rules of word building on page 10.

Build a medical word with **enter** + **cyst** + *-plasty:*

_____ / _____ / _____ / _____ / _____

Summarize the word building rules that apply in forming the above term. (Use *CF* to indicate *combining form.*)

Rule 3: _____

_____

Rule 2: _____

_____

---

leuk/o/cyt/o/penia
loo-kō-sī-tō-PĒ-nē-ă

Rule 3: CF links a root to another root to form a compound word.

Rule 2: CF links a suffix that begins with a consonant.

1–60 Build a medical word with **leuk** + **cyt** + *-penia:*

_____ / _____ / _____ / _____ / _____.

Summarize the word building rules that apply in forming the above term.

Rule 3: _____

_____

Rule 2: _____

_____

erythr/o/cyt/osis ĕ-rĭth-rō-sī-TŌ-sĭs	**1-61** Build a medical word with **erythr** + **cyt** + -osis: _____ / ____ / _____ / _____. Summarize the word building rules that apply in forming the above term. *Rule 3:* _____ _____ *Rule 1:* _____ _____
Rule 3: CF links a root to another root to form a compound word. **Rule 1:** Word root links a suffix that begins with a vowel.	
	1-62 You may or may not know the meaning of the suffixes covered in this chapter. It is not necessary for you to know all the meaning of the suffixes yet as these terms and definitions will be reviewed again. What is important now is that you understand how to identify the component parts (root, combining form, suffix) of a word.
root, suffix	For example, in the term *pancreat/itis*, **pancreat** is the _____; -*itis* is the _____.

In addition to word roots and CFs in **bold,** in subsequent frames, all suffixes that stand alone will be set in blue, type.

Prefixes

A *prefix* is a word element located at the beginning of a word. Substituting one prefix for another prefix changes the meaning of the word. A prefix usually indicates a number, time, position, or negation. Many prefixes found in medical terminology also are found in the English language. In this text, a prefix that stands alone is followed by a hyphen.

micro/cyte MĪ-krō-sīt	**1-63** In the term *macro/cyte*, *macro-* is a prefix meaning *large*; *-cyte* is a suffix meaning *cell*. A *macro/cyte* is a large cell. Form a new term meaning *small cell* by changing the prefix *macro-* to *micro-*: _____ / _____.
-al **post-** **nat**	**1-64** *Post/nat/al* refers the period after birth. Identify the elements that mean *pertaining to:* _____. *after, behind:* _____. *birth:* _____.
pre/nat/al prē-NĀ-tl	**1-65** Use *pre- (before)* to build a word meaning *pertaining to (the period) before birth:* _____ / _____ / _____
prefix	**1-66** A word element located at the beginning of a word is a _____.

intra- **post-** **peri-** **pre-**	**1–67** *Intra/muscul/ar, post/nat/al, peri/card/itis,* and *pre/operative* are medical terms that contain prefixes. Determine the prefix in this frame that means: *in, within:* _____. *after:* _____. *around:* _____. *before, in front of:* _____.
prefix **root** **suffix**	**1–68** Whenever a prefix stands alone, it is identified with a hyphen after it, as in *hyper-*. When it is part of a word, the prefix is not highlighted, but a slash separates it from the next element, as in *hyper/tension*. Analyze *hyper/insulin/ism* by identifying the elements. *hyper-* is a _____. *insulin* is a _____. *-ism* is a _____.
prefixes	**1–69** *Hypo-, intra-, super-,* and *homo-* are examples of word elements called _____.
post/operative pōst-ŎP-ĕr-ă-tĭv **after**	**1–70** *Pre/operative* designates the time before a surgery. By changing the prefix, you alter the meaning of the word. Build a word that designates the time after surgery. _____ / _____. Can you remember what *post-* in *post/operative* means? _____.
post-, after **after**	**1–71** You will recognize many prefixes in medical terms because they are the same ones found in the English language. In the term *post/mortem,* the prefix is _____ and means _____. *Post/mortem* means _____ death.
pre- **before, before**	**1–72** In the term *pre/mature,* the prefix is _____ and means _____. *Pre/mature* means _____ maturity.

Defining Medical Words

When defining a medical word, first define the suffix. Second, define the beginning of the word; finally, define the middle of the word. Here is an example using the term *osteoarthritis.*

oste/o/arthr/itis
(2)   (3)   (1)

1. Define the suffix first: *-itis* means *inflammation.*
2. Define the beginning of the word: *oste/o* means *bone.*
3. Define the middle of the word: *arthr* means *joint.*

Therefore, *oste/o/arthr/itis* is an inflammation of the bone and joint.

suffix	**1-73** The element that is defined first is the _____.
beginning	The element that is defined next is the _____ of the word.
last	The middle or rest of the word is defined _____.

	1-74 Use the technique for defining medical words, described above, to break the word *gastr/o/enter/itis* into its parts in order to define it.
-itis	Write the element that is defined first: _____
gastr/o	Write the element that is defined next: _____ / _____
enter	Write the element that is defined last: _____

	1-75 Appendix A, Glossary of Medical Word Elements on page 538 summarizes word elements and their meanings. Use this reference whenever you need to have an element defined. For example, look up the meaning of the CF enter/o and list it here.
intestine (usually small)	_____

	1-76 Define *gastr/o/enter/itis* using the technique for defining medical words as described above.
inflammation of the stomach and intestine (usually small intestine)	_____
	_____
	_____
	_____

In addition to word roots and CFs in **bold** and suffixes in blue, in subsequent frames, all prefixes that stand alone will be set in pink type.

Pronunciation Guidelines

Although pronunciation of medical words usually follows the same rules that govern pronunciation of English words, some medical terms may be difficult to pronounce when first encountered. Selected terms in this book include phonetic pronunciation. In addition, pronunciation guidelines can be found on the inside front cover of this book. Use them whenever you need help with the pronunciation of medical words. Locate and study the pronunciation guidelines before proceeding with Section Review 1–1.

Pronunciation Tools

At appropriate times in each chapter you will be directed to use the following pronunciation tools:

- Use the audio CD-ROM, *Listen and Learn*, to hear pronunciations of terms in the *Listen and Learn* sections of each chapter.
- *Visit Listen and Learn Online!* to hear pronunciation of selected medical words from medical reports sections.
- *Visit DavisPlus Online!* for a chapter's flash-card activity.

SECTION REVIEW 1-1

Review the pronunciation guidelines (located in the inside front cover of this book). Use them as reference when needed. Then, in the exercise below, underline one of the items within the parentheses to complete each sentence.

1. The diacritical mark ˘ is called a (breve, macron).

2. The diacritical mark ˉ is called a (breve, macron).

3. The macron (ˉ) above a vowel is used to indicate (short, long) vowel pronunciations.

4. The breve (˘) above a vowel is used to indicate the (short, long) vowel pronunciations.

5. When *pn* is in the middle of a word, pronounce (only *p, n, pn*). Examples are ortho*pn*ea, hyper*pn*ea.

6. The letters *c* and *g* have a (hard, soft) sound before the letters a and o. Examples are *c*ardiac, *c*ast, *g*astric, *g*onad.

7. When *pn* is at the beginning of a word, pronounce (only *p, n, pn*). Examples are *pn*eumonia, *pn*eumotoxin.

8. When *i* is at the end of a word (to form a plural), it is pronounced like (*eye, ee*). Examples are bronch*i*, fung*i*, nucle*i*.

9. For *ae* and *oe*, only the (first, second) vowel is pronounced. Examples are burs*ae*, pleur*ae*, r*oe*ntgen.

10. When *e* and *es* form the final letter or letters of a word, they are commonly pronounced as (combined, separate) syllables. Examples are syncop*e*, systol*e*, appendic*es*.

Competency Verification: Check your answers in Appendix B, Answer Key, page 548. If you are not satisfied with your level of comprehension, review the pronunciation guidelines (on the inside front cover of this book) and retake the review.

Correct Answers _____ × 10 = _____ % Score

Common Suffixes

In previous frames, you learned that a combining form (CF) is a word root + vowel and that the CF is the main part, or *foundation*, of a medical term. Examples of CFs are **gastr/o** (stomach), **dermat/o** (skin), and **nephr/o** (kidney). When you see **gastr/o** in a medical term, you will know the term refers to the stomach. You also learned that a suffix is an element located at the end of a word. The following sections introduce common surgical, diagnostic, and pathological suffixes as well as plural suffixes. Some of these elements have already been introduced in previous frames, but they are reinforced below.

Combinations of four elements are used to form medical words. These four elements are the word root, combining form, suffix, and prefix. Some words may also be used as suffixes. Other words may consist of just a prefix and a word root.

Surgical Suffixes

Common suffixes associated with surgical procedures, their meanings, and an example of a related term are presented in the table below. First, study the suffix as well as its meaning and practice pronouncing the term aloud. Then use the information to complete the meaning of the term. The first is completed for you. You may also refer to Appendix A: Glossary of Medical Word Elements, page 538. To build a working vocabulary of medical terms and understand how those terms are used in the health care industry, it is important that you complete these exercises.

Suffix	Term	Meaning
-centesis surgical puncture	arthr/o/**centesis** ăr-thrō-sĕn-TĒ-sĭs *arthr/o:* joint	<u>*surgical puncture of a joint*</u>
-clast to break	oste/o/**clast** ŎS-tē-ō-klăst *oste/o:* bone	 *Osteoclasts break down areas of old or damaged bone, while osteoblasts deposit new bone tissue in those areas.*
-desis binding, fixation (of a bone or joint)	arthr/o/**desis** ăr-thrō-DĒ-sĭs *arthr/o:* joint	
-ectomy excision, removal	append/**ectomy** ăp-ĕn-DĔK-tō-mē *append:* appendix	
-lysis separation; destruction; loosening	thromb/o/**lysis** thrŏm-BŎL-ĭ-sĭs *thromb/o:* blood clot	 *Drug therapy is usually used to dissolve a blood clot.*
-pexy fixation (of an organ)	mast/o/**pexy** MĂS-tō-pĕks-ē *mast/o:* breast	 *Mastopexy is performed to affix sagging breasts in a more elevated position, often improving their shape.*
-plasty surgical repair	rhin/o/**plasty** RĪ-nō-plăs-tē *rhin/o:* nose	
-rrhaphy suture	my/o/**rrhaphy** mī-OR-ă-fē *my/o:* muscle	
-stomy forming an opening (mouth)	trache/o/**stomy** trā-kē-ŎS-tō-mē *trache/o:* trachea (windpipe)	 *Tracheostomy may be performed to bypass an obstructed upper airway.*

(continued)

Suffix	Term	Meaning
-tome instrument to cut	oste/o/**tome** ŎS-tē-ō-tōm *oste/o:* bone	_____

-tomy
incision
	trache/o/**tomy**
	trā-kē–ŎT-ō–mē
	    trache/o: trachea
	        (windpipe)
		_____
		_____
		Tracheotomy may be performed to gain access to an air-way below a blockage.

-tripsy crushing	lith/o/**tripsy** LĬTH-ō-trĭp-sē *lith/o:* stone, calculus	_____

Pronunciation Help	**Long Sound** **Short Sound**	ā in rāte ă in ălone	ē in rēbirth ĕ in ĕver	ī in īsle ĭ in ĭt	ō in ōver ŏ in nŏt	ū in ūnite ŭ in cŭt

Diagnostic Suffixes

Common suffixes associated with diagnostic procedures, their meanings, and an example of a related term are presented in the table below. First, study the suffix as well as its meaning and practice pronouncing the term aloud. Then use the information to complete the meaning of the term. You may also refer to Appendix A: Glossary of Medical Word Elements, page 538. To build a working vocabulary of medical terms and understand how those terms are used in the health care industry, it is important that you complete these exercises.

Suffix	Term	Meaning

-gram
record, writing
	electr/o/cardi/o/**gram**
	ē-lĕk-trō-KĂR-dē-ō-grăm
	    electr/o: electricity
	    cardi/o: heart
		_____
		_____
		An electrocardiogram allows diagnosis of specific cardiac abnormalities.

-graph instrument for recording	cardi/o/**graph** KĂR-dē-ō-grăf *cardi/o:* heart	_____

-graphy
process of recording
	angi/o/**graphy**
	ăn-jē-ŎG-ră-fē
	    angi/o: vessel (usually
	        blood or lymph)
		_____

-meter instrument for measuring	pelv/i/**meter*** pĕl-VĬM-ĕ-tĕr *pelv/i:* pelvis	_____
-metry act of measuring	pelv/i/**metry*** pĕl-VĬM-ĕ-trē *pelv/i:* pelvis	_____

*The *i* in *pelv/i/meter* is an exception to the rule of using the connecting vowel *o*.

Suffix	Term	Meaning
-scope instrument for examining	endo/**scope** ĔN-dō-skōp *endo-:* in, within	_____ _____
-scopy visual examination	endo/**scopy** ĕn-DŎS-kō-pē *endo-:* in, within	_____ _____

Pronunciation Help	Long Sound Short Sound	ā in rāte ă in ălone	ē in rēbirth ĕ in ĕver	ī in īsle ĭ in ĭt	ō in ōver ŏ in nŏt	ū in ūnite ŭ in cŭt

Pathological Suffixes

Common suffixes associated with pathological (disease) conditions, their meanings, and an example of a related term are presented in the table below. First, study the suffix as well as its meaning and practice pronouncing the term aloud. Then use the information to complete the meaning of the term. You may also refer to Appendix A: Glossary of Medical Word Elements, page 538. To build a working vocabulary of medical terms and understand how those terms are used in the health care industry, it is important that you complete these exercises.

Suffix	Term	Meaning
-algia, -dynia pain	neur/**algia** nū-RĂL-jē-ă *neur:* nerve ot/o/**dynia** ō-tō-DĬN-ē-ă *ot/o:* ear	_____ _____ _____ _____
-cele hernia, swelling	hepat/o/**cele** hĕ-PĂT-ō-sēl *hepat/o:* liver	_____ _____
-ectasis dilation, expansion	bronchi/**ectasis** brŏng-kē-ĔK-tă-sĭs *bronchi:* bronchus (plural, bronchi)	_____ _____ *Bronchiectasis is associated with various lung conditions and is commonly accompanied by chronic infection.*
-edema swelling	lymph/**edema** lĭmf-ĕ-DĒ-mă *lymph:* lymph	_____ _____ *Lymphedema may be caused by a blockage of the lymph vessels.*

(continued)

Suffix	Term	Meaning
-emesis vomiting	hyper/**emesis** hī-pĕr-ĔM-ĕ-sĭs *hyper-:* excessive, above normal	_____ _____
-emia blood condition	an/**emia** ă-NĒ-mē-ă *an-:* without, not	_____ _____
-iasis abnormal condition (produced by something specific)	chol/e/lith/**iasis*** kō-lē-lĭ-THĪ-ă-sĭs *chol/e:* bile, gall *lith:* stone, calculus	_____ _____
-itis inflammation	gastr/**itis** găs-TRĪ-tĭs *gastr:* stomach	_____ _____
-lith stone, calculus	chol/e/**lith*** KŌ-lē-lĭth *cho/e:* bile, gall	_____ _____
-malacia softening	chondr/o/**malacia** kŏn-drō-mă-LĀ-shē-ă *chondr/o:* cartilage	_____ _____
-megaly enlargement	cardi/o/**megaly** kăr-dē-ō-MĔG-ă-lē *cardi/o:* heart	_____ _____
-oma tumor	neur/**oma** nū-RŌ-mă *neur:* nerve	_____ _____
-osis abnormal condition; increase (used primarily with blood cells)	cyan/**osis** sī-ă-NŌ-sĭs *cyan:* blue	_____ _____
-pathy disease	my/o/**pathy** mī-ŎP-ă-thē *my/o:* muscle	_____ _____
-penia decrease, deficiency	erythr/o/**penia** ĕ-rĭth-rō-PĒ-nē-ă *erythr/o:* red	_____ _____

*The *e* in *chol/e/lithiasis* and *chol/e/lith* is an exception to the rule of using the connecting vowel *o.*

Suffix	Term	Meaning
-phobia fear	hem/o/**phobia** hē-mō-FŌ-bē-ă *hem/o:* blood	_____ _____
-plegia paralysis	hemi/**plegia** hĕm-ē-PLĒ-jē-ă *hemi-:* one half	_____ _____ *Hemiplegia affects the right or left side of the body and is caused by a brain injury or stroke.*
-rrhage, -rrhagia bursting forth (of)	hem/o/**rrhage** HĔM-ĕ-rĭj *hem/o:* blood men/o/**rrhagia** mĕn-ō-RĀ-jē-ă *men/o:* menses, menstruation	_____ _____ _____
-rrhea discharge, flow	dia/**rrhea** dī-ă-RĒ-ă *dia-:* through, across	_____ _____
-rrhexis rupture	arteri/o/**rrhexis** ăr-tē-rē-ō-RĔK-sĭs *arteri/o:* artery	_____ _____
-stenosis narrowing, stricture	arteri/o/**stenosis** ăr-tē-rē-ō-stĕ-NŌ-sĭs *arteri/o:* artery	_____ _____
-toxic poison	hepat/o/**toxic** HĔP-ă-tō-tŏk-sĭk *hepat/o:* liver	_____ _____
-trophy nourishment, development	dys/**trophy** DĬS-trō-fē *dys-:* bad; painful; difficult	_____ _____

Pronunciation Help	Long Sound	ā in rāte	ē in rēbirth	ī in īsle	ō in ōver	ū in ūnite
	Short Sound	ă in ălone	ĕ in ĕver	ĭ in ĭt	ŏ in nŏt	ŭ in cŭt

Plural Suffixes

Because many medical words have Greek or Latin origins, there are a few unusual rules you need to learn to change a singular word into its plural form. When you begin learning these rules, you will find that they are easy to apply. You will also find that some English word endings have been adopted for commonly used medical terms. When a word changes from a singular to a plural form, the suffix of the word is the part that changes. A summary of the rules for changing a singular word into its plural form is located on the inside back cover of this book. Use it to complete Section Review 1–2 below and whenever you need help forming plural words.

SECTION REVIEW 1-2

Write the plural form for each of the following words and state the rule that applies. The first word is completed for you.

Singular	Plural	Rule
1. sarcoma săr-KŌ-mă	*sarcomata*	*Retain the* ma *and add* ta.
2. thrombus THRŎM-bŭs		
3. appendix ă-PĔN-dĭks		
4. diverticulum dī-vĕr-TĬK-ū-lŭm		
5. ovary Ō-vă-rē		
6. diagnosis dī-ăg-NŌ-sĭs		
7. lumen LŪ-mĕn		
8. vertebra VĔR-tĕ-bră		
9. thorax THŌ-răks		
10. spermatozoon spĕr-măt-ō-ZŌ-ŏn		

Competency Verification: Check your answers in Appendix B, Answer Key, page 553. If you are not satisfied with your level of comprehension, review the rules for changing a singular word into its plural form (on the inside back cover of this book) and retake the review.

Correct Answers _____ × 10 = _____ % Score

Common Prefixes

Common prefixes, their meanings, and an example of a related term are presented in the table below. First, study the prefix as well as its meaning and practice pronouncing the term aloud. Then use the information in the table below to complete the meaning of the term. You may also refer to Appendix A: Glossary of Medical Word Elements, page 538. To build a working vocabulary of medical terms and understand how those terms are used in the health care industry, it is important that you complete these exercises.

Prefix	Term	Meaning

a-*, an-**
 without, not
	a/mast/ia
	 ă-MĂS-tē-ă
	    mast: breast
	     -ia: condition
		_____
		 _____
		
		 Amastia may be the result of a congenital defect, an endocrine disorder, or mastectomy.

	an/esthesia ăn-ĕs-THĒ-zē-ă *-esthesia:* feeling	_____ _____

circum-, peri-
 around
	circum/duction
	 sĕr-kŭm-DŬK-shŭn
	   -duction: act of leading,
	        bringing,
	        conducting
		_____
		 _____

	peri/odont/al
	 pĕr-ē-ō-DŎN-tăl
	   odont: teeth
	    -al: pertaining to
		_____
		 _____

dia-, trans-
 through, across
	dia/rrhea (dī-ă-RĒ-ă):
	   flow through
	   -rrhea: discharge, flow
		_____
		 _____
		
		 Diarrhea is a condition of abnormally frequent discharge or flow of fluid fecal matter from the bowel.

	trans/vagin/al
	 trăns-VĂJ-ĭn-ăl
	   vagin: vagina
	    -al: pertaining to
		_____
		 _____

dipl-, diplo- double	**dipl**/opia dĭp-LŌ-pē-ă *-opia:* vision	_____ _____ *Diplobacteria reproduce in such a manner that they are joined together in pairs.*
	diplo/bacteri/al dĭp-lō-băk-TĒR-ē-ăl *bacteri:* bacteria *-al:* pertaining to	_____ _____

*The prefix *a-* is usually used before a consonant.** The prefix *an-* is usually used before a vowel.

(continued)

Prefix	Term	Meaning
endo-, intra- in, within	**endo**/crine ĔN-dō-krīn -crine: secrete	*Endocrine refers to a gland that secretes directly into the bloodstream.*
	intra/muscul/ar ĭn-tră-MŬS-kū-lăr *muscul:* muscle -ar: pertaining to	
homo-, homeo- same	**homo**/graft HŌ-mō-grăft -graft: transplantation	*A homograft is also called an allograft.*
	homeo/plasia hō-mē-ō-PLĀ-zē-ă -plasia: formation, growth	
hypo- under, below, deficient	**hypo**/derm/ic hī-pō-DĔR-mĭk *derm:* skin -ic: pertaining to	
macro- large	**macro**/cyte MĂK-rō-sīt -cyte: cell	
micro- small	**micro**/scope MĪ-krō-skōp -scope: instrument for examining	
mono-, uni- one	**mono**/cyte MŎN-ō-sīt -cyte: cell	
	uni/nucle/ar ū-nĭ-NŪ-klē-ăr *nucle:* nucleus -ar: pertaining to	
post- after, behind	**post**/nat/al pōst-NĀ-tăl *nat:* birth -al: pertaining to	

Prefix	Term	Meaning

pre-, pro-
before, in front of
	pre/nat/al
	prē-NĀ-tăl
	   nat: birth
	   -al: pertaining to
	pro/gnosis
	prŏg-NŌ-sĭs
	   -gnosis: knowing
		_____
		_____
		
		_____
		_____

primi-
first
	primi/gravida
	prī-mĭ-GRĂV-ĭ-dă
	   -gravida: pregnant
	           woman
		_____
		_____

retro- backward, behind	**retro**/version rĕt-rō-VĔR-shŭn *-version:* turning	_____ _____
super- upper, above	**super**/ior soo-PĒ-rē-or *-ior:* pertaining to	_____ _____

Pronunciation Help	Long Sound Short Sound	ā in rāte ă in ălone	ē in rēbirth ĕ in ĕver	ī in īsle ĭ in ĭt	ō in ōver ŏ in nŏt	ū in ūnite ŭ in cŭt

 Enhance your study and reinforcement of word elements with the power of *Davis Plus.* Visit *http://davisplus.fadavis.com/gylys/simplified* for this chapter's flash card activity. We recommend you complete the flash-card activity before continuing to the next chapter.

2 Body Structure

OBJECTIVES

Upon completion of this chapter, you will be able to:

- List and describe the basic structural units of the body.
- Describe the anatomical position of the body.
- Locate the body cavities and abdominopelvic regions of the body.
- Describe terms related to position, direction, and planes of the body and their applications during radiographic examinations.
- Describe common signs, symptoms, and diseases that may affect several body systems.
- Describe common diagnostic, medical, and surgical procedures related to several body systems.
- Recognize, define, pronounce, and spell terms correctly.
- Demonstrate your knowledge of this chapter by successfully completing the frames and reviews.

The human body consists of several structural and functional levels of organization. The complexity of each level increases from one to the next because the higher level incorporates the structures and functions of the previous level or levels. Eventually, all levels contribute to the structure and function of the entire organism (see Figure 2–1). The levels of organization from the least to the most complex are the:

- **Cellular level**, the smallest structural and functional unit of the body
- **Tissue level**, groups of cells that perform a specialized function
- **Organ level**, groups of tissues that perform a specific function
- **System level**, groups of organs that are interconnected or that have similar or interrelated functions
- **Organism level**, collection of body systems that makes up the most complex level—a living human being.

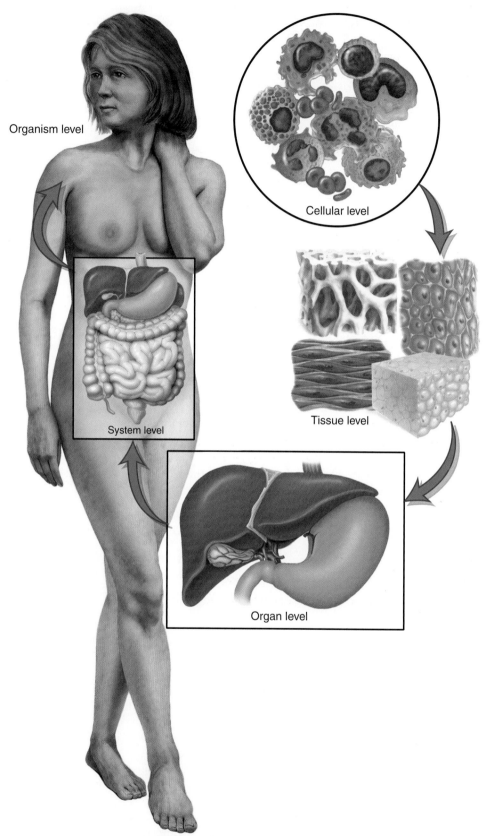

Organism level

Cellular level

Tissue level

System level

Organ level

Figure 2-1　Levels of structural organization of the human body shown from the basic unit of structure, the cellular level, to the most complex, the organism level—a living human being. The body system illustrated is the digestive system.

WORD ELEMENTS

This section introduces combining forms (CFs) related to the basic structural units of the body and those that describe a particular location, or direction in the body. Key suffixes are also summarized. Other word elements are defined in the right-hand column as needed. Review the table and pronounce each word in the word analysis column aloud before you begin to work in the frames.

Word Element	Meaning	Word Analysis
Combining Forms		

BASIC STRUCTURAL UNITS

chondr/o	cartilage	**chondr**/oma (kŏn-DRŌ-mă): tumor composed of cartilage *-oma:* tumor
cyt/o	cell	**cyt**/o/meter (sī-TŎM-ĕ-ter): instrument for counting and measuring cells *-meter:* instrument for measuring *The cells are counted and measured within a specified amount of fluid, such as blood, urine, or cerebrospinal fluid*
hist/o	tissue	**hist**/o/lysis (hĭs-TŎL-ĭ-sĭs): separation; destruction; or loosening of tissue *-lysis:* separation; destruction; loosening
nucle/o	nucleus	**nucle**/ar (NŪ-klē-ăr): pertaining to a nucleus *-ar:* pertaining to

DIRECTIONAL

anter/o	anterior, front	**anter**/ior (ăn-TĒ-rē-ōr): toward the front of the body, organ, or structure *-ior:* pertaining to
caud/o	tail	**caud**/ad (KAW-dăd): toward the tail; in a posterior direction *-ad:* toward
dist/o	far, farthest	**dist**/al (DĬS-tăl): pertaining to a point farthest from the center, a medial line, or the trunk; opposed to proximal *-al:* pertaining to
dors/o	back (of body)	**dors**/al (DŌR-săl): pertaining to the back or posterior of the body *-al:* pertaining to
infer/o	lower, below	**infer**/ior (ĭn-FĒ-rē-or): pertaining to below or lower; toward the tail *-ior:* pertaining to
later/o	side, to one side	**later**/al (LĂT-ĕr-ăl): pertaining to the side *-al:* pertaining to

Word Element	Meaning	Word Analysis
medi/o	middle	**medi**/al (MĒ-dē-ăl): pertaining to the middle *-al:* pertaining to
poster/o	back (of body), behind, posterior	**poster**/ior (pŏs-TĒ-rē-or): pertaining to or toward the rear or caudal end *-ior:* pertaining to
proxim/o	near, nearest	**proxim**/al (PRŎK-sĭm-ăl): nearest the point of attachment, center of the body, or point of reference *-al:* pertaining to
super/o*	upper, above	**super**/ior (soo-PĒ-rē-or): pertaining to above or higher; toward the head *-ior:* pertaining to
ventr/o	belly, belly side	**ventr**/al (VĔN-trăl): pertaining to the belly side or front of the body *-al:* pertaining to

SUFFIXES

Word Element	Meaning	Word Analysis
-ad	toward	medi/**ad** (MĒ-dē-ăd): toward the middle or center *medi/o-:* middle
-logist	specialist in the study of	hist/o/**logist** (hĭs-TŎL-ō-jĭst): specialist in the study of tissue *hist/o:* tissue
-logy	study of	cyt/o/**logy** (sī-TŎL-ō-jē): study of cells *cyt/o:* cell
-lysis	separation; destruction; loosening	cyt/o/**lysis** (sī-TŎL-ĭ-sĭs): destruction, dissolution, or separation of a cell *cyt/o:* cell
-toxic	poison	cyt/o/**toxic** (sī-tō-TŎKS-ĭk): substance that is detrimental or destructive to cells *cyt/o:* cell

*Super/o is used as a CF here, but it can also be used as a prefix, as in *supersonic*.

Listen and Learn, the audio CD-ROM included in this book, will help you master pronunciation of selected medical words. Use it to practice pronunciations of the above-listed medical terms and for instructions to complete the *Listen and Learn* exercise for this section.

SECTION REVIEW 2-1

For the following medical terms, first write the suffix and its meaning. Then translate the meaning of the remaining elements starting with the first part of the word. For example, the first word is completed for you.

Term	Meaning
1. dist/al	*-al: pertaining to; far, farthest*
2. poster/ior	
3. hist/o/logist	
4. dors/al	
5. anter/ior	
6. later/al	
7. medi/ad	
8. cyt/o/toxic	
9. proxim/al	
10. ventr/al	

Competency Verification: Check your answers in Appendix B, Answer Key, page 555. If you are not satisfied with your level of comprehension, review the vocabulary and retake the review.

Correct Answers _____ × 10 = _____ % Score

Basic Units of Structure

2-1 Cells are the smallest living units of structure and function in the human body. Every tissue and organ in the body is composed of cells. Review the illustration depicting the cellular level in Figure 2–1.

Note the darkened area in the center, the nucleus. It is the control center of the cell and is responsible for reproduction. This spherical unit contains genetic codes for maintaining life systems of the organism and for issuing commands for growth and reproduction.

nucle/o

CF for *nucleus* is: _____ / _____.

2-2 Any chemical substance, such as a drug that interferes with or destroys the cellular reproductive process in the nucleus, is referred to as a *nucle/o/toxic substance.* Examples of nucle/o/toxic drugs are those administered to cancer patients during chemotherapy.

Identify the elements in this frame that mean

-toxic

poison: _____

nucle/o

nucleus: _____ / _____

cell	**2-3** Recall that **cyt/o** and *-cyte* are used to form words that refer to a _____.
cyt/o/logy sī-TŎL-ō-jē	**2-4** A *cyt/o/logist* is usually a biologist who specializes in the study of cells, especially one who uses cyt/o/log/ic techniques to diagnose neoplasms. Using **cyt/o**, build a word that means *study of cells:* _____ / _____ / _____.
cyt/o/logist sī-TŎL-ă-jĭst **cyt/o/lysis** sī-TŎL-ĭ-sĭs	**2-5** Use **cyt/o** to form words that mean *specialist in the study of cells:* _____ / _____ / _____. *dissolution or destruction of a cell:* _____ / _____ / _____
-logist **hist/o**	**2-6** At the tissue level, the structural organization of the human body consists of groups of cells working together to carry out a specialized activity. (See Figure 2–1.) The medical scientist who specializes in the study of microscopic structures of tissues is called a *hist/o/logist*. Identify word elements in *hist/o/logist* that mean *specialist in the study of:* _____ *tissue:* _____ / _____
hist/o/logy hĭs-TŎL-ō-jē **cyt/o/logy** sī-TŎL-ō-jē	**2-7** Use *-logy* to form medical words that mean *study of tissue:* _____ / _____ / _____ *study of cells:* _____ / _____ / _____

When defining a medical word, first define the suffix. Second, define the beginning of the word; finally, define the middle of the word. Here is an example of the term

super/medi/al

(2)   (3)   (1)

1. Define the suffix first: *-al* means *pertaining to.*
2. Define the beginning of the word: *super-* means *upper, above.*
3. Define the middle of the word: *medi* means *middle.*

Directional Terms

The following frames introduce terms that describe regions of the body. Included are directional terms that describe a structure in relation to some defined center or reference point.

2–8 The suffixes *-ac, -al, -ar, -ic, -iac,* and *-ior* are adjective endings that mean *pertaining to.* You will find them used throughout this book. These suffixes help describe position, direction, body divisions, and body structures.

Use the adjective ending *-al* to form words that mean *pertaining to the*

dors/al
DŌR-săl

back (of body):   ___dors___ / _____

later/al
LĂT-ĕr-ăl

side, to one side: ___later___ / _____

ventr/al
VĔN-trăl

belly, belly side: ___ventr___ / _____

2–9 Practice building medical terms with **dors/o, later/o,** and **ventr/o.** Form medical terms that mean *pertaining to the*

dors/al
DŌR-săl

back (of body): _____ / _____

later/al
LĂT-ĕr-ăl

side, to one side: _____ / _____

ventr/al
VĔN-trăl

belly, belly side: _____ / _____

2–10 In Frame 2–8, six adjective suffixes that mean *pertaining to* were reviewed. Four additional adjective suffixes meaning *pertaining to* that are common in medical terms are *-ary, -eal, -ous,* and *-tic.* You may want to summarize these suffixes on a 5-inch × 3-inch index card and keep it in your book as a reference until you commit all of them to memory. However, if you are in doubt about meanings of any word elements, refer to Appendix A, Glossary of Medical Word Elements.

List the 10 adjective suffixes that mean *pertaining to* in alphabetical order.

-ac   _____

-al   _____

-ar   _____

-ary   _____

-eal   _____

-iac   _____

-ic   _____

-ior   _____

-ous   _____

-tic   _____

cardi/ac KĂR-dē-ăk	**2-11** Underline the suffixes in the following terms that mean *pertaining to.* cardi/ac
umbilic/al ŭm-BĬL-ĭ-kăl	umbilic/al
nucle/ar NŪ-klē-ăr	nucle/ar
pulmon/ary PŬL-mō-nĕ-rē	pulmon/ary
tox/ic TŎKS-ĭk	tox/ic
anter/ior ăn-TĒ-rē-or	anter/ior
cutane/ous kū-TĀ-nē-ŭs	cutane/ous
acous/tic ă-KOOS-tĭk	acous/tic

2-12 The human body is capable of being in many different positions, such as standing, kneeling, and lying down. To guarantee consistency in descriptions of location, the *anatomic/al position* is used as a reference point to describe the location or direction of a body structure. In anatomic/al position, the body is erect and the eyes are looking forward. The arms hang to the sides, with palms facing forward; the legs are parallel with the toes pointing straight ahead.

Review Figure 2–2 and study the terms to become acquainted with their usage in denoting positions of direction when the body is in the anatomic/al position. Refer to this figure to complete the following frames.

anatomic/al position ăn-ă-TŎM-ĭk-ăl	**2-13** When a person is standing upright facing forward, arms at the sides with palms forward, with the legs parallel and the feet slightly apart with the toes pointing forward, he or she is in the standard position called the _____ / ____ _____.

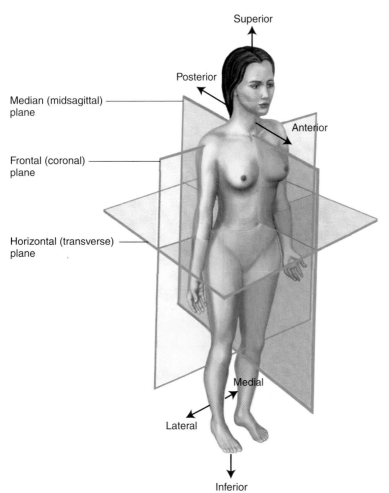

Figure 2-2 Body planes. (Note the body is in the anatomical position.)

<table>
<tr><td>

anter/ior, ventr/al
ăn-TĒ-rē-or, VĔN-trăl

poster/ior, dors/al
pŏs-TĒ-rē-or, DŌR-săl

</td><td>

2–14 Health care professionals use a common language of special terms when referring to body structures and their functions. However, their descriptions of any region or part of the human body assume that it is in anatomic/al position.

In anatomical position, the terms *anter/ior* and *ventr/al* refer to the front of the body or the front of any body structure. The terms *poster/ior* and *dors/al* refer to the back of the body or the back of any body structure. Identify the elements in this frame that refer to the

front of the body: _____ / _____ and _____ / _____

back of the body: _____ / _____ and _____ / _____

</td></tr>
</table>

<table>
<tr><td>

front

back

</td><td>

2–15 What position of the body do the terms *anter/ior* and *ventr/al* refer to?
_____ (of the body)
What position of the body do the terms *poster/ior* and *dors/al* refer to?
_____ (of the body)

</td></tr>
</table>

-ior **poster/o** **anter**	**2-16** The term *poster/o/anter/ior* refers to the back and front of the body. Identify the word elements in this frame that mean *pertaining to* _____ *back:* _____ / _____ *front:* _____
posterior, anterior pŏs-TĒ-rē-or, ăn-TĒ-rē-or *OR* **back, front**	**2-17** Directional terms are commonly used in radi/o/logy to describe the direction of the x-ray beam from its source and its point of exit. In an anter/o/poster/ior projection, the beam enters the body anteriorly and exits posteriorly. 　　A poster/o/anter/ior projection indicates that the beam enters the body on the _____ side and exits on the _____ side.
anter/ior ăn-TĒ-rē-or **poster/ior** pŏs-TĒ-rē-or	**2-18** Use *anter/ior* or *poster/ior* to complete the following statements, which refer to the position of body structures. The stomach is located on the _____ / _____ side of the body. The shoulder blades are located on the _____ / _____ side of the body.
infer/ior ĭn-FĒ-rē-or	**2-19** The term *inferior* in the English language refers to something of little or no importance. However, when used in a medical report, it designates a position or direction meaning *lower, below*. 　　Combine **infer/o** (lower, below) + *-ior* (pertaining to) to form a directional term that literally means *pertaining to lower or below*. _____ / _____
above	**2-20** In medical terms, the prefix *super-* designates an upper position. When you say "the head is superior to the stomach," you mean it is located above the stomach. When you say "the eyes are superior to the mouth," you mean they are located _____ the mouth.
side	**2-21** The word element **later/o** means *side, to one side*. A radiographic projection that enters through the left or right side of the body is referred to as a *later/al* projection. The term *later/al position* refers to the _____ (of the body).

 Review the three basic rules for building medical words.

Rule 1: Word root links a suffix that begins with a vowel.

Rule 2: CF (root + o) links a suffix that begins with a consonant.

Rule 3: CF (root + o) links a root to another root to form a compound word. (This rule holds true even if the next root begins with a vowel.)

later/al
LĂT-ĕr-ăl
anter/o/later/al
ăn-tĕr-ō-LĂT-ĕr-ăl
poster/o/later/al
pŏs-tĕr-ō-LĂT-ĕr-ăl

2–22   Here is a review of terms in radi/o/logy that specify direction of the x-ray beam from its source to its exit surface before striking the film. Build directional terms that mean

pertaining to the side or to one side (of the body): _____ / _____

pertaining to the anterior or front, and the side (of the body):
_____ / _____ / _____ / _____

pertaining to the posterior or back, and the side (of the body):
_____ / _____ / _____ / _____

---

medi

-al

2–23   The term *medi/al* is used to describe the midline of the body or a structure. The medi/al portion of the face contains the nose.
From the term *medi/al*, determine the

root meaning *middle* _____

suffix meaning *pertaining to* _____

-ad, medi
medi/ad
MĒ-dē-ăd

2–24   Suffix for *toward* is _____. Root for middle is _____.
Combine **medi** + *-ad* to form a word that means *toward the middle.*

_____ / _____

---

medi/ad
MĒ-dē-ăd

2–25   Use *-ad* to form a directional term that means *toward the middle (or center of the body).*

_____ / _____.

---

infer/ior
ĭn-FĒ-rē-or
infer/ior
ĭn-FĒ-rē-or

2–26   Anatomists use the term *infer/ior* to refer to a body structure located below another body structure or the lower part of a structure. For example, your chin is situated infer/ior to your mouth. (See Figure 2–2.) The rectum is the infer/ior portion of the colon.
To indicate that a structure is below another structure, use the

directional term _____ / _____.
To indicate the lower part of a structure, use the directional

term _____ / _____.

---

infer/ior
ĭn-FĒ-rē-or
later/al
LĂT-ĕr-ăl

2–27   Practice using the directional terms *later/al* and *infer/ior* to describe the following positions.

The legs are _____ / _____ to the trunk.

The eyes are _____ / _____ to the nose.

---

cephal/ad
SĔF-ă-lăd

2–28   Anatomists and health care professionals use the term *super/ior* to refer to a body structure that is above another body structure or toward the head, because the head is the most superior structure of the body. *Cephal/ad* is a term that refers to the direction toward the head.
When referring to the direction going toward the head, use the term

_____ / _____.

pertaining to **upper, above**	**2-29** Define the word elements in super/ior. *-ior:* _____ *super:* _____
super/ior soo-PĒ-rē-or **infer/ior** ĭn-FĔ-rē-or **super/ior** soo-PĒ-rē-or	**2-30** Use *super/ior* or *infer/ior* to complete the following statements that refer to the relative position of one body structure to another body structure. The chest is _____ / _____ to the stomach. The stomach is _____ / _____ to the lungs. The head is _____ / _____ to the neck.
caud/al KAWD-ăl	**2-31** The CF **caud/o** means *tail*. In this sense, *tail* designates a position toward the end of the body, away from the head. In humans, it also refers to an infer/ior position in the body or within a structure. Combine **caud** + *-al* to build a word that means *pertaining to the tail*. _____ / _____
proxim/al PRŎK-sĭm-ăl **dist/al** DĬS-tăl	**2-32** The terms *proxim/al* and *dist/al* are used as positional and directional terms. **Proxim/al** describes a structure as being *nearest* the point of attachment to the trunk or near the beginning of a structure. **Dist/al** describes a structure as being *far from* the point of attachment to the trunk or from the beginning of a structure. Identify the terms in this frame that mean *nearest the point of attachment:* _____ / _____ *farthest from the point of attachment:* _____ / _____
proxim/al PRŎK-sĭm-ăl **dist/al** DĬS-tăl	**2-33** The directional element **proxim/o** means *near or nearest the point of attachment;* **dist/o** means *far or farthest from the point of attachment.* The knee is proxim/al to the foot; the palm is dist/al to the elbow. (See Figure 2–2.) To describe a structure nearest the point of attachment, use the directional term _____ / _____. To describe a structure as being farthest from the point of attachment, use the directional term _____ / _____.
ad/duction ă-DŬK-shŭn	**2-34** Some directional terms, such as ab/duction and ad/duction indicate movement away from and toward the body. These are also types of movements produced by muscles (See Figure 10-2). The prefix *ab-* means from, *away from;* the suffix *-duction* means *act of leading, bringing, conducting.* Thus, ab/duction means *movement away from the body.* Can you determine the directional term in this frame that means *movement toward the body?* _____/_____

SECTION REVIEW 2-2

Using the following table, write the CF or suffix that matches its definition in the space provided to the left of the definition. There may be more than one word element that matches a definition.

Combining Form		Suffix	
caud/o	later/o	-ad	-lysis
cyt/o	medi/o	-al	-toxic
dist/o	proxim/o	-ior	
hist/o	ventr/o	-logist	
infer/o		-logy	

1. _____ tissue
2. _____ pertaining to
3. _____ middle
4. _____ near, nearest
5. _____ study of
6. _____ cell
7. _____ belly, belly side
8. _____ poison
9. _____ toward
10. _____ tail
11. _____ specialist in study of
12. _____ far, farthest
13. _____ lower, below
14. _____ separation; destruction; loosening
15. _____ side, to one side

Competency Verification: Check your answers in Appendix B, Answer Key, page 555. If you are not satisfied with your level of comprehension, go back to Frame 2–1 and rework the frames.

Correct Answers _____ × 6.67 = _____ % Score

WORD ELEMENTS

This section introduces word elements that describe a body structure. When these elements are attached to positional prefixes or suffixes, they form words that describe a region or position in the body. Review the following table and pronounce each word in the word analysis column aloud before you begin to work in the frames.

Word Element	Meaning	Word Analysis
Combining Forms		

BODY REGIONS

abdomin/o	abdomen	**abdomin**/al (ăb-DŎM-ĭ-năl): pertaining to the abdomen *-al:* pertaining to
cephal/o	head	**cephal**/ad (SĔF-ă-lăd): toward the head *-ad:* toward
cervic/o	neck; cervix uteri (neck of uterus)	**cervic**/al (SĔR-vĭ-kăl): pertaining to the neck of the body or the neck of the uterus *-al:* pertaining to
crani/o	cranium (skull)	**crani**/al (KRĀ-nē-ăl): pertaining to the cranium or skull *-al:* pertaining to
gastr/o	stomach	**gastr**/ic (GĂS-trĭk): pertaining to the stomach *-ic:* pertaining to
ili/o	ilium (lateral, flaring portion of hip bone)	**ili**/ac (ĬL-ē-ăk): pertaining to the ilium *-ac:* pertaining to
inguin/o	groin	**inguin**/al (ĬNG-gwĭ-năl): pertaining to the groin *-al:* pertaining to
lumb/o	loins (lower back)	**lumb**/ar (LŬM-băr): pertaining to the loin area or lower back *-ar:* pertaining to
pelv/i*	pelvis	**pelv**/i/meter (pĕl-VĬM-ĕ-tĕr): instrument for measuring the pelvis *-meter:* instrument for measuring
pelv/o		**pelv**/ic (PĔL-vĭc): pertaining to the pelvis *-ic:* pertaining to
spin/o	spine	**spin**/al (SPĪ-năl): pertaining to the spine or spinal column *-al:* pertaining to
thorac/o	chest	**thorac**/ic (thō-RĂS-ĭk): pertaining to the chest *-ic:* pertaining to

*The *i* in *pelv/i/meter* is an exception to the rule of using the connecting vowel *o*.

(continued)

Word Element	Meaning	Word Analysis
umbilic/o	umbilicus, navel	peri/**umbilic**/al (pĕr-ē-ŭm-BĬL-ĭ-kăl): pertaining to the area around the umbilicus *peri-:* around *-al:* pertaining to

Listen and Learn, the audio CD-ROM included with this book, will help you master pronunciation of selected medical words. Use it to practice pronunciations of the above-listed medical terms and for instructions to complete the *Listen and Learn* exercise for this section.

SECTION REVIEW 2-3

For the following medical terms, first write the suffix and its meaning. Then translate the meaning of the remaining elements starting with the first part of the word. The first word is completed for you.

Term	Meaning
1. ili/ac	*-ac: pertaining to; ilium (lateral, flaring portion of hip bone)*
2. abdomin/al	
3. inguin/al	
4. spin/al	
5. peri/umbilic/al	
6. cephal/ad	
7. gastr/ic	
8. thorac/ic	
9. cervic/al	
10. lumb/ar	

Competency Verification: Check your answers in Appendix B, Answer Key, page 556. If you are not satisfied with your level of comprehenion, review the vocabulary and retake the review.

Correct Answers _____ × 10 = _____ % Score

Body Planes and Cavities

To visualize structural arrangements of various organs, the body may be sectioned (cut) according to planes of reference. The three major planes are the frontal, median, and horizontal planes, as shown in Figure 2–2. In addition, body cavities, as shown in Figure 2–3, contain internal organs and are used as a point of reference to locate structures within body cavities.

Body Planes

2-35 Review Figures 2–2 and 2–3 carefully before proceeding with the next frame. You may refer to the two figures to complete the following frames.

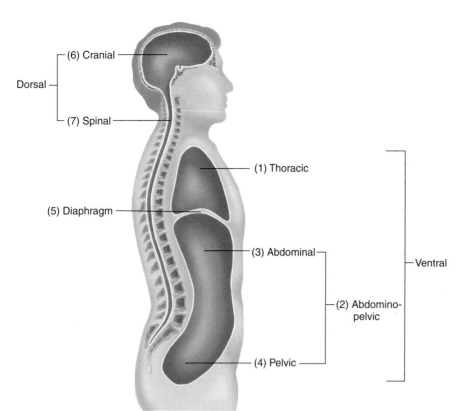

Figure 2-3 Body cavities. Ventral cavities (anterior) located in the front of the body; dorsal cavities (posterior) located in the back of the body.

Dorsal
(6) Cranial
(7) Spinal
(5) Diaphragm
(1) Thoracic
(3) Abdominal
(2) Abdomino-pelvic
(4) Pelvic
Ventral

	2-36 A body plane is an imaginary flat surface that divides the body into two sections. Different planes divide the body into different sections, such as front and back, left side and right side, and top and bottom. These planes serve as points of reference for describing the direction from which the body is being observed. Planes are particularly useful to describe views in which radiographic images are taken.
	An imaginary flat surface that divides the body into two sections is
body plane	a _____ _____.

	2-37 Examine Figure 2–2 and list the three major planes of the body.
median (midsagittal) mĭd-SĂJ-ĭ-tăl	_____ (_____)
frontal (coronal) kŏ-rō-năl	_____ (_____)
horizontal (transverse) trăns-VĔRS	_____ (_____)

 | When in doubt about the meaning of a word element, refer to Appendix A, page 538.

midsagittal plane mĭd-SĂJ-ĭ-tăl	**2–38** The *median (midsagittal) plane* lies exactly in the middle of the body and divides the body into two equal halves. (See Figure 2–2.) When the chest is divided into equal right and left sides, it is divided by the median plane, also known as the _____ _____.
median plane	**2–39** When the lungs are divided into equal right and left sides, they are divided by the midsagittal plane, also known as the _____ _____.
infer/ior, super/ior ĭn-FĒ-rē-or, soo-PĒ-rē-or	**2–40** The *horizontal (transverse) plane* runs across the body from the right side to the left side and divides the body into upper (superior) and lower (inferior) portions. Figure 2–2 shows the division of this plane. Recall the term *super/ior.* It is a point of reference that refers to a structure above or oriented toward a higher place. For example, the head is superior to the heart. *Infer/ior* is a point of reference that refers to a structure situated below or oriented toward a lower place. For example, the feet are inferior to the legs. Because the head is located superior to the heart, the heart is located _____ / _____ to the head. Because the feet are located inferior to the legs, the legs are located _____ / _____ to the feet.
transverse plane trăns-VĔRS	**2–41** The plane that divides the body into superior and inferior portions is the horizontal plane. This plane is also called the _____ _____.
cross-sectional	**2–42** Many different transverse planes exist at every possible level of the body, from head to foot. A trans/verse section is also called a *cross-sectional plane.* Some radiographic imaging devices produce cross-sectional images. Cross-sectioning of the body or of an organ along different planes results in different views. The horizontal, or *trans/verse*, plane is also known as the _____ plane.
-graph **radi/o** **trans-** **-verse**	**2–43** A radi/o/graph of the liver along a trans/verse plane results in a different view than a radiograph along the frontal plane. That is why a series of x-rays is commonly taken using different planes. Views along different planes result in a complete and comprehensive image of a body structure. Identify the elements in this frame that mean *process of recording:* _____ *radiation, x-ray; radius (lower arm bone on thumb side):* _____ / _____ *through, across:* _____ *turning:* _____
coronal plane CŎR-ŏ-năl	**2–44** Locate the frontal plane in Figure 2–2. The frontal plane is also called the _____ _____.

poster/ior pŏs-TĒ-rē-or	**2-45** The frontal (coronal) plane is commonly used to take an anter/o/poster/ior (AP) chest radiograph, indicating that the x-ray beam enters the body on the anterior side and exits the body on the _____ / _____ side. The radiograph produced shows a view from the front of the chest toward the back (of the body)
study of	**2-46** In the previous frame, you learned that _anter/o/poster/ior_ is used in radi/o/logy to describe the direction or path of an x-ray beam. The CF _radi/o_ means _radiation; x-ray; radius (lower arm bone on thumb side)_. The suffix _-logy_ means _____ _____.
radi/o/logy rā-dē-ŎL-ō-jē	**2-47** Use _radi/o_ to form a word that means _study of radiation or x-rays:_ _____ / ____ / _____.
AP	**2-48** Identify the abbreviation in Frame 2–45 that designates the path of an x-ray beam from the anterior to the posterior part of the body: _____.

Body Cavities

crani/al, spin/al KRĀ-nē-ăl, SPĪ-năl **thorac/ic,** **abdomin/o/pelv/ic** thō-RĂS-ĭk, ăb-dŏm-ĭ-nō-PĔL-vĭk	**2-49** The body contains two major cavities: the dorsal and ventral cavities. These cavities are hollow spaces that contain internal organs. They are further subdivided into two dors/al and two ventr/al cavities. (Note: The terms in Figure 2–3 are not broken down into their component parts.) In Figure 2–3, locate and name the dors/al cavities: _____ / _____, _____ / _____ ventr/al cavities: _____ / _____, _____ / ____ / _____ / _____

2-50 Let us continue to learn about the body cavities as you read and locate them in Figure 2–3. The (1) **thoracic cavity** contains the heart and lungs. The (2) **abdominopelvic cavity** contains organs of the digestive and reproductive systems and includes two subcavities: the (3) **abdominal** and (4) **pelvic cavities**. The abdomin/o/pelv/ic subdivision is useful because of the different types of organs present in each (digestive versus reproductive). Because there is no dividing wall between them, they are actually one large cavity, the abdominopelvic cavity.

super/ior soo-PĒ-rē-or **infer/ior** ĭn-FĒ-rē-or	**2-51** Use the terms *super/ior* and *infer/ior* to describe locations, or positions, of body cavities. The thoracic cavitiy is located _____ / _____ to the abdomino-pelvic cavity. The spinal cavity is located _____ / _____ to the cranial cavity.

	2-52 The (5) **diaphragm** is a dome-shaped muscle that plays an important role in breathing. It separates the thorac/ic cavity from the abdomin/o/pelv/ic cavity. Locate the diaphragm in Figure 2–3.

pelv **thorac** **abdomin**	**2-53** Let us review some of the elements in the previous frame. The root that refers to the pelvis is: _____ chest is: _____ abdomen is: _____

crani/al KRĀ-nē-ăl **spin/al** SPĪ-năl	**2-54** The *dorsal cavity* consists of the (6) **cranial** and (7) **spinal cavities**. These cavities contain the organs of the *nervous system:* the brain and spinal cord. The nervous system is one of the most complex systems of the body (see Chapter 9) and controls many vital activities of the body. Practice building words that refer to the body cavities by building a term that means *pertaining to the cranium (skull):* _____ / _____ *pertaining to the spine:* _____ / _____

crani/al KRĀ-nē-ăl **spin/al** SPĪ-năl	**2-55** As discussed earlier, the dors/al cavity includes the crani/al cavity, which is formed by the skull and contains the brain. The spin/al cavity, which is formed by the spine (backbone), contains the spinal cord. Refer to Figure 2–3 to complete the following frames. The body cavity surrounding the skull is the _____ / _____ cavity. spinal cord is the _____ / _____ cavity.

Abdominopelvic Quadrants and Regions

The abdominopelvic region is further divided into quadrants and regions. (See Figure 2–4.)

Abdominopelvic Quadrants

2-56 Because the abdomin/o/pelv/ic cavity is a large area and contains many organs, it is useful to divide it into smaller sections. One method divides the abdomin/o/pelv/ic cavity into quadrants. A second method divides the abdomin/o/pelv/ic cavity into regions. Physicians and health care professionals use quadrants or regions as a point of reference.

The larger division of the abdomin/o/pelv/ic cavity consists of four quadrants: right upper quadrant (RUQ), left upper quadrant (LUQ), right lower quadrant (RLQ), and left lower quadrant (LLQ). Locate these quadrants in Figure 2–4A.

2-57 After you have located and reviewed the quadrants, determine the meaning of the following abbreviations

right upper quadrant	RUQ: _____ _____ _____
left upper quadrant	LUQ: _____ _____ _____
right lower quadrant	RLQ: _____ _____ _____
left lower quadrant	LLQ: _____ _____ _____

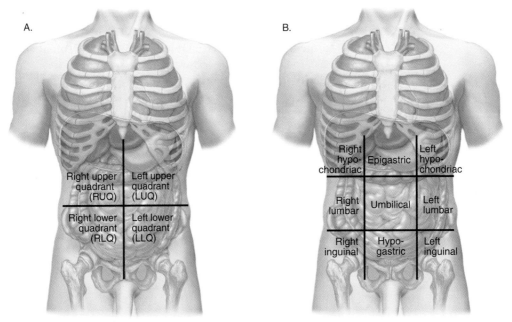

Figure 2-4   Abdominopelvic quadrants and regions. (A) Four quadrants of the abdomen. (B) Nine regions of the abdomen showing superficial organs.

	2-58 Quadrants are useful in describing the location in the body in which a surgical procedure will be performed. They also are useful in denoting incision sites or the location of abnormal masses such as tumors. A tumor located in the right lower quadrant will most likely be
RLQ	denoted in the medical record with the abbreviation _____.

	2-59 Quadrants may also be used to describe the location of a patient's symptoms. The physician may pinpoint a patient's abdominal pain in the RLQ. Such a finding could indicate a diagnosis of appendicitis, because the appendix is located in that quadrant. Pain in another quadrant, such as the LLQ, would indicate a different diagnosis. Identify the abbreviation for the:
RLQ	right lower quadrant: _____
LLQ	left lower quadrant: _____

	2-60 Locate the quadrant that contains a major part of the stomach.
left upper quadrant,	This quadrant is the _____ _____ _____ and
LUQ	its abbreviation is _____.

Abdominopelvic Regions

2-61 Whereas larger sections of the abdomin/o/pelv/ic cavity are divided into four quadrants, the smaller sections are divided into nine regions, each of which corresponds to a region near a specific point in the body. As with quadrants, body region designation is also used to describe the location of internal organs and the origin of pain. Review Figure 2–4B to see the location of various organs within these regions.

2–62 Now that you have examined the nine regions, let us review some of the terms within each region. These terms are commonly used to describe a location of organs within the abdominal cavity.

Although the CFs in the left-hand column below denote a body structure, when attached to directional elements, they form terms denoting specific regions of the abdomen. Study the meaning of each regional term, then divide each one in the right-hand column into its basic elements. The first term is completed for you.

hypo/chondr/iac
hī-pō-KŎN-drē-ăk

epi/gastr/ic
ĕp-ĭ-GĂS-trĭk

inguin/al
ĬNG-gwĭ-năl

lumb/ar
LŬM-băr

umbilic/al
ŭm-BĬL-ĭ-kăl

Combining Form	Meaning	Regions of the Abdomen
chondr/o	cartilage	h y p o / c h o n d r / i a c
gastr/o	stomach	e p i g a s t r i c
inguin/o	groin	i n g u i n a l
lumb/o	loins (lower back)	l u m b a r
umbilic/o	umbilicus, navel	u m b i l i c a l

2–63 Refer to Figure 2–4B to identify the terms in the regions that describe the following statements. The first one is completed for you.
The region located

near the groin: _inguin____ / _al_____

hypo/chondr/iac
hī-pō-KŎN-drē-ăk

umbilic/al
ŭm-BĬL-ĭ-kăl

hypo/gastr/ic
hī-pō-GĂS-trĭk

beneath the ribs: _____ / _____ / _____.

near the navel: _____ / _____.

below the stomach: _____ / _____ / _____.

2–64 Suffixes *-ac, -ic, -ous* and *-ior* mean *pertaining to.* Can you identify the parts of speech of these suffixes?

adjectives

_____

2–65 Use *gastr/o* to develop medical words that pertain to the area

hypo/gastr/ic
hī-pō-GĂS-trĭk

epi/gastr/ic
ĕp-ĭ-GĂS-trĭk

under or below the stomach: _____ / _____ / _____

above or on the stomach: _____ / _____ / _____

epi/gastr/ic ĕp-ĭ-GĂS-trĭk	**2-66** The epi/gastr/ic region may be the location of "heartburn" pain. Pain in this area could be symptomatic of many abnormal conditions, including indigestion or heart attack. The area of heartburn pain may be felt in the _____ / _____ / _____ region.
-iac **hypo-** **chondr**	**2-67** The right and left hypo/chondr/iac regions are located on each side of the epi/gastr/ic region and directly under the cartilage of the ribs. Identify the elements in hypo/chondr/iac that mean _pertaining to:_ _____ _under, below, deficient:_ _____ _cartilage:_ _____

Refer to Figure 2–4B to answer the following frames. If needed, use Appendix A, Glossary of Medical Word Elements.

loins (lower back)	**2-68** The lumbar regions consist of the middle right and middle left regions, located near the waistline of the body. The term _lumb/ar_ means _pertaining to the_ _____ (_____ _____).
lumb/o/abdomin/al lŭm-bō-ăb-DŎM-ĭ-năl	**2-69** Combine **lumb/o** + **abdomin** + _-al_ to form a term that means _pertaining to the loins and abdomen._ _____ / ____ / _____ / ____
umbilic/al region ŭm-BĬL-ĭ-kăl	**2-70** The center of the umbilic/al region marks the point where the umbilic/al cord of the mother entered the fetus. This is the navel or, in layman's terms, the "belly button." The region that lies between the right and left lumbar regions is designated as the _____ / _____.
umbilic/al ŭm-BĬL-ĭ-kăl	**2-71** CF **umbilic/o** refers to _umbilicus,_ or _navel._ The region that literally means _pertaining to the navel_ is _____ / _____.
inguin/al ĬNG-gwĭ-năl	**2-72** A hernia is a protrusion or projection of an organ through the wall of the cavity that normally contains it. A common type of hernia that may occur, particularly in males, is an inguin/al hernia. This hernia would be located in the right or left _____ / _____ region.
right inguin/al hernia ĬNG-gwĭ-năl HĔR-nē-ă	**2-73** Locate the right inguin/al region and the left inguin/al region in Figure 2–4B. A hernia on the right side of the groin is called a _____ _____ / _____ _____.

hypo/gastr/ic

hī-pō-GĂS-trĭk

2-74 The area between the right and the left inguin/al regions is called the *hypo/gastr/ic* region. This region contains the large intestine (colon), which is involved in the removal of solid waste from the body. Identify the name of the region below the stomach that literally means *pertaining to below the stomach.*

_____ / _____ / _____

SECTION REVIEW 2-4

Using the following table, write the combining form, suffix, or prefix that matches its definition in the space provided to the left of the definition. There may be more than one word element that matches a definition.

Combining Forms		Suffixes	Prefixes
abdomin/o	lumb/o	-ac	epi-
chondr/o	pelv/i, pelv/o	-ad	hypo-
crani/o	poster/o	-al	
gastr/o	spin/o	-ic	
inguin/o	thorac/o	-ior	
	umbilic/o		

1. _____ toward
2. _____ groin
3. _____ stomach
4. _____ pelvis
5. _____ cartilage
6. _____ above, on
7. _____ pertaining to
8. _____ loins, (lower back)
9. _____ chest
10. _____ under, below, deficient
11. _____ cranium (skull)
12. _____ spine
13. _____ umbilicus, navel
14. _____ back (of body), behind, posterior
15. _____ abdomen

Competency Verification: Check your answers in Appendix B, Answer Key, page 556. If you are not satisfied with your level of comprehension, go back to Frames 2–35 and reword the frames.

Correct Answers _____ × 6.67 = _____ % Score

Abbreviations

This section introduces body structure and abbreviations related to radiology and their meanings.

Abbreviation	Meaning	Abbreviation	Meaning
Body Structure and Related			
abd	abdomen	**LUQ**	left upper quadrant
ant	anterior	**PA**	posteroanterior; pernicious anemia; pulmonary artery; physician assistant
AP	anteroposterior	**RLQ**	right lower quadrant
Bx, bx	biopsy	**RUQ**	right upper quadrant
LAT, lat	lateral	**U&L, U/L**	upper and lower
LLQ	left lower quadrant		
Radiology			
CT	computed tomography	**PET**	positron emission tomography
CXR	chest x-ray, chest radiograph	**US**	ultrasound; ultrasonography
MRI	magnetic resonance imaging	**SPECT**	single photon emission computed tomography

Additional Medical Terms

The following are additional terms related to the structure of the body. Recognizing and learning these terms will help you understand the connection between a pathological condition, its diagnosis, and the rationale behind the method of treatment selected for a particular disorder.

Signs, Symptoms, and Diseases

adhesion ăd-HĒ-zhŭn	Band of scar tissue binding anatomical surfaces that are normally separate from each other *Adhesions most commonly form in the abdomen after abdominal surgery, inflammation, or injury.*
inflammation ĭn-flă-MĀ-shun	Protective response of body tissues to irritation, infection, or allergy *Signs of inflammation include redness, swelling, heat, and pain, commonly accompanied by loss of function.*

sepsis SĔP-sĭs	Body's inflammatory response to infection, in which there is fever, elevated heart and respiratory rate, and low blood pressure *Septicemia is a common type of sepsis.*

Diagnostic Procedures

endoscopy ĕn-DŎS-kō-pē *endo-:* in, within *-scopy:* visual examination	Visual examination of the interior of organs and cavities with a specialized lighted instrument called an *endoscope* *Endoscopy can also be used to obtain tissue samples for biopsy, perform surgery, and follow the course of a disease, as in the assessment of the healing of gastric ulcers. The cavity or organ examined dictates the name of the endoscopic procedure. A camera and video recorder are commonly used during this procedure to provide a permanent record. (See Figure 2–5.)*

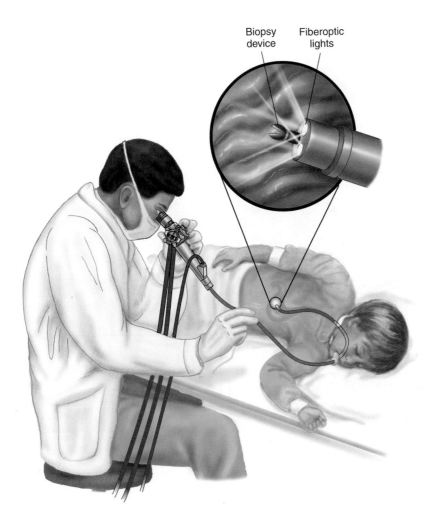

Biopsy device   Fiberoptic lights

Figure 2-5 Endoscopy.

fluoroscopy floo-or-ŎS-kō-pē *fluor/o:* luminous, fluorescence *-scopy:* visual examination	Radiographic procedure that uses a fluorescent screen instead of a photographic plate to produce a visual image from x-rays that pass through the patient, resulting in continuous imaging of the motion of internal structures and immediate serial images *Fluoroscopy is invaluable in diagnostic and clinical procedures. It permits the radiographer to observe organs, such as the digestive tract and heart, in motion. It is also used during biopsy surgery, nasogastric tube placement, and catheter insertion during angiography.*
magnetic resonance imaging (MRI) măg-NĔT-ĭc RĔZ-ĕn-ăns ĬM-ĭj-ĭng	Radiographic technique that uses electromagnetic energy to produce multiplanar cross-sectional images of the body *MRI does not require a contrast medium; however, one may be used to enhance visualization of internal structures. (See Figure 2–6E.) MRI is regarded as superior to CT for most central nervous system abnormalities, particularly abnormalities of the brainstem and spinal cord, and musculoskeletal and pelvic area abnormalities.*

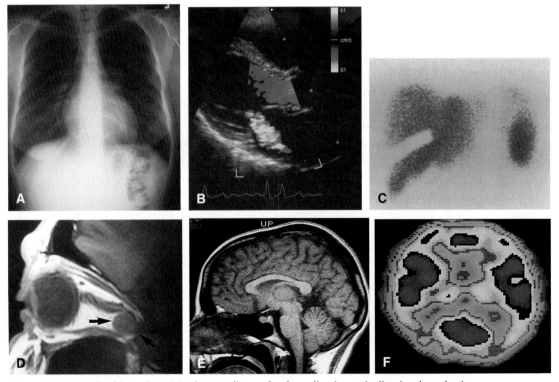

Figure 2-6 Medical imaging. (A) Chest radiograph of mediastinum indicating lymphatic enlargement in suspected lymphoma. (B) Ultrasonography of blood flow with color indicating direction. (C) Nuclear scan of the liver and spleen showing a heterogeneous uptake pattern characteristic of lymphoma. (D) CT scan of the eye in lateral view showing a tumor (arrows) below the optic nerve. (E) MRI scan of the midsagittal section of the head, showing extreme clarity of soft tissue. (F) PET scan of the brain in transverse section (frontal lobes at top). (A) From McKinnis, L. *Fundamentals of Orthopedic Radiology*, page 149. F.A. Davis, 1997, with permission. (B) Courtesy of Suzanne Wambold, PhD, University of Toledo. (C) From Pittiglio, D.H., and Sacher, R.A. *Clinical Hematology and Fundamentals of Hemostasis*, page 302. F.A. Davis, 1987, with permission. (D, E, F) From Mazziotta, J.C., and Gilman, S. *Clinical Brain imagining: Principles and Applications*, pages 27 and 298. Oxford University Press, 1992, with permission.

nuclear scan NŪ-klē-ăr	Diagnostic technique that produces an image of an organ or area by recording the concentration of a *radiopharmaceutical* (the combination of a radioactive substance called a *radionuclide* and another chemical) introduced into the body (ingested, inhaled, or injected) *A scanning device detects the shape, size, location, and function of the organ or structure under study. It provides information about the structure and the function of an organ or system. There is a variety of nuclear scans, such as bone scans, liver scans, and brain scans. (See Figure 2–6C.)*
radiography rā-dē-ŎG-ră-fē *radi/o:* radiation, x-ray; radius (lower arm bone on thumb side) *-graphy:* process of recording	Production of captured shadow images on photographic film through the action of ionizing radiation passing through the body from an external source *Soft body tissues, such as the stomach or liver, appear black or gray on the radiograph; dense body tissues, such as bone, appear white on the radiograph, making it useful in diagnosing fractures. Figure 2–6A is a chest radiograph showing widening of the mediastinum.*
radiopharmaceutical rā-dē-ō-fărm-ă-SŪ-tĭ-kăl *pharmaceutic:* drug, medicine *-al:* pertaining to	Drug that contains a radioactive substance which travels to an area or a specific organ that will be scanned *Types of radiopharmaceuticals include diagnostic, research, and therapeutic.*
scan	Technique for carefully studying an area, organ, or system of the body by recording and displaying an image of the area *A concentration of a radioactive substance that has an affinity for a specific tissue may be administered intravenously to enhance the image. The liver, brain, and thyroid can be examined; tumors can be located; and function can be evaluated by various scanning techniques.*

tomography tō-MŎG-ră-fē *tom/o:* to cut *-graphy:* process of recording	Radiographic technique that produces a film representing a detailed cross-section, or slice, of an area, tissue, or organ at a predetermined depth *Tomography is a valuable diagnostic tool for identifying space-occupying lesions, such as those found in the liver, brain, pancreas, and gallbladder. Types of tomography include computed tomography (CT), positron emission tomography (PET), and single photon emission computed tomography (SPECT).*
computed tomography (CT) kŏm-PŪ-tĕd tō-MŎG-ră-fē *tom/o:* to cut *-graphy:* process of recording	Radiographic technique that uses a narrow beam of x-rays that rotates in a full arc around the patient to acquire multiple views of the body that a computer interprets to produce cross-sectional images of that body part (See Figure 2–6D.) *CT scans are used to detect tumor masses, bone displacement, and accumulations of fluid. CT may be administered with or without a contrast medium.*
positron emission tomography (PET) PŎZ-ĭ-trŏn ē-MĬSH-ŭn tō-MŎG-ră-fē *tom/o:* to cut *-graphy:* process of recording	Radiographic technique combining computed tomography with radiopharmaceuticals that produces a cross-sectional (transverse) image of the dispersement of radioactivity (through emission of positrons) in a section of the body to reveal the areas where the radiopharmaceutical is being metabolized and where there is a deficiency in metabolism *PET is a type of nuclear scan used to diagnose disorders that involve metabolic processes. It can aid in the diagnosis of neurological disorders, such as brain tumors, epilepsy, stroke, Alzheimer disease, and abdominal and pulmonary disorders. (See Figure 2–6F.)*
single-photon emission computed tomography (SPECT) SĬNG-gŭl FŌ-tŏn ē-MĬ-shŭn cŏm-PŪ-tĕd tō-MŎG-ră-fē *tom/o:* to cut *-graphy:* process of recording	Type of nuclear imaging study that scans organs after injection of a radioactive tracer and employs a specialized gamma camera that detects emitted radiation to produce a three-dimensional image from a composite of numerous views *SPECT differs from PET in that the chemical substance stay in the bloodstream instead of being absorbed into the surrounding tissues. Organs commonly studied by SPECT scans include the brain, heart, lungs, liver, spleen, bones and, in some cases, joints.*
ultrasonography (US) ŭl-tră-sŏn-ŎG-ră-fē *-ultra:* excess, beyond *son:* sound *-graphy:* process of recording	Imaging technique that uses high-frequency sound waves (ultrasound) that bounce off body tissues and are recorded to produce an image of an internal organ or tissue *In contrast to other imaging techniques, US does not use ionizing radiation (x-ray). It is used to diagnose fetal development and internal structures of the abdomen, brain, and heart and musculoskeletal disorders. The record produced by US is called a sonogram or echogram. (See Figure 2–6B.)*
Doppler	Ultra high-frequency sound waves and Doppler technology are used to produce audible sound of blood flowing through an artery. *A transducer emits and then collects reflected sound waves. If the artery is blocked, little or no sound will be heard.*

Medical and Surgical Procedures

anastomosis ă-năs-tō-MŌ-sĭs	Connection between two vessels; surgical joining of two ducts, blood vessels, or bowel segments to allow flow from one to the other (See Figure 2–7.)

Chapter Review

Word Elements Summary

The following table summarizes CFs, suffixes, and prefixes related to body structure.

Word Element	Meaning	Word Element	Meaning
Combining Forms			
abdomin/o	abdomen	**inguin/o**	groin
anter/o	anterior, front	**later/o**	side, to one side
caud/o	tail	**lumb/o**	loins (lower back)
cephal/o	head	**medi/o**	middle
cervic/o	neck; cervix uteri (neck of uterus)	**nucle/o**	nucleus
chondr/o	cartilage	**pelv/o, pelv/i**	pelvis
crani/o	cranium (skull)	**poster/o**	back (of body), behind, posterior
cyt/o	cell	**proxim/o**	near, nearest
dist/o	far, farthest	**radi/o**	radiation, x-ray; radius (lower arm bone on thumb side)
dors/o	back (of body)	**spin/o**	spine
gastr/o	stomach	**super/o**	upper, above
hist/o	tissue	**thorac/o**	chest
ili/o	ilium (lateral, flaring portion of hip bone)	**umbilic/o**	umbilicus, navel
infer/o	lower, below	**ventr/o**	belly, belly side
Suffixes			
ADJECTIVE			
-ac, -al, -ar, -ary, -ous, -iac, -ic, -ior	pertaining to		
OTHER			
-ad	toward	**-lysis**	separation; destruction; loosening
-logist	specialist in study of	**-toxic**	poison
-logy	study of	**-verse**	turning

(continued)

Word Element	Meaning	Word Element	Meaning
Prefixes			
epi-	above, on	**super-**	upper, above
hypo-	under, below, deficient	**trans-**	through, across
medi-	middle		

 Enhance your study and reinforcement of word elements with the power of *Davis Plus.* Visit *http://davisplus.fadavis.com/gylys/simplified* for this chapter's flash-card activity. We recommend you complete the flash-card activity before completing the word elements review below.

Word Elements Review

After you review the previous Word Elements Summary, complete this activity by writing the meaning of each element or abbreviation in the space provided.

Word Element	Meaning	Word Element	Meaning
Combining Forms			
1. abdomin/o	_____	**11.** inguin/o	_____
2. anter/o	_____	**12.** later/o	_____
3. caud/o	_____	**13.** lumb/o	_____
4. cephal/o	_____	**14.** medi/o	_____
5. chondr/o	_____	**15.** nucle/o	_____
6. crani/o	_____	**16.** pelv/o	_____
7. cyt/o	_____	**17.** proxim/o	_____
8. dist/o	_____	**18.** thorac/o	_____
9. hist/o	_____	**19.** umbilic/o	_____
10. infer/o	_____	**20.** ventr/o	_____
Suffixes			
21. -ac, -al, -ar, -iac, -ic, -ior	_____	**24.** -lysis	_____
22. -ad	_____	**25.** -toxic	_____
23. -logist	_____		
Prefixes and Abbreviations			
26. CT	_____	**29.** MRI	_____
27. epi-	_____	**30.** RUQ	_____
28. hypo-	_____		

Competency Verification: Check your answers in Appendix A, Glossary of Medical Word Elements, page 538. If you are not satisfied with your level of comprehension, review the word elements and retake the review.

Correct Answers: _____ × 3.33 = _____ % Score

Vocabulary Review

In **figure A**, label the four abdominopelvic quadrants; in **figure B**, label the nine abdominopelvic regions.

Right upper quadrant (RUQ)
Left upper quadrant (LUQ)
Right lower quadrant (RLQ)
Left lower quadrant (LLQ)

A.

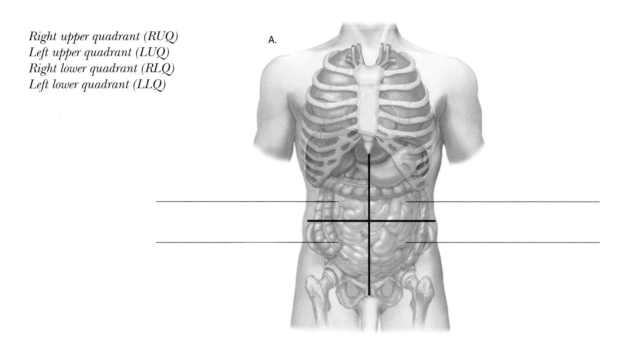

Right hypochondriac
Epigastric
Right lumbar
Right inguinal
Left hypochondriac
Umbilical
Left lumbar
Left inguinal
Hypogastric

B.

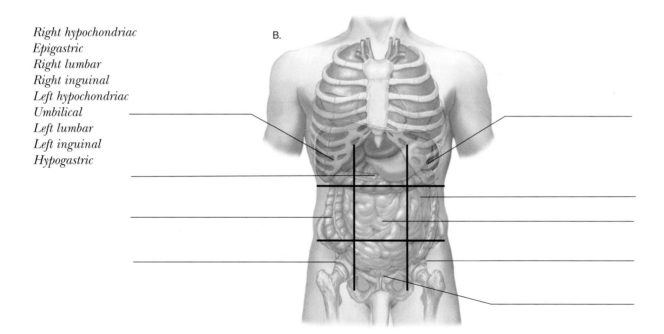

Competency Verification: Compare your answers by referring to Figure 2–4A and B, page 46.

3 Integumentary System

OBJECTIVES

Upon completion of this chapter, you will be able to:

- Describe the type of medical treatment the dermatologist provides.
- Identify the integumentary system structures by labeling the anatomical illustrations.
- Describe the primary functions of the integumentary system.
- Describe common diseases related to the integumentary system.
- Describe common diagnostic, medical, and surgical procedures related to the integumentary system.
- Apply your word-building skills by constructing various medical terms related to the integumentary system.
- Describe common abbreviations and symbols related to the integumentary system.
- Reinforce word elements and their meanings by completing the flash card activities.
- Recognize, define, pronounce, and spell terms correctly.
- Demonstrate your knowledge of this chapter by successfully completing the frames, reviews, and medical report evaluations.

Medical Specialty

Dermatology

Dermatology is the branch of medicine concerned with diagnosis and treatment of diseases involving the skin and the relationship of skin lesions to systemic diseases. The physician who specializes in diagnosis and treatment of skin diseases is called a **dermatologist**. The dermatologist's scope of practice includes the management of skin cancers, moles, and other skin tumors. This specialist also uses various techniques for the enhancement and correction of cosmetic skin defects and prescribes measures to maintain the skin in a state of health.

Anatomy and Physiology Overview

The integumentary system consists of the skin and its accessory organs: the hair, nails, sebaceous glands, and sweat glands. The skin is the largest organ in the body and protects the body from the external environment. It shields the body against injuries, infection, dehydration, harmful ultraviolet rays, and toxic compounds. Beneath the skin's surface is an intricate network of sensory receptors that register sensations of temperature, pain, and pressure. The millions of sensory receptors and a vascular network aid the functions of the entire body in maintaining *homeostasis,* a stable internal environment of the body. (See Figure 3–1.)

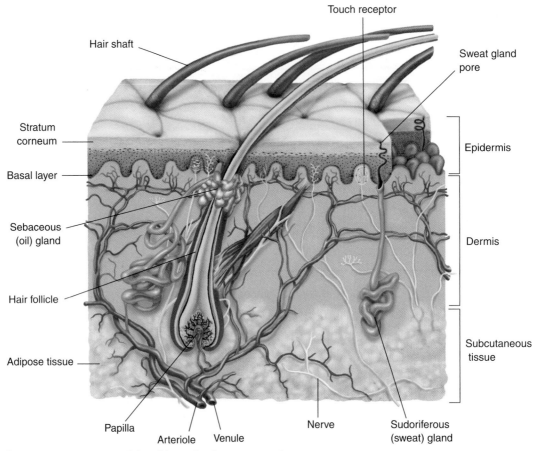

Figure 3-1 Structure of the skin and subcutaneous tissue.

WORD ELEMENTS

This section introduces combining forms (CFs) related to the integumentary system. Included are key suffixes; prefixes are defined in the right-hand column as needed. Review the following table, and pronounce each word in the word analysis column aloud before you begin to work the frames.

Word Elements	Meaning	Word Analysis
Combining Forms		
adip/o	fat	**adip/o/cele** (ĂD-ĭ-pō-sēl): hernia containing fat or fatty tissue *-cele:* hernia, swelling
lip/o		**lip/o/cyte** (LĬP-ō-sīt): fat cell *-cyte:* cell
steat/o		**steat/itis** (stē-ă-TĪ-tĭs): inflammation of fatty tissue *-itis:* inflammation

Word Elements	Meaning	Word Analysis
cutane/o	skin	**cutane**/ous (kū-TĀ-nē-ŭs): pertaining to the skin *-ous:* pertaining to
dermat/o		**dermat**/o/logist (dĕr-mă-TŎL-ō-jĭst): physician specializing in treating skin disorders *-logist:* specialist in study of
derm/o		hypo/**derm**/ic (hī-pō-DĔR-mĭk): under or inserted under the skin, as in a hypodermic injection *hypo-:* under, below, deficient *-ic:* pertaining to
hidr/o	sweat	**hidr**/aden/itis (hī-drăd-ĕ-NĪ-tĭs): inflammation of a sweat gland *aden:* gland *-itis:* inflammation *Do not confuse **hidr/o** (sweat) with **hydr/o** (water).*
sudor/o		**sudor**/esis (sū-dō-RĒ-sĭs): condition of profuse sweating; also called *diaphoresis* and *hyperhidrosis.* *-esis:* condition
ichthy/o	dry, scaly	**ichthy**/osis (ĭk-thē-Ō-sĭs): any of several dermatologic conditions characterized by noninflammatory dryness and scaling of the skin, commonly associated with other abnormalities of lipid metabolism *-osis:* abnormal condition; increase (used primarily with blood cells) *A mild form of ichthyosis, called winter itch, is commonly seen on the legs of older patients, especially during the dry winter months.*
kerat/o	horny tissue; hard; cornea	**kerat**/osis (kĕr-ă-TŌ-sĭs): any condition of the skin characterized by an overgrowth and thickening of skin *-osis:* abnormal condition; increase (used primarily with blood cells)
melan/o	black	**melan**/oma (mĕl-ă-NŌ-mă): malignant tumor of melanocytes that commonly begins in a darkly pigmented mole and can metastasize widely *-oma:* tumor *Melanomas are attributed to intense exposure to sunlight and commonly metastasize throughout the body.*
myc/o	fungus (plural, fungi)	dermat/o/**myc**/osis (dĕr-mă-tō-mī-KŌ-sĭs): fungal infection of the skin *dermat/o:* skin *-osis:* abnormal condition; increase (used primarily with blood cells)

(continued)

Word Elements	Meaning	Word Analysis
onych/o	nail	**onych/o**/malacia (ŏn-ĭ-kō-mă-LĀ-shē-ă): abnormal softening of the nails *-malacia:* softening
pil/o	hair	**pil/o**/nid/al (pī-lō-NĪ-dăl): growth of hair in a dermoid cyst or in a sinus opening on the skin *nid:* nest *-al:* pertaining to A *pilonidal cyst commonly develops in the sacral region (fourth segment of the lower spinal column) of the skin. The cystic tumor contains elements derived from the ectoderm, such as hair, skin, sebum, or teeth.*
trich/o		**trich/o**/pathy (trĭk-ŎP-ă-thē): any disease of the hair *-pathy:* disease
scler/o	hardening; sclera (white of eye)	**scler/o**/derma (sklĕr-ō-DĔR-mă): chronic disease with abnormal hardening of the skin caused by formation of new collagen *-derma:* skin
seb/o	sebum, sebaceous	**seb/o**/rrhea (sĕb-or-Ē-ă): increase in the amount and, commonly, an alteration of the quality of the fats secreted by the sebaceous glands *-rrhea:* discharge, flow
squam/o	scale	**squam/o**/ous (SKWĀ-mŭs): covered with scales; scalelike *-ous:* pertaining to
xer/o	dry	**xer/o**/derma (zē-rō-DĔR-mă): chronic skin condition characterized by excessive roughness and dryness *-derma:* skin *Xeroderma is a mild form of ichthyosis.*
Suffixes		
-derma	skin	py/o/**derma** (pī-ō-DĔR-mă): any pyogenic infection of the skin *py/o:* pus
-oid	resembling	derm/**oid** (DĔR-moyd): resembling skin *derm:* skin
-phoresis	carrying, transmission	dia/**phoresis** (dī-ă-fō-RĒ-sĭs): condition of profuse sweating, also called *sudoresis* and *hyperhidrosis* *dia-:* through, across
-plasty	surgical repair	dermat/o/**plasty** (DĔR-mă-tō-plăs-tē): surgical repair of the skin *dermat/o:* skin

Word Elements	Meaning	Word Analysis
-therapy	treatment	cry/o/**therapy** (krī-ō-THĔR-ă-pē): treatment using cold as a destructive medium *cry/o:* cold *Warts and actinic keratosis are some of the common skin disorders treated with cryotherapy.*

Pronunciation Help						
Pronunciation Help	**Long Sound**	ā in rāte	ē in rēbirth	ī in īsle	ō in ōver	ū in ūnite
	Short Sound	ă in ălone	ĕ in ĕver	ĭ in ĭt	ŏ in nŏt	ŭ in cŭt

 Listen and Learn, the audio CD-ROM included in this book, will help you master pronunciation of selected medical words. Use it to practice pronunciations of the above-listed medical terms and for instructions to complete the *Listen and Learn* exercise for this section.

SECTION REVIEW 3-1

For the following medical terms, first write the suffix and its meaning. Then translate the meaning of the remaining elements starting with the first part of the word. The first word is an example that is completed for you.

Term	Meaning
1. hypo/derm/ic	*-ic: pertaining to; under, below, deficient; skin*
2. melan/oma	
3. kerat/osis	
4. cutane/ous	
5. lip/o/cyte	
6. onych/o/malacia	
7. scler/o/derma	
8. dia/phoresis	
9. dermat/o/myc/osis	
10. cry/o/therapy	

Competency Verification: Check your answers in Appendix B, Answer Key, page 556. If you are not satisfied with your level of comprehension, review the vocabulary and retake the review.

Correct Answers _____ × 10 = _____ % Score

 Throughout the frames in this book, prefixes that stand alone are pink; word roots and CFs that stand alone are **bold**; and suffixes that stand alone are blue.

Skin and Accessory Organs

The skin is a sensory organ that also provides protection for the body. The accessory organs of the skin include the hair, nails, sebaceous glands, and sweat glands.

Skin

3-1 The skin is considered an organ and is composed of two layers of tissue: the outer epidermis, which is visible to the naked eye, and the inner layer, the dermis.

Identify and label the (1) **epidermis** and the (2) **dermis** in Figure 3–2.

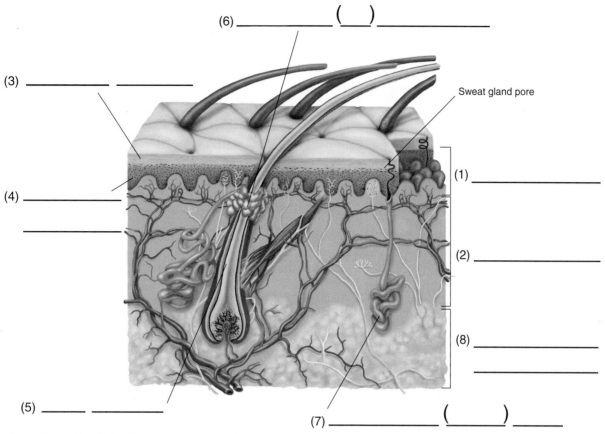

(6) _____ (_) _____

(3) _____ _____

Sweat gland pore

(4) _____

_____

(1) _____

(2) _____

(8) _____

_____

(5) _____ _____

(7) _____ (_____) _____

Figure 3-2 Identifying integumentary structures.

	3-2 The epi/derm/is forms the protective covering of the body and does not have a blood or nerve supply. It is dependent on the dermis's network of capillaries for nourishment. As oxygen and nutrients flow out of the capillaries in the dermis, they pass through tissue fluid, supplying nourishment to the deeper layers of the epidermis.
epi/derm/is ĕp-ĭ-DĔR-mĭs **derm/is** DĔR-mĭs	When you talk about the outer layer of skin, you are referring to the _____ / _____ / _____ . When you talk about the deeper layer of skin, consisting of nerve and blood vessels, you are talking about the _____ / _____ .
	3-3 The epi/derm/is is thick on the palms of the hands and the soles of the feet but relatively thin over most other areas. Identify the element in *epi/derm/is* that means
epi- **-is**	*above or upon:* _____ *a part of speech (noun):* _____
	3-4 The CF **derm/o** refers to the *skin*. *Derm/o/pathy* is a disease of
skin	the _____ .

-pathy **derm/o**	**3-5** Identify the elements in *derm/o/pathy* that mean *disease:*_____ *skin:* _____ / _____

3-6 Although the epidermis is composed of several layers, the (3) **stratum corneum** and the (4) **basal layer** are of greatest importance.

The stratum corneum is composed of dead, flat cells, which convert to keratin that continually flakes away. Its thickness is correlated with normal wear of the area it covers. Only the basal layer is composed of living cells. It is where new cells are continuously being reproduced. Label the two structures in Figure 3–2.

3-7 As new cells form in the basal layer, they move toward the stratum corneum to replace the cells that have been sloughed off. Eventually they die and become filled with a hard protein material called *keratin*. The relatively waterproof characteristic of keratin prevents body fluids from evaporating and moisture from entering the body. The entire process by which a cell forms in the basal layers, rises to the surface, becomes keratinized, and sloughs off takes about 1 month.

Check the basal layer in Figure 3–1 to see the single row of newly formed cells in the deepest layer of the epi/derm/is.

skin **study, skin**	**3-8** In addition to **derm/o,** two other CFs for *skin* are **cutane/o** and **dermat/o.** *Cutane/ous* means pertaining to the _____. *Dermat/o/logy* is the_____ of the _____.
dermat/o/logist dĕr-mă-TŎL-ō-jĭst	**3-9** A physician who specializes in treating skin diseases is called a _____ / _____ / _____.
dermat/itis dĕr-mă-TĪ-tĭs	**3-10** Use **dermat** to build a word meaning *inflammation of the skin.* _____ / _____
skin **skin**	**3-11** The prefix *sub-* means *under* or *below;* the prefix *hypo-* means *under, below, deficient.* A sub/cutane/ous injection occurs beneath the _____. A hypo/derm/ic needle is inserted under the _____.
skin	**3-12** Sub/cutane/ous literally means *pertaining to under the* _____.
skin	**3-13** When you see the terms *derm/a, derm/is,* and *derm/oid,* you will know the roots refer to the _____.

3-14   As discussed previously, suffixes *-al, -ic, -ior,* and *-ous* are adjective endings that mean *pertaining to*. Terms such as *derm/al* and *derm/ic* mean

skin   *pertaining to the _____.*

3-15   In the basal layer, specialized cells, called *melan/o/cytes,* produce a black pigment called *melanin*. Production of melanin increases with exposure to strong ultraviolet light. This exposure creates a suntan that provides a protective barrier from damaging effects of the sun. The number of melan/o/cytes is about the same in all races, but skin color differences are attributed to production of melanin. In people with dark skin, melan/o/cytes continuously produce large amounts of melanin. In people with light skin, melan/o/cytes produce less melanin.

melan/o/cyte
MĔL-ăn-ō-sīt

melan/oma
mĕl-ă-NŌ-mă

The CF **melan/o** refers to the color black. Build a word that literally means

black cell: _____ / _____ / _____

black tumor: _____ / _____

When defining a medical word, first define the suffix. Second, define the beginning of the word; finally, define the middle of the word. Here is an example of a term

dermat/o / myc / osis
   (2)   (3)   (1)

3-16   The term *derm/is* is a noun that means *pertaining to the skin*. Identify the part of speech in

adjective   *derm/ic:* _____

adjective   *derm/al* _____

3-17   Label Figure 3–2 as you learn about the parts of the dermis. The second layer of skin, the derm/is, contains the (5) **hair follicle**, (6) **sebaceous (oil) gland,** and (7) **sudoriferous (sweat) gland.**

---

inflammation, skin   **3-18**   Dermat/itis is an _____ of the _____.

---

disease, skin   **3-19**   *Derm/o/pathy* is a disease of the skin; *dermat/o/pathy* is also a _____ of the _____.

---

epi/derm/is, derm/is
ĕp-ĭ-DĔR-mĭs, DĔR-mĭs

3-20   The two layers of the skin are the
_____ / _____ / _____ and _____ / _____.

aden/oma ăd-ĕ-NŌ-mă	**3-21** An aden/oma is a benign (not malignant) neo/plasm in which the tumor cells form glands or glandlike structures. The tumor is usually well circumscribed, tending to compress rather than infiltrate or invade adjacent tissue. Build a word that means *tumor composed of glandular tissue:* _____ / _____
adip/ectomy ăd-ĭ-PĔK-tō-mē	**3-22** *Lip/o* and ***adip/o*** are CFs that mean *fat.* A *lip/ectomy* is excision of fat or adipose tissue. Use ***adip/o*** to form another surgical term that means *excision of fat:* _____ / _____
adip/o, lip/o **steat/o**	**3-23** *Adip/oma* and *lip/oma* are terms that mean *fatty tumor.* Both are benign tumors consisting of fat cells. The CFs in this frame that mean *fat* are _____ / _____ and _____ / _____. A third CF that refers to fat is _____ / _____.
	3-24 The dermis is attached to underlying structures of the skin by (8) **subcutaneous tissue.** Identify and label the layer of subcutaneous tissue in Figure 3–2.
sub/cutane/ous sŭb-kū-TĀ-nē-ŭs **lip/o/cytes** LĬP-ō-sītz	**3-25** Sub/cutane/ous tissue forms lip/o/cytes, also known as *fat cells.* Determine words in this frame that mean *pertaining to under or below the skin:* _____ / _____ / _____ *fat cells:* _____ / _____ / _____
cell **tumor**	**3-26** Whereas a *lip/o/cyte* is a fat _____, an *adip/oma* is a fatty _____.

Competency Verification: Check your labeling of Figure 3–2 in Appendix B, Answer Key, page 557.

	3-27 *Suction lip/ectomy,* also called *lip/o/suction,* is removal of sub/cutane/ous fat tissue using a blunt-tipped cannula (tube) introduced into the fatty area through a small incision. Suction is applied and fat tissue is removed. Locate the sub/cutane/ous tissue in Figure 3–1.
sub/cutane/ous sŭb-kū-TĀ-nē-ŭs **lip/ectomy** *or* **lip/o/suction** lĭ-PĔK-tō-mē, LĬP-ō-sŭk-shŭn	**3-28** Identify terms in Frame 3-27 that mean *under the skin:* _____ / _____ / _____ *excision of fat:* _____ / _____ *or* _____ / _____ / _____.

	3-29 Lip/o/suction is used primarily to remove or reduce localized areas of fat around the abdomen, breasts, legs, face, and upper arms, where skin is contractile enough to redrape in a normal manner, and is performed for cosmetic reasons.
fat	*Lip/o/suction* literally means *suction of* _____ .

derm/o, dermat/o, **cutane/o**	**3-30** List three CFs that refer to the skin: _____ / _____, _____ / _____, and _____ / _____.

dermat/o/plasty DĔR-mă-tō-plăs-tē	**3-31** Use *dermat/o* to form a word meaning *surgical repair (of) skin.* _____ / _____ / _____

	3-32 The noun suffixes *-logy* and *-logist* contain the same root, **log/o**, which means *study of.* The *y* at the end of a term means *condition, process* and denotes a noun ending. The definitions of both suffixes are easier to remember if you analyze their components: *-logy* means *study of; -logist* means *specialist in study of.*
log	The root in each suffix that means *study of* is _____ .
-ist	The element in the suffix *logist* that means *specialist* is _____ .
-y	The element in the suffix *-logy* that means *condition or process* is _____ .

dermat/o/logy dĕr-mă-TŎL-ō-jē **dermat/o/logist** dĕr-mă-TŎL-ō-jĭst	**3-33** Refer to Frame 3-32 and use *dermat/o* to develop words that mean *study of the skin:* _____ / _____ / _____ *specialist who treats skin disorders:* _____ / _____ / _____

dermat/oma dĕr-mă-TŌ-mă **dermat/o/pathy** dĕr-mă-TŎP-ă-thē **dermat/o/logy** dĕr-mă-TŎL-ō-jē	**3-34** Use *dermat/o* to practice forming words that mean *tumor of the skin:* _____ / _____ *disease of the skin:* _____ / _____ / _____ *study of the skin:* _____ / _____ / _____

dermat/o/logist dĕr-mă-TŎL-ō-jĭst	**3-35** A physician specializing in treating diseases of the stomach is a *gastr/o/logist.* A physician specializing in treating diseases of the skin is a _____ / _____ / _____ .

dermat/o/logy dĕr-mă-TŎL-ō-jē	**3-36** The medical specialty concerned with treatment of stomach diseases is *gastr/o/logy.* The medical specialty concerned with treatment of skin diseases is _____ / _____ / _____ .

hardening	**3–37** *Scler/osis* is an abnormal condition of _____.

skin	**3–38** *Scler/o/derma*, a chronic hardening and thickening of the skin, is caused by new collagen formation. It is characterized by inflammation that ultimately develops into fibrosis (scarring), then sclerosis (hardening) of tissues. Systemic scler/o/derma can be defined as hardening of the _____.

system/ic scler/osis sĭs-TĔM-ĭk sklĕ-RŌ-sĭs **hardening**	**3–39** System/ic scler/osis, a form of scler/o/derma, is characterized by formation of thickened collagenous fibrous tissue, thickening of the skin, and adhesion to underlying tissues. The disease progresses to involve tissues of the heart, lungs, muscles, genit/o/urin/ary tract, and kidneys. A form of scler/o/derma that causes fibr/osis and scler/osis of multiple body systems is known as _____ / _____ _____ / _____. If you check *scler/o* in Appendix A, Glossary of Medical Word Elements, you will see that *scler/o* means *hardening; sclera (white of eye)*. In the integumentary system, however, it specifically refers to _____.

horny tissue or hard **cornea**	**3–40** The CF *kerat/o* means *horny tissue, hard,* and *cornea*. (The cornea of the eye is covered in Chapter 11.) When *kerat/o* is used in discussions of the skin, it refers to: _____ _____ or _____. When *kerat/o* is used in discussions of the eye, it refers to the _____.

kerat/osis kĕr-ă-TŌ-sĭs	**3–41** *Kerat/osis*, a skin condition, is characterized by hard, horny tissue. A person with a skin lesion in which there is overgrowth and thickening of the epidermis most likely would be diagnosed with _____ / _____.

tumor	**3–42** A *kerat/oma* is a horny _____, also called *kerat/osis*.

sub/cutane/ous sŭb-kū-TĀ-nē-ŭs	**3–43** Sub/cutane/ous surgery is performed through a small opening in the skin. In this frame, the word meaning *under the skin* is _____ / _____ / _____ (adjective ending).

Accessory Organs of the Skin

	3–44 Accessory organs of the skin include the sebaceous (oil) glands, sudoriferous (sweat) glands, hair, and nails. Refer to Figure 3–1 to complete this frame.
sebaceous sē-BĀ-shŭs	Oil-secreting glands of the skin are called _____ *glands.*
sudoriferous sū-dŏr-ĬF-ĕr-ŭs	Sweat glands are called _____ *glands.*

	3–45 Sebaceous glands are found in all areas of the body that have hair. The oily material, called *sebum,* is secreted by the sebaceous gland. It keeps hair and skin soft and pliable and inhibits growth of bacteria on the skin. Increased activity of sebaceous glands at puberty may block the hair follicle and form blackheads **(comedos).** As bacteria feed on the sebum, they release irritating substances that produce inflammation. Large numbers of bacteria produce infection, forming whiteheads **(pustules).**
	Identify the medical term for
comedos KŎM-ē-dōs	*blackheads:* _____
pustules PŬS-tūlz	*whiteheads:* _____

sebaceous sē-BĀ-shŭs	**3–46** Comedos and pustules are the result of hypersecretion of sebum by the _____ (oil) glands.

	3–47 Sweat glands that are not associated with hair follicles open to the surface of the skin through pores, as illustrated in Figure 3–1. These glands are stimulated by temperature increases or emotional stress and produce perspiration that evaporates on the surface of the skin and provides a cooling effect.
sudoriferous sū-dŏr-ĬF-ĕr-ŭs	Sweat, or perspiration, is produced by the _____ (sweat) glands.

hidr/osis hī-DRŌ-sĭs	**3–48** The CF for *sweat* is **hidr/o.** Use *-osis* to form a word that means *abnormal condition of sweat:* _____ / _____

	3–49 The term *diaphoresis* denotes a condition of profuse or excessive sweating. The following two terms also refer to sweating. The term *hidr/aden/itis* means
sweat	*hidr:* _____
gland	*aden:* _____
inflammation	*-itis:* _____ The term *hyper/hidr/osis* means
excessive, above normal	*hyper-:* _____, _____ _____
sweat	*hidr:* _____
abnormal condition	*-osis:* _____ _____

sweat, water	**3-50** Although *hidr/o* and *hydr/o* sound alike, they have different meanings. *Hidr/o* refers to _____. *Hydr/o* refers to _____.
an/hidr/osis ăn-hī-DRŌ-sĭs	**3-51** *An/hidr/osis* is an abnormal condition characterized by inadequate perspiration. When a person suffers from an absence of sweating, you would say they have a condition called _____ / _____ / _____.
cutane/ous kū-TĀ-nē-ŭs	**3-52** Combine *cutane* + *-ous* to build a medical word that means *pertaining to the skin*. _____ / _____
derm/o/pathy dĕr-MŎP-ă-thē	**3-53** Use *derm/o* to form a medical term that means *disease of the skin*. _____ / ____ / _____
myc/osis mī-KŌ-sĭs	**3-54** The CF *myc/o* refers to a *fungus* (plural, *fungi*). Combine *myc/o* + *-osis* to form a word that means *abnormal condition caused by fungi*. _____ / _____
skin	**3-55** *Dermat/o/myc/osis*, a fungal infection of the skin, is caused by dermatophytes, yeasts, and other fungi. When you see this term in a medical report, you will know it refers to a fungal infection of the _____.
dermat/itis dĕr-mă-TĪ-tĭs	**3-56** Form a medical word that means *an inflammation of the skin*. _____ / _____
fungus FŬN-gŭs	**3-57** *Myc/o/dermat/itis*, an inflammation of the skin, is caused by a _____.
trich/o/pathy trĭk-ŎP-ă-thē **trich/osis** trĭ-KŌ-sĭs	**3-58** The CF *trich/o* refers to the *hair*. Construct medical terms that mean *disease of the hair:* _____ / ____ / _____ *abnormal condition of the hair:* _____ / _____
trich/o/myc/osis trĭk-ō-mī-KŌ-sĭs	**3-59** Combine *trich/o* + *myc* + *-osis* to form a medical term that means *an abnormal condition of the hair caused by a fungus*. _____ / ____ / _____ / _____
hair	**3-60** Another CF for hair is *pil/o*. Whenever you see *pil/o* or *trich/o* in a word, you will know it refers to the _____.

pil/o **-oid**	**3-61** *Pil/o/cyst/ic* refers to a *derm/oid cyst containing hair.* The element in this frame that means *hair* is _____ / _____. The element in this frame that means *resembling* is _____.

3-62 Label the structures of the fingernail in Figure 3–3 as you read the following material. Each nail is formed in the (1) **nail root** and is composed of keratin, a hard fibrous protein, which is also the main component of hair. As the nail grows from a (2) **matrix** of active cells beneath the (3) **cuticle,** it stays attached and slides forward over the epithelial layer called the (4) **nail bed.** Most of the (5) **nail body** appears pink because of the underlying blood vessels. The (6) **lunula** is the crescent-shaped area at the base of the nail. It has a whitish appearance because the vascular tissue underneath does not show through.

Here is a review of the three basic rules of word building:

Rule 1: Word root links a suffix that begins with a vowel.

Rule 2: Combining form (root + **o**) links a suffix that begins with a consonant.

Rule 3: Combining form (root + **o**) links a root to another root to form a compound word. (This rule holds true even if the next root begins with a vowel.)

onych/oma ŏn-ĭ-KŌ-mă **onych/o/pathy** ŏn-ĭ-KŎP-ăth-ē	**3-63** The CF *onych/o* refers to the *nail*(s). Form medical words that mean *tumor of the nail (or nailbed):* _____ / _____ *disease of the nail:* _____ / _____ / _____
onych/o/malacia ŏn-ĭ-kō-mă-LĀ-shē-ă	**3-64** The term **malacia** means *abnormal softening of tissue.* This term is also used in words as a suffix. Build a word with *-malacia* that means *softening of the nail(s):* _____ / _____ / _____.

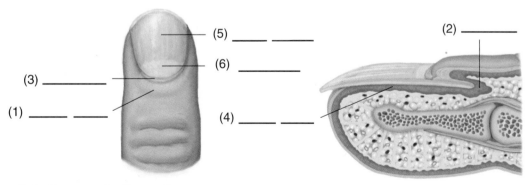

Figure 3-3   Structure of a fingernail.

onych/o **myc** **-osis**	**3–65** Nails become white, opaque, thickened, and brittle when a person has a disease called *onych/o/myc/osis*. Identify elements in *onych/o/myc/osis* that mean *nail:* _____ / _____ *fungus:* _____ *abnormal condition:* _____
nail(s)	**3–66** When you see the term *onych/o/myc/osis* in a medical chart, you will know it means an infection of the _____ caused by a fungus.
xer/o	**3–67** The noun suffix *-derma* denotes *skin*. A person with excessive dryness of skin has a condition called *xer/o/derma*. From *xer/o/derma*, identify the CF that means *dry:* _____ / _____.
hernia, swelling	**3–68** The suffix *-cele* refers to a _____ or _____.
lip/o/cele LĬP-ō-sēl	**3–69** A hernia containing fat or fatty tissue is called an *adip/o/cele* or _____ / _____ / _____.

Competency Verification: Check your labeling of Figure 3–3 in Appendix B, Answer Key, page 557.

SECTION REVIEW 3-2

Using the following table, write the CF, suffix, or prefix that matches its definition in the space provided to the left of the definition. There may be more than one word element that matches a definition.

Combining Forms		Suffixes	Prefixes
adip/o	pil/o	-cele	epi-
cutane/o	scler/o	-derma	hypo-
derm/o	steat/o	-logist	
dermat/o	trich/o	-malacia	
hidr/o	xer/o	-osis	
lip/o		-pathy	
onych/o		-rrhea	

1. _____ disease
2. _____ dry
3. _____ fat
4. _____ discharge, flow
5. _____ hair
6. _____ hardening; sclera (white of eye)
7. _____ hernia, swelling
8. _____ nail
9. _____ skin
10. _____ softening
11. _____ specialist in study of
12. _____ above, upon
13. _____ abnormal condition; increase (used primarily with blood cells)
14. _____ sweat
15. _____ under, below, deficient

Competency Verification: Check your answers in Appendix B, Answer Key, page 557. If you are not satisfied with your level of comprehension, go back to Frame 3–1 and rework the frames.

Correct Answers _____ × 6.67 = _____ Score

 When defining a medical word, first define the suffix. Second, define the beginning of the word. Finally, define the middle of the word. Here is an example using the term

sub / cutane / ous
(2)   (3)   (1)

Combining Forms Denoting Color

Skin

3-70 Examine the CFs and their meanings that denote color in the left-hand column of the table below. Examples of medical terms with their definitions are provided in the middle column. In the far right-hand column of this frame, use a slash to break down each word into its basic elements.

Combining Form	Medical Term	Word Breakdown
albin/o: white	albinism: *white condition*	a l b i n i s m
cyan/o: blue	cyanoderma: *blue skin*	c y a n o d e r m a
erythr/o: red	erythroderma: *red skin*	e r y t h r o d e r m a
leuk/o: white	leukoderma: *white skin*	l e u k o d e r m a
melan/o: black	melanoderma: *black skin*	m e l a n o d e r m a
xanth/o: yellow	xanthoma: *yellow tumor*	x a n t h o m a

albin/ism
ĂL-bĭn-ĭzm

cyan/o/derma
sī-ă-nō-DĔR-mă

erythr/o/derma
ĕ-rĭth-rō-DĔR-mă

leuk/o/derma
loo-kō-DĔR-mă

melan/o/derma
mĕl-ăn-ō-DĔR-mă

xanth/oma
zăn-THŌ-mă

3-71 The *-a* ending in *cyan/o/derma*, *erythr/o/derma*, *leuk/o/derma*, and *melan/o/derma* designates that these words are (adjectives, nouns)

nouns

_____.

3-72 Use *-derma* to build medical words that mean

erythr/o/derma
ĕ-rĭth-rō-DĔR-mă

melan/o/derma
mĕl-ăn-ō-DĔR-mă

xanth/o/derma
zăn-thō-DĔR-mă

xer/o/derma
zē-rō-DĔR-mă

skin that is red: _____ / _____ / _____

skin that is black: _____ / _____ / _____

skin that is yellow: _____ / _____ / _____

skin that is dry: _____ / _____ / _____

Cells

3-73 You have already learned that a cell is the smallest basic unit of the human organism and that every tissue and organ in the human body is made up of cells. *Cyt/o/logy* is the study of _____.

The word elements **cyt/o** and *-cyte* are used to build words that refer to a _____.

cells

cell

cells	**3-74** *Cyt/o/logy* is the study of _____.
erythr/o/cyte ĕ-RĬTH-rō-sīt **leuk/o/cyte** LOO-kō-sīt **melan/o/cyte** MĔL-ăn-ō-sīt **xanth/o/cyte** ZĂN-thō-sīt	**3-75** Use *-cyte* (cell) to form words that mean *cell that is red:* _____ / _____ / _____ *cell that is white:* _____ / _____ / _____ *cell that is black:* _____ / _____ / _____ *cell that is yellow:* _____ / _____ / _____
-penia **leuk/o** **cyt/o**	**3-76** Leuk/o/cyt/o/penia, an abnormal decrease in white blood cells (WBCs), may be caused by an adverse drug reaction, radiation poisoning, or a path/o/logic/al condition. The term *leuk/o/cyt/o/penia* is formed from the suffix that means *decrease or deficiency:* _____ The CF that means *white* _____ / _____ The CF that means *cell:* _____ / _____
leuk/o/cyt/o/penia loo-kō-sī-tō-PĒ-nē-ă	**3-77** Deficiency in white blood cell production may be a sign of a path/ o/log/ic condition known as *leuk/o/penia* or _____ / _____ / _____ / _____ / _____
WBC	**3-78** Abbreviation for *white blood cell*, *white blood count* is _____.
blood	**3-79** The suffix *-emia* is used in words to mean *blood condition*. *Xanth/emia*, an occurrence of yellow pigment in the blood, literally means *yellow* _____.
xanth/omas zăn-THŌ-măs	**3-80** High cholesterol levels may cause small yellow tumors called _____ / _____.
blood **white**	**3-81** Leuk/emia is a progressive malignant disease of the blood forming organs. It is characterized by proliferation and development of immature leuk/o/cytes in the blood and bone marrow. *Leuk/emia* literally means *white* _____. Leuk/o/cytes are _____ blood cells.
leuk/emia loo-KĒ-mē-ă	**3-82** A disease of unrestrained growth of immature white blood cells is called _____ / _____.

3-83 Activity of melan/o/cytes (produce melanin) is genetically regulated and inherited. Local accumulations of melanin are seen in pigmented moles and freckles. Environmental and physiological factors also play a role in skin color. Locate the basal layer in Figure 3–1.

---

albin/ism
ĂL-bĭn-ĭzm

3-84 Absence of pigment in the skin, eyes, and hair is most likely due to an inherited inability to produce melanin. This lack of melanin results in the condition called *albin/ism*. A person with this condition is called an *albino*.
Deficiency or absence of pigment in the skin, hair, and eyes due to an

abnormality in production of melanin is known as _____ / _____.

---

melanin
MĔL-ă-nĭn

3-85 The number of melan/o/cytes is about the same in all races. Differences in skin color are attributed to production of melanin. In people with dark skin, melan/o/cytes continuously produce large amounts of melanin. In

people with light skin, melan/o/cytes produce less _____.

---

melan/o/cyte
mĕl-ĂN-ō-sīt

melan/oma
mĕl-ă-NŌ-mă

3-86 Melan/oma is a malignant neo/plasm (new growth) that originates in the skin and is composed of melan/o/cytes.
Form medical words that literally mean

black cell: _____ / _____ / _____

black tumor: _____ / _____

---

melan/oma
mĕl-ă-NŌ-mă

3-87 The lesion of melan/oma is characterized by its asymmetry, irregular border, and lack of uniform color. Malignant melan/oma is the most dangerous form of skin cancer because of its tendency to metastasize rapidly.
The medical term that literally means *black tumor* is

_____ / _____.

---

cyan/o/derma
sī-ă-nō-DĔR-mă

3-88 Cyan/osis, also called *cyan/o/derma*, is caused by deficiency of oxygen and an excess of carbon dioxide in the blood. A person who is rescued from drowning exhibits a dark bluish or purplish discoloration of the skin.
This condition is known as *cyan/osis* or _____ / _____ / _____.

---

cyan/osis
sī-ă-NŌ-sĭs

erythr/osis
ĕr-ĭ-THRŌ-sĭs

melan/osis
mĕl-ăn-Ō-sĭs

xanth/osis
zăn-THŌ-sĭs

3-89 Use *-osis* to develop medical words that mean

abnormal condition of blue (skin): _____ / _____

abnormal condition of red (skin): _____ / _____

abnormal condition of black (pigmentation): _____ / _____

abnormal condition of yellow (skin): _____ / _____

increase **leuk/o/cyt/osis** loo-kō-sī-TŌ-sĭs	**3-90** The suffix *-osis* is used in words to mean abnormal condition. However, when *-osis* is used in a word related to blood, it means *increase*. The complete meaning of *-osis* is *abnormal condition; increase (used primarily with blood cells)*. The term *erythr/o/cyt/osis* is an _____ in red blood cells. Use **leuk/o** (white) to build a term that means *increase in white blood cells:* _____ / _____ / _____ / _____.
melan/oma mĕl-ă-NŌ-mă	**3-91** Skin cancer is the most common type of cancer. The rate of skin cancer has increased, mainly due to increased exposure to ultraviolet rays in sunlight. Sun exposure, especially excessive tanning of the skin, can cause the lethal black tumor called _____ / _____.
carcin/oma kăr-sĭ-NŌ-mă	**3-92** Basal cell carcin/oma is a type of skin cancer that affects the basal cell layer of the epidermis. (See Figure 3–4.) Metastasis is rare, but local invasion destroys underlying and adjacent tissue. This condition occurs most frequently on areas of the skin exposed to the sun. A type of skin cancer that affects the basal layer is called basal cell _____ / _____.
AIDS **Kaposi sarc/oma** KĂP-ō-sē săr-KŌ-mă	**3-93** The CF **sarc/o** means flesh (connective tissue). Kaposi sarc/oma, a malignant skin tumor commonly associated with patients who are diagnosed with acquired immune deficiency syndrome (AIDS), is usually fatal. Initially, the tumor appears as a purplish brown lesion. The abbreviation for acquired immune deficiency syndrome is _____. The type of skin cancer associated with the AIDS virus is _____ _____ / _____.
death	**3-94** The CF **necr/o** is used in words to denote *death* or *necr/osis*. *Necr/o/tic* is a word that means *pertaining to necr/osis or* _____.

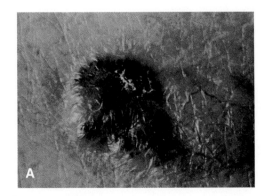

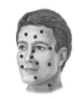

Figure 3-4   (A) Basal cell carcinoma (late stage). (B) Common sites of basal cell carcinoma. (From Goldsmith, LA, Lazarus, GS, and Tharp, MD. *Adult and Pediatric Dermatology: A Color Guide to Diagnosis and Treatment*. Philadelphia: FA Davis, 1997, page 144, with permission.)

dead	**3-95** The term *necr/osis* is used to denote the death of areas of tissue or bone surrounded by healthy tissue. *Cellular necr/osis* means that the cells are _____.
dead	**3-96** *Necr/o/cyt/osis* also means that cells are _____.
necr/osis nĕ-KRŌ-sĭs	**3-97** Bony necr/osis occurs when dead bone tissue results from the loss of blood supply (for example, after a fracture). The term that means *abnormal condition of death* is _____ / _____.
gangrene GĂNG-grēn	**3-98** Gangrene is a form of necr/osis associated with loss of blood supply. Before healing can take place, the dead matter must be removed. When there is an injury to blood flow, a form of necr/osis may develop that is known as _____.
self **self** **self**	**3-99** In the English language, an *auto/graph* is a signature written by oneself. In medical words, *auto-* is used as a prefix and means *self, own.* *Auto/hypnosis* is *hypnosis of one's* _____. *Auto/examination* is an *examination of one's* _____. An *auto/graft* is *skin transplanted from one's* _____.
auto/grafts AW-tō-grăfts	**3-100** A *graft* is tissue transplanted or implanted in a part of the body to repair a defect. Grafts done with tissue transplanted from the patient's own skin are called _____ / _____.
derm/a/tome DĔR-mă-tōm	**3-101** A *derm/a/tome** is an instrument used to incise or cut. When there is a need to graft a thin slice of skin, the physician asks for an instrument called a _____ / _____ / _____.
auto/graft AW-tō-grăft	**3-102** Skin transplanted from another person does not survive very long. Thus, a graft is typically performed using tissue transplanted from the patient's own skin. This surgical procedure is called an _____ / _____.

---

*The use of *a* as the connecting vowel is an exception to the rule of using an *o.*

SECTION REVIEW 3-3

Using the following table, write the CF, suffix, or prefix that matches its definition in the space provided to the left of the definition. There may be more than one word element that matches a definition.

Combining Forms		Suffixes		Prefixes
cyan/o	melan/o	-cyte	-osis	auto-
cyt/o	necr/o	-derma	-pathy	
erythr/o	xanth/o	-emia	-penia	
leuk/o		-oma	-rrhea	

1. _____ black

2. _____ blue

3. _____ blood condition

4. _____ cell

5. _____ decrease, deficiency

6. _____ disease

7. _____ discharge, flow

8. _____ red

9. _____ self, own

10. _____ skin

11. _____ tumor

12. _____ white

13. _____ yellow

14. _____ death, necrosis

15. _____ abnormal condition; increase (used primarily with blood cells)

Competency Verification: Check your answers in Appendix B, Answer Key, page 557. If you are not satisfied with your level of comprehension, go back to Frame 3–70 and rework the frames.

Correct Answers _____ × 6.67 = _____ % Score

Abbreviations

This section introduces abbreviations related to the integumentary system and their meanings. Included are abbreviations contained in the medical report activities that follow.

Abbreviation	Meaning	Abbreviation	Meaning
AIDS	acquired immune deficiency syndrome	**ID**	intradermal
BCC	basal cell carcinoma	**IM**	intramuscular
Bx, bx	biopsy	**IMP**	impression (synonymous with *diagnosis*)
cm	centimeter (1/100 of a meter)	**PE**	physical examination
Derm	dermatology	**subcu, Sub-Q, subQ**	subcutaneous (injection)
FH	family history	**ung**	ointment
FS	frozen section	**WBC**	white blood cell, white blood count
I&D	incision and drainage; irrigation and debridement	**XP, XDP**	xeroderma pigmentosum

Additional Medical Terms

The following are additional terms related to the integumentary system. Recognizing and learning these terms will help you understand the connection between common signs, symptoms, and diseases and their diagnoses, as well as the rationale behind methods of treatment selected for a particular disorder.

Signs, Symptoms, and Diseases

abrasion ă-BRĀ-zhŭn	Scraping, or rubbing away of a surface, such as skin, by friction *Abrasion may be the result of trauma, such as a skinned knee, therapy, as in dermabrasion of the skin for removal of scar tissue, or normal function, such as wearing down of a tooth by mastication.*

abscess
ĂB-sĕs
  furuncle
  FŪ-rŭng-kl
  carbuncle
  KĂR-bŭng-kl
	Localized collection of pus at the site of an infection (characteristically a staphylococcal infection)
	Abscess that originates in a hair follicle; also called *boil*
	
	Cluster of furuncles in the subcutaneous tissue
	An abscess can occur in any body part. Treatment includes oral antibiotics and I&D to drain the purulent material. (See Figure 3–5.)

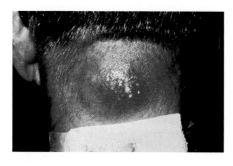

Figure 3-5   Abscess that has formed a furuncle in hair follicles of the neck. Large furuncles with connecting channels to the skin surface form a carbuncle. (From Goldsmith, LA, Lazarus, GS, and Tharp, MD. *Adult and Pediatric Dermatology: A Color Guide to Diagnosis and Treatment.* Philadelphia: FA Davis, 1997, page 364, with permission.)

acne ĂK-nē	Inflammatory disease of sebaceous follicles of the skin, marked by comedos (blackheads), papules, and pustules *Acne is especially common in puberty and adolescence. It usually affects the face, chest, back, and shoulders.*
alopecia ăl-ō-PĒ-shē-ă	Absence or loss of hair, especially of the head; also known as *baldness*
comedo KŎM-ē-dō	Discolored, dried sebum plugging an excretory duct of the skin; also called *blackhead*
cyst sĭst **sebaceous** sē-BĀ-shŭs	Closed sac or pouch in or under the skin with a definite wall that contains fluid, semifluid, or solid material *The cyst may enlarge as sebum collects and may become infected.* A cyst filled with sebum (fatty material) from a sebaceous gland
eczema ĔK-zĕ-mă	Redness of the skin caused by swelling of the capillaries *Eczematous rash may result from various causes, including allergies, irritating chemicals, drugs, scratching or rubbing the skin, or sun exposure. It may be acute or chronic. (See Figure 3–6.)*

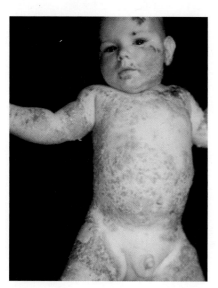

Figure 3-6   Scattered eczema of the trunk of an infant. (From Goldsmith, LA, Lazarus, GS, and Tharp, MD. *Adult and Pediatric Dermatology: A Color Guide to Diagnosis and Treatment.* Philadelphia: FA Davis, 1997, page 243, with permission.)

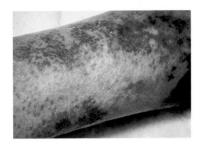

Figure 3-7 Ecchymosis. (From Harmening, DM. *Clinical Hematology and Fundamentals of Hemostasis,* 4th edition., Philadelphia: FA Davis, 2001, page 489, with permission.)

hemorrhage HĔM-ĕ-rĭj	Loss of a large amount of blood in a short period, externally or internally *Hemorrhage may be arterial, venous, or capillary.*
contusion kŏn-TOO-zhŭn	Hemorrhage of any size under the skin in which the skin is not broken; also known as a *bruise*
ecchymosis ĕk-ĭ-MŌ-sĭs	Skin discoloration consisting of a large, irregularly formed hemorrhagic area with colors changing from blue-black to greenish brown or yellow; commonly called a *bruise* (See Figure 3–7.)
petechia pē-TĒ-kē-ă	Minute, pinpoint hemorrhagic spot of the skin *A petechia is a smaller version of an ecchymosis.*
hematoma hēm-ă-TŌ-mă	Elevated, localized collection of blood trapped under the skin that usually results from trauma
hirsutism HŬR-sūt-ĭzm	Condition characterized by excessive growth of hair or presence of hair in unusual places, especially in women
impetigo ĭm-pĕ-TĪ-gō	Bacterial skin infection characterized by isolated pustules that become crusted and rupture
psoriasis sō-RĪ-ă-sĭs	Chronic skin disease characterized by itchy red patches covered with silvery scales (See Figure 3–8.) *Psoriasis runs in families and may be brought on by anxiety. Topical corticosteroids, vitamin D, ultraviolet light exposure, and saltwater immersion are among the many methods that have been used effectively to treat the condition.*
scabies SKĀ-bēz	Contagious skin disease transmitted by the itch mite

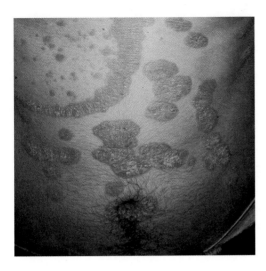

Figure 3-8   Psoriasis. (From Goldsmith, LA, Lazarus, GS, and Tharp, MD. *Adult and Pediatric Dermatology: A Color Guide to Diagnosis and Treatment.* Philadelphia: FA Davis, 1997, page 258, with permission.)

skin lesions LĒ-zhŭn	Areas of pathologically altered tissue caused by disease, injury, or a wound due to external factors or internal disease *Evaluation of skin lesions, injuries, or changes to tissue helps establish the diagnosis of skin disorders. Lesions are described as primary or secondary.*
primary lesions	Initial reaction to pathologically altered tissue that may be flat or elevated
secondary lesions	Result from the changes that take place in the primary lesion due to infection, scratching, trauma, or various stages of a disease *Lesions are also described by their appearance, color, location, and size as measured in centimeters. Review the primary and secondary lesions illustrated in Figure 3–9.*
tinea TĬN-ē-ă	Fungal infection whose name commonly indicates the body part affected; also called *ringworm* *Examples of tinea include tinea barbae (beard), tinea corporis (body), tinea pedis (athlete's foot), tinea versicolor (skin), and tinea cruris (jock itch).*
ulcer ŬL-sĕr	Lesion of the skin or mucous membranes marked by inflammation, necrosis, and sloughing of damaged tissues (See Figure 3–9.) *Ulcers may be the result of trauma, caustic chemicals, intense heat or cold, arterial or venous stasis, cancers, drugs, and infectious agents.*
pressure ulcer	Skin ulceration caused by prolonged pressure, usually in a person who is bedridden; also known as *decubitus ulcer* or *bedsore* *Pressure ulcers are most commonly found in skin overlying a bony projection, such as the hip, ankle, heel, shoulder, and elbow.*
urticaria ŭr-tĭ-KĀ-rē-ă	Allergic reaction of the skin characterized by eruption of pale-red elevated patches that are intensely itchy; also called *wheals* or *hives*

PRIMARY LESIONS

FLAT LESIONS
Flat, discolored, circumscribed lesions of any size

Macule
Flat, pigmented, circumscribed area less than 1 cm in diameter.
Examples: freckle, flat mole, or rash that occurs in rubella.

ELEVATED LESIONS

Solid

Fluid-filled

Papule
Solid, elevated lesion less than 1 cm in diameter that may be the same color as the skin or pigmented.
Examples: nevus, wart, pimple, ringworm, psoriasis, eczema.

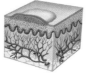

Vesicle
Elevated, circumscribed, fluid-filled lesion less than 0.5 cm in diameter.
Examples: poison ivy, shingles, chickenpox.

Nodule
Palpable, circumscribed lesion; larger and deeper than a papule (0.6 to 2 cm in diameter); extends into the dermal area.
Examples: intradermal nevus, benign or malignant tumor.

Pustule
Small, raised, circumscribed lesion that contains pus; usually less than 1 cm in diameter.
Examples: acne, furuncle, pustular psoriasis, scabies.

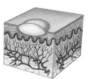

Tumor
Solid, elevated lesion larger than 2 cm in diameter that extends into the dermal and subcutaneous layers.
Examples: lipoma, steatoma, dermatofibroma, hemangioma.

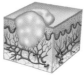

Bulla
A vesicle or blister larger than 1 cm in diameter.
Examples: second degree burns, severe poison oak, poison ivy.

Wheal
Elevated, firm, rounded lesion with localized skin edema (swelling) that varies in size, shape, and color; paler in the center than its surrounding edges; accompanied by itching.
Examples: hives, insect bites, urticaria.

SECONDARY LESIONS

DEPRESSED LESIONS
Depressed lesions caused by loss of skin surface

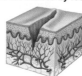

Excoriations
Linear scratch marks or traumatized abrasions of the epidermis.
Examples: scratches, abrasions, chemical or thermal burns.

Fissure
Small slit or cracklike sore that extends into the dermal layer; could be caused by continuous inflammation and drying.

Ulcer
An open sore or lesion that extends to the dermis and usually heals with scarring.
Examples: pressure sore, basal cell carcinoma.

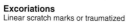

Figure 3-9 Primary and secondary lesions.

verruca vĕ-ROO-kă	Rounded epidermal growths caused by a virus; also called *wart* *Types of warts include plantar warts, juvenile warts, and venereal warts. Warts may be removed by cryosurgery, electrocautery, or acids; however, they may regrow if virus remains in the skin.*
vitiligo vĭt-ĭl-Ī-gō	Localized loss of skin pigmentation characterized by milk-white patches; also called *leukoderma* (See Figure 3–10.)

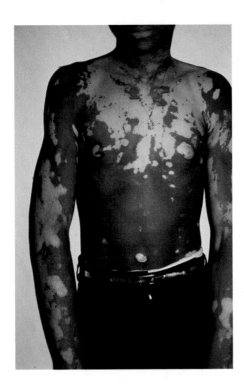

Fig 3-10 **Vitiligo.** (From Goldsmith, LA, Lazarus, GS, and Tharp, MD. *Adult and Pediatric Dermatology: A Color Guide to Diagnosis and Treatment.* Philadelphia: FA Davis, 1997, page 121, with permission.)

Diagnostic Procedures

biopsy BĪ-ŏp-sē	Removal of a small piece of living tissue from an organ or other part of the body for microscopic examination to confirm or establish a diagnosis, estimate prognosis, or follow the course of a disease *Types of biopsy include aspiration biopsy, needle biopsy, punch biopsy, shave biopsy, and frozen section.*
skin test	Method for determining induced sensitivity (allergy) by applying or inoculating a suspected allergen or sensitizer into the skin and determining sensitivity (allergy) to the specific antigen by an inflammatory skin reaction to it *The most commonly used skin tests are the intradermal, patch, and scratch tests. (See Figure 3–11.)*

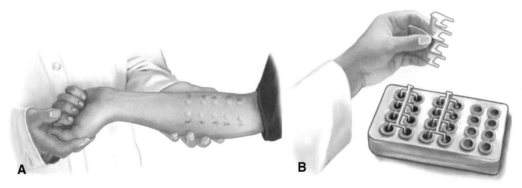

Figure 3-11 Skin tests. (A) Intradermal allergy test reactions. (B) Scratch (prick) skin test kit for allergy testing.

Medical and Surgical Procedures

cryosurgery krī-ō-SĔR-jĕr-ē	Use of subfreezing temperature, commonly with liquid nitrogen, to destroy abnormal tissue cells, such as unwanted, cancerous, or infected tissue
debridement dā-brēd-MŎN or dĭ-BRĒD-mĕnt	Treatment that involves removal of foreign material and dead or damaged tissue, especially in a wound, and is used to promote healing and prevent infection
electrodesiccation ē-lĕk-trō-dĕs-ĭ-KĀ-shŭn	Process in which high-frequency electrical sparks are used to dehydrate and destroy diseased tissue
incision and drainage (I&D)	Incision of a lesion, such as an abscess, followed by the drainage of its contents
skin graft	Surgical procedure to transplant healthy tissue by applying it to an injured site *Human, animal, or artificial skin is used to provide a temporary covering or permanent layer of skin over a wound or burn.*
allograft ĂL-ō-grăft	Transplantation of healthy tissue from one person to another person; also called *homograft* *In an allograft, the skin donor is usually a cadaver. This type of skin graft is temporary and is used to protect the patient against infection and fluid loss. The allograft is frozen and stored in a skin bank until needed.*
autograft AW-tō-grăft	Transplantation of healthy tissue from one site to another site in the same individual
synthetic sĭn-THĔT-ĭk	Transplantation of artificial skin produced from collagen fibers arranged in a lattice pattern *With a synthetic skin graft, the recipient's body does not reject the synthetic skin (produced artificially) and healing skin grows into it as the graft gradually disintegrates.*
xenograft ZĔN-ō-grăft	Transplantation (dermis only) from a foreign donor (usually a pig) and transferred to a human; also called *heterograft* *A xenograft is used as a temporary graft to protect the patient against infection and fluid loss.*

skin resurfacing	Procedure that repairs damaged skin, acne scars, fine or deep wrinkles, or tattoos or improves skin tone irregularities through the use of topical chemicals, abrasion, or laser
	In cosmetic surgery, skin resurfacing may involve dermabrasion, chemical peels, cutaneous lasers, and other techniques.
chemical peel	Use of chemicals to remove outer layers of skin to treat acne scarring and general keratoses as well as cosmetic purposes to remove fine wrinkles on the face; also called *chemabrasion*
cutaneous laser kū-TĀ-nē-ŭs *cutane: skin* *-ous: pertaining to*	Any of several laser treatments employed for cosmetic and plastic surgery *Cutaneous laser includes treatment of pigmented lesions, wrinkles, vascular malformations, and other cosmetic skin surface irregularities.*
dermabrasion DĔRM-ă-brā-zhŭn	Removal of acne scars, nevi, tattoos, or fine wrinkles on the skin through the use of sandpaper, wire brushes, or other abrasive materials on the epidermal layer

Pharmacology

antibiotics ăn-tĭ-bī-ŎT-ĭks	Agents that kill bacteria that cause skin infections
antifungals ăn-tĭ-FŬNG-găls	Agents that kill fungi that infect the skin
antipruritics ăn-tĭ-proo-RĬT-ĭks	Agents that reduce severe itching
corticosteroids kor-tĭ-kō-STĒR-oyds	Anti-inflammatory agents that treat skin inflammation

Pronunciation Help	**Long Sound** **Short Sound**	ā in rāte ă in ălone	ē in rēbirth ĕ in ĕver	ī in īsle ĭ in ĭt	ō in ōver ŏ in nŏt	ū in ūnite ŭ in cŭt

Additional Medical Terms Review

Match the medical term(s) below with the definitions in the numbered list.

alopecia	dermabrasion	scabies
biopsy	eczema	tinea
comedo	electrodesiccation	urticaria
cryosurgery	petechia	verruca
debridement	furuncle	vitiligo

1. _____ is a rounded epidermal growth caused by a virus.

2. _____ is localized loss of skin pigmentation characterized by appearance of milk-white patches.

3. _____ is a fungal skin disease, commonly called *ringworm*, whose name indicates the body part affected.

4. _____ is an abscess that originates in a hair follicle; also called *boil*.

5. _____ is a general term for an itchy red rash that may become crusted, thickened, or scaly.

6. _____ is an allergic reaction of the skin characterized by eruption of pale red elevated patches that are intensely itchy; also called *hives*.

7. _____ refers to excision of a small piece of living tissue from an organ or other part of the body for microscopic examination.

8. _____ refers to use of revolving wire brushes or sandpaper to remove superficial scars on the skin.

9. _____ refers to the procedure in which diseased tissue is dehydrated and destroyed by high-frequency electrical sparks.

10. _____ refers to use of liquid nitrogen to destroy or eliminate abnormal tissue cells.

11. _____ refers to removal of foreign material and dead or damaged tissue, especially in a wound.

12. _____ is a contagious skin disease transmitted by the itch mite.

13. _____ is absence or loss of hair, especially of the head; baldness.

14. _____ is a blackhead.

15. _____ is a minute hemorrhagic spot on the skin that is a smaller version of ecchymosis.

Competency Verification: Check your answers in Appendix B, Answer Key, page 557. If you are not satisfied with your level of comprehension, review the additional medical terms section and retake the review.

Correct Answers _____ × 6.67 = _____ % Score

Primary and Secondary Lesions Review

Identify and label the following skin lesions using the terms listed below.

bulla	macule	pustule	vesicle
excoriations	nodule	tumor	wheal
fissure	papule	ulcer	

PRIMARY LESIONS

FLAT LESIONS
Flat, discolored, circumscribed lesions of any size

Flat, pigmented, circumscribed area less than 1 cm in diameter.
Examples: freckle, flat mole, or rash that occurs in rubella.

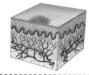

ELEVATED LESIONS

Solid   *Fluid-filled*

Solid, elevated lesion less than 1 cm in diameter that may be the same color as the skin or pigmented.
Examples: nevus, wart, pimple, ringworm, psoriasis, eczema.

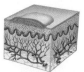

Elevated, circumscribed, fluid-filled lesion less than 0.5 cm in diameter.
Examples: poison ivy, shingles, chickenpox.

Palpable, circumscribed lesion; larger and deeper than a papule (0.6 to 2 cm in diameter); extends into the dermal area.
Examples: intradermal nevus, benign or malignant tumor.

Small, raised, circumscribed lesion that contains pus; usually less than 1 cm in diameter.
Examples: acne, furuncle, pustular psoriasis, scabies.

Solid, elevated lesion larger than 2 cm in diameter that extends into the dermal and subcutaneous layers.
Examples: lipoma, steatoma, dermatofibroma, hemangioma.

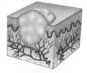

A vesicle or blister larger than 1 cm in diameter.
Examples: second degree burns, severe poison oak, poison ivy.

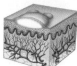

Elevated, firm, rounded lesion with localized skin edema (swelling) that varies in size, shape, and color; paler in the center than its surrounding edges; accompanied by itching.
Examples: hives, insect bites, urticaria.

SECONDARY LESIONS

DEPRESSED LESIONS
Depressed lesions caused by loss of skin surface

Linear scratch marks or traumatized abrasions of the epidermis.
Examples: scratches, abrasions, chemical or thermal burns.

Small slit or cracklike sore that extends into the dermal layer; could be caused by continuous inflammation and drying.

An open sore or lesion that extends to the dermis and usually heals with scarring.
Examples: pressure sore, basal cell carcinoma.

Competency Verification: Check your answers by referring to Figure 3–9, page 90. Review material that you did not answer correctly.

Medical Record Activities

Medical reports included in the following activities reflect common real-life clinical scenarios using medical terminology to document patient care.

MEDICAL RECORD ACTIVITY 3-1

Compound Nevus

Terminology

Terms listed in the table below come from the medical report *Compound Nevus* that follows. Use a medical dictionary such as *Taber's Cyclopedic Medical Dictionary,* the appendices of this book, or other resources to define each term. Then practice the pronunciations aloud for each term.

Term	Definition
circumscribed SĔR-kŭm-skrībd	
crusting KRŬST-ĭng	
lesion LĒ-zhŭn	
melanoma mĕl-ă-NŌ-mă	
nevus NĒ-vŭs	
trauma TRAW-mă	
vermilion border vĕr-MĬL-yŏn	

Listen and Learn Online! will help you master pronunciations of selected medical words from this medical record activity. Visit *http://davisplus.fadavis.com/gylys/simplified* to find instructions on completing the *Listen and Learn Online!* exercise for this section and to practice pronunciations.

Reading

Practice pronunciation of medical terms by reading the following medical report aloud.

Compound Nevus

A 29-year-old married white woman was referred for surgical treatment of a nevus of the right lower lip. The patient has had a small nevus located at the vermilion border of her lower lip all of her life, but recently it has enlarged and has become irritated with crusting and bleeding due to local trauma.

The lesion was evaluated initially about 1 month ago during a period of trauma, but it could not be removed at that time because the patient had a prominent upper respiratory infection. Subsequently, there has been healing of the local inflammatory component, and the nevus is clear at this time.

Examination reveals a brownish lesion with a flat, irregular border that is fairly circumscribed, measuring 0.5 cm in the greatest diameter, and located just at the edge of the vermilion border on the right side of the lower lip.

IMPRESSION: Compound nevus, lower lip, rule out melanoma.

Evaluation

Review the medical report above to answer the following questions. Use a medical dictionary such as *Taber's Cyclopedic Medical Dictionary* and other resources if needed.

1. What is a nevus?

_____

_____

2. Locate the vermilion border on your lip. Where is it located?

_____

_____

3. Was the lesion limited to a certain area?

_____

_____

4. In the impression, the pathologist has ruled out melanoma. What does this mean?

_____

_____

5. Is melanoma a dangerous condition? If so, explain why.

_____

_____

MEDICAL RECORD ACTIVITY 3-2

Psoriasis

Terminology

Terms listed in the table below come from the medical report *Psoriasis* that follows. Use a medical dictionary such as *Taber's Cyclopedic Medical Dictionary,* the appendices of this book, or other resources to define each term. Then practice the pronunciations aloud for each term.

Term	Definition
Bartholin gland BĂR-tō-lĭn	_____
colitis kō-LĪ-tĭs	_____
diabetes mellitus dī-ă-BĒ-tēz MĔ-lĭ-tŭs	_____
diaphoresis dī-ă-fō-RĒ-sĭs	_____
Dx	_____
enteritis ĕn-tĕr-Ī-tĭs	_____
erythematous ĕr-ĭ-THĔM-ă-tŭs	_____
FH	_____
histiocytoma hĭs-tē-ō-sī-TŌ-mă	_____
macules MĂK-ūlz	_____
papules PĂP-ūlz	_____
pruritus proo-RĪ-tŭs	_____
psoriasis sō-RĪ-ă-sĭs (See Figure 3–8.)	_____
sclerosed sklĕ-RŌST	_____
sinusitis sī-nŭs-Ī-tĭs	_____
syncope SĬN-kō-pē	_____
vulgaris vŭl-GĀ-rĭs	_____

 Listen and Learn Online! will help you master pronunciations of selected medical words from this medical report activity. Visit *http://davisplus.fadavis.com/gylys/simplified* to find instructions on completing the *Listen and Learn Online!* exercise for this section and to practice pronunciations.

Reading

Practice pronunciation of medical terms by reading the following medical report aloud.

Psoriasis

Patient is a 24-year-old white woman who has experienced intermittent psoriasis in various stages of severity since her early teens. Since May, her condition has become more troublesome because of an increase of symptoms after being exposed to the sun. Her past history indicates she had chronic sinusitis of 3 years' duration. Her Bartholin gland was excised in 20XX. She has had pruritus of the scalp and abdominal regions. There is no FH of psoriasis. An uncle has had diabetes mellitus since age 43. Patient has occasional abdominal pains accompanied by diaphoresis and/or syncope. PE showed the patient to have psoriatic involvement of the scalp, external ears, trunk, and, to a lesser degree, legs. There are many scattered erythematous (light ruby), thickened plaques covered by thick, yellowish white scales. A few areas on the legs and arms show multiple, sclerosed, brown macules and papules.

DIAGNOSES: 1. Psoriasis vulgaris.
2. Multiple histiocytomas.
3. Abdominal pain, by history.
4. Rule out colitis, regional enteritis.

Evaluation

Review the medical report above to answer the following questions. Use a medical dictionary such as *Taber's Cyclopedic Medical Dictionary* and other resources if needed.

1. What causes psoriasis?

_____

_____

2. On what parts of the body does psoriasis typically occur?

_____

_____

3. How is psoriasis treated?

_____

_____

4. What is a histiocytoma?

_____

_____

Chapter Review

Word Elements Summary

The following table summarizes CFs, suffixes, and prefixes related to the integumentary system.

Word Element	Meaning	Word Element	Meaning
Combining Forms			
adip/o, lip/o, steat/o	fat	**myc/o**	fungus
cutane/o, derm/o, dermat/o	skin	**necr/o**	death, necrosis
cyt/o	cell	**onych/o**	nail
hidr/o, sudor/o	sweat	**pil/o, trich/o**	hair
hydr/o	water	**scler/o**	hardening; sclera (white of eye)
ichthy/o	dry, scaly	**squam/o**	scale
kerat/o	horny tissue; hard; cornea	**xer/o**	dry
Combining Forms for Color			
cyan/o	blue	**melan/o**	black
erythr/o, erythemat/o	red	**xanth/o**	yellow
leuk/o	white		
Suffixes			
SURGICAL			
-plasty	surgical repair	**-tome**	instrument to cut
DIAGNOSTIC, SYMPTOMATIC, AND RELATED			
-cele	hernia, swelling	**-oma**	tumor
-cyte	cell	**-osis**	abnormal condition; increase (used primarily with blood cells)
-derma	skin	**-pathy**	disease
-emia	blood condition	**-penia**	decrease, deficiency
-esis	condition	**-phagia**	swallowing, eating
-itis	inflammation	**-phoresis**	carrying, transmission
-logist	specialist in study of	**-rrhea**	discharge, flow

Word Element	Meaning	Word Element	Meaning
-logy	study of	**-therapy**	treatment
-malacia	softening		
ADJECTIVE			
-al, -ous	pertaining to		
Prefixes			
auto-	self, own	**hypo-**	under, below, deficient
epi-	above, on	**sub-**	under, below

 Enhance your study and reinforcement of word elements with the power of *Davis Plus.* Visit *http://davisplus.fadavis.com/gylys/simplified* for this chapter's flash-card activity. We recommend you complete the flash-card activity before completing the word elements review below.

Word Elements Review

After you review the Word Elements Summary, complete this activity by writing the meaning of each element in the space provided.

Word Element	Meaning	Word Element	Meaning
Combining Forms			
1. adip/o, lip/o, steat/o	_____	8. myc/o	_____
2. cutane/o, derm/o, dermat/o	_____	9. necr/o	_____
3. cyt/o	_____	10. onych/o	_____
4. hidr/o, sudor/o	_____	11. pil/o, trich/o	_____
5. hydr/o	_____	12. scler/o	_____
6. ichthy/o	_____	13. squam/o	_____
7. kerat/o	_____	14. xer/o	_____
Combining Forms of Color			
15. cyan/o	_____	18. melan/o	_____
16. erythr/o	_____	19. xanth/o	_____
17. leuk/o	_____		
Suffixes			
SURGICAL			
20. -plasty	_____	21. -tome	_____
DIAGNOSTIC, SYMPTOMATIC, AND RELATED			
22. -cele	_____	30. -oma	_____
23. -cyte	_____	31. -osis	_____
24. -emia	_____	32. -pathy	_____
25. -esis	_____	33. -penia	_____
26. -itis	_____	34. -phagia	_____
27. -logist	_____	35. -phoresis	_____
28. -logy	_____	36. -rrhea	_____
29. -malacia	_____	37. -therapy	_____
Prefixes			
38. auto-	_____	40. sub-	_____
39. epi-	_____		

Competency Verification: Check your answers in Appendix A, Glossary of Medical Word Elements, page 538. If you are not satisfied with your level of comprehension, review the word elements and retake the review.

Correct Answers: _____ × 2.5 = _____ % Score

Vocabulary Review

Match the medical term(s) below with the definitions in the numbered list.

autograft	Kaposi sarcoma	onychomalacia	subcutaneous
diaphoresis	leukemia	onychomycosis	suction lipectomy
ecchymosis	lipocele	papules	trichopathy
erythrocyte	melanoma	pressure ulcers	xanthoma
hirsutism	onychoma	pustule	xeroderma

1. _____ means beneath the skin.

2. _____ is a condition in which a person sweats excessively; profuse perspiration.

3. _____ refers to any disease of the hair.

4. _____ is a transplantation of healthy tissue from one site to another site in the same individual

5. _____ is a type of malignant skin tumor associated with AIDS.

6. _____ refers to excision of subcutaneous fat tissue by use of a blunt-tipped cannula (tube), done for cosmetic reasons.

7. _____ is a fungal infection of the nails.

8. _____ are caused by prolonged pressure against an area of skin from a bed or chair.

9. _____ refers to excessive production of white blood cells; literally means white blood.

10. _____ is a black-and-blue mark on the skin; a bruise.

11. _____ is a benign tumor of the nail bed.

12. _____ means excessive body hair, especially in women.

13. _____ is an elevated lesion containing pus, as seen in acne, furuncles, and psoriasis.

14. _____ is a medical term for warts, moles, and pimples.

15. _____ is a red blood cell.

16. _____ means excessive dryness of skin.

17. _____ is a black tumor.

18. _____ refers to a hernia that contains fat or fatty cells.

19. _____ refers to a tumor containing yellow material.

20. _____ is an abnormal softening of the nail or nailbed.

Competency Verification: Check your answers in Appendix B, Answer Key, page 558. If you are not satisfied with your level of comprehension, review the chapter vocabulary and retake the review.

Correct Answers: _____ × 5 = _____ % Score

4 Respiratory System

OBJECTIVES

Upon completion of this chapter, you will be able to:

- Describe the type of medical treatment the pulmonologist provides.
- Identify respiratory structures by labeling them on anatomical illustrations.
- Describe the primary functions of the respiratory system.
- Describe common diseases related to the respiratory system.
- Describe common diagnostic, medical, and surgical procedures related to the respiratory system.
- Apply your word-building skills by constructing medical terms related to the respiratory system.
- Describe common abbreviations and symbols related to the respiratory system.
- Reinforce word elements by completing flash card activities.
- Recognize, define, pronounce, and spell terms correctly.
- Demonstrate your knowledge of this chapter by successfully completing the frames, reviews, and medical report evaluations.

Medical Specialty

Pulmonology

The medical specialty of **pulmonology**, also called *pulmonary medicine*, is the branch of medicine concerned with the diagnosis and treatment of diseases involving the structures of the lower respiratory tract, including the lungs, their airways and blood vessels, and the chest wall (thoracic cage). Medical doctors who treat respiratory disorders are called *pulmonologists*. Respiratory disorders include but are not limited to asthma, emphysema, chronic bronchitis, lung disease, and pulmonary vascular disease. Pulmonologists also care for patients requiring specialized ventilator support and lung transplantation. In general, they are specialized to diagnose and manage pulmonary disorders and acute and chronic respiratory failure. Diagnosis and management of pulmonary disorders may include pulmonary function tests, arterial blood gas analysis, chest x-rays, and chemical or microbiological tests.

Anatomy and Physiology Overview

The respiratory system consists of the upper and lower respiratory tracts. The upper tract includes the nose, pharynx, larynx, and trachea. The lower tract includes the left and right bronchi, bronchioles, alveoli, and the lungs. (See Figure 4-1.) The main function of the respiratory system is to perform pulmonary ventilation of the body. Respiratory structures, along with the structures of the cardiovascular system, transport oxygen and remove carbon dioxide (waste product) from the cells of the body. This process is accomplished by events of respiration, exchanging oxygen and carbon dioxide between the environmental air and the blood circulating through the lungs. Secondary functions of the respiratory system include warming air as it passes into the body and assisting in the speech function (providing air for the larynx and the vocal cords).

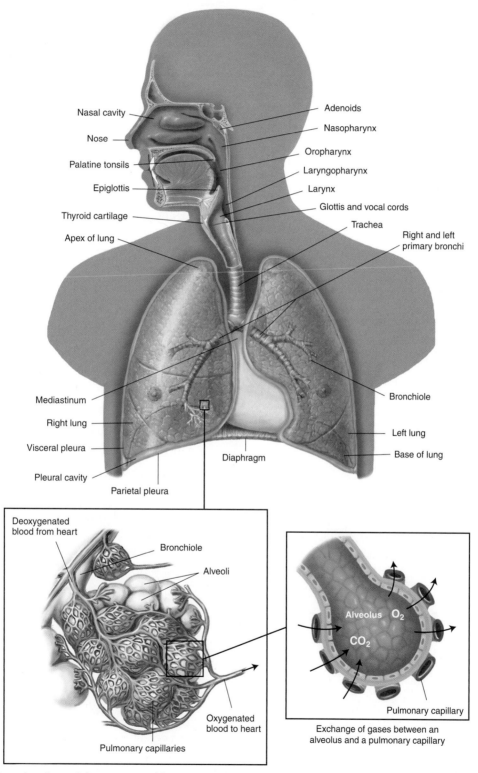

Figure 4-1 Anterior view of the upper and lower respiratory tracts.

WORD ELEMENTS

This section introduces combining forms (CFs) related to the respiratory system. Included are key suffixes; prefixes are defined in the right-hand column as needed. Review the following table and pronounce each word in the word analysis column aloud before you begin to work the frames.

Word Element	Meaning	Word Analysis
Combining Forms		

UPPER RESPIRATORY TRACT

Word Element	Meaning	Word Analysis
adenoid/o	adenoids	**adenoid**/ectomy (ăd-ĕ-noyd-ĔK-tō-mē): excision of the adenoids *-ectomy:* excision, removal
laryng/o	larynx (voice box)	**laryng**/o/scope (lăr-ĬN-gō-skōp): instrument for examining the larynx *-scope:* instrument for examining
nas/o	nose	**nas**/al (NĀ-zl): pertaining to the nose *-al:* pertaining to
rhin/o		**rhin**/o/rrhea (rī-nō-RĒ-ă): watery discharge from the nose *-rrhea:* discharge, flow *Allergies and a common cold commonly cause rhinorrhea. It may also be caused by flow of cerebrospinal fluid from the nose after an injury to the head.*
pharyng/o	pharynx (throat)	**pharyng**/itis (făr-ĭn-JĪ-tĭs): inflammation of the pharynx, usually due to infection *-itis:* inflammation
tonsill/o	tonsils	peri/**tonsill**/ar (pĕr-ĭ-TŎN-sĭ-lăr): pertaining to area surrounding the tonsils *peri-:* around *-ar:* pertaining to
trache/o	trachea (windpipe)	**trache**/o/stomy (trā-kē-ŎS-tō-mē): creation of an opening into the trachea *-stomy:* forming an opening (mouth) *Tracheostomy is performed to provide and secure an open airway.*

LOWER RESPIRATORY TRACT

Word Element	Meaning	Word Analysis
alveol/o	alveolus (plural, alveoli)	**alveol**/ar (ăl-VĒ-ō-lăr): pertaining to alveoli *-ar:* pertaining to

Word Element	Meaning	Word Analysis
bronchi/o	bronchus (plural, bronchi)	**bronchi**/ectasis (brŏng-kē-ĔK-tă-sĭs): dilation of a bronchus or bronchi *-ectasis:* dilation, expansion *Bronchiectasis can be caused by damaging effects of a long-standing infection.*
bronch/o		**bronch**/o/scope (BRŎNG-kō-skōp): curved, flexible tube with a light for visual examination of the bronchi *-scope:* instrument for examining *A bronchoscope is used to examine the bronchi or secure a specimen for biopsy or culture. It is also used to aspirate secretions or a foreign body from the respiratory tract.*
bronchiol/o	bronchiole	**bronchiol**/itis (brŏng-kē-ō-LĪ-tĭs): inflammation of the bronchioles *-itis:* inflammation
pleur/o	pleura	**pleur**/itic (ploo-RĬT-ĭk): pertaining to pleurisy *-itic:* pertaining to
pneum/o	air; lung	**pneum**/ectomy (nū-MĔK-tō-mē): excision of all or part of a lung *-ectomy:* excision, removal
pneumon/o		**pneumon**/ia (nū-MŌ-nē-ă): acute inflammation and infection of alveoli, which fill with pus or products of the inflammatory reaction *-ia:* condition *Pneumonia is most commonly caused by inhaled pneumonococci and less commonly by staphylococci, fungi, or viruses.*
pulmon/o	lung	**pulmon**/o/logist (pŭl-mŏ-NŎL-ŏ-jĭst): physician who specializes in treating pathological conditions of the lungs *-logist:* specialist in study of
thorac/o	chest	**thorac**/o/pathy (thō-răk-ŎP-ă-thē): disease of the thorax or the organs it contains *-pathy:* disease

SUFFIXES

-algia	pain	pleur/**algia** (ploo-RĂL-jē-ă): pain in the pleura *pleur:* pleura
-dynia		thorac/o/**dynia** (thō-răk-ō-DĬN-ē-ă): pain in the chest *thorac:* chest

(continued)

Word Element	Meaning	Word Analysis
-ectasis	dilation, expansion	atel/**ectasis** (ăt-ĕ-LĔK-tă-sĭs): abnormal condition characterized by collapse of alveoli *atel:* incomplete; imperfect *Atelectasis is characterized by collapse of alveoli, preventing respiratory exchange of carbon dioxide and oxygen in a part of the lungs.*
-osis	abnormal condition; increase (used primarily with blood cells)	cyan/**osis** (sī-ă-NŌ-sĭs): bluish discoloration of the skin and mucous membranes *cyan:* blue *Cyanosis is caused by deficiency of oxygen in the blood.*
-osmia	smell	an/**osmia** (ăn-ŎZ-mē-ă): loss or impairment of the sense of smell, which usually occurs as a temporary condition *an-:* without, not
-oxia	oxygen	hyp/**oxia** (hī-PŎKS-ē-ă): abnormally low level of oxygen at the cellular level *hyp-:* under, below, deficient *Because tissues have a decreased amount of oxygen, cyanosis can result.*
-phagia	swallowing, eating	aer/o/**phagia** (ĕr-ō-FĂ-jē-ă): swallowing air *aer/o:* air
-pnea	breathing	a/**pnea** (ăp-NĒ-ă): temporary cessation of breathing *a-:* without, not *Apnea may be a serious symptom, especially in patients with other potentially life-threatening conditions. Some types of apnea include newborn, cardiac, and sleep.*
-spasm	involuntary contraction, twitching	pharyng/o/**spasm** (făr-ĬN-gō-spăzm): spasm of muscles in the pharynx *pharyng/o:* pharynx (throat)
-thorax	chest	py/o/**thorax** (pī-ō-THŌ-răks): accumulation of pus in the thorax *py/o:* pus

Pronunciation Help						
	Long Sound	ā in rāte	ē in rēbirth	ī in īsle	ō in ōver	ū in ūnite
	Short Sound	ă in ălone	ĕ in ĕver	ĭ in ĭt	ŏ in nŏt	ŭ in cŭt

 Listen and Learn, the audio CD-ROM included in this book, will help you master pronunciation of selected medical words. Use it to practice pronunciations of the above-listed medical terms and for instructions to complete the *Listen and Learn* exercise for this section.

SECTION REVIEW 4-1

For the following medical terms, first write the suffix and its meaning. Then translate the meaning of the remaining elements starting with the first part of the word. The first word is completed for you.

Term	Meaning
1. laryng/o/scope	*-scope: instrument for examining; larynx (voice box)*
2. py/o/thorax	
3. hyp/oxia	
4. trache/o/stomy	
5. a/pnea	
6. pulmon/o/logist	
7. pneumon/ia	
8. rhin/o/rrhea	
9. an/osmia	
10. pneum/ectomy	

Competency Verification: Check your answers in Appendix B, Answer Key, page 559. If you are not satisfied with your level of comprehension, review the vocabulary and retake the review.

Correct Answers _____ × 10 = _____ % Score

Respiratory System

Upper Respiratory Tract

nose, stomach

4-1 External openings of the nose are referred to as *nostrils* or *nares* (singular, naris). *Nas/o/gastr/ic* refers to the nose and stomach. This term is used to describe procedures and devices associated with the nose and the stomach, such as *nas/o/gastr/ic feeding* and *nas/o/gastr/ic suction.* When you see the term *nas/o/gastr/ic tube,* you will know it refers to a device inserted into the _____ and into the _____.

pharynx (throat)
FĂR-ĭnks

4-2 When the term *tube* is used in association with a medical procedure, it usually refers to a catheter. A catheter is a hollow, flexible tube inserted into a vessel or body cavity. Its purpose is to withdraw or instill fluids into a body cavity or vessel. A *pharyng/eal suction catheter* is a rigid tube used to suction the pharynx when the physician performs a visual examination or therapeutic procedure of the throat.

The CF *pharyng/o* means _____ (_____).

nas/o, rhin/o	**4-3** CFs for nose are _____ / _____ and _____ / _____.

para/nas/al păr-ă-NĀ-săl	**4-4** The prefix *para-* is a directional element that means *near, beside, beyond.* The para/nas/al sinuses are hollow spaces within the skull that open into the nasal cavities. They are lined with *ciliated epithelium,* which is continuous with the mucosa of the nasal cavities. The term in this frame that means *near* or *beside the nose* is _____ / _____ / _____.

rhin/o/plasty RĪ-nō-plăs-tē **rhin/o/tomy** rī-NŎT-ō-mē	**4-5** Both **rhin/o** and **nas/o** refer to the nose. As a general rule, **nas/o** is not used to build surgical terms. However, if you are in doubt about which element to use, consult a medical dictionary. Form operative terms that mean *surgical repair of the nose:* _____ / _____ / _____ *incision of the nose:* _____ / _____ / _____

rhin/o/rrhea rī-nō-RĒ-ă	**4-6** *Rhin/o/rrhea* is a discharge from the nose. Sneezing, tearing, and a runny nose are common symptoms of a cold. Build a term that means *discharge from the nose:* _____ / _____ / _____

rhin/o/rrhagia rī-nō-RĂ-jē-ă **rhin/o/rrhea** rī-nō-RĒ-ă	**4-7** Whereas *rhin/o/rrhea* refers to a runny nose, *rhin/o/rrhagia* refers to nosebleed. Profuse bleeding from the nose is charted with the Dx _____ / _____ / _____. A runny discharge from the nose is charted with the Dx _____ / _____ / _____.

rhin/itis rī-NĪ-tĭs **rhin/o/logist** rī-NŎL-ă-jĭst	**4-8** Practice building other medical terms with **rhin/o**. Inflammation of the nose is called _____ / _____. A physician who specializes in diseases of the nose is a _____ / _____ / _____.

> **!** When in doubt about the meaning of a word element, refer to Appendix A, Glossary of Medical Word Elements.

air; lung	**4-9** Air enters the nose and passes through the (1) **nasal cavity**, where fine hairs catch many of the dust particles that we inhale. Label the nasal cavity in Figure 4-2. CFs *pneum/o* and *pneumon/o* mean _____; _____.

A.

(1) _____ _____

(2) _____ (_____)

(3) _____ (_____)

(4) _____

(6) _____ and _____

(5) _____ (_____)

_____ _____

(7) _____

(8) _____ _____

(11) _____ _____

(12) _____

(9) _____

Alveolus O$_2$

CO$_2$

(10) _____ _____

B.

Figure 4-2   Identifying the upper and lower respiratory tracts.

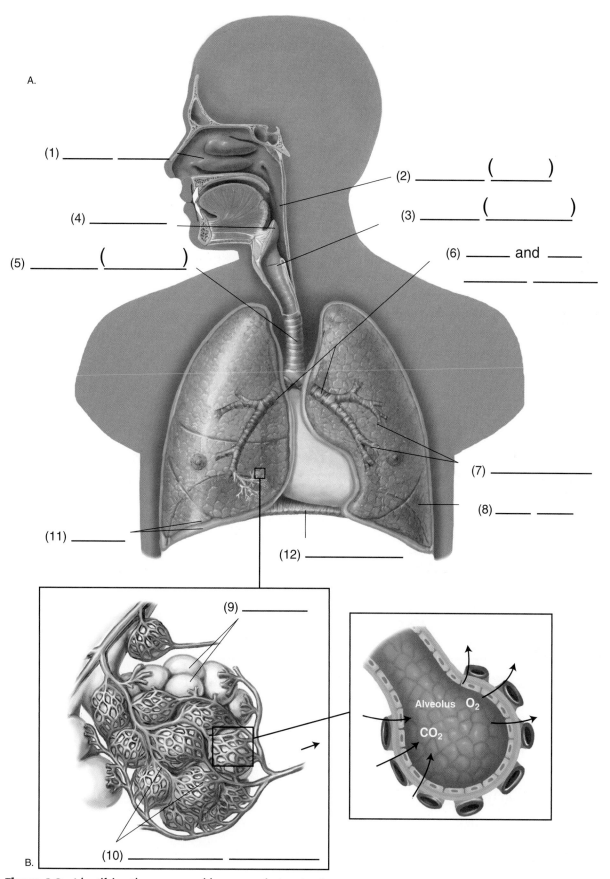

aer/o/phagia ĕr-ō-FĀ-jē-ă	**4-10** Swallowing air is not unusual for infants. It can occur as they suck on a nipple to obtain milk, water, or any liquid substance. Doing so commonly causes gaseous discomfort, which is relieved when the infant is burped. Combine **aer/o** + *-phagia* to form a medical term that means *swallowing air:* _____ / _____ / _____.
air	**4-11** The suffix *-therapy* is used in words to mean *treatment. Aer/o/ therapy* is treatment of diseases by use of _____.
water	**4-12** *Hydr/o/therapy* is treatment of diseases by use of _____.
air, water	**4-13** Combining air and water to treat a disease or injury is also a form of therapy. *Aer/o/hydr/o/therapy* is treatment by application of _____ and _____.
aer/o/therapy ĕr-ō-THĔR-ă-pē **hydr/o/therapy** hī-drō-THĔR-ă-pē **aer/o/hydr/o/therapy** ĕr-ō-hī-drō-THĔR-ă-pē	**4-14** Use *-therapy* to develop words meaning treatment with *air:* _____ / _____ / _____ *water:* _____ / _____ / _____ *air and water:* _____ / _____ / _____ / _____ / _____
	4-15 After passing through the nasal cavity, air reaches the (2) **pharynx (throat)**. Label the pharynx in Figure 4-2.
pharyng/o **myc** **-osis**	**4-16** From the term *pharyng/o/myc/osis*, determine the elements that mean *pharynx (throat):* _____ / _____ *fungus:* _____ *abnormal condition:* _____
pharynx *or* **throat** FĂR-ĭnks	**4-17** Pharyng/o/myc/osis is a fungal disease of the _____.
pharynx FĂR-ĭnks	**4-18** The suffix *-plegia* means *paralysis. Pharyng/o/plegia* and *pharyng/o/paralysis* are used to describe muscle paralysis of the _____.

cancer
KĂN-sĕr

4-19 Smoking, drinking alcohol, and chewing tobacco can cause cancer (CA) of the pharynx. Patients with pharyng/eal CA may require some type of plastic surgery.

When you see CA in a medical chart, you will know it is an abbreviation for _____.

pharyng/itis
făr-ĭn-JĪ-tĭs

pharyng/o/plasty
făr-ĬN-gō-plăs-tē

pharyng/o/tomy
făr-ĭn-GŎT-ō-mē

pharyng/o/tome
făr-ĬN-gō-tōm

pharyng/o/spasm
făr-ĬN-gō-spăzm

4-20 Use *pharyng/o* to form medical words that mean

inflammation of the pharynx (throat): _____ / _____

surgical repair of the pharynx (throat):
_____ / _____ / _____

incision of the pharynx (throat): _____ / _____ / _____

instrument to incise the pharynx (throat):
_____ / _____ / _____

involuntary contraction or twitching of the pharynx (throat):
_____ / _____ / _____

pharyng/o/cele
făr-ĬN-gō-sēl

4-21 Use *-cele* to build a word that literally means *hernia or swelling of the pharynx:* _____ / _____ / _____

stricture, pharynx
STRĬK-chūr, FĂR-ĭnks

4-22 *Pharyng/o/stenosis* is a narrowing, or _____ of the _____.

4-23 The (3) **larynx (voice box)** is responsible for sound production and makes speech possible. Label the larynx in Figure 4-2.

laryng/o

4-24 From the term *laryng/itis* (inflammation of the larynx), construct the CF for *larynx:* _____ / _____

laryng/o/scope
lăr-ĬN-gō-skōp

4-25 Combine *laryng/o* + *-scope* to form a word that means *instrument to view the larynx:* _____ / _____ / _____

laryng/ectomy
lăr-ĭn-JĔK-tō-mē

4-26 When laryng/eal CA is detected in its early stages, a partial laryng/ectomy may be recommended. For extensive CA of the larynx, the entire larynx is removed. In either case, when excision of the larynx is performed, the surgery is called a _____ / _____.

laryng/o/spasm
lăr-ĬN-gō-spazm

4-27 Spasms of the laryng/eal muscles cause a closure that impedes breathing.

Use *-spasm* to build a medical term meaning *spasm of the larynx:* _____ / _____ / _____

-stenosis

laryng/o

4–28   Laryng/o/stenosis is a stricture of the larynx.

Determine the elements that mean

narrowing, stricture: _____

larynx: _____ / _____

---

laryng/itis
lăr-ĭn-JĪ-tĭs

laryng/o/scope
lăr-ĬN-gō-skōp

laryng/o/scopy
lăr-ĭn-GŎS-kō-pē

laryng/o/stenosis
lăr-ĭn-gō-stĕ-NŌ-sĭs

4–29   Form medical words that mean

inflammation of larynx: _____ / _____

instrument to view or examine the larynx:

_____ / _____ / _____

visual examination of larynx: _____ / _____ / _____

narrowing or stricture of larynx:

_____ / _____ / _____

4–30   Label the structures in Figure 4-2 as you continue to read the material in this frame. A small leaf-shaped cartilage called the (4) **epiglottis** is located in the super/ior portion of the larynx. During swallowing, it closes off the larynx so that foods and liquids are directed into the esophagus. If anything but air passes into the larynx, a cough reflex attempts to expel the material to avoid a serious blockage of breathing.

When defining a medical word, first define the suffix. Second, define the beginning of the word; finally, define the middle of the word. Here is an example of the term

bronch / o / pneumon / itis
(2)   (3)   (1)

S E C T I O N   R E V I E W   4-2

Using the following table, write the CF, suffix, or prefix that matches its
definition in the space provided to the left of the definition. There may be
more than one word element that matches a definition.

Combining Forms		Suffixes		Prefixes
aer/o	pharyng/o	-cele	-stenosis	a-
hydr/o	rhin/o	-ectasis	-stomy	an-
laryng/o	trache/o	-phagia	-therapy	neo-
myc/o		-plegia	-tome	para-
nas/o		-scopy	-tomy	

1. _____ air

2. _____ near, beside; beyond

3. _____ fungus

4. _____ dilation, expansion

5. _____ forming an opening (mouth)

6. _____ incision

7. _____ instrument to cut

8. _____ larynx (voice box)

9. _____ hernia, swelling

10. _____ new

11. _____ nose

12. _____ paralysis

13. _____ pharynx (throat)

14. _____ narrowing, stricture

15. _____ swallowing, eating

16. _____ trachea (windpipe)

17. _____ treatment

18. _____ without, not

19. _____ visual examination

20. _____ water

Competency Verification: Check your answers in Appendix B, Answer Key, page 559. If you are not
satisfied with your level of comprehension, go back to Frame 4-1 and rework the frames.

Correct Answers _____ × 5 = _____ % Score

Lower Respiratory Tract

bronchi/oles BRŎNG-kē-ōlz	**4–31** Continue to label structures in Figure 4-2, page 111, as you read the following material. The (5) **trachea (windpipe)** is a cylindrical tube composed of smooth muscle embedded with a series of 16 to 20 C-shaped rings of cartilage. The trachea extends downward into the thoracic cavity, where it divides to form the (6) **right** and **left primary bronchi** (singular, bronchus). Each bronchus enters a lung and continues to subdivide into increasingly finer, smaller branches known as (7) *bronchioles.* The diminutive suffix *–ole* means *small, minute.* Thus, smaller segments of the bronchus are called _____ / _____.
bronchus BRŎNG-kŭs	**4–32** The continuous branching of bronchi and bronchi/oles from the trachea throughout the lungs resembles an inverted tree. The trachea resembles the trunk, and the branching of bronchi and bronchi/oles that become smaller and smaller resembles the branches. Thus, the term *bronchi/al tree* is commonly used to describe air passages in the lungs. Refer to Figure 4-1 to examine these structures. The singular form of *bronchi* is _____.
cartilage KĂR-tĭ-lĭj	**4–33** The trachea's cartilaginous rings provide necessary rigidity to keep air passage open at all times. The CF **chondr/o** refers to *cartilage.* *Chondr/itis* is an inflammation of _____.
chondr/o/plasty KŎN-drō-plăs-tē **chondr/o/pathy** kŏn-DRŎP-ă-thē **chondr/oma** kŏn-DRŌ-mă	**4–34** Form medical words that mean *surgical repair of cartilage:* _____ / _____ / _____ *disease of cartilage:* _____ / _____ / _____ *tumor (or tumorlike growth) of cartilage:* _____ / _____
trache/o/stomy trā-kē-ŎS-tō-mē **trache/o/stomy** trā-kē-ŎS-tō-mē	**4–35** On its way to the lungs, air passes from the larynx to the trachea, or *windpipe.* In a life-threatening situation, when trache/al obstruction causes cessation of breathing, a trache/o/stomy is performed through the neck into the trachea to gain access below the blockage. (See Figure 4-3.) When an emergency situation warrants creation of an opening into the trachea, the procedure performed is _____ / _____ / _____. The surgical procedure that means *forming an opening (mouth) into the trachea* is _____ / _____ / _____.
trache/o/malacia trā-kē-ō-mă-LĀ-shē-ă	**4–36** Softening of trache/al cartilage may be caused by pressure of the left pulmonary artery on the trachea. Use *-malacia* to form a word that literally means *softening of the trachea:* _____ / _____ / _____

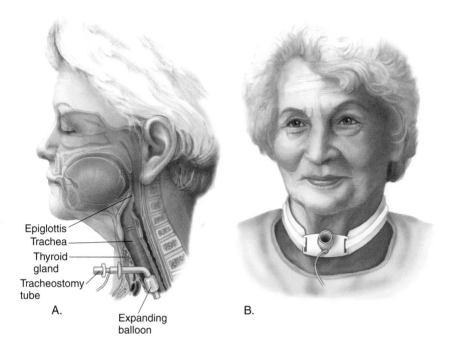

Epiglottis
Trachea
Thyroid
gland
Tracheostomy
tube

A.

Expanding
balloon

B.

Figure 4-3 Tracheostomy.
(A) Lateral view with
tracheostomy tube in place.
(B) Frontal view.

---

trache/o/pathy
trā-kē-ŎP-ă-thē

trache/o/plasty
TRĀ-kē-ō-plăs-tē

trache/o/stenosis
trā-kē-ō-stĕn-Ō-sĭs

trache/o/tomy
trā-kē-ŎT-ō-mē

4–37 Use *trache/o* to develop medical terms that mean

disease of the trachea: _____ / _____ / _____

surgical repair of the trachea:

_____ / _____ / _____

narrowing or stricture of the trachea:

_____ / _____ / _____

incision of the trachea: _____ / _____ / _____

---

trachea, larynx
TRĀ-kē-ă, LĂR-inks

4–38 Trache/o/laryng/o/tomy is an incision of the

_____ and _____.

4–39 Label the left lung in Figure 4-2 as you continue to read the material in this frame. Then review the position of the trachea to see how it branches into a right and left primary bronchus. Each primary *bronchus (plural, bronchi)* leads to a separate lung, the right and the (8) **left lung**. Structures of the bronchi and alveoli are part of the lungs, which are the organs of *respiration* (act of breathing).

---

bronchi
BRŎNG-kē

4–40 Change the singular form of *bronchus* to a plural form:

_____

---

bronch/o/spasm
BRŎNG-kō-spăzm

4–41 Patients with asthma experience wheezing caused by bronch/ial spasms. The medical term for this condition is *bronchi/o/spasm* or

_____ / _____ / _____.

---

bronchi/ectasis
brŏng-kē-ĔK-tă-sĭs

4-42 Chronic dilation of bronchi is called *bronchi/ectasis*. Chronic pneumon/ia or flu may result in dilation of bronchi. The medical term for this condition is _____ / _____.

bronch/itis
brŏng-KĪ-tĭs
bronch/o/spasm
BRŎNG-kō-spăzm

bronch/o/stenosis
brŏng-kō-stĕn-Ō-sĭs

4-43 Use *bronch/o* to build medical words that mean

inflammation of bronchi: _____ / _____

involuntary contraction or twitching of the bronchus:

_____ / _____ / _____

narrowing or stricture of bronchi:

_____ / _____ / _____

4-44 Structurally, each primary bronchus is similar to that of the trachea, but as they subdivide into finer branches, the amount of cartilage in the walls decreases and finally disappears as it forms bronchi/oles. As cartilage diminishes, a layer of smooth muscle surrounding the tube becomes more prominent. Smooth muscles in the walls of bronchi/oles are designed to constrict or dilate the airways to maintain unobstructed air passages. Bronchi/oles eventually distribute air to the (9) **alveoli** (singular, *alveolus*), small clusters of grapelike air sacs of the lungs. Each alveolus is surrounded by a network of microscopic (10) **pulmonary capillaries.** Label the alveoli and pulmonary capillaries in Figure 4-2.

erythr/o/cytes
ĕ-RĬTH-rō-sītz

oxygen
carbon dioxide

4-45 The thin walls of the alveoli permit an exchange of gases between the alveolus and the surrounding capillaries. Blood flowing through the capillaries accepts oxygen (O_2) from the alveolus, while depositing carbon dioxide (CO_2) into the alveolus. Erythr/o/cytes in the blood carry O_2 to all parts of the body and CO_2 to the lungs for exhalation.

The medical term for red blood cells is

_____ / _____ / _____.

The abbreviation O_2 means _____.

The abbreviation CO_2 means _____ _____.

micro/scope
MĪ-krō-skōp

4-46 Macro/scopic structures are visible to the naked eye. Micro/scopic structures, such as the alveoli, are visible only through the use of a micro/scope.

Micro/scopic capillaries are visible to the eye through the use of a magnifying instrument called a _____ / _____.

alveoli
ăl-VĒ-ō-lī

4-47 If a lung disorder destroys or damages enough alveol/ar sacs, there is less surface area for gas exchange, and breathlessness results. Clusters of air sacs at the end of the bronchi/al tree are called

_____ (plural).

4-48 Abbreviations O_2 and CO_2 are commonly seen in laboratory reports. Whenever you are in doubt about an abbreviation, refer to Appendix E, a list of common abbreviations and symbols.

O_2

The abbreviation for oxygen is _____.

CO_2

The abbreviation for carbon dioxide is _____.

4-49 Process of gas exchange between the atmosphere and body cells is called *respiration* and it occurs in two phases. ***External respiration*** occurs each time we *inhale* (breathe in) air. This process results in a gas exchange (O_2 loading and CO_2 unloading) between air-filled chambers of the lungs and the blood in the pulmonary capillaries. (See Figure 4-2, structure 10.) ***Internal (cellular) respiration*** is exchange of gases (O_2 unloading and CO_2 loading) between the blood and body tissue cells. This process occurs in body tissues when O_2 (carried in blood from the lungs to nourish the body's cells) is exchanged for CO_2. The CO_2 travels in the bloodstream to the lungs and is *exhaled* through the mouth or nose.

You may have to read this frame a few times to understand the process of respiration. Nevertheless, see if you can differentiate between the two types of respiration and also identify the symbols for oxygen and carbon dioxide.

external respiration

Gas exchange between the body and the outside environment is called

_____ _____.

internal respiration

Gas exchange at the cellular level between the blood and body tissue cells is called _____ _____.

4-50 The CFs ***pneum/o*** and ***pneumon/o*** mean *air; lung.*

inflammation, lung(s)
ĭn-flă-MĀ-shŭn

Pneumon/itis is an _____ of the _____.

4-51 Pneumon/ia, an acute inflammation and infection of the lungs in which alveoli fill with secretions, is the fifth leading cause of death in the United States.

Analyze pneumon/ia by defining the word elements:

air, lung

pneumon/o means _____ or _____.

condition

-ia means _____ (noun ending).

4-52 In patients with lung cancer, it may be necessary to remove part or all of the lung.

Use ***pneumon/o*** to form a word that means *excision of a lung:*

pneumon/ectomy
nū-mōn-ĔK-tō-mē

_____ / _____

4-53 The suffix *-cele* means *hernia, swelling.* A hernial protrusion of lung tissue may be caused by a partial airway obstruction.

Use ***pneumon/o*** to form a word that means *herniation of the lung:*

pneumon/o/cele
nū-MŌN-ō-sēl

_____ / _____ / _____

pneumon/osis nū-mōn-Ō-sĭs **pneumon/o/pathy** nū-mō-NŎP-ăth-ē **pneumon/ectomy** nū-mōn-ĔK-tō-mē	**4-54** Use *pneumon/o* to build medical words that mean *abnormal condition of the lungs:* _____ / _____ *disease of the lung:* _____ / _____ / _____ *excision of a lung:* _____ / _____
lung(s)	**4-55** The suffix *-centesis* is used in words to denote a *surgical puncture*. *Pneum/o/centesis* is a surgical puncture to aspirate the _____.
	4-56 If you are not sure what *aspirate* means in the previous frame, take a few minutes to use your medical dictionary to define the term. _____ _____
pneumon/o/centesis nū-mō-nō-sĕn-TĒ-sis	**4-57** Lung abscess, an abnormal localized collection of fluid, may be caused by pneumonia. Therapeutic treatment with pneum/o/centesis may be required. Construct another word that means *surgical puncture of a lung*. _____ / _____ / _____
lung(s), air **black** **abnormal condition**	**4-58** Pneumon/o/melan/osis is an abnormal condition of black lung caused by inhalation of black dust (a disease common among coal miners), which is also called *pneumomelanosis* or *pneumoconiosis*. Analyze *pneumon/o/melan/osis* by defining the word elements: *pneumon/o* means: _____ or _____ *melan/o* means: _____ *-osis* means: _____ _____
oxygen **carbon dioxide**	**4-59** The lungs are divided into five lobes: three lobes in the right lung and two lobes in the left lung. Both lungs supply blood with O_2 inhaled from the environment and dispose of waste CO_2 in the exhaled air. O_2 refers to _____. CO_2 refers to _____ _____.
excision *or* **removal** ĕk-SĬ-zhŭn	**4-60** Lung CA patients may undergo a *lob/ectomy*, which is a(n) _____ of a lobe.
lob/o	**4-61** From *lob/ar* (pertaining to the lobe), construct the CF for *lobe*: _____ / ____

lob/itis lō-BĪ-tĭs **lob/o/tomy** lō-BŎT-ō-mē **lob/ectomy** lō-BĚK-tō-mē	**4-62** Develop medical words that mean *inflammation of a lobe:* _____ / _____ *incision of a lobe:* _____ / ____ / _____ *excision of a lobe:* _____ / _____
	4-63 Each lung is enclosed in a double-folded membrane called the (11) ***pleura***. Label the pleura in Figure 4-2.
inflammation	**4-64** *Pleur/itis* is an _____ of the pleura.
pleur/o	**4-65** From *pleur/o/dynia*, identify the CF for *pleura:* _____ / ____
pleur/o/dynia, **pleur/algia** ploo-rō-DĬN-ē-ă, ploo-RĂL-jē-ă	**4-66** Pain in the pleura is known as _____ / ____ / _____ or _____ / _____.
pneumon/o *or* **pneum/o**	**4-67** *Pleur/o/pneumon/ia* is pleurisy complicated with pneumonia. The CF for *air or lung* is _____ / ____.
pleur/itis ploo-RĪ-tĭs **pleur/o/cele** PLOO-rō-sēl	**4-68** Form medical words that mean *inflammation of the pleura:* _____ / _____ *hernia or swelling of the pleura:* _____ / ____ / _____
inflammation, pleura PLOO-ră	**4-69** *Pleurisy* is an inflammation of the pleura. *Pleur/itis* is also an _____ of the _____.
inflammation, pleura PLOO-ră	**4-70** Whenever you see *pleur/isy* or *pleur/itis*, you will know it means _____ of the _____.
pleur/o/dynia ploo-rō-DĬN-ē-ă	**4-71** The suffixes *-algia* and *-dynia* refer to pain. The *pleura* commonly becomes inflamed when a person has pneumonia. This condition may cause pleur/algia, which is also called _____ / ____ / _____.

without, not **slow** **bad; painful; difficult** **good, normal** **rapid** **breathing**	**4–72** Prefixes *a-*, *brady-*, *dys-*, *eu-*, and *tachy-* are commonly attached to *-pnea* to describe various types of breathing conditions. Write the meanings of each of the following elements. *a-:* _____, _____ *brady-:* _____ *dys-:* _____; _____; _____ *eu-:* _____, _____ *tachy-:* _____ *-pnea:* _____
a/pnea ăp-NĒ-ă	**4–73** *A/pnea* is a temporary loss of breathing that results in brief or prolonged absence of spontaneous respiration. It is a serious symptom, especially in patients with other potentially life-threatening conditions. Causes include respiratory arrest or respiratory failure. A term that literally means *without breathing* is _____ / _____.
a/pnea ăp-NĒ-ă	**4–74** When a/pnea occurs in premature infants, the immature central nervous system (CNS) fails to maintain a consistent respiratory rate. Thus, there are occasional long pauses between periods of regular breathing. An infant whose mother used cocaine during pregnancy is also likely to develop life-threatening a/pnea. When there is temporary cessation of breathing, the event is documented in the medical record as _____ / _____.
CPAP **OSA**	**4–75** Another type of a/pnea, obstructive sleep apnea (OSA), may be due to enlarged tonsils that cause an airway obstruction. Treatment includes use of a continuous positive airway pressure (CPAP) machine. (See Figure 4-4.) Provide the abbreviation that means *continuous positive airway pressure:* _____ *obstructive sleep apnea:* _____
a/pnea ăp-NĒ-ă **dys/pnea** dĭsp-NĒ-ă	**4–76** Because of airway obstruction, OSA patients stop breathing multiple times each night. A/pnea is followed by a gasping breath that often awakens the patient and results in sleep deprivation, fatigue, and difficulty concentrating during the day. This condition occurs most commonly in middle-aged, obese men who snore excessively. Build a medical term that means *without or not breathing:* _____ / _____ *painful or difficult breathing:* _____ / _____

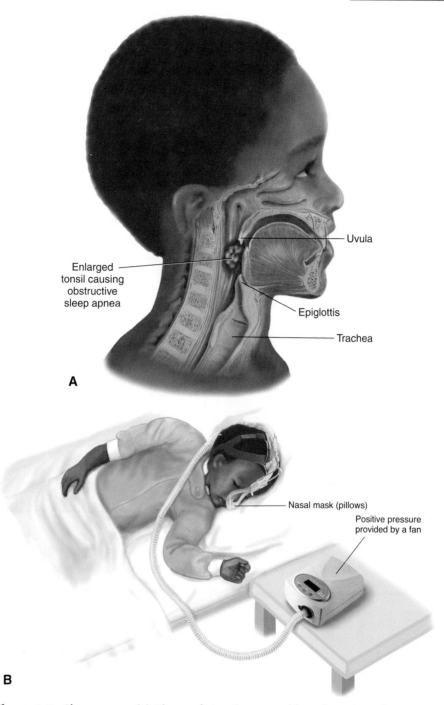

Figure 4-4 Sleep apnea. (A) Airway obstruction caused by enlarged tonsils eventually leads to obstructive sleep apnea. (B) Continuous positive airway pressure (CPAP) machine used to treat sleep apnea.

dys/pnea
dĭsp-NĒ-ă

4–77 Dys/pnea is normal when due to vigorous work or athletic activity. Dys/pnea can also occur as a result of various disorders of the respiratory system, such as pleurisy. A patient with pleurisy may experience

_____ / _____.

eu- **-pnea**	**4-78** *Eu/pnea* is normal breathing, as distinguished from *dys/pnea* and *a/pnea*. From *eu/pnea*, determine word elements that mean *good, normal:* _____ *breathing:* _____

a/pnea ăp-NĒ-ă **dys/pnea** dĭsp-NĒ-ă **eu/pnea** ūp-NĒ-ă **tachy/pnea** tăk-ĭp-NĒ-ă	**4-79** Here is a review of forming words with *-pnea*. Construct medical words that mean *without breathing:* _____ / _____ *difficult or labored breathing:* _____ / _____ *normal breathing:* _____ / _____ *rapid breathing:* _____ / _____

-pnea **orth/o**	**4-80** Orth/o/pnea is a condition in which there is labored breathing in any posture except in the erect sitting or standing position. Identify word elements in this frame that mean *breathing:* _____ *straight:* _____ / _____

thorac/o/tomy thō-răk-ŎT-ō-mē	**4-81** The CF *thorac/o* means *chest*. Form a word that means *incision of the chest:* _____ / _____ / _____

thorac/o/centesis thō-răk-ō-sĕn-TĒ-sĭs	**4-82** To remove fluid from the thorac/ic cavity, a surgical puncture of the chest is performed. This procedure is called *thoracentesis*, or _____ / _____ / _____. (See Figure 4-5).

thoracentesis thō-ră-sĕn-TĒ-sĭs	**4-83** Fluid commonly builds up around the lung(s) in patients with CA or pneumonia. To remove fluid from the thorac/ic cavity, the physician performs the surgical procedure called *thorac/o/centesis*, also known as _____.

	4-84 The (12) **diaphragm** is a muscular partition that separates the lungs from the abdominal cavity and aids in the process of breathing. The CF **phren/o** refers to the *diaphragm*. Label the *diaphragm* in Figure 4-2.

phren/o	**4-85** The CF **phren/o** also refers to the *mind*. When you want to build words that refer to the diaphragm or mind, use the CF _____ / _____.

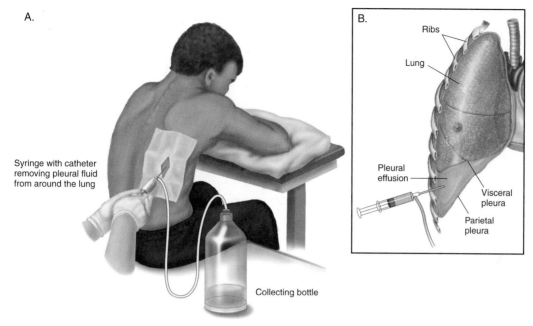

A.

Syringe with catheter removing pleural fluid from around the lung

Collecting bottle

B.

Ribs

Lung

Pleural effusion

Visceral pleura

Parietal pleura

Figure 4-5 Thoracentesis.

diaphragm DĪ-ă-frăm	**4–86** Whereas *phren/o/logy* is the study of the mind, *phren/o/ptosis* refers to a prolapse or downward displacement of the _____.
phren/o/spasm FRĚN-ō-spăzm	**4–87** Involuntary contraction or twitching of the diaphragm is documented in the medical record as _____ / ____ / _____.

Competency Verification: Check your labeling of Figure 4-2 with Appendix B, Answer Key, page 559.

inspiration *or* **inhalation** ĭn-spĭ-RĀ-shŭn, ĭn-hă-LĀ-shŭn **expiration** *or* **exhalation** ĕks-pĭ-RĀ-shŭn, ĕks-hă-LĀ-shŭn	**4–88** Identify words in Figure 4-6 that mean *process of breathing air into the lungs:* _____ *out of the lungs:* _____
inter/cost/al ĭn-tĕr-KŎS-tăl	**4–89** During inspiration, the diaphragm and the inter/cost/al muscles contract. As their name implies, the muscles between adjacent ribs are known as the _____ / _____ / _____ muscles.

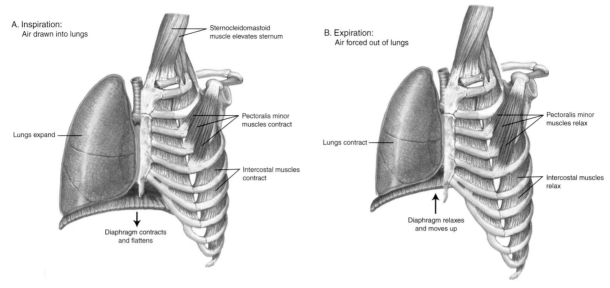

A. Inspiration:
Air drawn into lungs

Sternocleidomastoid
muscle elevates sternum

B. Expiration:
Air forced out of lungs

Pectoralis minor
muscles contract

Pectoralis minor
muscles relax

Lungs expand

Lungs contract

Intercostal muscles
contract

Intercostal muscles
relax

Diaphragm contracts
and flattens

Diaphragm relaxes
and moves up

Figure 4-6 Position of the diaphragm during inspiration (A) and expiration (B).

descends **ascends**	**4-90** Examine Figure 4-6A and B and use the terms *ascends* or *descends* to complete this frame. During inspiration (or inhalation), the diaphragm _____. During expiration (or exhalation), the diaphragm _____.
air	**4-91** Recall *aer/o* is the CF for _____.
aer/o/phobia ĕr-ō-FŌ-bē-ă	**4-92** Aer/o/phobia is a fear of air, drafts of air, airborne influences, or "bad air" (body odor). The medical word that means *fear of air* is _____ / _____ / _____.
hem/o/phobia hē-mō-FŌ-bē-ă	**4-93** Combine **hem/o** and *-phobia* to form a word that means *fear of blood*. _____ / _____ / _____.
muc/o **myc/o**	**4-94** Although the CFs **muc/o** and **myc/o** look similar, they have different meanings. Determine the CF that means *mucus:* _____ / _____ *fungus:* _____ / _____
air, lung **fungus** **abnormal condition**	**4-95** Analyze *pneumon/o/myc/osis* by defining the word elements. **pneumon/o:** _____ or _____ **myc:** _____ *-osis:* _____ _____

chronic bronch/itis
brŏng-KĪ-tĭs

4–96 Chronic bronch/itis is an inflammation of the bronchi that persists for a long time. This pulmon/ary disease is commonly caused by cigarette smoking and is characterized by increased production of mucus and obstruction of respiratory passages.

Bronch/itis may be of short duration, but when it persists for a long time, it may be a more serious pulmon/ary disease called

_____ _____ / _____.

bronchi/al
BRŎNG-kē-ăl

bronch/itis
brŏng-KĪ-tĭs

4–97 Chronic bronch/itis results in expectoration of mucus, sputum, or fluids by coughing or spitting.

Use *bronchi/o* to build a term that means *pertaining to the bronchi:*

_____ / _____

Use *bronch/o* to build a term that means *inflammation of the bronchi:*

_____ / _____

laryng/itis
lăr-ĭn-JĪ-tĭs

4–98 The larynx contains the organ of sound called *vocal cords.* When vocal cords become inflamed from overuse or infection, laryng/itis occurs. This condition results in hoarseness and difficulty speaking.

The medical term for *inflamed larynx* is _____ / _____.

bronch/o

pneumon

-ia

4–99 *Pneumon/ia* is lung inflammation caused by bacteria, a virus, or chemical irritants. Some pneumon/ias affect only one lobe of the lung (lobar pneumon/ia). Others, such as bronch/o/pneumon/ia, involve the lungs and bronchi/oles.

Identify elements in *bronch/o/pneumon/ia* that mean

bronchus: _____ / _____

air; lung: _____

condition: _____

bronch/o/pneumon/ia
brong-kō-nū-MŌ-nē-ă

4–100 A type of pneumon/ia that involves the lungs and bronchi/oles is called _____ / _____ / _____ / _____.

-oles

4–101 In Frame 4-99, the diminutive element that means *small* or *minute* is _____.

**compromised,
immunocompromised**
ĭm-ū-nō-KŎM-pră-mīzd

4–102 *Pneumocystis* pneumon/ia (PCP) is closely associated with a compromised immune system, particularly in patients with acquired immune deficiency syndrome (AIDS). PCP is caused by a fungus that resides in or on the normal flora (potentially path/o/gen/ic organisms that reside in, but are harmless to, healthy individuals). The fungus becomes an aggressive path/o/gen in immunocompromised persons.

Identify two terms in this frame that refer to an immune system incapable of resisting path/o/gen/ic organisms: _____ or

_____

PCP **AIDS**	**4-103** Identify the abbreviation for Pneumocystis *pneumon/ia:* _____ *acquired immune deficiency syndrome:* _____
***Pneumocystis* pneumonia** nū-mō-SĬS-tĭs nū-MŌ-nē-ă	**4-104** A type of pneumonia seen in patients with AIDS is _____ _____.
emphys/ema ĕm-fĭ-SĒ-mă	**4-105** The CF *emphys/o* means *to inflate*. The suffix *-ema* means *state of; condition. Emphys/ema* is a chronic disease characterized by overexpansion and destruction of alveoli, and is commonly associated with cigarette smoking. Destruction of alveoli occurs in the respiratory disease known as _____ / _____.
COPD **asthma, emphys/ema** ĂZ-mă, ĕm-fĭ-SĒ-mă	**4-106** Chronic obstructive pulmonary disease (COPD), a group of respiratory disorders, is characterized by a chronic, partial obstruction of the bronchi and lungs. Three major disorders included in COPD are asthma, chronic bronch/itis, and emphys/ema. (See Figure 4-7.) The abbreviation for *chronic obstructive pulmonary disease* is _____. Three major path/o/logic/al conditions associated with COPD are chronic bronch/itis, _____, and _____ / _____.
bronch/itis brong-KĪ-tĭs	**4-107** Chronic bronch/itis, an inflammation of the mucous membranes lining the bronchial airways, is characterized by increased mucus production resulting in a chronic productive cough. (see Figure 4-7A.) Cigarette smoking, environmental irritants, allergic response, and infectious agents cause this condition. The medical term that means *inflammation of bronchi* is _____ / _____.
dys/pnea dĭsp-NĒ-ă	**4-108** Asthma is a respiratory condition characterized by recurrent attacks of labored or difficult breathing accompanied by wheezing. (See Figure 4-7C.) The medical term for painful or difficult breathing is _____ / _____.
metastasize *or* **metastasis** mĕ-TĂS-tă-sīz, mĕ-TĂS-tă-sĭs	**4-109** Lung CA, associated with smoking, is the leading cause of cancer-related deaths in men and women in the United States. It usually spreads rapidly and metastasizes to other parts of the body, making it difficult to diagnose and treat in its early stages. When CA spreads to other parts of the body, the medical term used to describe that condition is _____.

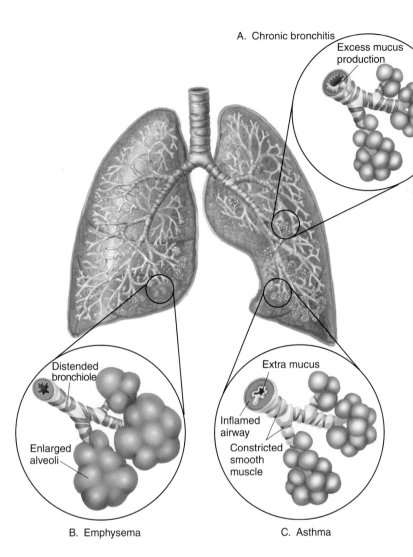

A. Chronic bronchitis

Excess mucus production

Distended bronchiole

Enlarged alveoli

B. Emphysema

Extra mucus

Inflamed airway

Constricted smooth muscle

C. Asthma

Figure 4-7 COPD. (A) Chronic bronchitis with inflamed airways and excessive mucus. (B) Emphysema with distended bronchioles and alveoli. (C) Asthma with narrowed bronchial tubes and swollen mucous membranes.

4–110 Tuberculosis (TB), an infectious disease, produces small lesions, or *tubercles*, in the lungs. If left untreated, it infects the bones and organs of the entire body. An increase in TB is attributed to the increasing prevalence of AIDS.

The abbreviation *TB* refers to _____.

The name *tuberculosis* is derived from small lesions that appear in the lungs called _____.

tuberculosis
tū-bĕr-kū-LŌ-sĭs
tubercles
TŪ-bĕr-klz

S E C T I O N   R E V I E W   4-3

Using the table below, write the CF, suffix, or prefix that matches its definition in the space provided to the left of the definition. There may be more than one word element that matches a definition.

Combining Forms		Suffixes		Prefixes	
bronchi/o	orth/o	-cele	-pnea	a-	micro-
bronch/o	pleur/o	-centesis	-scope	brady-	tachy-
chondr/o	pneum/o	-ectasis	-spasm	dys-	
hem/o	pneumon/o	-osis	-stenosis	eu-	
melan/o	thorac/o	-phobia		macro-	
myc/o					

1. _____ abnormal condition; increase (used primarily with blood cells)

2. _____ slow

3. _____ bad; painful; difficult

4. _____ black

5. _____ breathing

6. _____ bronchus (plural, bronchi)

7. _____ blood

8. _____ chest

9. _____ dilation, expansion

10. _____ fear

11. _____ fungus

12. _____ good, normal

13. _____ hernia, swelling

14. _____ instrument for examining

15. _____ involuntary contraction, twitching

16. _____ large

17. _____ rapid

18. _____ air; lung

19. _____ pleura

20. _____ small

21. _____ straight

22. _____ narrowing, stricture

23. _____ surgical puncture

24. _____ without, not

25. _____ cartilage

Competency Verification: Check your answers in Appendix B, Answer Key, page 559. If you are not satisfied with your level of comprehension, go back to Frame 4-31 and rework the frames.

Correct Answers _____ × 4 = _____ % Score

Abbreviations

This section introduces respiratory system-related abbreviations and their meanings. Included are abbreviations contained in the medical report activities that follow.

Abbreviation	Meaning	Abbreviation	Meaning
ABGs	arterial blood gases	IPPB	intermittent positive-pressure breathing
AIDS	acquired immune deficiency syndrome	IRDS	infant respiratory distress syndrome
ARDS	acute respiratory distress syndrome	MRI	magnetic resonance imaging
CA	cancer; chronological age; cardiac arrest	NMT	nebulized mist treatment
CF	cystic fibrosis	O_2	oxygen
COPD	chronic obstructive pulmonary disease	OSA	obstructive sleep apnea
CO_2	carbon dioxide	PCP	*Pneumocystis* pneumonia; primary care physician; phencyclidine (hallucinogen)
CPAP	continuous positive airway pressure	PFT	pulmonary function test
CPR	cardiopulmonary resuscitation	PND	paroxysmal nocturnal dyspnea
CT	computed tomography	RD	respiratory disease
DPT	diphtheria, pertussis, tetanus	SIDS	sudden infant death syndrome
Dx	diagnosis	SOB	shortness of breath
FEV_1	forced expiratory volume in one second	TB	tuberculosis
FVC	forced vital capacity	URI	upper respiratory infection
HF	heart failure	VC	vital capacity
HMD	hyaline membrane disease		

Additional Medical Terms

The following are additional terms related to the respiratory system. Recognizing and learning these terms will help you understand the connection between common signs, symptoms, and diseases and their diagnoses as well as the rationale behind methods of medical and surgical treatments selected for a particular disorder.

Signs, Symptoms, and Diseases

abnormal breath sounds	Abnormal breathing sounds heard during inhalation or expiration, with or without a stethoscope
crackles KRĂK-ălz	Fine crackling or bubbling sounds, commonly heard during inspiration when there is fluid in the alveoli; also called *rales*
	Crackles are commonly associated with bronchitis, pneumonia, and heart failure (HF). Crackles that do not clear after a cough may indicate pulmonary edema or fluid in the alveoli due to HF or acute respiratory distress syndrome (ARDS).
friction rub	Dry, grating sound heard with a stethoscope during auscultation (listening for sounds within the body)
	A friction rub over the pleural area may be a sign of lung disease; however, when heard over the liver and splenic areas, it is normal.
rhonchi RONG-kē	Loud, coarse or snoring sounds heard during inspiration or expiration that is caused by obstructed airways
stridor STRĪ-dor	High-pitched, musical sound made on inspiration that is caused by an obstruction in the trachea or larynx
	Stridor is characteristic of the upper respiratory disorder called croup.
wheezes HWĒZ-ĕz	Continuous high-pitched whistling sounds, usually during expiration, that are caused by narrowing of an airway
	Wheezes occur in such conditions as asthma, croup, hay fever, and emphysema.
acidosis ăs-i-DŌ-sĭs	Excessive acidity of blood due to an accumulation of acids or an excessive loss of bicarbonate
	Respiratory acidosis is caused by abnormally high levels of carbon dioxide (CO_2) in the body.
acute respiratory distress syndrome (ARDS) ă-KŪT RĔS-pĭ-ră-tō-rē dĭs-TRĔS SĬN-drōm	Respiratory insufficiency marked by progressive hypoxia *ARDS is due to severe inflammatory damage that causes abnormal permeability of the alveolar-capillary membrane. As a result, the alveoli fill with fluid, which interferes with gas exchange.*
anoxia ăn-ŎK-sē-ă *an:* without, not *-oxia:* oxygen	Total absence of oxygen in body tissues *Anoxia is caused by a lack of O_2 in inhaled air or by obstruction that prevents O_2 from reaching the lungs.*

atelectasis ăt-ĕ-LĚK-tă-sĭs *atel:* incomplete; imperfect *-ectasis:* dilation, expansion	Collapse of lung tissue, preventing respiratory exchange of oxygen (O_2) and carbon dioxide (CO_2) *Atelectasis can be caused by obstruction of foreign bodies, excessive secretions, or pressure on the lung from a tumor. In fetal atelectasis, the lungs fail to expand normally at birth.*
consolidation kŏn-sŏl-ĭ-DĀ-shŭn	Process of becoming solid, especially in connection with the lungs *Solidification of the lungs is caused by a pathological engorgement of lung tissues that occurs in acute pneumonia.*
coryza kō-RĪ-ză	Acute inflammation of nasal passages accompanied by profuse nasal discharge; also called a *cold*
croup croop	Acute respiratory syndrome that occurs primarily in children and infants and is characterized by laryngeal obstruction and spasm, barking cough, and stridor
cystic fibrosis (CF) SĬS-tĭk fĭ-BRŌ-sĭs *cyst:* bladder *-ic:* pertaining to *fibr:* fiber, fibrous tissue *-osis:* abnormal condition; increase used primarily with blood cells)	Genetic disease of exocrine glands characterized by excessive secretions of thick mucus that do not drain normally, causing obstruction of passageways (including pancreatic and bile ducts and bronchi) *CF leads to chronic airway obstruction, recurrent respiratory infection, bronchiectasis and, eventually, respiratory failure.*
empyema ĕm-pī-Ē-mă	Pus in a body cavity, especially in the pleural cavity (pyothorax) *Empyema is usually the result of a primary infection in the lungs.*
epiglottitis ĕp-ĭ-glŏt-Ī-tĭs *epiglott:* epiglottis *-itis:* inflammation	In acute form, a severe, life-threatening infection of the epiglottis and surrounding area that occurs most commonly in children between ages 2 and 12 *In the classic form, epiglottitis involves a sudden onset of fever, dysphagia, inspiratory stridor, and severe respiratory distress that commonly requires intubation or tracheotomy to open the obstructed airway.*
epistaxis ĕp-ĭ-STĂK-sĭs	Hemorrhage from the nose; also called *nosebleed*

hypoxemia hī-pŏks-Ē-mē-ă *hyp:* under, below, deficient *ox:* oxygen *-emia:* blood	Deficiency of oxygen in the blood, usually a sign of respiratory impairment
hypoxia hī-PŎKS-ē-ă *hyp:* under, below, deficient *ox:* oxygen *-ia:* condition	Deficiency of oxygen in body tissues, usually a sign of respiratory impairment *In hypoxia, body tissues have a decreased amount of oxygen, which results in cyanosis.*
influenza ĭn-floo-ĔN-ză	Acute, contagious respiratory infection characterized by sudden onset of fever, chills, headache, and muscle pain
lung cancer LŬNG KĂN-sĕr	Pulmonary malignancy commonly attributable to cigarette smoking *Lung cancer comprises various malignant neoplasms that may appear in the trachea, bronchi, or air sacs of the lungs. Survival rates are low in lung cancer, due to rapid metastasis and late detection.*
pertussis pĕr-TŬS-ĭs	Acute infectious disease characterized by a "whoop"-sounding cough; also called *whooping cough* *Immunization of infants as part of the diphtheria, pertussis, tetanus (DPT) vaccine prevents the spread of pertussis.*
pleural effusion PLOO-răl ě-FŪ-zhŭn *pleur:* pleura *-al:* pertaining to	Abnormal presence of fluid in the pleural cavity *The fluid may contain blood (hemothorax), serum (hydrothorax), or pus (pyothorax). Treatment includes a surgical puncture of the chest using a hollow-bore needle (thoracentesis, thoracocentesis) to remove excess fluid(See Figure 4-5).*
pneumothorax nū-mō-THŌ-răks *pneum/o:* air; lung *-thorax:* chest	Collection of air in the pleural cavity, causing the complete or partial collapse of a lung *Pneumothorax can occur with pulmonary disease (emphysema, lung cancer, or tuberculosis) when pulmonary lesions rupture near the pleural surface, allowing communication between an alveolus or bronchus and the pleural cavity. It may also be the result of an open chest wound or a perforation of the chest wall that permits entrance of air. (See Figure 4-8.)*
sudden infant death syndrome (SIDS)	Completely unexpected and unexplained death of an apparently well, or virtually well, infant; also called *crib death* *SIDS is the most common cause of death between the second week and first year of life.*

A.

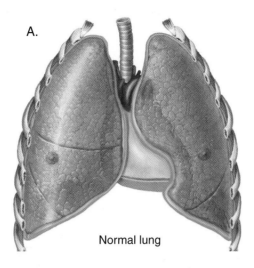

Normal lung

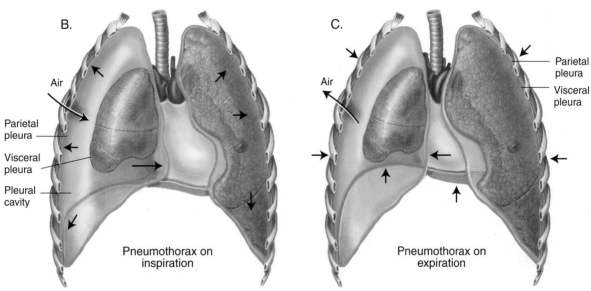

Figure 4-8 Pneumothorax. (A) Normal lung. (B) Pneumothorax on inspiration. Outside air rushes in due to disruption of chest wall and parietal pleura; the mediastinal contents shift to the side opposite the injury compressing the uninjured lung. (C) Pneumothorax on expiration. Lung air rushes out due to disruption of visceral pleura; the mediastinal contents move toward the center.

Diagnostic Procedures

arterial blood gas (ABG)
ăr-TĒ-rē-ăl
  arteri: artery
    -al: pertaining to
	Measurement of oxygen (O_2) and carbon dioxide (CO_2) content of arterial blood by various methods
	
	ABG analysis is used to assess adequacy of ventilation and oxygenation and the acid-base status of the body.

bronchoscopy brŏng-KŎS-kō-pē *bronch/o:* bronchus (plural, *bronchi*) *-scopy:* visual examination	Visual examination of the interior bronchi using a bronchoscope, a flexible fiberoptic instrument with a light, which can be inserted through the nose or mouth (See Figure 4–9.) *Bronchoscopy may be performed to remove obstructions, obtain a biopsy specimen, or observe directly for pathological changes.*
chest x-ray	Radiograph of the chest taken from the anteroposterior (AP), posteroanterior (PA), or lateral projections *Chest x-ray is used to diagnose atelectasis, tumors, pneumonia, emphysema, and many other lung diseases.*
computed tomography (CT) cŏm-PŪ-tĕd tō-MŎG-ră-fē *tom/o:* to cut *-graphy:* process of recording	Radiographic technique that uses a narrow beam of x-rays that rotates in a full arc around the patient to acquire multiple views of the body that a computer interprets to produce cross-sectional images of that body part *CT scanning is used to detect lesions in the lungs and thorax, blood clots, and pulmonary embolism (PE). CT scan may be performed with or without a contrast medium.*
magnetic resonance imaging (MRI) măg-NĔT-ĭc RĔZ-ĕn-ăns ĬM-ĭj-ĭng	Radiographic technique that uses electromagnetic energy to produce multiplanar cross-sectional images of the body *In the respiratory system, MRI is used to produce a scan of the chest and lungs. MRI does not require a contrast medium, but it may be used to enhance visualization of internal structures.*
pulmonary function tests (PFTs) PŬL-mō-nĕ-rē	Variety of tests to determine the capacity of the lungs to exchange oxygen (O_2) and carbon dioxide (CO_2) efficiently *Respiratory function is assessed by measuring the capacity of the lungs and the volume of air during inhalation and exhalation.*
forced vital capacity (FVC)	Measurement of the amount of air that can be forcefully exhaled from the lungs after the deepest inhalation
forced expiratory volume in one second (FEV_1)	Measurement of the volume of air that can be forcefully exhaled during the first second of measuring the FVC
spirometry spī-RŎM-ĕ-trē *spir/o:* to breathe *-metry:* act of measuring	Measurement of FVC and FEV_1 producing a tracing on a graph *Spirometry measures the breathing capacity of the lungs and produces a tracing on a graph.*

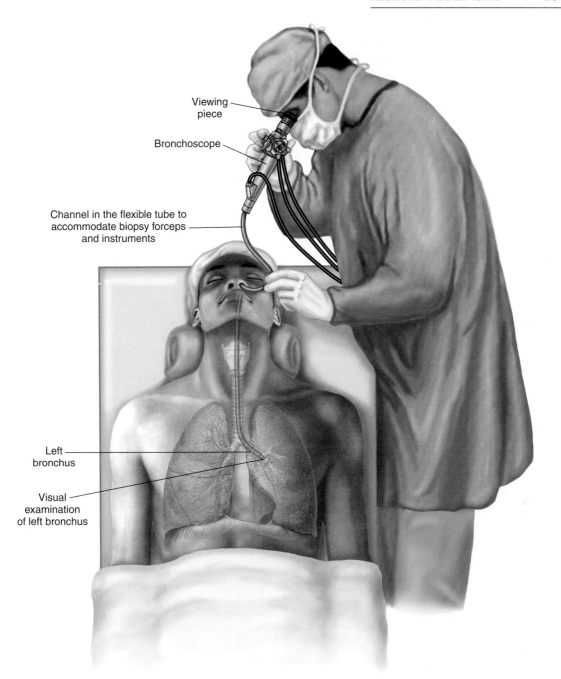

Viewing
piece

Bronchoscope

Channel in the flexible tube to
accommodate biopsy forceps
and instruments

Left
bronchus

Visual
examination
of left bronchus

Figure 4-9 Bronchoscopy of the left bronchus.

Medical and Surgical Procedures

postural drainage PŎS-chur-ăl DRĀN-ăj	Use of body positioning to assist in removal of secretions from specific lobes of the lung, bronchi, or lung cavities

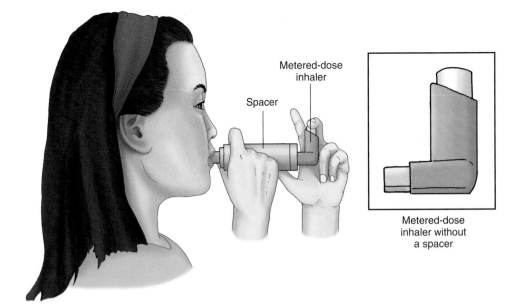

Spacer

Metered-dose inhaler

Metered-dose inhaler without a spacer

Figure 4-10   Inhaler with spacer.

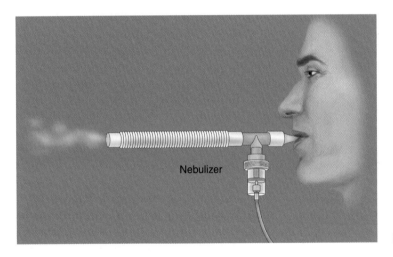

Nebulizer

Figure 4-11   Nebulizer.

Pharmacology

bronchodilators brŏng-kō-DĪ-lā-tŏrz	Drugs used to increase airflow by dilating constricted airways through relaxation of the smooth muscles that surround the bronchioles and bronchi *Bronchodilators are used to treat asthma, emphysema, chronic obstructive pulmonary disease (COPD), and exercise-induced bronchospasm. Most bronchodilators provide metered dosages of the medication and may employ a spacer as a reservoir for the medication. (See Figure 4-10.)*
corticosteroids kor-tĭ-kō-STĔR-oyds	Hormonal agents that reduce tissue edema and inflammation associated with chronic lung disease
nebulized mist treatment (NMT) NĔB-ū-līzd	Therapy that uses a device to produce a fine spray (nebulizer) that delivers medication directly into the lungs (See Figure 4-11.)

Additional Medical Terms Review

Match the medical term(s) below with the definitions in the numbered list.

acidosis	coryza	hypoxia	pleural effusion
ARDS	crackle	influenza	pneumothorax
atelectasis	cystic fibrosis	lung cancer	rhonchi
bronchodilators	epiglottitis	MRI	SIDS
consolidation	epistaxis	pertussis	stridor

1. _____ is a high-pitched breathing sound resembling the blowing of wind, caused by obstruction of air passages.

2. _____ refers to nosebleed.

3. _____ is a contagious respiratory infection characterized by onset of fever, chills, headache, and muscle pain.

4. _____ is excessive acidity of blood due to an accumulation of acids or excessive loss of bicarbonate.

5. _____ is acute inflammation of nasal passages accompanied by profuse nasal discharge; a cold.

6. _____ is a genetic disorder of exocrine glands characterized by excessive production of mucus, causing severe congestion within the lungs and pancreas

7. _____ refers to pulmonary malignancy commonly attributed to cigarette smoking.

8. _____ is an abnormal presence of fluid in the pleural cavity.

9. _____ refers to accumulation of air in the pleural cavity.

10. _____ is an adventitious lung sound produced by air passing over retained airway secretions; formerly called *rale.*

11. _____ are used to dilate bronchial walls to increase airflow.

12. _____ is a form of restrictive lung disease that follows severe infection or trauma in young and previously healthy individuals.

13. _____ uses electromagnetic energy to produce multiplanar cross-sectional images of the body.

14. _____ refers to a collapsed lung.

15. _____ is a severe life-threatening infection of the epiglottis that occurs most commonly in children.

16. _____ is an acute infectious disease characterized by an explosive cough; also called *whooping cough.*

17. _____ Process of becoming solid, especially in connection with the lungs

18. _____ refers to the unexpected and unexplained death of an apparently well, or virtually well, infant.

19. _____ is a deficiency of oxygen in the tissues

20. _____ refers to abnormal chest sounds resembling snoring, produced in obstructed airways.

Competency Verification: Check your answers in Appendix B, Answer Key, page 559. If you are not satisfied with your level of comprehension, review the pathological, diagnostic, and therapeutic terms and retake the review.

Correct Answers: _____ × 5 = _____ % Score

Medical Record Activities

Medical reports included in the following activities reflect common real-life clinical scenarios using medical terminology to document patient care.

MEDICAL RECORD ACTIVITY 4-1

Upper Airway Obstruction

Terminology

Terms listed in the table below come from the medical report *Upper Airway Obstruction* that follows. Use a medical dictionary such as *Taber's Cyclopedic Medical Dictionary,* the appendices of this book, or other resources to define each term. Then practice reading the pronunciations aloud for each term.

Term	Definition
anesthesia ăn-ĕs-THĒ-zē-ă	
biopsy BĪ-ŏp-sē	
carcinoma kăr-sĭ-NŌ-mă	
diagnosis dī-ăg-NŌ-sĭs	
expired	
fascia FĂSH-ē-ă	
hemorrhage HĔM-ĕ-rĭj	
lymph node lĭmf nōd	
meatus mē-Ā-tŭs	
metastatic mĕt-ă-STĂT-ĭk	
necropsy NĔK-rŏp-sē	
needle biopsy BĪ-ŏp-sē	

Term	Definition
node nōd	
papillary PĂP-ĭ-lăr-ē	
pneumonia nū-MŌ-nē-ă	
polyp PŎL-ĭp	
polypectomy pŏl-ĭ-PĔK-tō-mē	
pulmonary PŬL-mō-nĕ-rē	
snare snār	
submaxillary sŭb-MĂK-sĭ-lār-ē	

Listen and Learn Online! will help you master pronunciations of selected medical words from this medical record activity. Visit *http://davisplus.fadavis.com/gylys/simplified* to find instructions on completing the *Listen and Learn Online!* exercise for this section and to practice pronunciations.

Reading

Practice pronunciation of medical terms by reading the following medical report aloud.

Upper Airway Obstruction

A 55-year-old white man was seen 2 years ago because of upper airway obstruction due to large polyps in the right nasal cavity. On examination, a large polypoid mass was observed to fill most of the right nasal cavity. The mass originated in the middle meatus. With the use of a nasal snare, polypectomy was performed to remove several sections. There was a slight hemorrhage. On the next day, a 4 × 3–cm oval soft mass was excised from beneath the left submaxillary region, with the patient under local anesthesia. The mass was just beneath the superficial fascia and appeared to be an enlarged lymph node unconnected with the nasal disease.

The pathological diagnosis of the nasal growth was low-grade papillary carcinoma. The diagnosis of the lymph node was metastatic carcinoma. A chest film was taken that indicated the presence of pulmonary densities attributed to unresolved pneumonia. Also, a needle biopsy of the enlarged liver nodes yielded no results.

After discharge from the hospital, the patient expired at home, and no necropsy was obtained.

Evaluation

Review the medical report above to answer the following questions. Use a medical dictionary such as *Taber's Cyclopedic Medical Dictionary* and other resources if needed.

1. What types of patients are at risk for nasal polyps?

_____

_____

2. When is a polypectomy indicated?

_____

_____

3. Were the patient's nasal polyps cancerous?

_____

_____

4. What contributed to the patient's death?

_____

_____

5. Why was a biopsy of the liver performed?

_____

_____

6. What does "patient expired at home" mean?

_____

_____

MEDICAL RECORD ACTIVITY 4-2

Bronchoscopy

Terminology

Terms listed in the table below come from the medical report *Bronchoscopy* that follows. Use a medical dictionary such as *Taber's Cyclopedic Medical Dictionary*, the appendices of this book, or other resources to define each term. Then practice reading the pronunciations aloud for each term.

Term	Definition
acid-fast bacilli bă-SĬL-ī	_____
bronchopulmonary brŏng-kō-PŬL-mō-nă-rē	_____
bronchoscope BRŎNG-kō-skōp	_____

Term	Definition
brush biopsies BĬ-ŏp-sēz	_____
carina kă-RĬ-nă	_____
culture and sensitivity	_____
cytology sī-TŎL-ō-jē	_____
endobronchial ĕn-dō-BRŎNG-kē-ăl	_____
fluoroscopic FLŌR-ō-skŏp-ĭk	_____
friable FRĬ-ă-bl	_____
Legionella LĒ-jĭ-nĕl-ă	_____
lesion LĒ-zhŭn	_____
mucosal mū-KŌS-ăl	_____
needle aspiration ăs-pĭ-RĀ-shŭn	_____
transbronchial trăns-BRŎNG-kē-ăl	_____
transnasally trăns-NĀ-zlē	_____

Listen and Learn Online! will help you master pronunciations of selected medical words from this medical record activity. Visit *http://davisplus.fadavis.com/gylys/simplified* to find instructions on completing the *Listen and Learn Online!* exercise for this section and to practice pronunciations.

Reading

Practice pronunciation of medical terms by reading the following medical report aloud.

Bronchoscopy

The bronchoscope was passed transnasally. The vocal cords, larynx, and trachea were normal. The main carina was sharp. All bronchopulmonary segments were visualized. There was an endobronchial friable mucosal lesion seen in the left lower lobe bronchus, partially occluding the entire left lower lobe bronchus. No other endobronchial lesions or bleeding sites were noted.

Under fluoroscopic control, transbronchial biopsies of this left lower lung area were obtained, as well as transbronchial needle aspiration, bronchial brush biopsies, and bronchial brush washings for cytology evaluation. Sterile brush cultures for culture and sensitivity, acid-fast bacilli, fungus, and *Legionella* were also done.

The patient tolerated the procedure well.

Evaluation

Review the medical record to answer the following questions. Use a medical dictionary such as *Taber's Cyclopedic Medical Dictionary* and other resources if needed.

1. What does "bronchoscope was inserted transnasally" mean?

_____

_____

2. What was seen in the left lower bronchus?

_____

_____

3. What kinds of biopsies were obtained during the bronchoscopy?

_____

_____

4. What type of radiographic procedure was used to enhance visualization to obtain biopsies for cytology evaluation?

_____

_____

5. What condition results from the bacterium *Legionella?*

_____

_____

Chapter Review

Word Elements Summary

The following table summarizes CFs, suffixes, and prefixes related to the respiratory system.

Word Element	Meaning	Word Element	Meaning
Combining Forms			
adenoid/o	adenoids	**pharyng/o**	pharynx (throat)
alveol/o	alveolus (plural, alveoli)	**pleur/o**	pleura
atel/o	incomplete, imperfect	**pneum/o, pneumon/o**	air; lung
bronch/o, bronchi/o	bronchus (plural, bronchi)	**pulmon/o**	lung
chondr/o	cartilage	**sinus/o**	sinus, cavity
epiglott/o	epiglottis	**spir/o**	to breathe
laryng/o	larynx (voice box)	**thorac/o**	chest
nas/o, rhin/o	nose	**tonsill/o**	tonsils
or/o	mouth	**trache/o**	trachea (windpipe)
ox/o	oxygen		
Other Combining Forms			
acid/o	acid	**hepat/o**	liver
aer/o	air	**hydr/o**	water
arteri/o	artery	**melan/o**	black
carcin/o	cancer	**muc/o**	mucus
cyst/o	bladder	**my/o**	muscle
fibr/o	fiber, fibrous tissue	**myc/o**	fungus
gastr/o	stomach	**orth/o**	straight
hem/o	blood	**tom/o**	to cut
Suffixes			
SURGICAL			
-centesis	surgical puncture	**-rrhaphy**	suture
-ectomy	excision, removal	**-tome**	instrument to cut
-plasty	surgical repair	**-tomy**	incision

(continued)

Word Element	Meaning	Word Element	Meaning
DIAGNOSTIC, SYMPTOMATIC, AND RELATED			
-algia, -dynia	pain	-phagia	swallowing, eating
-cele	hernia, swelling	-phobia	fear
-ectasis	dilation, expansion	-plasm	formation, growth
-emia	blood condition	-plegia	paralysis
-graphy	process of recording	-pnea	breathing
-itis	inflammation	-rrhagia	bursting forth (of)
-logist	specialist in study of	-scope	instrument for examining
-malacia	softening	-scopy	visual examination
-metry	act of measuring	-spasm	involuntary contraction, twitching
-oma	tumor	-stenosis	narrowing, stricture
-osis	abnormal condition, increase (used primarily with blood cells)	-therapy	treatment
-pathy	disease	-thorax	chest
ADJECTIVE			
-al, -ic, -ous	pertaining to		
NOUN			
-ia	condition	-ist	specialist
PREFIXES			
an-	without, not	macro-	large
epi-	above, upon	micro-	small
eu-	good, normal	neo-	new
hyp-, hypo-	under, below, deficient	peri-	around

Enhance your study and reinforcement of word elements with the power of *Davis Plus.* Visit *http://davisplus.fadavis.com/gylys/simplified* for this chapter's flash-card activity. We recommend you complete the flash-card activity before completing the word elements review below.

Word Elements Review

After you review the Word Elements Summary, complete this activity by writing the meaning of each element in the space provided.

Word Element	Meaning	Word Element	Meaning
Combining Forms			
1. atel/o	_____	**8.** pleur/o	_____
2. bronch/o, bronchi/o	_____	**9.** pneum/o, pneumon/o	_____
3. chondr/o	_____	**10.** pulmon/o	_____
4. nas/o, rhin/o	_____	**11.** spir/o	_____
5. or/o	_____	**12.** thorac/o	_____
6. ox/o	_____	**13.** tonsill/o	_____
7. pharyng/o	_____	**14.** trache/o	_____
OTHER COMBINING FORMS			
15. acid/o	_____	**21.** melan/o	_____
16. aer/o	_____	**22.** muc/o	_____
17. carcin/o	_____	**23.** myc/o	_____
18. fibr/o	_____	**24.** my/o	_____
19. hem/o	_____	**25.** tom/o	_____
20. hydr/o	_____		
Suffixes			
SURGICAL			
26. -centesis	_____	**40.** -oma	_____
27. -emia	_____	**41.** -osis	_____
28. -metry	_____	**42.** -pathy	_____
29. -plasty	_____	**43.** -phagia	_____
30. -rrhaphy	_____	**44.** -phobia	_____
31. -thorax	_____	**45.** -plasm	_____
32. -tome	_____	**46.** -plegia	_____
33. -tomy	_____	**47.** -pnea	_____
34. -algia, -dynia	_____	**48.** -rrhagia	_____
35. -cele	_____	**49.** -scope	_____
36. -ectasis	_____	**50.** -scopy	_____
37. -itis	_____	**51.** -spasm	_____
38. -logist	_____	**52.** -stenosis	_____
39. -malacia	_____	**53.** -therapy	_____

(continued)

Word Element	Meaning	Word Element	Meaning
Prefixes			
54. epi-	_____	**58.** micro-	_____
55. eu-	_____	**59.** neo-	_____
56. hypo-	_____	**60.** peri-	_____
57. macro-	_____		

Competency Verification: Check your answers in Appendix A, Glossary of Medical Word Elements, page 538. If you are not satisfied with your level of comprehension, review the word elements and retake the review.

Correct Answers: _____ × 2 = _____ % Score

Vocabulary Review

Match the medical terms with the definitions in the numbered list.

aerophagia	atelectasis	diagnosis	pyothorax
anosmia	catheter	pharyngoplegia	rhinoplasty
apnea	chondroma	pleurisy	TB
aspirate	COPD	*Pneumocystis*	thoracentesis
asthma	croup	pneumothorax	tracheostomy

1. _____ refers to presence of pus in the chest.

2. _____ is surgical puncture of the chest to remove fluid.

3. _____ is a respiratory condition marked by recurrent attacks of difficult or labored breathing accompanied by wheezing.

4. _____ is an acute respiratory syndrome of childhood characterized by laryngeal obstruction and spasm, barking cough, and stridor.

5. _____ is a surgical procedure that creates an opening through the neck into the trachea.

6. _____ refers to use of scientific methods and medical skill to establish the cause and nature of a person's illness.

7. _____ is temporary cessation of breathing.

8. _____ refers to swallowing air.

9. _____ refers to using suction to remove fluids from a body cavity.

10. _____ is a cartilaginous tumor.

11. _____ is an abnormal condition characterized by collapse of alveoli.

12. _____ is loss or impairment of sense of smell.

13. _____ is paralysis of pharyngeal muscles.

14. _____ is inflammation of the pleura.

15. _____ is a type of pneumonia seen in patients with AIDS and in debilitated children.

16. _____ is a hollow, flexible tube that can be inserted into a vessel or cavity of the body to withdraw or instill fluids.

17. _____ refers to surgical repair or plastic surgery of the nose.

18. _____ is an infectious disease that produces small lesions or tubercles in the lungs.

19. _____ refers to a group of respiratory disorders characterized by chronic bronchitis, asthma, and emphysema.

20. _____ is presence of air in the pleural cavity.

Competency Verification: Check your answers in Appendix B, Answer Key, page 561. If you are not satisfied with your level of comprehension, review the chapter vocabulary and retake the review.

Correct Answers: _____ × 5 _____ % Score

5 Cardiovascular and Lymphatic Systems

OBJECTIVES

Upon completion of this chapter, you will be able to:

- Describe the type of medical treatment the cardiologist, vascular surgeon, and immunologist provide.
- Identify cardiovascular and lymphatic systems structures by labeling them on anatomical illustrations.
- Describe the primary functions of the cardiovascular system and lymphatic systems.
- Describe common diseases related to the cardiovascular and lymphatic systems.
- Describe common diagnostic, medical, and surgical procedures related to the cardiovascular and lymphatic systems.
- Apply your word-building skills by constructing various medical terms related to the cardiovascular and lymphatic systems.
- Describe common abbreviations and symbols related to the cardiovascular and lymphatic systems.
- Reinforce word elements and their meanings by completing the flash card activities.
- Recognize, define, pronounce, and spell terms correctly.
- Demonstrate your knowledge of this chapter by successfully completing the frames, reviews, and medical report evaluations.

Medical Specialties

Cardiology

The medical specialty of **cardiology** encompasses the treatment of heart disease. Generally, three types of cardiology specialists provide medical care: the *cardiologist,* the *pediatric cardiologist,* and the *cardiothoracic surgeon.* While the **cardiologist** specializes in treating adults, the **pediatric cardiologist** specializes in treating infants, children, and teenagers. The cardiologist and pediatric cardiologists provide nonsurgical treatments to detect, prevent, and treat heart and vascular diseases, while the **cardiothoracic surgeon** performs surgeries to treat cardiovascular disorders. Some of these critical, lifesaving surgeries include coronary artery bypass, valve replacement or repairs, heart transplants, and repairs of complex heart problems present from birth (congenital heart disease). An **interventional cardiologist** performs other invasive procedures, such as angioplasty, pacemaker insertion, and implantable cardioverter defibrillator insertion. The physician who further specializes in surgical treatment of blood vessels and vascular disorders is a **vascular surgeon**.

Immunology

Immunology is the medical specialty that encompasses the study of the various elements of the immune system and their functions. The immune system is the body's defense against cancer and foreign invaders, such as bacteria and viruses. The ability to fight off disease and protect the body depends on an adequate functioning immune response. An *immunologist* is the medical specialist who studies and treats the body's defense mechanism against invasion of foreign substances that cause diseases. The **immunologist** is consulted when the immune system breaks down and the body loses its ability to recognize antigens or its ability to mount an attack against them. Our immune system also has the ability to react in a manner disadvantageous to our own body by way of *allergic* and *autoimmune diseases*. Thus, immunologists treat patients with immunodeficiency diseases, such as AIDS; immune complex diseases, such as malaria and viral hepatitis; autoimmune diseases, such as lupus; transplanted cells and organs; allergies; and various cancer types related to the immune system.

Anatomy and Physiology Overview

The *cardiovascular (CV) system* is composed of the heart, which is essentially a muscular pump, and an extensive network of blood vessels. The main purpose of the CV system, also called the *circulatory system,* is to deliver oxygen, nutrients, and other essential substances to body cells and remove waste products of cellular metabolism. This process is carried out by a complex network of blood vessels that includes arteries, capillaries, and veins—all of which are connected to the heart. A healthy CV system is vital to a person's survival. A CV system that does not provide adequate circulation deprives tissues of oxygen and nutrients and fails to remove waste, resulting in irreversible changes to cells that could be life-threatening.

The lymphatic system is closely linked to the CV system. It depends on the pumping action of the heart to circulate its substances throughout the body. The lymphatic system consists of a network of vessels and nodes, and a few specialized organs including the tonsils, thymus, and spleen. (See Figure 5–1.)

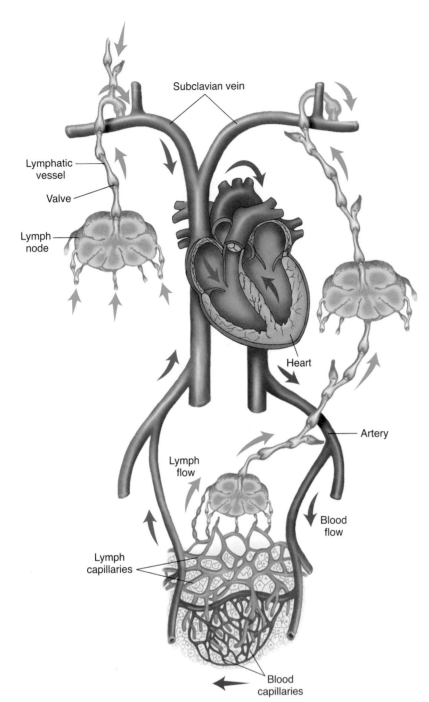

Subclavian vein

Lymphatic vessel

Valve

Lymph node

Heart

Artery

Lymph flow

Blood flow

Lymph capillaries

Blood capillaries

Figure 5-1 Interrelationship of the cardiovascular system with the lymphatic system. Blood flows from the heart to blood capillaries and back to the heart. Lymph capillaries collect tissue fluid, which is returned to the blood. The arrows indicate direction of flow of the blood and lymph.

WORD ELEMENTS

This section introduces combining forms (CFs), suffixes, and prefixes related to the cardiovascular system, along with each element's meaning, an example, and additional analysis of key elements in the example. Review the following table and pronounce each word in the word analysis column aloud before you begin to work in the frames.

Word Element	Meaning	Word Analysis
Combining Forms		
angi/o	vessel (usually blood or lymph)	**angi/o**/graphy (ăn-jē-ŎG-ră-fē): process of recording blood vessels *-graphy:* process of recording *Angiography is an x-ray visualization of internal anatomy of the heart and blood vessels after the intravascular introduction of a contrast medium. It is used as a diagnostic aid to visualize blood vessel and heart abnormalities.*
aneurysm/o	widening, widened blood vessel	**aneurysm/o**/rrhaphy (ăn-ū-rĭz-MŌR-ă-fē): suture of a blood vessel *-rrhaphy:* suture *Aneurysmorrhaphy closes the area of dilation and weakness in the wall of an artery. This condition may result from a congenital defect or a damaged vessel wall due to arteriosclerosis.*
aort/o	aorta	**aort/o**/stenosis (ā-or-tō-stĕn-Ō-sĭs): narrowing of the aorta *-stenosis:* narrowing, stricture
arteri/o	artery	**arteri/o**/scler/osis (ăr-tē-rē-ō-sklĕ-RŌ-sĭs): abnormal hardening of arterial walls *scler:* hardening; sclera (white of eye) *-osis:* abnormal condition; increase (used primarily with blood cells) *Arteriosclerosis results in a decreased blood supply, especially to the cerebrum and lower extremities.*
arteriol/o	arteriole	**arteriol**/itis (ăr-tēr-ē-ō-LĪ-tĭs): inflammation of an arteriole *-itis:* inflammation
ather/o	fatty plaque	**ather**/oma (ăth-ĕr-Ō-mă): fatty degeneration or thickening of the larger arterial walls, as in atherosclerosis *-oma:* tumor
atri/o	atrium	**atri/o**/ventricul/ar (ā-trē-ō-vĕn-TRĬK-ū-lăr): pertaining to the atrium and the ventricle *ventricul:* ventricle (of heart or brain) *-ar:* pertaining to

(continued)

Word Element	Meaning	Word Analysis
cardi/o	heart	**cardi**/o/megaly (kăr-dē-ō-MĔG-ă-lē): enlargement of the heart; also called *megalocardia* *-megaly:* enlargement
coron/o		**coron**/ary (KOR-ō-nă-rē): pertaining to the heart *-ary:* pertaining to
phleb/o	vein	**phleb**/itis (flĕb-Ī-tĭs): inflammation of a vein *-itis:* inflammation
ven/o		**ven**/ous (VĒ-nŭs): pertaining to the veins or blood passing through them *-ous:* pertaining to
thromb/o	blood clot	**thromb**/o/lysis (thrŏm-BŎL-ĭ-sĭs): breaking up of a thrombus *-lysis:* separation; destruction; loosening
varic/o	dilated vein	**varic**/ose (VĂR-ĭ-kōs): pertaining to a dilated vein *-ose:* pertaining to; sugar
vas/o	vessel; vas deferens; duct	**vas**/o/spasm (VĂS-ō-spăzm): spasm of a blood vessel *-spasm:* involuntary contraction, twitching
vascul/o	vessel	**vascul**/ar (VĂS-kū-lăr): pertaining to or composed of blood vessels *-ar:* pertaining to
ventricul/o	ventricle (of heart or brain)	intra/**ventricul**/ar (ĭn-tră-vĕn-TRĬK-ū-lăr): within a ventricle *-ar:* pertaining to
Suffixes		
-cardia	heart condition	tachy/**cardia** (tăk-ē-KĂR-dē-ă): rapid heart rate *tachy-:* rapid
-gram	record, writing	electr/o/cardi/o/**gram** (ē-lĕk-trō-KĂR-dē-ō-grăm): record of electrical activity of the heart *electr/o:* electricity *cardi/o:* heart
-graph	instrument for recording	electr/o/cardi/o/**graph** (ē-lĕk-trō-KĂR-dē-ō-grăf): instrument for recording electrical activity of the heart *electr/o:* electricity *cardi/o:* heart

Word Element	Meaning	Word Analysis
-graphy	process of recording	electr/o/cardi/o/**graphy** (ē-lĕk-trō-kăr-dē-ŎG-ră-fē): process of recording electrical activity of the heart *electr/o:* electricity *cardi/o:* heart *Electrocardiography is a noninvasive test that records the electrical activity of the heart during contractions and rest. It is used to diagnose abnormal cardiac rhythm and the presence of heart muscle (myocardial) damage.*
-stenosis	narrowing, stricture	arteri/o/**stenosis** (ăr-tē-rē-ō-stĕ-NŌ-sĭs): narrowing of an artery *arteri/o:* artery *Narrowing of an artery may be caused by fatty plaque buildup, scar tissue, or a blood clot.*
-um	structure, thing	endo/cardi/**um** (ĕn-dō-KĂR-dē-ŭm): structure within the heart *endo-:* in, within *cardi:* heart

Pronunciation Help	Long Sound	ā in rāte	ē in rēbirth	ī in īsle	ō in ōver	ū in ūnite
	Short Sound	ă in ălone	ĕ in ĕver	ĭ in ĭt	ŏ in nŏt	ŭ in cŭt

 Listen and Learn, the audio CD-ROM included in this book, will help you master pronunciation of selected medical words. Use it to practice pronunciations of the above-listed medical terms and for instructions to complete the *Listen and Learn* exercise for this section.

S E C T I O N   R E V I E W   5-1

For the following medical terms, first write the suffix and its meaning. Then translate the meaning of the remaining elements starting with the first part of the word. The first word is completed for you.

Term	Meaning
1. endo/cardi/um	*-um: structure, thing; in, within; heart*
2. cardi/o/megaly	
3. aort/o/stenosis	
4. tachy/cardia	
5. phleb/itis	
6. thromb/o/lysis	
7. vas/o/spasm	
8. ather/oma	
9. electr/o/cardi/o/graphy	
10. atri/o/ventricul/ar	

Competency Verification: Check your answers in Appendix B, Answer Key, page 561. If you are not satisfied with your level of comprehension, review the vocabulary and complete the review again.

Correct Answers _____ × 10 = _____ % Score

Cardiovascular System

Walls of the Heart

5-1   The heart is a four-chambered muscular organ located in the mediastin/um, the area of the chest between the lungs. Its primary purpose is to pump blood through the arteries, veins, and capillaries. The walls of the heart are composed of the (1) **endocardium**, (2) **myocardium**, and (3) **pericardium**. Review the structures of the heart and label its three layers in Figure 5–2.

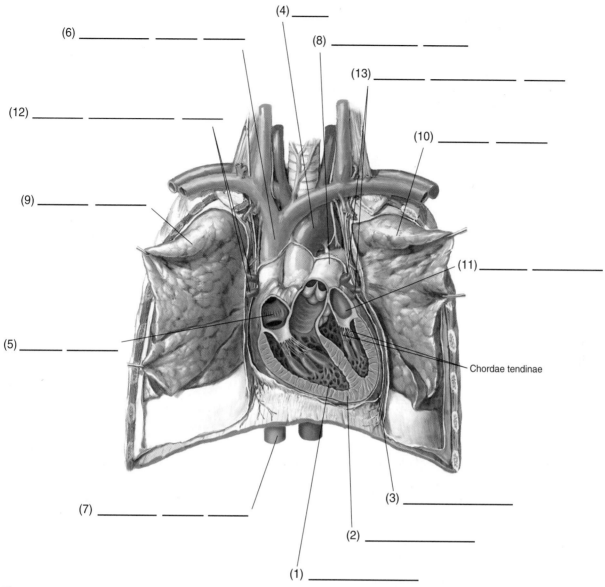

(6) _____ _____ _____

(4) _____

(8) _____ _____ _____

(13) _____ _____ _____

(12) _____ _____ _____

(10) _____ _____

(9) _____ _____

(5) _____ _____ _____

(11) _____ _____

Chordae tendinae

(7) _____ _____ _____

(3) _____

(2) _____

(1) _____

Figure 5-2 Heart structures.

5-2 The *endo/cardi/um*, the inner membranous layer, lines the interior of the heart and the heart valves. The *my/o/cardi/um*, the middle muscular layer, is composed of a special type of muscle arranged in such a way that the contraction of muscle bundles results in squeezing or wringing of the heart chambers to eject blood from the chambers. The *peri/cardi/um*, a fibrous sac, surrounds and encloses the entire heart.

When we talk about the muscular layer of the heart, we are referring to the

_____ / _____ / _____ / _____. When we talk about the fibrous sac that encloses the entire heart, we are referring to the

_____ / _____ / _____.

my/o/cardi/um
mī-ō-KĂR-dē-ŭm

peri/cardi/um
pĕr-ĭ-KĂR-dē-ŭm

peri/card/itis
pĕr-ĭ-kăr-DĪ-tĭs

peri/cardi/o/centesis
pĕr-ĭ-kăr-dē-ō-sĕn-TĒ-sĭs

5-3   The prefix *peri-* means around. *Peri/card/itis* is an inflammation or infection of the pericardial sac with an accumulation of pericardial fluid. When the fluid presses on the heart and prevents it from beating, the condition is known as *cardi/ac tamponade*. If necessary, peri/cardi/o/centesis may be performed.

Build medical terms that mean

inflammation around the heart: _____ / _____ / _____.

surgical puncture around the heart:

_____ / _____ / _____ / _____.

---

peri/cardi/ectomy
pĕr-ĭ-kăr-dē-ĔK-tō-mē

5-4   The surgical procedure meaning *excision of all or part of the peri/cardi/um* is _____ / _____ / _____.

---

peri/cardi/o/rrhaphy
pĕr-ĭ-kăr-dē-OR-ă-fē

5-5   Suturing a wound in the peri/cardi/um is called

_____ / _____ / _____ / _____.

---

my/o/cardi/um
mī-ō-KĂR-dē-ŭm

5-6   Cross-striations of *cardi/ac* muscle provide the mechanics of squeezing blood out of the heart chambers to maintain the flow of blood in one direction. Identify the *muscul/ar* layer of the heart responsible for this function.

_____ / _____ / _____ / _____

---

endo/cardi/um
ĕn-dō-KĂR-dē-ŭm

peri/cardi/um
pĕr-ĭ-KĂR-dē-ŭm

my/o/cardi/um
mī-ō-KĂR-dē-ŭm

5-7   Review the three layers of the heart by completing the following statements:

The layer that lines the heart and the heart valves is known as the

_____ / _____ / _____.

The fibrous sac surrounding the entire heart and composed of two membranes separated by fluid is called the

_____ / _____ / _____.

The middle specialized muscular layer is called the

_____ / _____ / _____ / _____.

Circulation and Heart Structures

5-8   The circulatory system is commonly divided into the *cardiovascular system,* which consists of the heart and blood vessels, and the *lymphatic system,* which consists of lymph vessels, lymph nodes, and lymphoid organs (spleen, thymus, and tonsils). Review Figure 5–1 to see the interrelationship of the cardiovascular system with the lymphatic system.

5-9 Some of the main vessels associated with circulation are illustrated in Figure 5–2. Observe the locations and label the structures as you read the following material. The (4) **aorta,** the largest blood vessel in the body, is the main trunk of systemic circulation. It starts and arches out at the left ventricle. Deoxygenated blood enters the (5) **right atrium** via two large veins, the *vena cavae* (singular, vena cava). The (6) **superior vena cava** conveys blood from the upper portion of the body (head and arms); the (7) **inferior vena cava** conveys blood from the lower portion of the body (legs).

---

deoxygenated
dē-ŎK-sĭ-jĕn-ā-tĕd

5-10 Blood in the veins except for pulmonary veins has a low oxygen content (deoxygenated) and a relatively high concentration of carbon dioxide. In contrast to the bright red color of the oxygenated blood in the arteries, deoxygenated blood has a dark blue to purplish color.
The term in this frame that means *low oxygen content* is

_____.

5-11 Label Figure 5–2 as you continue to identify and learn about the structures and functions of the circulatory system. The (8) **pulmonary trunk** is the only artery that carries deoxygenated blood. As deoxygenated blood is pumped from the right ventricle, it enters the pulmonary trunk. The pulmonary trunk runs diagonally upward, then divides abruptly to form the branches of the *right* and *left pulmonary arteries.* Each branch conveys deoxygenated blood to the lungs. The (9) **right lung** has three lobes; the (10) **left lung** has two lobes. Oxygen-rich blood returns to the heart via four pulmonary veins, which deposit the blood into the (11) **left atrium**. There are two (12) **right pulmonary veins** and two (13) **left pulmonary veins**.

Competency Verification: Check your labeling of Figure 5–2 in Appendix B, Answer Key, page 561.

5-12 Internally, the heart is composed of four chambers. The upper chambers are the (1) **right atrium (RA)** and (2) **left atrium (LA)**. The lower chambers are the (3) **right ventricle (RV)** and (4) **left ventricle (LV)**. Locate and label the chambers of the heart in Figure 5–3.

---

atri/al
Ā-trē-ăl

5-13 The CF *atri/o* refers to the *atrium.* A term that means *pertaining to the atrium* is _____ / _____.

---

atrium, left
Ā-trē-ŭm

5-14 The heart consists of two upper chambers, the right _____ and the _____ atrium.

---

ventricul/o/tomy
vĕn-trĭk-ū-LŎT-ō-mē

5-15 The CF *ventricul/o* means *ventricle (of heart or brain).* A ventricle is a small cavity, such as the right and left ventricles of the heart or one of the cavities filled with cerebrospinal fluid in the brain.
Incisions are sometimes performed into these cavities. An incision of a ventricle is known as a

_____ / _____ / _____.

atrium Ă-trē-ŭm **ventricle** VĔN-trĭk-l	**5–16** The term *atri/o/ventricul/ar (AV)* refers to the atrium and the ventricle. It also pertains to a connecting conduction event between the atria and ventricles. The singular form of *atria* is _____; the singular form of *ventricles* is _____.
ventricul/ar vĕn-TRĬK-ū-lăr	**5–17** Flutter is an a/rrhythm/ia in which there is very rapid but regular rhythm (250–300 beats per minute) of the atria or ventricles. The heart chambers do not have time to completely fill with blood before the next contraction. Flutter can progress to fibrillation. When the flutter occurs in the atrium, it is called an *atri/al flutter.* When the flutter occurs in the ventricle, it is called a _____ / _____ *flutter.*
a/rrhythm/ia ă-RĬTH-mē-ă **my/o/cardi/um** mī-ō-KĂR-dē-ŭm	**5–18** Flutter that progresses to fibrillation (a/rrhythm/ia in which there is a rapid, uncoordinated quivering of the my/o/cardi/um) can affect the atria or the ventricles. Write the term that means *without rhythm:* _____ / _____ / _____ *muscular layer of the heart:* _____ / ____ / _____ / _____
RV **LV**	**5–19** Write the abbreviations for the two lower chambers of the heart. right ventricle: _____ left ventricle: _____
atria Ā-trē-ă **cardia** KĂR-dē-ă **septa** SĔP-tă **bacteria** băk-TĒ-rē-ă	**5–20** The rule for forming plural words from singular words that end in *-um* is to drop *-um* and add *-a*. Practice modifying the singular terms below to their plural forms. **Singular** **Plural** atrium _____ cardium _____ septum _____ bacterium _____

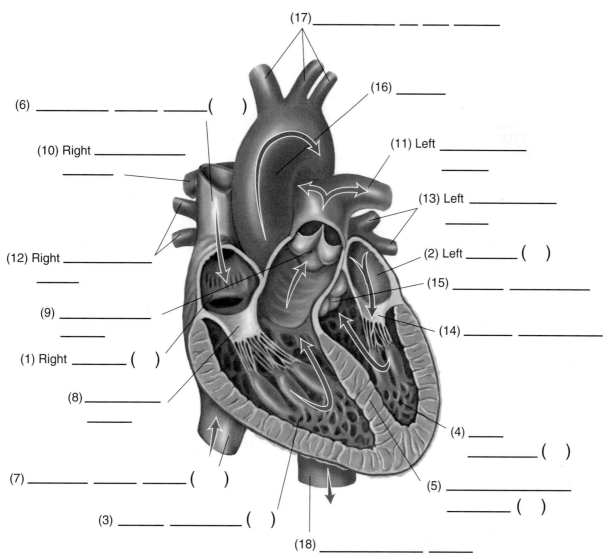

(17) _____ __ __ _____

(16) _____

(6) _____ _____ _____ (   )

(10) Right _____ _____

(11) Left _____ _____

(13) Left _____ _____

(12) Right _____ _____

(2) Left _____ (   )

(15) _____ _____

(9) _____ _____

(14) _____ _____

(1) Right _____ (   )

(8) _____ _____

(7) _____ _____ _____ (   )

(4) _____ _____ (   )

(3) _____ _____ (   )

(5) _____ _____ (   )

(18) _____ _____

Figure 5-3   Internal structures of the heart. Red arrows designate oxygen-rich blood flow; blue arrows designate oxygen-poor blood flow.

5–21   A wall or partition dividing a body space or cavity is known as a *septum* (plural, *septa*). Some *septa* are membranous; others are composed of bone or cartilage. Each is named according to its location in the body. In the heart, there are several septa, one of which is the *interventricular septum (IVS)*, the partition that divides the LV from the RV. Label the (5) **interventricular septum (IVS)** in Figure 5–3.

5–22   The ventricles are separated by a thick muscular IVS, whereas the atria are separated by a thinner muscular *interatrial septum (IAS)*. The abbreviation of the septum situated between the

IVS

IAS

ventricles is: _____.

atria is: _____.

bacterium
băk-TĒ-rē-ŭm

septum
SĔP-tŭm

atrium
Ā-trē-ŭm

cardium
KĂR-dē-ŭm

5-23 Form singular words from the following plural words. Apply the rule that was covered in Frame 5–20.

Plural	Singular
bacteria	_____
septa	_____
atria	_____
cardia	_____

---

rapid

5-24 The prefix *tachy-* is used in words to mean *rapid*.

Tachy/cardia is a heart rate that is _____.

---

rapid eating

5-25 *Tachy/pnea* refers to rapid breathing; *tachy/phagia* refers to *rapid swallowing* or _____ _____.

---

brady/cardia
brād-ē-KĂR-dē-ă

5-26 The prefix *brady-* is used in words to mean *slow*. People with symptoms of brady/cardia commonly have difficulty pumping an adequate supply of blood to the tissues of the body.
The medical term that literally means *slow heart* is _____ / _____.

---

brady/pnea
brād-ĭp-NĒ-ă

brady/phagia
brād-ē-FĂ-jē-ă

5-27 Form medical words that literally mean

slow breathing: _____ / _____.

slow eating: _____ / _____.

---

tachy/pnea
tăk-ĭp-NĒ-ă

tachy/phagia
tăk-ē-FĂ-jē-ă

5-28 Construct medical words that mean

rapid breathing: _____ / _____

rapid eating: _____ / _____.

RA

LA

RV

LV

IVS

5-29 Review the chambers and structures of the heart (see Figure 5–3) by writing the abbreviation for the

right atrium: _____.

left atrium: _____.

right ventricle: _____.

left ventricle: _____.

interventricular septum: _____.

Blood Flow Through the Heart

5–30 Although general circulatory information was discussed previously, this section covers in greater detail the specific structures involved in the flow of blood through the heart. The heart's double pump serves two distinct circulations: *pulmonary circulation,* which is the short loop of blood vessels that runs from the heart to the lungs and back to the heart; *systemic circulation* routes blood through a long loop to all parts of the body before returning it to the heart.

Continue to label Figure 5–3 as you read the following information. The right atrium receives oxygen-poor blood from all tissues except those of the lungs. The blood from the head and arms is delivered to the RA through the (6) **superior vena cava (SVC)**. The blood from the legs and torso is delivered to the RA through the (7) **inferior vena cava (IVC)**.

---

inferior superior	**5–31** Determine the directional words in Frame 5–30 that mean *below (another structure):* _____. *above (another structure):* _____.

---

superior inferior	**5–32** Refer to Figure 5–3 and use the words superior or inferior to complete this frame. The left atrium is _____ to the left ventricle. The right ventricle is _____ to the right atrium.

5–33 Blood flows from the right atrium through the (8) **tricuspid valve** and into the right ventricle. The leaflets (cusps) are shaped so that they form a one-way passage, which keeps the blood flowing in only one direction. Label the tricuspid valve in Figure 5–3.

---

tri/cuspid valve trī-KŬS-pĭd	**5–34** The prefix *tri-* means three. The valve that has *three* leaflets or flaps is the _____ / _____ _____.

---

three	**5–35** In the English language, a tri/angle is a figure that has _____ sides.

---

two	**5–36** The prefix *bi-* refers to two. A bi/cuspid valve has _____ leaflets or flaps.

---

three	**5–37** In the English language, a bi/cycle has two wheels; a tri/cycle has _____ wheels.

---

two, three	**5–38** By relating *bi-* and *tri-* to words in the English language, these prefixes should not be difficult to recall that *bi-* means _____ and *tri-* means _____.

5-39 The ventricles are the pumping chambers of the heart. As the right ventricle contracts to pump oxygen-deficient blood through the (9) **pulmonary valve** into the pulmonary artery, the tri/cuspid valve remains closed, preventing a backflow of blood into the right atrium. When the blood passes through the pulmonary trunk, also known as the *main pulmonary artery,* it branches into the (10) **right pulmonary artery** and the (11) **left pulmonary artery**. The pulmonary arteries carry the oxygen-deficient blood to the lungs. Label the structures introduced in this frame in Figure 5–3.

---

artery
ĂR-tĕr-ē

5-40 The CF *arteri/o* refers to an *artery*. Arteri/al bleeding is bleeding from an _____.

---

arteries
ĂR-tĕr-ēs

5-41 Arteri/al circulation is movement of blood through the _____.

---

arteri/o/scler/osis
ăr-tē-rē-ō-sklĕ-RŌ-sĭs

5-42 Arteri/o/scler/osis is a disease characterized by thickening and loss of elasticity of arteri/al walls. A person with a disease or abnormal condition of arteri/al hardening has _____ / ____ / _____ / _____.

---

stone
artery
ĂR-tĕr-ē

5-43 The suffix *-lith* refers to a stone or calculus. An *arteri/o/lith,* also called an *arteri/al calculus,* is a calculus, or _____, in an _____.

---

artery
ĂR-tĕr-ē

5-44 An arteri/al spasm is a spasm of an _____.

---

arteri/o/rrhexis
ăr-tē-rē-ō-RĔK-sĭs

arteri/o/rrhaphy
ăr-tē-rē-OR-ă-fē

arteri/o/pathy
ăr-tē-rē-ŎP-ă-thē

arteri/o/spasm
ăr-TĒ-rē-ō-spăzm

5-45 Develop medical words that mean

rupture of an artery: _____ / ____ / _____.

suture of an artery: _____ / ____ / _____.

disease of an artery: _____ / ____ / _____.

involuntary contraction or twitching of an artery:
_____ / ____ / _____.

5-46 The right and left pulmonary arteries leading to the lungs branch and subdivide until ultimately they form capillaries around the alveoli. Carbon dioxide is passed from the blood into the alveoli and expelled out of the lungs. Oxygen inhaled by the lungs is passed from the alveoli into the blood. (Refer to Chapter 4 to review the alveolar structure.)

The left pulmonary artery is identified in Figure 5–3 as number

11

_____.

The right pulmonary artery is identified in Figure 5–3 as number

10

_____.

5-47 Oxygenated blood leaves the lungs and returns to the heart via the (12) **right pulmonary veins** and (13) **left pulmonary veins**. The four pulmonary veins empty into the LA. The LA contracts to force blood through the (14) **mitral valve** into the LV. Label the structures in Figure 5–3.

---

two

5-48 The mitral valve, located between the LA and LV, is a bi/cuspid, or bi/leaflet, valve, which means that the number of leaflets or flaps that the mitral valve has is _____.

---

left atrium
Ā-trē-ŭm

left ventricle
VĔN-trĭk-l

inter/ventricul/ar septum
ĭn-tĕr-vĕn-TRĬK-ū-lăr SĔP-tum

inter/atri/al septum
ĭn-tĕr-Ā-trē-ăl SĔP-tŭm

5-49 Write the meaning for the following abbreviations:

LA: _____ _____.

LV: _____ _____.

IVS: _____ / _____ / _____ _____.

IAS: _____ / _____ / _____ _____.

---

vein
vān

5-50 **Ven/o** is a combining form meaning _____.

---

vein
vān

5-51 *Phleb/o* is another CF for *vein*. Phleb/o/tomy is a procedure used to draw blood from a _____.

---

phleb/o/rrhaphy
flĕb-ŎR-ă-fē

phleb/o/rrhexis
flĕb-ō-RĔK-sĭs

phleb/o/stenosis
flĕb-ō-stĕ-NŌ-sĭs

5-52 Use **phleb/o** to construct words meaning

suture of a vein: _____ / _____ / _____.

rupture of a vein: _____ / _____ / _____.

stricture or narrowing of a vein: _____ / _____ / _____.

ven/o/scler/osis vēn-ō-sklĕ-RŌ-sĭs **ven/o/tomy** vē-NŎT-ō-mē **ven/o/spasm** VĒ-nō-spăzm	**5-53** Use **ven/o** to form words meaning *hardening of a vein:* _____ / _____ / _____/ _____. *incision of a vein:* _____ / _____ / _____. *contraction or twitching of a vein:* _____ / _____ / _____.
blood	**5-54** **Hemat/o** and **hem/o** mean _____.
hemat/o/logy hē-mă-TŎL-ō-jē **hemat/o/logist** hē-mă-TŎL-ō-jĭst	**5-55** Use **hemat/o** to form words meaning *study of blood:* _____ / _____ / _____ *specialist in the study of blood:* _____ / _____ / _____
lymph vessels	**5-56** The CF **angi/o** means *vessel (usually blood or lymph).* An angioma is a tumor consisting primarily of blood or _____ _____.
hemangi/oma hē-măn-jē-Ō-mă	**5-57** **Hem/o** and **angi/o** can be combined into a new element that also means blood vessel. Use **hemangi/o** *(blood vessel)* to develop a word meaning *tumor of blood vessels:* _____ / _____.
expansion	**5-58** Hemangi/ectasis is a dilation or _____ of a blood vessel.
	5-59 Label the structures in Figure 5–3 as you continue to learn about the heart. Contractions of the LV send oxygenated blood through the (15) **aortic valve** and into the (16) **aorta**. The three ascending (17) **branches of the aorta** transport blood to the head and arms. The (18) **descending aorta** transports the blood to the legs and torso.
aort/o/pathy ā-ŏr-TŎP-ă-thē	**5-60** The aorta is the largest artery of the body and originates at the LV of the heart. The combining form **aort/o** refers to the *aorta.* Any disease of the aorta is called _____ / _____ / _____.

5–61 Aortic stenosis, a narrowing or stricture of the aortic valve, may be due to congenital malformation or fusion of the cusps. The stenosis obstructs the flow of blood from the LV into the aorta, causing decreased cardi/ac output and pulmon/ary vascul/ar congestion. Treatment usually requires surgical repair.

Identify the terms in this frame that mean

pertaining to the lungs: _____ / _____ .

pertaining to a vessel: _____ / _____ .

pertaining to the heart: _____ / _____ .

pulmon/ary
PŬL-mō-nĕ-rē

vascul/ar
VĂS-kū-lăr

cardi/ac
KĂR-dē-ăk

---

artery, small vein

5–62 The suffixes *-ole* and *-ule* refer to small, minute.

An *arteri/ole* is a small _____; a *ven/ule* is a _____
_____ .

---

arteries
ĂR-tĕr-ēz

arteri/oles
ăr-TĒ-rē-ōls

5–63 Arteries are large vessels that convey blood away from the heart; they branch into smaller vessels called *arteri/oles*. The arteri/oles deliver blood to adjoining minute vessels called *capillaries*. (See Figure 5–1.)

Large vessels that transport blood away from the heart are called

_____ .

Smaller vessels that are formed from arteries are called

_____ / _____ .

---

arteri/oles
ăr-TĒ-rē-ōls

5–64 Arteries convey blood to adjacent smaller vessels called

_____ / _____ . (See Figure 5–1.)

---

capillaries
KĂP-ĭ-lă-rēz

5–65 Arteri/oles are thinner than arteries and carry blood to extending minute vessels called _____ . (See Figure 5–1.)

---

arteri/o/scler/osis
ăr-tē-ō-sklĕ-RŌ-sĭs

5–66 As a person ages, the arteries lose elasticity, thicken, become weakened, and deteriorate. Deterioration of arterial walls is also due to constant high pressure needed to transport blood throughout the body. The medical term for an *abnormal condition of artery hardening* is known as:

_____ / _____ / _____ / _____ .

---

arteri/o/scler/osis
ăr-tē-rē-ō-sklĕ-RŌ-sĭs

5–67 High blood pressure and high-fat diets contribute greatly to early arteri/o/scler/osis. A healthy diet can decrease the risk for hardening of the arteries, also called

_____ / _____ / _____ / _____ .

superior vena cava VĒ-nă KĂ-vă **inferior vena cava** VĒ-nă KĂ-vă	**5-68** Capillaries carry blood from arteri/oles to ven/ules. Ven/ules form a collecting system to return oxygen-deficient blood to the heart through two large veins, the SVC and the IVC. Define the following abbreviations SVC: _____ _____ _____. IVC: _____ _____ _____.
6, 7	**5-69** In Figure 5–3, the SVC is number _____; the IVC is number _____.
arteri/o/spasm ăr-TĒ-rē-ō-spăzm	**5-70** Combine *arteri/o* and *-spasm* to form a word meaning *arterial spasm:* _____ / _____ / _____.
        varic/ose VĂR-ĭ-kōs **incompetent** **competent**	**5-71** Normal veins have competent (healthy) valves whose ven/ous walls are strong enough to withstand the later/al pressure of blood that is exerted upon them. Blood flows through competent valves in one direction, which is toward the heart. In varic/ose veins, also known as *varicosities*, dilatation (dilation) of veins from long periods of pressure prevents complete closure of the valves. When damaged (incompetent) valves do not close completely, there is a backflow of blood in the veins. In turn, incompetent valves create varicosities which contribute to enlarged and twisted superficial veins. (See Figure 5–4.) The medical term in this frame meaning *pertaining to a dilated vein* is: _____ / _____ *damaged* is: _____ *healthy* is: _____.
   varic/ose VĂR-ĭ-kōs	**5-72** Whereas competent valves prevent a backflow of blood into the veins, incompetent valves result in blood collecting in the veins. The accumulated blood causes dilation and distention of the veins, a condition known as *varic/ose veins*. (See Figure 5–4.) The term in this frame meaning *pertaining to a dilated vein:* _____ / _____

Competency Verification: Check your labeling of Figure 5–3 in Appendix B, Answer Key, page 562.

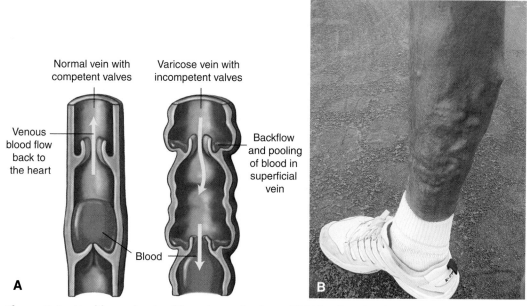

Normal vein with competent valves

Varicose vein with incompetent valves

Venous blood flow back to the heart

Backflow and pooling of blood in superficial vein

Blood

A

B

Figure 5-4   Healthy and unhealthy veins and valves. (A) Valve function in competent and incompetent valves. (B) Varicose veins.

Heart Valves

5-73   Label Figure 5–5 as you read the material about the heart valves and their cusps, also called flaps. Four heart valves maintain the flow of blood in one direction through the heart. The (1) **tricuspid valve** and the (2) **mitral valve** are situated between the upper and lower chambers and are attached to the heart walls by fibrous strands called (3) **chordae tendineae**. The (4) **pulmonary valve** and the (5) **aortic valve** are located at the exits of the ventricles.

Heart valves are composed of thin, fibrous cusps, covered by a smooth membrane called *endocardium,* and reinforced by dense connective tissue. The aortic, pulmonary, and tricuspid valves contain (6) **three cusps;** the mitral valve contains (7) **two cusps.** The purpose of the cusps is to open and permit blood to flow through and seal shut to prevent backflow. The opening and closing of the cusps takes place with each heartbeat.

---

mitral valve
MĪ-trăl

5-74   To classify a heart abnormality, it is important to identify the part of the organ in which the disorder occurs. A mitral valve murmur is caused by an incompetent, or faulty, valve. This type of murmur occurs in the valvular structure of the heart known as the _____ _____.

---

valve

5-75   Replacement surgery can be performed to replace a damaged heart valve. When the tri/cuspid valve is damaged, it is replaced at the level of the tri/cuspid _____.

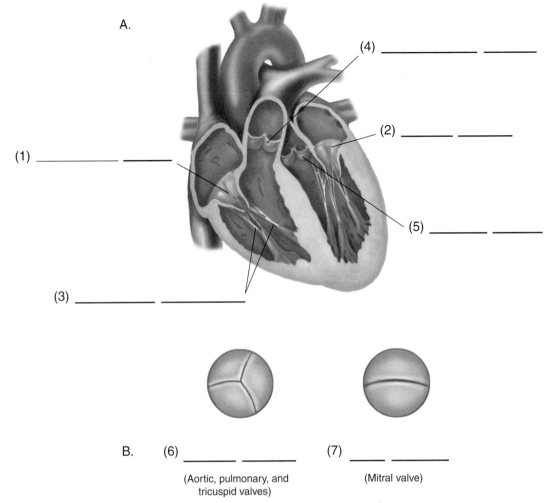

A.

(4) _____ _____

(2) _____ _____

(1) _____ _____

(5) _____ _____

(3) _____ _____

B.   (6) _____ _____   (7) _____ _____

(Aortic, pulmonary, and   (Mitral valve)
tricuspid valves)

Figure 5-5   Heart structures depicting valves and cusps. (A) Heart valves.
(B) Valve cusps.

cardi/o/rrhaphy kăr-dē-OR-ă-fē	**5–76** When valve replacement is performed, the heart must be opened. After the valve is inserted, sutures are required to repair the incision. The surgical procedure that literally means *suture of the heart* is _____ / _____ / _____.

Competency Verification: Check your labeling of Figure 5–5 in Appendix B, Answer Key, page 562.

SECTION REVIEW 5-2

Using the following table, write the CF, suffix, or prefix that matches its definition in the space provided to the left of the definition. There may be more than one word element that matches a definition.

Combining Forms		Suffixes		Prefixes
aort/o	my/o	-ectasis	-rrhaphy	bi-
arteri/o	phleb/o	-ole	-rrhexis	brady-
atri/o	scler/o	-osis	-spasm	epi-
cardi/o	ven/o	-pathy	-stenosis	peri-
hem/o	ventricul/o	-phagia	-ule	tachy-
hemat/o		-pnea		tri-

1. _____ abnormal condition; increase (used primarily with blood cells)

2. _____ above, on

3. _____ aorta

4. _____ around

5. _____ artery

6. _____ atrium

7. _____ blood

8. _____ breathing

9. _____ disease

10. _____ dilation, expansion

11. _____ hardening; sclera (white of eye)

12. _____ heart

13. _____ involuntary contraction, twitching

14. _____ muscle

15. _____ rapid

16. _____ rupture

17. _____ slow

18. _____ small, minute

19. _____ suture

20. _____ narrowing, stricture

21. _____ swallowing, eating

22. _____ three

23. _____ two

24. _____ vein

25. _____ ventricle (of heart or brain)

Competency Verification: Check your answers in Appendix B, Answer Key, page 562. If you are not satisfied with your level of comprehension, go back to Frame 5–1 and rework the frames.

Correct Answers _____ × 4 = _____ % Score

Conduction Pathway of the Heart

	5-77 Primary responsibility for initiating the heartbeat rests with the (1) **sinoatrial (SA) node**, also known as the pacemaker of the heart. The SA node is a small region of specialized cardiac muscle tissue located on the posterior wall of the (2) **right atrium (RA)**. Label the two structures in Figure 5–6.
SA **RA**	**5-78** Write the abbreviations for sinoatrial: _____. right atrium: _____.
electricity	**5-79** The CF **electr/o** refers to *electricity*. *Electric/al* and *electr/ic* both mean *pertaining to* _____.
	5-80 The electric/al current generated by the heart's pacemaker causes the atrial walls to contract and forces the flow of blood into the ventricles. The wave of electricity moves to another region of the myo/cardi/um called the (3) *atrioventricular (AV) node*. Label the structure in Figure 5–6 to learn about the conduction pathway of the heart.
atri/o/ventricul/ar ā-trē-ō-vĕn-TRĬK-ū-lăr **electric/al** **atri/al** Ā-trē-ăl	**5-81** Identify the words in Frame 5–80 that mean *pertaining to the atrium and ventricles:* _____ / _____ / _____ / _____. *pertaining to electricity:* _____ / _____. *pertaining to the atrium:* _____ / _____.
AV **SA**	**5-82** Write the abbreviations for atri/o/ventricul/ar: _____. sino/atri/al: _____.
	5-83 The AV node instantaneously transmits impulses to the (4) **bundle of His**, a bundle of specialized fibers that transmits those impulses to the right and left (5) **bundle branches**. Label the structures in Figure 5–6.
	5-84 From the right and left bundle branches, impulses travel through the (6) **Purkinje fibers** to the rest of the ventricul/ar my/o/cardi/um and bring about ventricul/ar contraction. Label the Purkinje (pŭr-KĬN-jē) fibers in Figure 5–6.

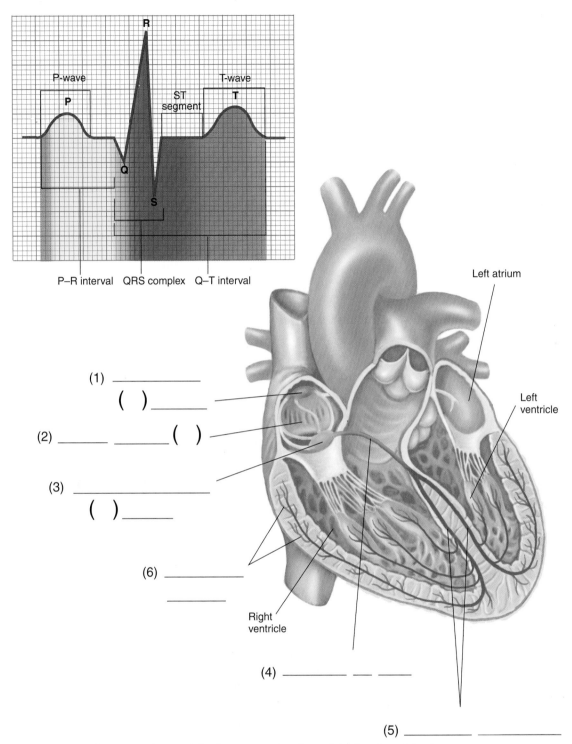

Figure 5-6 Conduction pathway of the heart. Anterior view of the interior of the heart. The electrocardiogram tracing is one normal heartbeat.

5–85 Use your medical dictionary to define *contraction*.

_____

_____

_____

_____

Competency Verification: Check your labeling of Figure 5–6 in Appendix B, Answer Key, page 562.

Cardiac Cycle and Heart Sounds

diastole
dī-ĂS-tō-lē

5–86 The cardi/ac cycle refers to the events of one complete heartbeat. Each contraction, or systole, of the heart is followed by a period of relaxation, or diastole. This cycle occurs 60 to 100 times per minute in the normal functioning heart.

The normal period of heart contraction is called *systole;* the normal period of heart relaxation is called _____.

systole
SĬS-tō-lē

diastole
dī-ĂS-tō-lē

systole
SĬS-tō-lē

5–87 When the heart is in the phase of relaxation, it is in diastole.

When the heart is in the contraction phase, it is in _____.

The pumping action of the heart consists of contraction and relaxation of the myocardial layer of the heart wall. During relaxation, *diastole,* blood fills the ventricles. The contraction that follows, *systole,* propels the blood out of the ventricles and into the circulation.

Write the medical term relating to the cardi/ac cycle that is in the phase of

relaxation: _____.

contraction: _____.

-graphy
-gram

5–88 Recall the suffixes that mean

process of recording: _____.

record, writing: _____.

heart

5–89 Electr/o/cardi/o/graphy is the process of recording electric/al activity generated by the _____.

record
heart

5–90 An electr/o/cardi/o/gram is a _____ of electric/al activity generated by the _____. (See Figure 5–6.)

electr/o/cardi/o/gram
ē-lĕk-trō-KĂR-dē-ō-grăm

5–91 *ECG* and *EKG* are abbreviations for *electr/o/cardi/o/gram.* To evaluate an abnormal cardi/ac rhythm, such as tachy/cardia, an *EKG* may be helpful.

The abbreviations *ECG* and *EKG* refer to

_____ / _____ / _____ / _____ / _____.

| tachy-
brady- | **5–92** The prefix that means *rapid* is _____; the prefix that means *slow* is _____. |

| rapid
slow | **5–93** Tachy/cardia is a heart rate that is _____; brady/cardia is a heart rate that is _____. |

 The following summary provides a brief, general interpretation of an ECG. A more comprehensive explanation of ECG abnormalities is beyond the scope of this book. Refer to Figure 5–6 as you read the text that follows.

A normal heart rhythm, or *sinus rhythm*, shows five waves on the ECG strip, which represent electrical changes as they spread through the heart. The waves are known as *P wave*, *QRS waves*, and *T wave*.

The **P** wave represents atrial depolarization, conduction of an electrical impulse through the atria. These electrical changes cause atrial contraction. The **QRS** waves, commonly referred to as the QRS complex, represent ventricular depolarization, conduction of electrical impulses through the ventricle by way of the bundle of His and the Purkinje fibers. These electrical changes cause ventricular contraction. The **T** wave represents the electrical recovery and relaxation of the ventricles (during diastole).

| electr/o/cardi/o/gram
ē-lĕk-trō-KĂR-dē-ō-grăm | **5–94** Although the heart itself generates the heartbeat, factors such as hormones, drugs, and nervous system stimulation also can influence the heart rate.
To evaluate a patient's heart rate, a physician may order an *EKG*, which is an abbreviation for _____ / ____ / _____ / ____ / _____. |

| micro/cardia
mī-krō-KĂR-dē-ă | **5–95** Micro/cardia, an abnormal smallness of the heart, is a condition that is not usually compatible with a normal life.
A person diagnosed with an underdeveloped heart suffers from the condition called _____ / _____. |

| enlargement, heart | **5–96** Megal/o/cardia is an enlargement of the heart. Cardi/o/megaly also means _____ of the _____. |

| cardi/o/megaly,
megal/o/cardia
kăr-dē-ō-MĔG-ă-lē,
mĕg-ă-lō-KĂR-dē-ă | **5–97** In patients with high blood pressure, the heart must work extremely hard. As a result, it enlarges, similar to any other muscle in response to excessive activity or exercise.
A patient who develops an enlarged heart has a condition called _____ / ____ / _____ or _____ / ____ / _____. |

5–98 Use your medical dictionary to define *angina pectoris* and *lumen*.

_____

_____

_____

_____

	5–99 Coronary artery disease (CAD) affects the arteries and may cause various pathological conditions, including a reduced flow of oxygen and nutrients to the myocardium. (See Figure 5–7.) The most common type of CAD is coronary ather/o/scler/osis. It is now the leading cause of death in the Western world. Identify the word elements in this frame that mean
-osis	*abnormal condition:* _____.
scler	*hardening:* _____.
ather/o	*fatty plaque:* _____ / _____.

	5–100 Arteri/o/scler/osis is a thickening, hardening, and loss of elasticity of arteri/al walls, which results in decreased blood supply. Thus, arteri/o/scler/osis is commonly referred to as *hardening of the arteries.* When the physician diagnoses a hardening of the arteries, the condition is recorded in the medical chart as
arteri/o/scler/osis ăr-tē-rē-ō-sklĕ-RŌ-sĭs	_____ / _____ / _____ / _____.

	5–101 *Ather/o/scler/osis,* a type of *arteri/o/scler/osis,* is characterized by an accumulation of plaque within the arterial wall. (See Figure 5–7.) Both conditions develop over a long period and usually occur together. Review the word elements used to denote coronary artery disease.
ather/o	fatty plaque: _____ / _____
arteri/o	artery: _____ / _____
scler/o	hardening: _____ / _____
my/o	muscle: _____ / _____
cardi	heart: _____.

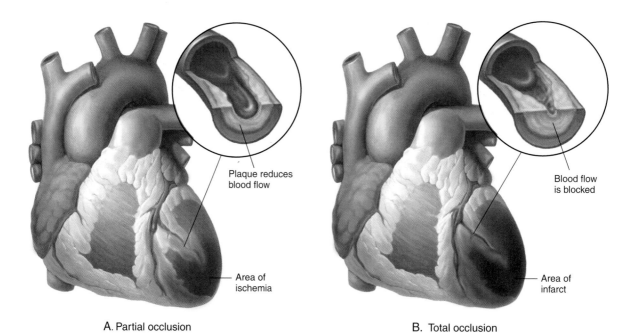

A. Partial occlusion   B. Total occlusion

Figure 5-7 Coronary artery disease. (A) Partial occlusion. (B) Total occlusion.

arteri/o/scler/osis
ăr-tē-rē-ō-sklĕ-RŌ-sĭs

ather/o/scler/osis
ăth-ĕr-ō-sklĕ-RŌ-sĭs

5-102 Build medical words that mean

abnormal condition of arterial hardening:
_____ / _____ / _____ / _____.

abnormal condition of fatty plaque hardening:
_____ / _____ / _____ / _____.

---

excision *or* removal

5-103 The CF *necr/o* refers to *death or necrosis.* Necr/ectomy is an
_____ of dead tissue.

---

necr/o/phobia
nĕk-rō-FŌ-bē-ă

5-104 Use *-phobia* to form a word meaning fear of death:
_____ / _____ / _____.

---

cardi/ac
KĂR-dē-ăk

necr/osis
nĕ-KRŌ-sĭs

5-105 Necr/osis of the my/o/cardi/um occurs when there is insufficient blood supply to the heart. Eventually, such a condition may result in cardi/ac failure and death of the my/o/cardi/um.
Identify the words in this frame that mean

pertaining to the heart: _____ / _____.

abnormal condition of tissue death: _____ / _____.

5-106 A my/o/cardi/al infarction (MI), or *infarct,* is caused by occlusion of one or more coronary arteries. *MI* is a medical emergency requiring immediate attention. Using your medical dictionary, define *infarct.*

_____

_____

_____

---

thromb/us
THRŎM-bŭs

5-107 The CF *thromb/o* is used in words to refer to a *blood clot;* the suffix *-us* means *condition, structure.*
Combine *thromb/o* and *-us* to form a word that means *condition of a blood clot:* _____ / _____.

---

thromb/ectomy
thrŏm-BĔK-tō-mē

5-108 *Thromb/osis* is a condition in which a stationary blood clot obstructs a blood vessel at the site of its formation.
The surgical excision of a blood clot is called
_____ / _____.

thrombi THRŎM-bī **anti-**	**5-109** Anti/coagulants are agents that prevent or delay blood coagulation; they are used in the prevention and treatment of a thrombus. The plural form of *thrombus* is _____. The element in this frame meaning *against* is _____.
thromb/o/genesis thrŏm-bō-JĚN-ĕ-sĭs	**5-110** Use *-genesis* to form a word meaning *producing or forming a blood clot:* _____ / _____ / _____.
clot	**5-111** If the anti/coagulant does not dissolve the clot, it may be surgically removed. A *thromb/ectomy* is an excision of a blood _____.
anti/coagulant ăn-tī-kō-ĂG-ū-lănt	**5-112** To prevent blood coagulation, the physician uses an agent known as an _____ / _____.
thromb/o/lysis thrŏm-BŎL-ĭ-sĭs	**5-113** Use the surgical suffix *-lysis* to form a word meaning *destruction or dissolving of a thrombus:* _____ / _____ / _____.
thromb/o/lysis thrŏm-BŎL-ĭ-sĭs	**5-114** The surgical procedure to destroy or remove a clot is *thromb/ectomy* or _____ / _____ / _____.
aneurysm ĂN-ū-rĭzm	**5-115** An *aneurysm* is an abnormal dilation of the vessel wall due to a weakness that causes the vessel to balloon and potentially rupture. (See Figure 5–8.) A ballooning out of the wall of the aorta is called an *aort/ic* _____.
aorta ā-ŎR-tă	**5-116** If a *cerebr/al* aneurysm ruptures, the *hem/o/rrhage* occurs in the cerebrum or brain. If an *aort/ic* aneurysm ruptures, the *hem/o/rrhage* occurs in the _____.

Fusiform   Saccular   Dissecting

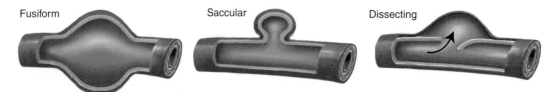

Figure 5-8 Aneurysms.

5-117 Identify the words in Frame 5–116 that mean

aort/ic	*pertaining to the aorta:* _____ / _____.
ă-ŎR-tĭk	
hem/o/rrhage	*bursting forth (of) blood:* _____ / _____ / _____.
HĔM-ĕ-rĭj	
cerebr/al	*pertaining to the cerebrum:* _____ / _____.
SĔR-ĕ-brăl	
aneurysm	*dilation of a vessel caused by weakness:* _____.
ĂN-ū-rĭzm	

Lymphatic System

The lymphatic system consists of lymph, lymph vessels, lymph nodes, and three organs—the tonsils, thymus, and spleen. The lymphatic system has three main functions and is responsible for:

1. draining excess interstitial fluid from tissue spaces and returning it to circulating blood

2. protecting the body by defending against foreign or harmful agents, such as bacteria, viruses, and cancerous cells

3. absorbing and transporting digested fats to venous circulation. These are provided by aggregations of lymphatic tissue known as *Peyer patches* that are present in the lining of the ileum (small intestine).

The fluid (lymph) circulating through the lymphatic system comes from the blood. It contains white blood cells (leukocytes) responsible for immunity as well as monocytes and lymphocytes. As certain constituents of blood plasma filtrate through tiny capillaries into the spaces between cells, it becomes interstitial fluid. Most interstitial fluid is absorbed from the interstitial (or *intercellular*) spaces by thin-walled vessels called *lymph capillaries*. At this point of absorption, interstitial fluid becomes lymph and is passed through lymphatic tissue called *lymph nodes*. The nodes are found in clusters in such areas as the neck (cervic/al lymph nodes), under the arm (axill/ary lymph nodes), the pelvis (ili/ac lymph nodes), and the groin (inguin/al lymph nodes). The nodes act as filters against foreign materials. Eventually, lymph reaches large lymph vessels in the upper chest and reenters the bloodstream. (See Figure 5–1.)

WORD ELEMENTS

This section introduces CFs, suffixes, and prefixes related to the lymphatic system, along with each element's meaning, an example, and additional analysis of key elements in the example. Review the following table and pronounce each word in the word analysis column aloud before you begin to work in the frames.

Word Element	Meaning	Word Analysis
Combining Forms		
aden/o	gland	**aden/o**/pathy (ă-dĕ-NŎP-ă-thē): disease of a gland *-pathy:* disease
agglutin/o	clumping, gluing	**agglutin**/ation (ă-gloo-tĭ-NĀ-shŭn): process of cells clumping together *-ation:* process (of)

(continued)

Word Element	Meaning	Word Analysis
immun/o	immune, immunity, safe	**immun**/o/gen (ĭ-MŪ-nō-jĕn): producing immunity *-gen:* forming, producing, origin *An immunogen is a substance capable of producing an immune response.*
lymph/o	lymph	**lymph**/o/poiesis (lĭm-fō-poy-Ē-sĭs): formation of lymphocytes or of lymphoid tissue *-poiesis:* formation, production
lymphaden/o	lymph gland (node)	**lymphaden**/itis (lĭm-făd-ĕn-Ī-tĭs): inflammation of a lymph gland (node) *-itis:* inflammation
lymphangi/o	lymph vessel	**lymphangi**/oma (lĭm-făn-jē-Ō-mă): tumor composed of lymphatic vessels *-oma:* tumor
phag/o	swallowing, eating	**phag**/o/cyte (FĂG-ō-sīt): cell that swallows and eats (cellular debris) *-cyte:* cell *A phagocyte surrounds, engulfs, and digests microorganisms and cellular debris.*
splen/o	spleen	**splen**/o/megaly (splĕ-nō-MĔG-ă-lē): enlargement of the spleen *-megaly:* enlargement
thym/o	thymus gland	**thym**/oma (thī-MŌ-mă): tumor of the thymus gland, usually a benign tumor *-oma:* tumor

Suffix

-phylaxis	protection	**ana**/phylaxis (ăn-ă-fĭ-LĂK-sĭs): against protection *ana-:* against; up; back *Anaphylaxis is an extreme allergic reaction characterized by a rapid decrease in blood pressure, breathing difficulties, hives, and abdominal cramps.*

Pronunciation Help	Long Sound	ā in rāte	ē in rēbirth	ī in īsle	ō in ōver	ū in ūnite
	Short Sound	ă in ălone	ĕ in ĕver	ĭ in ĭt	ŏ in nŏt	ŭ in cŭt

 Listen and Learn, the audio CD-ROM included in this book, will help you master pronunciation of selected medical words. Use it to practice pronunciations of the above-listed medical terms and for instructions to complete the *Listen and Learn* exercise for this section.

SECTION REVIEW 5-3

For the following medical terms, first write the suffix and its meaning. Then translate the meaning of the remaining elements starting with the first part of the word. The first word is an example that is completed for you.

Term	Meaning
1. agglutin/ation	*-ation: process (of); clumping, gluing*
2. thym/oma	
3. phag/o/cyte	
4. lymphaden/itis	
5. splen/o/megaly	
6. aden/o/pathy	
7. ana/phylaxis	
8. lymphangi/oma	
9. lymph/o/poiesis	
10. immun/o/gen	

Competency Verification: Check your answers in Appendix B, Answer Key, page 562. If you are not satisfied with your level of comprehension, review the vocabulary and retake the review.

Correct Answers _____ × 10 = _____ % Score

Lymphatic Structures

5-118 Similar to blood capillaries, (1) **lymph capillaries** are thin-walled tubes that carry lymph from the tissue spaces to larger (2) **lymph vessels**. Label these structures in Figure 5–9.

---

lymph/oma
lĭm-FŌ-mă

lymph/o/cyte
LĬM-fō-sīt

lymph/o/poiesis
lĭm-fō-poy-Ē-sĭs

5-119 *Lymph/oma* is a malignant tumor of lymph nodes and lymph tissue. Two main kinds of lymphomas are *Hodgkin disease* and *non-Hodgkin lymphoma*. These disorders are covered in the pathology section of this chapter.
Use *lymph/o* to build terms that mean

tumor composed of lymph tissue: _____ / _____

cell present in lymph tissue: _____ / _____ / _____.

formation or production of lymph: _____ / _____ / _____.

vessels	**5-120** Recall that *angi/o* is used in words to denote a *vessel (usually blood or lymph)*. *Angio/card/itis* is an inflammation of the heart and blood _____.
lymphangi/o	**5-121** Combine *lymph/o* and *angi/o* to form a new element meaning *lymph vessel:* _____ / _____.
lymphangi/oma lĭm-făn-jē-Ō-mă	**5-122** Use *lymphangi/o* to form a word meaning *tumor composed of lymph vessels:* _____ / _____.
angi/o/rrhaphy ăn-jē-OR-ă-fē **angi/o/plasty** ĂN-jē-ō-plăs-tē **angi/o/rrhexis** ăn-jē-ō-RĔK-sĭs	**5-123** Use *angi/o* to develop medical words meaning *suture of a vessel:* _____ / _____ / _____ *surgical repair of a vessel:* _____ / _____ / _____ *rupture of a vessel:* _____ / _____ / _____
chest	**5-124** Similar to veins, lymph vessels contain valves that keep lymph flowing in one direction, toward the thorac/ic cavity. *Thorac/ic* means *pertaining to the* _____.
	5-125 The (3) **thoracic duct** and the (4) **right lymphatic duct** carry lymph into veins in the upper thoracic region. Label these two ducts in Figure 5–9.
lymph/oid LĬM-foyd	**5-126** Use *-oid* to form a word meaning *resembling lymph:* _____ / _____.
lymph/o/pathy lĭm-FŎP-ă-thē	**5-127** The word meaning *any disease of the lymphat/ic system* is _____ / _____ / _____.
lymph/o/cytes LĬM-fō-sīts	**5-128** Small round structures called *lymph nodes* not only produce lymph/o/cytes, but also filter and purify lymph by removing such harmful substances as bacteria and cancerous cells. Lymph cells are known as _____ / _____ / _____.
	5-129 The major lymph node sites are the (5) **cervical nodes**, (6) the **axillary nodes**, and (7) the **inguinal nodes**. Label the three major lymph node sites in Figure 5–9.

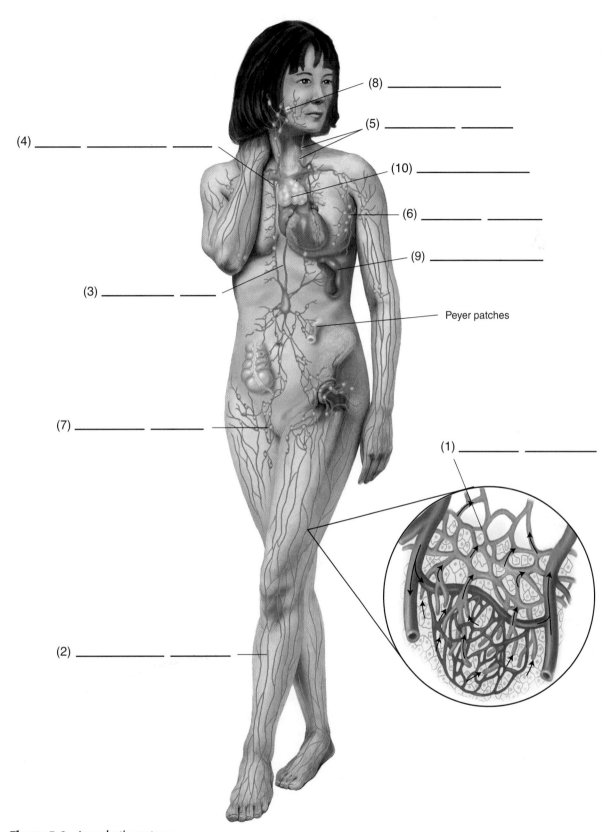

(8) _____

(5) _____   _____

(4) _____ _____ _____

(10) _____

(6) _____ _____

(9) _____

Peyer patches

(3) _____ _____

(7) _____ _____

(1) _____ _____

(2) _____ _____

Figure 5-9 Lymphatic system.

cervic/al
SĔR-vĭ-kăl

axill/ary
ĂK-sĭ-lăr-ē

inguin/al
ĬNG-gwĭ-năl

5-130 Write the name of the lymph node located in the

neck: _____ / _____.

armpit: _____ / _____.

groin (depression between the thigh and trunk):

_____ / _____.

Tonsil, Spleen, and Thymus

5-131 The (8) **tonsil** is a small mass of lymphoid tissue in the mucous membranes of the pharynx and base of the tongue. Tonsils consist of several masses and are the first line of defense from the external environment. They act as a filter to protect against bacteria and other harmful substances that may enter the body through the nose or mouth. Label the tonsil in Figure 5–9.

5-132 The (9) **spleen** is located in the left upper quadrant (LUQ) of the abdomen and behind the stomach. It is the largest lymphatic organ in the body. Although the spleen is not essential to life, it plays an important role in the immune response by filtering blood in much the same way that lymph nodes filter lymph. Label the spleen in Figure 5–9.

5-133 Path/o/gens of all types are filtered from the circulating blood by the macro/phages of the spleen. The spleen also removes and destroys old red blood cells (RBCs) from circulation. The spleen contains ven/ous sinuses that serve as a storage reservoir for blood. In emergencies, such as hem/o/rrhage, the spleen can release blood back into the general circulation. Identify the terms in the frame that refers to

path/o/gen
păth-ō-JĔN

hem/o/rrhage
HĔM-ĕ-rĭj

ven/ous
VĒ-nŭs

macro/phage
MĂK-rō-fāj

micro/organ/ism capable of producing disease: _____ / _____ / _____

loss of large amounts of blood in a short period:

_____ / _____ / _____

pertaining to a vein: _____ / _____

phag/o/cyt/ic cell in the spleen: _____ / _____

5-134 The (10) **thymus**, also an endocrine gland, is a lymphatic organ. It is located near the middle of the chest (mediastinum) just beneath the sternum. Label the thymus in Figure 5–9.

immun/o

5-135 During fetal life and childhood, the thymus is quite large, but becomes smaller with age as it completes most of its essential work during childhood. The thymus plays an important role in the body's ability to protect itself against disease (immunity), especially during the early years of growth.

What is the CF meaning *immune, immunity, safe?* _____ / _____

T cells

5-136 The thymus secretes a hormone called *thymosin,* which stimulates the red bone marrow to produce T lymph/o/cytes, or *T cells.* T cells are important in the immune process. They originate in the bone marrow but migrate and mature in the thymus. Upon maturation, T cells enter the blood and circulate throughout the body, providing a mechanism of defense against disease because the cells attack and destroy foreign or abnormal cells.

Specific lymph/o/cytes that attack foreign agents such as viruses are known as *T lympho/cytes* or _____.

---

cyt/o/tox/ic
sī-tō-TŎKS-ĭk

CA

5-137 Some T cells are called *killer cells* because they secrete immun/o/logic/ally essential chemical compounds that destroy foreign cells. **Killer T lymph/o/cytes,** also known as **cyt/o/toxic T lymph/o/cytes,** are so named because they are capable of destroying specific cells. The killer cells also play a significant role in the body's resistance to proliferation of cancer (CA) cells.

Specialized cells that provide surveillance against CA cells are called *killer T lymph/o/cytes,* or _____ / _____ / _____ / _____ *T lymph/o/cytes.*

The abbreviation for cancer is: _____.

---

cyt/o/tox/ic
sī-tō-TŎKS-ĭk

lymph/o/cyte
LĬM-fō-sīt

5-138 **Cyt/o/tox/ic T lymph/o/cytes** defend against viral and fung/al infections. They are also responsible for transplant rejection reactions and for immun/o/logic/al surveillance against cancer.

Identify the terms in this frame that mean

pertaining to cells that are poisonous:

_____ / _____ / _____ / _____

cell present in lymph tissue: _____ / _____ / _____

Competency Verification: Check your labeling of Figure 5–9 in Appendix B, Answer Key, page 563.

SECTION REVIEW 5-4

Using the following table, write the CF or suffix that matches its definition in the space provided to the left of the definition. There may be more than one word element that matches a definition.

Combining Forms		Suffixes	
angi/o	lymph/o	-al	-megaly
aort/o	my/o	-cyte	-pathy
cardi/o	necr/o	-ic	-plasty
cerebr/o	thromb/o	-gram	-rrhexis
electr/o		-graphy	-stenosis
hem/o		-lysis	

1. _____ aorta
2. _____ blood
3. _____ blood clot
4. _____ cell
5. _____ cerebrum
6. _____ death, necrosis
7. _____ disease
8. _____ electricity
9. _____ enlargement
10. _____ heart
11. _____ lymph
12. _____ muscle
13. _____ process of recording
14. _____ record, writing
15. _____ pertaining to
16. _____ rupture
17. _____ separation; destruction; loosening
18. _____ narrowing, stricture
19. _____ surgical repair
20. _____ vessel (usually blood or lymph)

Competency Verification: Check your answers in Appendix B, Answer Key, page 563. If you are not satisfied with your level of comprehension, go back to Frame 5–118 and rework the frames.

Correct Answers _____ × 5 = _____ % Score

Abbreviations

This section introduces cardiovascular and lymphatic systems-related abbreviations and their meanings. Included are abbreviations contained in the medical record activities that follow.

Abbreviation	Meaning	Abbreviation	Meaning
Cardiovascular			
AED	automatic external defibrillator	**HF**	heart failure
		IAS	Interatrial septum
AICD	automatic implantable cardioverter defibrillator	**ICD**	implantable cardioverter defibrillator
AS	aortic stenosis	**IVC**	inferior vena cava
ASD	atrial septal defect	**IVS**	interventricular septum
ASHD	arteriosclerotic heart disease	**LA**	left atrium
AV	atrioventricular; arteriovenous	**LDL**	low-density lipoprotein
BBB	bundle-branch block		
BP	blood pressure	**LV**	left ventricle
CA	cancer; chronological age; cardiac arrest	**MI**	myocardial infarction
CABG	coronary artery bypass graft	**MVP**	mitral valve prolapse
CAD	coronary artery disease	**RA**	right atrium
CC	cardiac catheterization; chief complaint	**RBC**	red blood cell(s)
CHB	complete heart block	**RV**	right ventricle
CHF	congestive heart failure	**SA**	sinoatrial (node)
CV	cardiovascular	**SOB**	shortness of breath
CVA	cerebrovascular accident; costovertebral angle	**SVC**	superior vena cava
DVT	deep vein thrombosis (also called *deep venous thrombosis*)	**TIA**	transient ischemic attack
ECG, EKG	electrocardiogram; electrocardiography	**US**	ultrasound; ultrasonography
ELISA	enzyme-linked immunosorbent assay (test to detect anti-HIV antibodies)		

(continued)

Abbreviation	Meaning	Abbreviation	Meaning
ELT	endovenous laser ablation; endoluminal laser ablation	VSD	ventricular septal defect
HDL	high-density lipoprotein	WBC	white blood cell(s)
Lymphatic			
AIDS	acquired immune deficiency syndrome	HSV	herpes simplex virus
EBV	Epstein-Barr virus	KS	Kaposi sarcoma
HIV	human immunodeficiency virus	PCP	*Pneumocystis* pneumonia; primary care physician; phencyclidine (hallucinogen)

Additional Medical Terms

The following are additional terms related to the cardiovascular and lymphatic systems. Recognizing and learning these terms will help you understand the connection between common signs, symptoms, and diseases and their diagnoses as well as the rationale behind methods of treatment selected for a particular disorder.

Signs, Symptoms, and Diseases

Cardiovascular System

aneurysm ĂN-ū-rĭzm	Localized dilation of the wall of a blood vessel, usually an artery, due to a congenital defect or weakness in the vessel wall (See Figure 5–8.) *An aneurysm may rupture, causing hemorrhage, or thrombi may form in the dilation and give rise to emboli that may obstruct smaller vessels.*
angina pectoris ăn-JĪ-nă pĕk-TŌ-rĭs	Mild to severe pain or pressure in the chest caused by ischemia; also called *angina* *Angina usually results from atherosclerosis of the coronary arteries. It can occur while resting or during exercise and is a warning sign of an impending myocardial infarction (MI).*

arrhythmia
ă-RĬTH-mē-ă
 	
    a-: without, not
rrhythm: rhythm
   -ia: condition
	Irregularity or loss of rhythm of the heartbeat; also called *dysrhythmia*
	
	Arrhythmias occur when the electrical impulses that stem from the conduction system of the heart do not function properly, causing the heart to deviate from the normal pattern heartbeat. Two common types are of arrhythmia are flutter and fibrillation.

fibrillation fĭ-brĭl-Ā-shŭn	Irregular, random contraction of heart fibers *Fibrillation commonly occurs in the atria or ventricles of the heart and is usually described by the part that is contracting abnormally, such as atrial fibrillation or ventricular fibrillation. Cardioversion is a medical procedure performed with a defibrillator. It is used to treat life-threatening arrhythmias, such as ventricular fibrillations, and restore the heart to normal sinus rhythm.*

arteriosclerosis
ăr-tē-rē-ō-sklĕ-RŌ-sĭs
 	
arteri/o: artery
  scler: hardening,
        sclera (white
        of eye)
  -osis: abnormal
        condition;
        increase (used
        primarily with
        blood cells)
	Thickening, hardening, and loss of elasticity of arterial walls; also called *hardening of the arteries* (See Figure 5–7.)
	
	Arteriosclerosis results in altered function of tissues and organs.

atherosclerosis
ăth-ĕ-rō-sklĕ-RŌ-sĭs
 	
ather/o: fatty plaque
  scler: hardening, sclera
        (white of eye)
  -osis: abnormal
        condition;
        increase (used
        primarily with
        blood cells)
	Most common form of arteriosclerosis, caused by accumulation of fatty substances within the arterial walls, resulting in partial and, eventually, total occlusion (See Figure 5–7.)
	
	Atherosclerosis of the internal carotid artery results from a piece of plaque that may travel and block the lumina of blood vessels that supply blood to the brain. (See Figure 5–10.)

bruit brwē	Soft blowing sound heard on auscultation caused by turbulent blood flow
coronary artery disease (CAD) KŌR-ō-nă-rē ĂR-tĕr-ē *coron:* heart *-ary:* pertaining to	Abnormal condition that affects the heart's arteries and produces various pathological effects, especially reduced flow of oxygen and nutrients to the myocardium *The most common form of CAD is coronary atherosclerosis. It is now the leading cause of death in the Western world. (See Figure 5–7.)*

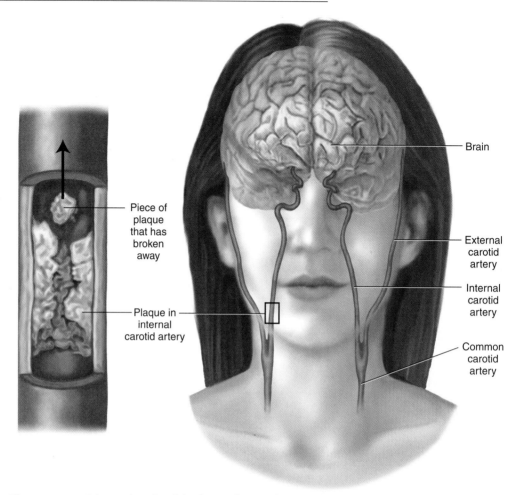

Brain

External carotid artery

Internal carotid artery

Common carotid artery

Piece of plaque that has broken away

Plaque in internal carotid artery

Figure 5-10 Atherosclerosis of the internal carotid artery. Pieces of plaque break free, travel to the brain, and block blood vessels that supply blood to the brain.

deep vein thrombosis (DVT) dēp vān thrŏm-BŌ-sĭs *thromb:* blood clot *-us:* condition; structure	Formation of a blood clot in a deep vein of the body, occurring most commonly in the iliac and femoral veins
embolus ĔM-bō-lŭs *embol:* embolus (plug) *-us:* condition; structure	Mass of undissolved matter — commonly a blood clot, fatty plaque, or air bubble — that travels through the bloodstream and becomes lodged in a blood vessel *Emboli may be solid, liquid, or gaseous. Occlusion of vessels from emboli usually results in the development of infarcts.*

heart block	Interference with normal conduction of electrical impulses that control activity of the heart muscle
	Heart block is usually specified by the location of the block and the type.
first-degree	Atrioventricular (AV) block in which the atrial electrical impulses are delayed by a fraction of a second before being conducted to the ventricles
	First-degree AV block is recognized on ECG by a prolonged PR interval. (See Figure 5–6.) There is no specific treatment for first-degree AV block, but the condition is monitored because it may precede higher degrees of block.
second-degree	AV block in which occasional electrical impulses from the SA node fail to be conducted to the ventricles
	Because of the dropped beats, the QRS complexes are dropped periodically, usually every second, third, or fourth beat. (See Figure 5–6.)
third-degree	AV block in which electrical impulses from the atria fail to reach the ventricles; also called *complete heart block* (CHB)
	In right- or left-bundle branch block, electrical impulses are unable to travel down the right or left bundle of His. (See Figure 5–6.) Treatment for second- or third-degree heart block consists of atropine (a drug used to increase heart rate) or pacemaker insertion.

heart failure (HF)	Condition in which the heart cannot pump enough blood to meet the metabolic requirement of body tissues; formerly called *congestive heart failure (CHF)*
	Heart failure may result from myocardial infarction, ischemic heart disease, and cardiomyopathy. It may also be caused by the dysfunction of organs other than the heart, especially the lungs, kidneys, and liver.

hypertension hī-pĕr-TĔN-shŭn *hyper:* excessive, above normal *-tension:* to stretch	Consistently elevated blood pressure that is higher than 119/79 mm Hg, causing damage to the blood vessels and, ultimately, the heart

ischemia ĭs-KĒ-mē-ă *isch:* to hold, back *-emia:* blood	Inadequate supply of oxygenated blood to a body part due to an interruption of blood flow (See the ischemic area of an occluded coronary artery in Figure 5–7.)
	Some causes of ischemia are arterial embolism, atherosclerosis, thrombosis, and vasoconstriction.

mitral valve prolapse (MVP) MĪ-trăl vălv PRŌ-lăps	Condition in which the leaflets of the mitral valve prolapse into the left atrium during systole, resulting in incomplete closure and backflow of blood
murmur MĔR-mĕr	Abnormal sound heard on auscultation, caused by defects in the valves or chambers of the heart
myocardial infarction (MI) mī-ō-KĂR-dē-ăl ĭn-FĂRK-shŭn *my/o:* muscle *cardi:* heart *-al:* pertaining to	Necrosis of a portion of cardiac muscle caused by partial or complete occlusion of one or more coronary arteries; also called *heart attack* (see Figure 5–7).
patent ductus arteriosus PĂT-ĕnt DŬK-tŭs ăr-tē-rē-Ō-sĭs	Failure of the ductus arteriosus to close after birth, resulting in an abnormal opening between the pulmonary artery and the aorta
Raynaud phenomenon rā-NŌ	Numbness in fingers or toes due to intermittent constriction of arterioles in the skin *Raynaud phenomenon is typically caused by exposure to cold temperatures or emotional stress. It may also be an indicator of some other, more serious problem.*
rheumatic heart disease rū-MĂT-ĭk	Streptococcal infection that causes damage to the heart valves and heart muscle, most commonly in children and young adults
stroke STRŌK	Damage to part of the brain due to interruption of its blood supply caused by bleeding within brain tissue or, more commonly, blockage of an artery, also called *cerebrovascular accident* (CVA) *When brain cells affected by stroke are deprived of oxygen, they cease to function. Movement, vision, and speech may be impaired.*
thrombus THRŎM-bŭs *thromb:* blood clot *us:* condition; structure	Aggregation of platelets, fibrin, clotting factors, and the cellular elements of the blood attached to the interior wall of a vein or artery, sometimes occluding the lumen of the vessel; also called *blood clot*
transient ischemic attack (TIA) TRĂN-zhĕnt ĭs-KĒ-mĭk	Temporary interference in the blood supply to the brain that causes no permanent brain damage

varicose veins VĂR-ĭ-kōs VĀNZ *varic:* dilated vein *-ose:* pertaining to; sugar	Swollen superficial veins that are visible through the skin and usually occur in the legs *Varicose veins commonly appear blue, bulging, and twisted. If left untreated, varicose veins can cause aching and feelings of fatigue as well as skin changes. Because the blood pools (collects), there is an increased risk of clot formation (thrombosis). Treatment consists of sclerosing chemicals (sclerotherapy), and surgical interventions such as endovenous laser ablation (ELT) of the greater saphenous veins with microphlebectomies of lesser saphenous veins.(See Figure 5–4.)*

Lymphatic System

acquired immune deficiency syndrome (AIDS) ă-KWĬRD ĭm-ŪN dē-FĬSH-ĕn-sē SĬN-drōm	Deficiency of cellular immunity induced by infection with the human immunodeficiency virus (HIV), characterized by increasing susceptibility to infections, malignancies, and neurological diseases *HIV is transmitted from person to person in cell-rich body fluids (notably blood and semen) through sexual contact, sharing of contaminated needles (as by intravenous drug abusers), or other contact with contaminated blood (as in accidental needle sticks among health care workers).*
Hodgkin disease HŎJ-kĭn	Malignant disease characterized by painless, progressive enlargement of lymphoid tissue (usually first evident in cervical lymph nodes), splenomegaly, and the presence of unique Reed-Sternberg cells in the lymph nodes
Kaposi sarcoma KĂP-ō-sē săr-KŌ-mă *sarc:* flesh (connective tissue) *-oma:* tumor	Malignancy of connective tissue, including bone, fat, muscle, and fibrous tissue *Kaposi sarcoma is closely associated with AIDS and is commonly fatal because the tumors readily metastasize to various organs.*
lymphadenitis lĭm-făd-ĕn-Ī-tĭs *lymph:* lymph *aden:* gland *-itis:* inflammation	Inflammation and enlargement of the lymph nodes, usually as a result of infection
mononucleosis mŏn-ō-nū-klē-Ō-sĭs *mono-:* one *nucle:* nucleus *-osis:* abnormal condition; increase (used primarily with blood cells)	Acute infection caused by the Epstein-Barr virus (EBV) and characterized by a sore throat, fever, fatigue, and enlarged lymph nodes
non-Hodgkin lymphoma non-HŎJ-kĭn lĭm-FŌ-mă *lymph:* lymph *-oma:* tumor	Any of a heterogeneous group of malignant tumors involving lymphoid tissue except for Hodgkin disease; previously called *lymphosarcoma*

Diagnostic Procedures

Cardiovascular System

cardiac catheterization (CC) KĂR-dē-ăk kăth-ĕ-tĕr-ĭ-ZĀ-shŭn *cardi:* heart *-ac:* pertaining to	Insertion of a catheter into the heart through a vein or artery, usually of an arm (brachial approach) or leg (femoral approach) to provide evaluation of the heart (See Figure 5–11.) *During CC, the cardiologist may also inject a contrast medium and take x-rays (angiography). Cardiac catheterization is used mainly in diagnosing and evaluating congenital, rheumatic, and coronary artery lesions, including myocardial infarction.*
cardiac enzyme studies KĂR-dē-ăk ĔN-zīm	Battery of blood tests performed to determine the presence of cardiac damage
echocardiography ĕk-ō-kăr-dē-ŎG-ră-fē *echo-:* a repeated sound *cardi/o:* heart *-graphy:* process of recording	Use of ultrasound to evaluate the heart and great vessels and diagnose cardiovascular lesions

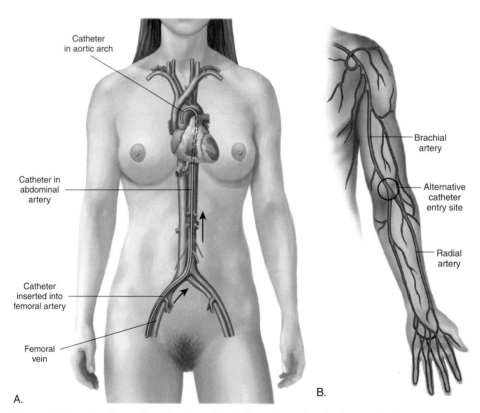

Catheter in aortic arch

Catheter in abdominal artery

Catheter inserted into femoral artery

Femoral vein

Brachial artery

Alternative catheter entry site

Radial artery

A.

B.

Figure 5-11 Cardiac catheterization. (A) Catheter insertion in femoral vein or artery. (B) Catheter insertion in brachial or radial artery.

electrocardiography (ECG, EKG) ē-lĕk-trō-kăr-dē-ŎG-ră-fē *electr/o:* electricity *cardi/o:* heart *-graphy:* process of recording	Creation and study of graphic records (electrocardiograms) produced by electric activity generated by the heart muscle; also called *cardiography* *ECG is analyzed by a cardiologist and is valuable in diagnosing cases of abnormal heart rhythm and myocardial damage.*
Holter monitor HŌL-ter MŎN-ĭ-tĕr	Monitoring device worn by a patient that records prolonged electrocardiograph readings (usually 24 hours) on a portable tape recorder while the patient conducts normal daily activities *Holter monitoring provides a record of cardiac arrhythmia that would not be discovered by means of an ECG of only a few minutes' duration. The patient keeps an activity diary to compare daily events with electrocardiograph tracings. (See Figure 5–12.)*
stress test	ECG taken under controlled exercise stress conditions (typically using a treadmill) while measuring the amount of oxygen consumption *A stress test may show abnormal ECG tracings that do not appear during an ECG taken when the patient is resting.*
nuclear	ECG that utilizes a radioisotope to evaluate coronary blood flow *In a nuclear stress test, the radioisotope is injected at the height of exercise. The area not receiving sufficient oxygen is visualized by decreased uptake of the isotope.*
troponin I TRŌ-pō-nĭn	Blood test that measures protein released into the blood by damaged heart muscle (not skeletal muscle) *The troponin I test is a highly sensitive and specific indicator of recent myocardial infarction (MI).*

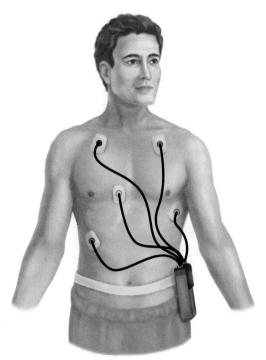

Figure 5-12 Holter monitor.

ultrasonography (US) ŭl-tră-sŏn-ŎG-răf-ē *ultra-:* excess, beyond *son/o:* sound *-graphy:* process of recording	Imaging technique that records high-frequency sound waves bouncing off body tissues and uses a computer to process those waves to produce an image of an internal organ or tissue (See Figure 2-5B.) *Doppler ultrasonography measures blood flow in blood vessels. It allows the examiner to hear characteristic alterations in blood flow caused by vessel obstruction in various parts of an extremity.*

Lymphatic System

bone marrow aspiration biopsy ăs-pĭ-RĀ-shŭn BĪ-ŏp-sē	Removal of living bone marrow tissue, usually taken from the sternum or iliac crest, for microscopic examination *Bone marrow aspiration biopsy evaluates hematopoiesis by revealing the number, shape, and size of red blood cells (RBCs), white blood cells (WBCs), and platelet precursors.*
ELISA	Blood test used to screen for an antibody to the AIDS virus *Positive outcome on this test indicates probably virus exposure and is confirmed with the **Western blot** test, which is more specific.*
lymphangiography lĭm-făn-jē-ŎG-ră-fē *lymph:* lymph *angi/o:* vessel (usually blood or lymph) *-graphy:* process of recording	Radiographic examination of lymph glands and lymphatic vessels after an injection of a contrast medium *Lymphangiography is used to show the path of lymph flow as it moves into the chest region.*
tissue typing	Technique used to determine the histocompatibility of tissues used in grafts and transplants with the recipient's tissues and cells; also known as *histocompatibility testing*

Medical and Surgical Procedures

Cardiovascular System

angioplasty ĂN-jē-ō-plăs-tē *angi/o:* vessel (usually blood or lymph) *-plasty:* surgical repair	Any endovascular procedure that reopens narrowed blood vessels and restores forward blood flow, usually using balloon dilation
coronary artery bypass graft (CABG) KOR-ō-nă-rē ĂR-tĕr-ē *coron:* heart *-ary:* pertaining to	Procedure in which a surgeon removes one or more of a patient's peripheral veins and then sutures each end of the vein onto the coronary artery to route blood flow around a blockage in a coronary artery, thus increasing blood flow to the heart (See Figure 5–13.) *Generally, the saphenous vein from the leg or the right or left internal mammary artery from the chest wall are used in CABG.*

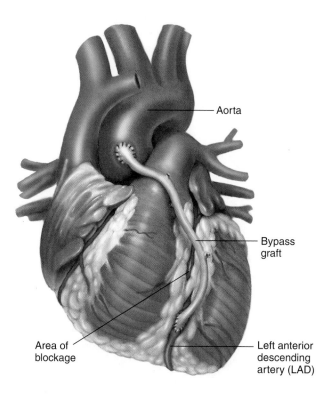

Aorta

Bypass
graft

Area of
blockage

Left anterior
descending
artery (LAD)

Figure 5-13 Coronary artery bypass graft.

cardioversion căr-dē-ō-VĔR-zhŭn *cardi/o:* heart *-version:* turning	Delivery of brief discharges of electricity that pass across the chest to stop a cardiac arrhythmia and restore normal sinus rhythm; also called *defibrillation* *A defibrillator is the electrical device used for cardioversion.*
defibrillator dē-FĬB-rĭ-lā-tĕr	Device designed to administer a defibrillating electric shock to restore normal sinus rhythm *There are two types of defibrillators: automatic implantable cardioverter-defibrillators (AICDs) and automatic external defibrillators (AEDs).*
automatic implantable cardioverter-defibrillator (AICD) căr-dē-ō-VĔR-tĕr dē-FĬB-rĭ-lā-tĕr	Surgically implanted defibrillator that automatically detects and corrects potentially fatal arrhythmias, such as ventricular fibrillations; also called *implantable cardioverter-defibrillator (ICD)*. (See Figure 5–14.) *An AICD is implanted, usually in the chest, in a patient who is at high risk for developing a serious arrhythmia. It has leads (wires) that go to the heart, sense its rhythm, and deliver an electrical shock if needed.*
automatic external defibrillator (AED) dē-FĬB-rĭ-lā-tĕr	Portable computerized defibrillator that analyzes the patient's heart rhythm and delivers an electrical shock to stimulate a heart in cardiac arrest *An AED is kept on emergency response vehicles and in public places, such as recreation facilities, and is designed to be used by trained first-responder personnel or laypeople.z*

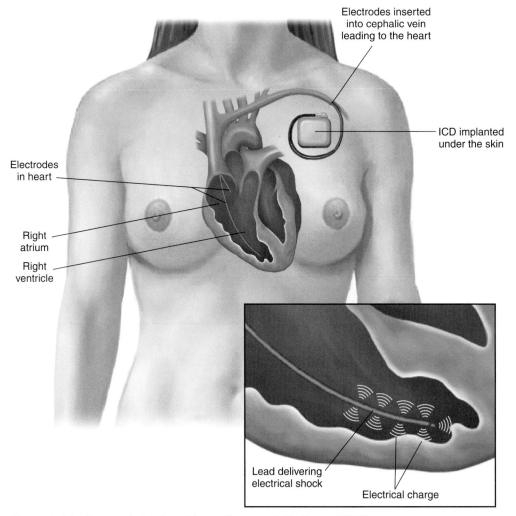

Electrodes inserted into cephalic vein leading to the heart

ICD implanted under the skin

Electrodes in heart

Right atrium

Right ventricle

Lead delivering electrical shock

Electrical charge

Figure 5-14 Automatic implantable cardioverter-defibrillator (AICD).

endarterectomy ĕnd-ăr-tĕr-ĔK-tō-mē 　end-: in, within 　arter: artery 　-ectomy: excision, 　　removal	Surgical removal of the lining of an artery *Endarterectomy is performed on almost any major artery that is diseased or blocked, such as the carotid or femoral artery.*
carotid endarterectomy	Surgical removal of plaque and thromboses from an occluded carotid artery (See Figure 5–10.) *Carotid endarterectomy can reduce the risk of stroke when it is performed on a patient with moderate or severe stenoses of the artery, with or without a history of transient ischemic attacks (TIAs).*
sclerotherapy sklĕr-ō-THĔR-ă-pē 　*scler/o:* hardening; 　　sclera (white 　　of eye) 　*-therapy:* treatment	Chemical injection into a varicose vein that causes inflammation and formation of fibrous tissue, which closes the vein (see Figure 5–4) *When a vein closes, it can no longer fill with blood. In a few weeks the treated varicose vein fades.*

valvuloplasty VĂL-vū-lō-plăs-tē	Plastic or restorative surgery on a valve, especially a cardiac valve *A special type of valvuloplasty, called balloon valvuloplasty, involves insertion of a balloon catheter to open a stenotic heart valve. Inflation of the balloon decreases the constriction.*

Lymphatic System

lymphangiectomy lĭm-făn-jē-ĔK-tō-mē *-ectomy:* excision	Removal of a lymph vessel

Pharmacology

statins STĂ-tĭnz	Drugs that reduce cholesterol levels by decreasing levels of low-density lipoproteins and triglycerides, and slightly increasing levels of high-density lipoproteins

thrombolytic therapy thrŏm-bō-LĬT-ĭk THĔR-ă-pē	Administration of drugs to dissolve a blood clot

Pronunciation Help	**Long Sound** **Short Sound**	ā in rāte ă in ălone	ē in rēbirth ĕ in ĕver	ī in īsle ĭ in ĭt	ō in ōver ŏ in nŏt	ū in ūnite ŭ in cŭt

Additional Medical Terms Review

Match the medical term(s) below with the definitions in the numbered list.

AIDS	fibrillation	lymphangiography	TIA
arrhythmia	HF	mononucleosis	troponin I
atherosclerosis	Hodgkin disease	Raynaud phenomenon	valvuloplasty
bruit	Holter monitor	rheumatic heart disease	varicose veins
CABG	hypertension	stroke	
DVT	ischemia	thrombolytic therapy	
embolus	lymphadenitis	tissue typing	

1. _____ are swollen, distended veins most commonly seen in the lower legs.

2. _____ is an acute infection caused by Epstein-Barr virus (EBV) and characterized by a sore throat, fever, fatigue, and enlarged lymph nodes.

3. _____ refers to administration of drugs to dissolve a blood clot.

4. _____ is a mass of undissolved matter present in a blood vessel.

5. _____ is inflammation and enlargement of the lymph nodes.

6. _____ refers to formation of a blood clot in a deep vein of the body.

7. _____ refers to blood pressure that is consistently higher than normal.

8. _____ is irregularity or loss of heart rhythm.

9. _____ refers to temporary interference of blood supply to the brain without permanent damage.

10. _____ is a soft blowing sound caused by turbulent blood flow.

11. _____ refers to partial brain damage due to interruption of its blood supply, commonly caused by blockage of an artery.

12. _____ is a streptococcal infection that causes damage to heart valves and heart muscle.

13. _____ is heart disease caused by an accumulation of fatty substances within the arterial walls.

14. _____ is a small portable device worn on a patient during normal activity to obtain a record of cardiac arrhythmia.

15. _____ is numbness in fingers or toes due to intermittent constriction of arterioles in the skin.

16. _____ refers to decreased supply of oxygenated blood to a body part due to an interruption of blood flow.

17. _____ refers to malignant solid tumors of the lymphatic system.

18. _____ is a transmissible infection caused by human immunodeficiency virus (HIV).

19. _____ is a condition in which the heart cannot pump enough blood to meet the metabolic requirement of body tissues.

20. _____ means irregular, random contraction of heart fibers.

21. _____ refers to plastic or restorative surgery on a valve, especially a cardiac valve.

22. _____ is a radiographic examination of lymph glands and lymphatic vessels after an injection of a contrast medium.

23. _____ also is known as histocompatibility testing.

24. _____ refers to blood test that measures protein that is released into the blood by damaged heart muscle.

25. _____ refers to surgery that involves bypassing one or more blocked coronary arteries to restore blood flow.

Competency Verification: Check your answers in Appendix B, Answer Key, page 563. If you are not satisfied with your level of comprehension, review the additional medical terms and retake the review.

Correct Answers _____ × 4 = _____ % Score

Medical Record Activities

The following medical reports reflect common, real-life clinical scenarios using medical terminology to document patient care.

MEDICAL RECORD ACTIVITY 5-1

Myocardial Infarction

Terminology

Terms listed in the table below come from the medical report *Myocardial Infarction* that follows. Use a medical dictionary such as *Taber's Cyclopedic Medical Dictionary,* the appendices of this book, or other resources to define each term. Then practice reading the pronunciations aloud for each term.

Term	Definition
apnea ăp-NĒ-ă	
desiccated dĕs-ĭ-KĀ-tĕd	
dyspnea dĭsp-NĒ-ă	
EKG	
fibrillation fĭ-brĭl-Ā-shŭn	
malaise mă-LĀZ	
myocardial infarction mī-ō-KĂR-dē-ăl ĭn-FĂRK-shŭn	
ST segment-T wave (See Figure 5–5.)	
syncope SĬN-kō-pē	
tachycardia tăk-ē-KĂR-dē-ă	
thyroidectomy thī-royd-ĔK-tō-mē	

Listen and Learn Online! will help you master pronunciations of selected medical words from this medical record activity. Visit *http://davisplus.fadavis.com/gylys/simplified* to find instructions on completing the *Listen and Learn Online!* exercise for this section and to practice pronunciations.

Reading

Practice pronunciation of medical terms by reading the following medical report aloud.

Myocardial Infarction

A 70-year-old white woman presented to the hospital for evaluation of a syncopal episode. She states that most recently she has experienced generalized malaise, increased shortness of breath while at rest, and dyspnea followed by periods of apnea and syncope.

Her past history includes recurrent episodes of thyroiditis, which led her to have a thyroidectomy 6 years ago while she was under the care of Dr. Knopp. At the time of surgery, the results of her EKG were interpreted as sinus tachycardia with nonspecific ST segment-T wave changes. The tachycardia was attributed to preoperative anxiety and thyroiditis. Postoperatively, under the direction of Dr. Knopp, the patient was treated with a daily dose of 50 mg of desiccated thyroid and has been symptom-free until this admission.

On clinical examination, the patient's radial pulse was found to be irregular, and the EKG showed uncontrolled atrial fibrillation with evidence of a recent myocardial infarction.

Evaluation

Review the medical record to answer the following questions. Use a medical dictionary such as *Taber's Cyclopedic Medical Dictionary* and other resources if needed.

1. What symptoms did the patient experience before admission to the hospital?

_____

_____

2. What was found during clinical examination?

_____

_____

3. What is the danger of atrial fibrillation?

_____

_____

4. Did the patient have prior history of heart problems? If so, describe them.

_____

_____

5. Was the patient's prior heart problem related to her current one?

_____

_____

MEDICAL RECORD ACTIVITY 5-2

Cardiac Catheterization

Terminology

Terms listed in the table below come from the medical report *Cardiac Catheterization* that follows. Use a medical dictionary such as *Taber's Cyclopedic Medical Dictionary,* the appendices of this book, or other resources to define each term. Then practice reading the pronunciations aloud for each term.

Term	Definition
angiography ăn-jē-ŎG-ră-fē	
angioplasty ĂN-jē-ō-plăs-tē	
catheter KĂTH-ĕ-tĕr	
heparin HĔP-ă-rĭn	
lidocaine LĪ-dō-kān	
sheath SHĒTH	
ST elevations	
stenosis stĕ-NŌ-sĭs	

Listen and Learn Online! will help you master pronunciations of selected medical words from this medical record activity. Visit *http://davisplus.fadavis.com/gylys/simplified* to find instructions on completing the *Listen and Learn Online!* exercise for this section and to practice pronunciations.

Reading

Practice pronunciation of medical terms by reading the following medical report aloud.

Cardiac Catheterization

PROCEDURE: Patient was prepared and draped in a sterile fashion and 20 mL of 1% lidocaine was infiltrated into the right groin. A No. 6 French Cordis right femoral arterial sheath was placed and a No. 6 French JL-5 and JR-4 catheter was used to engage the left and right coronary. A No. 6 French pigtail was used for left ventricular angiography. Angioplasty was performed, and further dictation is under the angioplasty report. There were minor irregularities, with a maximal 25% stenosis just after the first diagonal. The remainder of the vessel was free of significant disease.

A 0.014, high-torque, floppy, extrasupport, exchange-length wire was used to cross the stenosis in the distal right coronary artery. A 3.5 × 20–mm Track Star balloon was inflated in the right coronary artery in the distal portion. The initial stenosis was 50% to 75% with an ulcerated plaque, and the final stenosis was 20% with no significant clot seen in the region. The patient had significant ST elevations in the inferior leads and severe throat tightness and shortness of breath. This would resolve immediately with the inflation of the balloon. The catheters were removed, and the sheath was changed to a No. 8 French Arrow sheath. The patient will be on heparin over the next 12 hours.

IMPRESSION: 1. Two-vessel coronary artery disease with a 75% obtuse marginal and a 75% right coronary artery lesion.
2. Normal left ventricular function.
3. Successful angioplasty to right coronary artery with initial stenosis of 75% and a final stenosis of 20%.

Evaluation

Review the medical record to answer the following questions. Use a medical dictionary such as *Taber's Cyclopedic Medical Dictionary* and other resources if needed.

1. What coronary arteries were under examination?

_____

_____

2. Which surgical procedure was used to clear the stenosis?

_____

_____

3. What symptoms did the patient exhibit before balloon inflation?

_____

_____

4. Why was the patient put on heparin?

_____

_____

Chapter Review

Word Elements Summary

The following table summarizes CFs, suffixes, and prefixes related to the cardiovascular and lymphatic systems.

Word Element	Meaning	Word Element	Meaning
Cardiovascular and Lymphatic Combining Forms			
angi/o	vessel (usually blood or lymph)	**isch/o**	hold back
aneurysm/o	a widening, a widened blood vessel	**lymph/o**	lymph
aort/o	aorta	**phleb/o, ven/o**	vein
arteri/o	artery	**rrhythm/o**	rhythm
ather/o	fatty plaque	**thromb/o**	blood clot
atri/o	atrium	**varic/o**	dilated vein
cardi/o, coron/o	heart	**vas/o**	vessel; vas deferens; duct
electr/o	electric	**vascul/o**	vessel
embol/o	embolus (plug)	**ventricul/o**	ventricle (of heart or brain)
Other Combining Forms			
aden/o	gland	**necr/o**	death, necrosis
cerebr/o	cerebrum	**sarc/o**	flesh (connective tissue)
hem/o	blood	**scler/o**	hardening; sclera (white of eye)
my/o	muscle		
Suffixes			
SURGICAL			
-ectomy	excision, removal	**-rrhaphy**	suture
-lysis	separation; destruction; loosening	**-tomy**	incision
-plasty	surgical repair		
DIAGNOSTIC, SYMPTOMATIC, AND RELATED			
-cardia	heart condition	**-pathy**	disease
-cyte	cell	**-phagia**	swallowing, eating

(continued)

Word Element	Meaning	Word Element	Meaning
-ectasis	dilation, expansion	-phobia	fear
-emia	blood	-phylaxis	protection
-genesis	forming, producing, origin	-pnea	breathing
-gram	record, writing	-poiesis	formation, production
-graphy	process of recording	-rrhexis	rupture
-lith	stone, calculus	-spasm	involuntary contraction, twitching
-lysis	separation; destruction; loosening	-stenosis	narrowing, stricture
-malacia	softening		
-megaly	enlargement	-tension	to stretch
-oid	resembling	-therapy	treatment
-ole, -ule	small, minute	-um	structure, thing
-oma	tumor	-version	turning
-osis	abnormal condition; increase (used primarily with blood cells)		

ADJECTIVE

-al, -ic, -ary	pertaining to, relating to	-ose	pertaining to; sugar

NOUN

-ia	condition	-us	condition, structure

Prefixes			
a-	without, not	epi-	above, upon
anti-	against	micro-	small
bi-	two	peri-	around
brady-	slow	tachy-	rapid
echo-	a repeated sound	trans-	across, through
endo-	in, within	tri-	three

Enhance your study and reinforcement of word elements with the power of *Davis Plus.* Visit *http://davisplus.fadavis.com/gylys/simplified* for this chapter's flash-card activity. We recommend you complete the flash-card activity before completing the word elements review below.

Word Elements Review

After you review the Word Elements Summary, complete this activity by writing the meaning of each element in the space provided.

Word Element	Meaning	Word Element	Meaning
Combining Forms			
1. angi/o	_____	**10.** isch/o	_____
2. aneurysm/o	_____	**11.** lymph/o	_____
3. aort/o	_____	**12.** phleb/o, ven/o	_____
4. arteri/o	_____	**13.** rrhythm/o	_____
5. ather/o	_____	**14.** thromb/o	_____
6. atri/o	_____	**15.** varic/o	_____
7. cardi/o, coron/o	_____	**16.** vas/o	_____
8. electr/o	_____	**17.** vascul/o	_____
9. embol/o	_____	**18.** ventricul/o	_____
OTHER COMBINING FORMS			
19. aden/o	_____	**23.** necr/o	_____
20. cerebr/o	_____	**24.** sarc/o	_____
21. hem/o	_____	**25.** scler/o	_____
22. my/o	_____		
Suffixes			
SURGICAL			
26. -ectomy	_____	**29.** -rrhaphy	_____
27. -lysis	_____	**30.** -tomy	_____
28. -plasty	_____		
DIAGNOSTIC, SYMPTOMATIC, AND RELATED			
31. -cardia	_____	**43.** -osis	_____
32. -ectasis	_____	**44.** -pathy	_____
33. -emia	_____	**45.** -phagia	_____
34. -genesis	_____	**46.** -phobia	_____
35. -gram	_____	**47.** -pnea	_____
36. -graphy	_____	**48.** -rrhexis	_____
37. -lith	_____	**49.** -stenosis	_____
38. -malacia	_____	**50.** -tension	_____
39. -megaly	_____	**51.** -therapy	_____
40. -oid	_____	**52.** -um	_____
41. -ole, -ule	_____	**53.** -version	_____
42. -oma	_____		

(continued)

Word Element	Meaning	Word Element	Meaning
ADJECTIVE			
54. -ose	_____		
NOUN			
55. -ia	_____	**56.** -us	_____
Prefixes			
57. a-	_____	**62.** endo-	_____
58. anti-	_____	**63.** epi-	_____
59. bi-	_____	**64.** peri-	_____
60. brady-	_____	**65.** tachy-	_____
61. echo-	_____		

Competency Verification: Check your answers in Appendix A, Glossary of Medical Word Elements, page 538. If you are not satisfied with your level of comprehension, review the word elements and retake the review.

Correct Answers _____ ×1.53 = _____ % Score

Chapter 5 Vocabulary Review

Match the medical term(s) with the definitions in the numbered list.

agglutination	arteriosclerosis	ECG	pacemaker
anaphylaxis	capillaries	hemangioma	phagocyte
aneurysm	cardiomegaly	malaise	systole
angina pectoris	desiccated	MI	tachyphagia
arterioles	diastole	myocardium	tachypnea

1. _____ refers to the muscular layer of the heart.

2. _____ means rapid breathing.

3. _____ is a disease characterized by an abnormal hardening of the arteries.

4. _____ is a cell that engulfs and digests cellular debris.

5. _____ refers to the contraction phase of the heart.

6. _____ refers to the relaxation phase of the heart.

7. _____ is a record of the electrical impulses of the heart.

8. _____ means a vague feeling of bodily discomfort, which may be the first indication of an infection or disease.

9. _____ means dried thoroughly; rendered free from moisture.

10. _____ means enlarged heart.

11. _____ refers to weakness in the vessel wall that balloons and eventually bursts.

12. _____ is severe pain and constriction about the heart caused by an insufficient supply of oxygenated blood to the heart.

13. _____ is necrosis of an area of muscular heart tissue after cessation of blood supply.

14. _____ is a process of cells clumping together.

15. _____ means rapid eating or swallowing.

16. _____ is an allergic reaction characterized by a rapid decrease in blood pressure.

17. _____ are the smallest vessels of the circulatory system.

18. _____ is a tumor composed of blood vessels.

19. _____ are small arteries.

20. _____ maintains primary responsibility for initiating the heartbeat.

Competency Verification: Check your answers in Appendix B, Answer Key, page 564. If you are not satisfied with your level of comprehension, review the chapter vocabulary and retake the review.

Correct Answers _____ × 5 = _____ % Score

6 Digestive System

OBJECTIVES

Upon completion of this chapter, you will be able to:

- Describe the type of medical treatment the gastroenterologist provides.
- Identify digestive structures by labeling them on anatomical illustrations.
- Describe primary functions of the digestive system.
- Describe common diseases related to the digestive system.
- Describe common diagnostic, medical, and surgical procedures procedures related to the digestive system.
- Apply your word-building skills by constructing medical terms related to the digestive system.
- Describe common abbreviations and symbols related to the digestive system.
- Reinforce word elements by completing the flash card activities.
- Recognize, define, pronounce, and spell terms correctly.
- Demonstrate your knowledge of this chapter by successfully completing the frames, reviews, and medical report evaluations.

Medical Specialty

Gastroenterology

The medical practice of **gastroenterology** encompasses treatment of diseases affecting the **digestive system.** The physician who specializes in treating disorders of the **digestive system** is called a *gastroenerologist.*

During the initial office visit, the health care provider interviews the patient to gather personal and general health information. The physician usually performs a physical examination to assess the patient's health status. All of this information is documented on a history and physical examination record, which becomes a part of the patient's medical record. When the initial evaluation is complete, a range of diagnostic tests may be used to further evaluate the gastrointestinal (GI) tract.

One of the most commonly used diagnostic tools in assessing GI problems is the procedure known as *endoscopy.* This procedure involves the use of a flexible lighted instrument to examine the lining of the digestive tract. It is also commonly used to inspect the esophagus, stomach, intestines, and bile ducts. Endoscopic examinations have made it possible to identify various pathological conditions, including cancers, at an early stage. In addition to endoscopy, x-rays, blood tests, and tissue biopsies may be used to establish or verify the initial findings of the physical examination.

Anatomy and Physiology Overview

The primary function of the digestive system, also known as the *gastrointestinal (GI) system,* is to break down food, prepare it for absorption, and eliminate waste substances. The digestive system consists of a digestive tube, called the *GI tract* or *alimentary canal.* It includes the esophagus, stomach, intestines, and several accessory organs—the liver, gallbladder, and pancreas. The GI tract, extending from the oral cavity (mouth) to the anus, varies in size and structure in several distinct regions. It terminates at the anus, where solid wastes are eliminated from the body by means of defecation. (See Figure 6–1.)

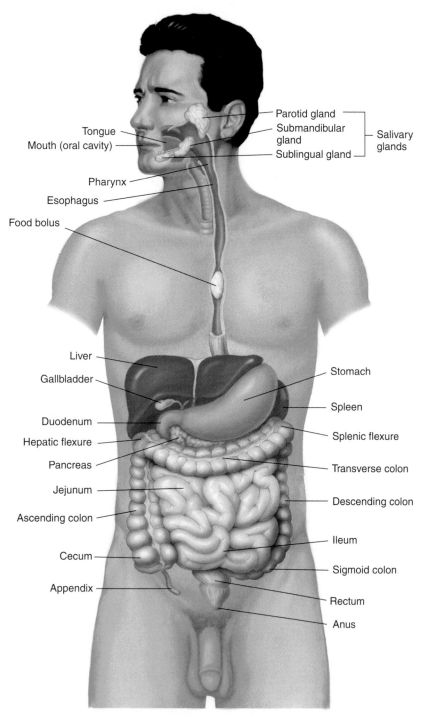

Figure 6-1   Organs of the digestive system (anterior view).

(continued)

WORD ELEMENTS

This section introduces combining forms (CFs) related to the oral cavity, esophagus, pharynx, and stomach. Included are key suffixes; prefixes are defined in the right-hand column as needed. Review the following table and pronounce each word in the word analysis column aloud before you begin to work the frames.

Word Element	Meaning	Word Analysis
Combining Forms		

ORAL CAVITY

dent/o	teeth	**dent**/ist (DĔN-tĭst): specialist who diagnoses and treats diseases and disorders of the oral cavity (teeth and gums) *-ist:* specialist
odont/o		orth/**odont**/ist (ŏr-thō-DŎN-tĭst): dental specialist in prevention and correction of abnormally positioned or misaligned teeth *orth:* straight *-ist:* specialist
gingiv/o	gum(s)	**gingiv**/itis (jĭn-jĭ-VĪ-tĭs): inflammation of gums *-itis:* inflammation
gloss/o	tongue	hypo/**gloss**/al (hī-pō-GLŎS-ăl): pertaining to under the tongue *hypo-:* under, below, deficient *-al:* pertaining to
lingu/o		sub/**lingu**/al (sŭb-LĬNG-gwăl): pertaining to under the tongue *sub-:* under, below *-al:* pertaining to
or/o	mouth	**or**/al (OR-ăl): pertaining to the mouth *-al:* pertaining to
stomat/o		**stomat**/o/pathy (stō-mă-TŎP-ă-thē): disease of the mouth *-pathy:* disease
ptyal/o	saliva	**ptyal**/ism (TĪ-ă-lĭzm): condition of excessive salivation *-ism:* condition
sial/o	saliva, salivary gland	**sial**/o/rrhea (sī-ă-lō-RĒ-ă): excessive flow of saliva; also called *hypersalivation* or *ptyalism* *-rrhea:* discharge, flow

ESOPHAGUS, PHARYNX, AND STOMACH

esophag/o	esophagus	**esophag**/o/scope (ē-SŎF-ă-gō-skōp): instrument for examining the esophagus *-scope:* instrument for examining

Word Element	Meaning	Word Analysis
pharyng/o	pharynx (throat)	**pharyng/o**/tonsill/itis (fă-rĭng-gō-tŏn-sĭ-LĪ-tĭs): inflammation of the pharynx and tonsils *tonsill:* tonsils *-itis:* inflammation
gastr/o	stomach	**gastr/o**/scopy (găs-TRŎS-kō-pē): visual examination of the stomach *-scopy:* visual examination *The gastroscope is a flexible, fiberoptic instrument used to inspect the interior of the stomach.*
pylor/o	pylorus	**pylor/o**/tomy (pī-lor-ŎT-ō-mē): incision of the pylorus (sphincter in lower portion of the stomach) *-tomy:* incision *Pylorotomy is usually performed to remove an obstruction.*

Suffixes

-algia	pain	gastr/**algia** (găs-TRĂL-jē-ă): pain in the stomach *gastr:* stomach
-dynia		gastr/o/**dynia** (găs-trō-DĬN-ē-ă): pain in the stomach *gastr/o:* stomach
-emesis	vomiting	hyper/**emesis** (hī-pĕr-ĔM-ĕ-sĭs): excessive vomiting *hyper-:* excessive, above normal
-megaly	enlargement	gastr/o/**megaly** (găs-trō-MĔG-ă-lē): enlargement of the stomach *gastr/o:* stomach
-orexia	appetite	an/**orexia** (ăn-ō-RĔK-sē-ă): loss of appetite *an-:* without, not *Anorexia can result from various conditions, such as adverse effects of medication as well as other physical or psychological causes.*
-pepsia	digestion	dys/**pepsia** (dĭs-PĔP-sē-ă): difficult or painful digestion; also called *indigestion* *dys-:* bad; painful; difficult *Dyspepsia is a feeling of epigastric discomfort after eating.*
-phagia	swallowing, eating	dys/**phagia** (dĭs-FĀ-jē-ă): difficulty swallowing or eating *dys-:* bad; painful; difficult
-rrhea	discharge, flow	dia/**rrhea** (dī-ă-RĒ-ă): discharge or flow of watery stools from the bowel *dia-:* through, across

Listen and Learn, the audio CD-ROM included in this book, will help you master pronunciation of selected medical words. Use it to practice pronunciations of the above-listed medical terms and for instructions to complete the *Listen and Learn* exercise for this section.

SECTION REVIEW 6-1

For the following medical terms, first write the suffix and its meaning. Then translate the meaning of the remaining elements starting with the first part of the word. The first word is an example that is completed for you.

Term	Meaning
1. gingiv/itis	*-itis: inflammation; gum(s)*
2. dys/pepsia	_____
3. pylor/o/tomy	_____
4. dent/ist	_____
5. esophag/o/scope	_____
6. gastr/o/scopy	_____
7. dia/rrhea	_____
8. hyper/emesis	_____
9. an/orexia	_____
10. sub/lingu/al	_____

Competency Verification: Check your answers in Appendix B, Answer Key, page 564. If you are not satisfied with your level of comprehension, review the vocabulary and retake the review.

Correct Answers _____ × 10 = _____ % Score

Upper GI Tract

The upper GI tract consists of the oral cavity, esophagus, pharynx, and stomach.

Oral Cavity

6-1 Label the structures in Figure 6–2 as you read the material in the following frames. Chemical and mechanical processes of digestion begin in the (1) **oral cavity** (mouth) when food is chewed to make it easier to swallow.

---

stomat/o

or/o

6-2 The CFs for the mouth are *or/o* and *stomat/o*.

From *stomat/itis*, construct the CF for *mouth*: _____ / _____

From *or/al*, construct the CF for *mouth*: _____ / _____

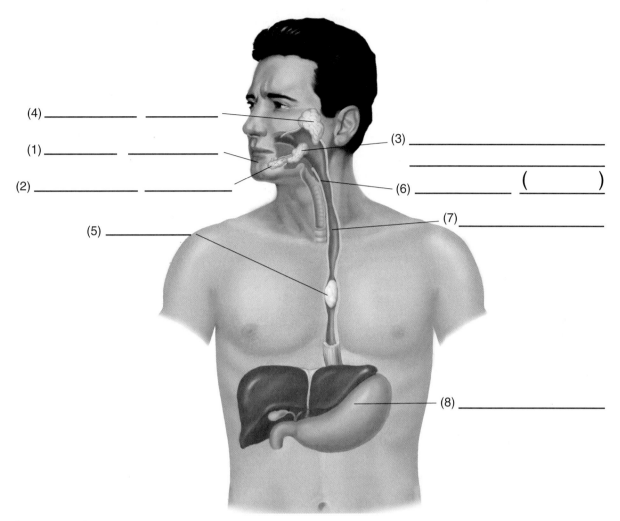

(4) _____ _____

(1) _____ _____

(2) _____ _____

(5) _____

(3) _____

_____

(6) _____ (_____)

(7) _____

(8) _____

Figure 6-2 The upper GI tract.

stomat/itis stō-mă-TĪ-tĭs	**6–3** The suffix -*itis* refers to inflammation. It is used in all body systems to describe an inflammation of a particular organ. Use **stomat/o** to form a word that means *inflammation of the mouth*: _____ / _____
pain, mouth **pain, mouth**	**6–4** The suffixes -*dynia* and -*algia* refer to pain. *Stomat/o/dynia* is a _____ in the _____. *Stomat/algia* is a _____ in the _____.
combining form *or* combining vowel	**6–5** The suffixes -*dynia* and -*algia* are used interchangeably. Because -*algia* begins with a vowel, use a word root to link the suffix. Because -*dynia* begins with a consonant, use a _____ _____ to link the suffix.

stomat/o/dynia, stomat/algia stō-mă-tō-DĬN-ē-ă, stō-mă-TĂL-jē-ă	**6-6** Use *stomat/o* to develop a word that means *pain in the mouth*. _____ / ____ / _____ *or* _____ / _____
	6-7 There are three pairs of salivary glands: the (2) **sublingual gland,** the (3) **submandibular gland,** and the (4) **parotid gland.** The salivary glands, whose primary function is to secrete saliva into the oral cavity, is richly supplied with blood vessels and nerves. Label the salivary glands in Figure 6–2.
sial/o	**6-8** During the chewing process, salivary secretions begin the chemical breakdown of food. The CF *sial/o* means *saliva, salivary glands.* From *sial/ic* (pertaining to saliva), construct the CF for *saliva* or *salivary gland.* _____ / ____
sial/itis sī-ă-LĪT-tĭs	**6-9** Use *sial/o* + *-itis* to form a word that means inflammation of a salivary gland. _____ / _____
-rrhea	**6-10** The suffix *-rrhea* is used in words to mean *discharge* or *flow.* From *sial/o/rrhea*, write the element that means *discharge, flow.* _____
saliva **flow** **saliva** **condition**	**6-11** *Sial/o/rrhea*, more commonly called *ptyal/ism* or *hyper/salivation*, refers to excessive secretion of saliva. Analyze *sial/o/rrhea* by defining the elements: *sial/o* refers to salivary glands or _____; *-rrhea* refers to discharge or _____; *ptyal/o* refers to _____; *-ism* refers to _____.
tongue	**6-12** The CF *lingu/o* means tongue. The prefix *sub-* means under. Sub/lingu/al means pertaining to under or below the _____.
jaw	**6-13** The CF *maxill/o* means *jaw.* Sub/maxill/ary is a directional term that means *under the* _____.
below **below** **above**	**6-14** Refer to Figure 6–1 and use the directional terms *below* or *above* to complete this frame. The *sub/lingu/al* gland is located _____ the tongue. The *sub/mandibul/ar* gland is located _____ the parotid gland. The tongue is located _____ the esophagus.

lingu/o	**6-15** From *sub/lingu/al*, construct the CF for *tongue*. _____ / _____
pertaining to, tongue	**6-16** *Lingu/o/dent/al* means _____ _____ *the* _____ *and teeth*.
dent	**6-17** From *lingu/o/dent/al*, determine the root for *teeth*. _____
abnormal condition, mouth	**6-18** The suffix *-osis* means *abnormal condition, increase (used primarily with blood cells)*. *Stomat/osis* literally means _____ _____ *of the* _____.
stomat/osis stō-mă-TŌ-sĭs **stomat/itis** stō-mă-TĪ-tĭs	**6-19** Use *stomat/o* to form medical words that mean *abnormal condition of the mouth:* _____ / _____ *inflammation of the mouth:* _____ / _____
myc	**6-20** *Stomat/o/myc/osis* is an abnormal condition of a mouth fungus. From *stomat/o/myc/osis*, identify the root that means *fungus*. _____
abnormal condition, fungus	**6-21** *Myc/osis* literally means _____ _____ of a _____.
abnormal condition **fungus**	**6-22** Whenever you see *-osis* in a word, you will know it means _____ _____ *or increase (used primarily with blood cells)*. Whenever you see *myc/o* in a word, you will know it refers to _____.
myc/osis mī-KŌS-sĭs	**6-23** Two types of mycoses are athlete's foot and thrush. Change the plural form *mycoses* to its singular form. _____ / _____
-logist	**6-24** The CF *log/o* means *study of*. Combine *log/o* and *-ist* to form a new suffix that means *specialist in study of*. _____

gastr/o/logist
găs-TRŎL-ō-jĭst

enter/o/logist
ĕn-tĕr-ŎL-ō-jĭst

gastr/o/enter/o/logist
găs-trō-ĕn-tĕr-ŎL-ō-jĭst

6-25 Recall *-logist* means *specialist in study of.* Specialists who treat digestive disorders are the *gastr/o/logist, enter/o/logist,* and *gastr/o/enter/o/logist.*

Build medical words that mean *specialist who treats*

stomach disorders: _____ / _____ / _____

intestin/al disorders: _____ / _____ / _____

stomach and intestin/al disorders:
_____ / _____ / _____ / _____ / _____

---

gastr/o/logy
găs-TRŎL-ō-jē

gastr/o/enter/o/logist
găs-trō-ĕn-tĕr-ŎL-ō-jĭst

6-26 Use *-logy* or *-logist* to form medical words that mean

study of stomach: _____ / _____ / _____

specialist in study of stomach and intestines:
_____ / _____ / _____ / _____ / _____

---

gastr/o/logist
găs-TRŎL-ō-jĭst

6-27 The specialist who diagnoses and treats stomach disorders is a
_____ / _____ / _____.

---

bowel movement

fasting blood sugar

diagnosis
dī-ăg-NŌ-sĭs

gastr/o/intestin/al
găs-trō-ĭn-TĔS-tĭn-ăl

6-28 Standardized abbreviations are commonly used in medical reports and insurance claims. Abbreviations are summarized at the end of each chapter and in Appendix E, Abbreviations. If needed, use one of those references to complete this frame.

BM: _____ _____

FBS: _____ _____ _____

Dx: _____

GI: _____ / _____ / _____ / _____

---

dent/o, odont/o

6-29 Most of us take our teeth for granted. We do not think about the important mechanical function they perform in the first step of the digestive process—breaking food down into smaller pieces.

The CFs for *teeth* are _____ / _____ and _____ / _____.

---

teeth, gums

6-30 A *dent/ist* specializes in the prevention, Dx, and treatment of diseases of the teeth and gums. Dentistry is the branch of medicine dealing with the care of the _____ and _____.

---

pain, tooth

odont/algia
ō-dŏn-TĂL-jē-ă

6-31 *Odont/algia* literally means _____ in a _____.

A toothache is another word for *odont/o/dynia* or _____ / _____.

specialist, teeth	**6-32** An *orth/odont/ist* is a dent/al specialist who corrects abnormal position and misalignment of the teeth. *Orth/o* means *straight. Orth/odont/ist* literally means _____ *in straight* _____.
odont **orth** **-ist**	**6-33** From *orth/odont/ist*, determine the root for *teeth:* _____ root for *straight:* _____ element that means *specialist:* _____
orth/odont/ist ŏr-thō-DŎN-tĭst	**6-34** Crooked, or misaligned, teeth require dental services of an _____ / _____ / _____ to correct the deformity.
orth/odont/ist ŏr-thō-DŎN-tĭst	**6-35** Being fitted for braces to straighten teeth requires a dent/al specialist known as an _____ / _____ / _____.
specialist **around** **teeth**	**6-36** Another dent/al specialist, the *peri/odont/ist*, treats abnormal conditions of tissues surrounding the teeth. (Use Appendix A, Glossary of Medical Word Elements, whenever you need help to work the frames.) The suffix *-ist* refers to _____. The prefix *peri-* refers to _____. The root **odont** refers to _____.
gingiv/o	**6-37** *Gingiv/itis,* a general term for *inflammation of gums,* is usually caused by accumulation of food particles in crevices between the gums and teeth. From *gingiv/itis,* construct the CF for *gums.* _____ / ____
gingiv/itis jĭn-jĭ-VĪ-tĭs	**6-38** Form a word that means *inflammation of gums.* _____ / _____
inflammation, teeth **inflammation, gums**	**6-39** Primary symptoms of gingiv/itis are bleeding gums. This condition can lead to a more serious disorder, *peri/odont/itis.* Gingiv/itis is best prevented by correct brushing of teeth and proper gum care. *Peri/odont/itis* is an _____ around the _____. *Gingiv/itis* means _____ of the _____.

gingiv/osis jĭn-jĭ-VŌ-sĭs **dent/ist** DĔN-tĭst **orth/odont/ist** ŏr-thō-DŎN-tĭst	**6-40** Develop words that mean *abnormal condition of gums:* _____ / _____ *specialist in teeth:* _____ / _____ *specialist in straightening teeth:* _____ / _____ / _____
tooth **pain, tooth**	**6-41** *Dent/algia* is a toothache. Literally, it means *pain in a* _____. *Dent/o/dynia* also means _____ in a _____.

Esophagus, Pharynx, and Stomach

	6-42 Continue labeling Figure 6–2 as you read the material in this frame. After food is chewed, it is formed into a round, sticky mass called a (5) **bolus.** The bolus is pushed by the tongue into the (6) **pharynx (throat)**, where it begins its descent down the (7) **esophagus** to the (8) **stomach.**
esophagus ē-SŎF-ă-gŭs	**6-43** In the stomach, undigested food is mixed with gastric juices to break it down further into a liquid mass called *chyme.* Name the structure that transports food from the mouth to the stomach. _____

Competency Verification: Check your labeling of Figure 6–2 with the answers in Appendix B, Answer Key, page 565.

esophag/o	**6-44** Esophag/itis can be caused by excessive acid production in the stomach. From esophag/itis, construct the CF for esophagus. _____ / ____
muc/ous MŪ-kŭs	**6-45** An ulcer is a lesion of the skin or muc/ous membrane marked by inflammation, necr/osis, and sloughing of damaged tissue. Various aggravations may produce ulcers, including trauma, drugs, infectious agents, smoking, and alcohol. A term that means pertaining to mucus is _____ / _____.
necr/osis nĕ-KRŌ-sĭs	**6-46** An insufficient blood supply may result in necr/osis of the ulcerated tissue. The CF **necr/o** means *death, necrosis.* An abnormal condition of (tissue) death is called _____ / _____.

gastr/ic ulcers GĂS-trĭk	**6–47** Peptic ulcers are open sores or lesions on the mucous membrane that lines the stomach or duodenum. They usually develop in the highly acidic regions of the stomach or duodenum. Peptic ulcers that occur in the small intestine are called *duoden/al ulcers;* peptic ulcers that occur in the stomach are called _____ / _____ _____.
gastr/itis găs-TRĪ-tĭs	**6–48** Gastr/ic ulcers may cause severe pain and inflammation of the stomach. A medical term that means *inflammation of the stomach* is _____ / _____.
gastr/algia găs-TRĂL-jē-ă	**6–49** *Gastr/o/dynia* is the medical term for *pain in the stomach.* Another term that means *pain in the stomach* is _____ / _____.
stomach	**6–50** Gastr/o/megaly and megal/o/gastr/ia mean enlargement of the _____.
megal/o/gastr/ic mĕg-ă-lō-GĂS-trĭk	**6–51** In *megal/o/gastr/ia* the suffix *-ia* is a noun ending that denotes a *condition.* Use *-ic* to change this word to an adjective. _____ / ____ / _____ / _____
endo/scopy ĕn-DŎS-kō-pē	**6–52** Endo/scopy is a visual examination of a hollow organ or cavity using a rigid or flexible fiberoptic tube and lighted optical system. (See Figure 2-5.) The term in this frame that means *visual examination in* or *within (an organ)* is _____ / _____.
duoden/o/scopy dū-ŏd-ĕ-NŎS-kō-pē	**6–53** An *endo/scope* is used to perform endo/scopy. The organ being examined dictates the name of the endoscop/ic procedure — for example, visual examination of the esophagus is *esophag/o/scopy,* of the stomach is *gastr/o/scopy,* and of the duodenum is *duoden/o/scopy.* Endo/scopy is used for bi/opsy, aspirating fluids, and coagulating bleeding areas. A laser can also be passed through the endo/scope for endoscopic surgeries. A camera or video recorder is commonly used during endo/scop/ic procedures to provide a permanent record for later reference. When the physician examines the duodenum, the endoscopic procedure is called _____ / ____ / _____.
esophag/o/scopy ē-sŏf-ă-GŎS-kō-pē	**6–54** Gastr/o/scopy is visual examination of the stomach. Build another term with *-scopy* that means *visual examination of the esophagus.* _____ / ____ / _____.

esophag/o/gastr/o/ duoden/o/scopy ĕ-SŎF-ă-gō-găs-trō-dū-ŏd-ĕ-NŎS-kō-pē	**6-55** Upper GI endoscopy, also referred to as *EGD*, includes visualization of the esophagus, stomach, and duodenum. Use Appendix E to define *EGD*. _____ / ____ / _____ / ____ / _____ / ____ / _____
gastr/ectomy găs-TRĔK-tō-mē	**6-56** Surgery is the branch of medicine concerned with diseases and trauma requiring an operative procedure. Surgery to remove all or part of the stomach is called _____ / _____.
mouth	**6-57** The suffix *-plasty* is used in words to mean *surgical repair*. *Stomat/o/plasty* is a surgical repair of the _____.
esophag/o/plasty ē-SŎF-ă-gō-plăs-tē **gastr/o/plasty** GĂS-trō-plăs-tē	**6-58** Form medical words that mean *surgical repair of the* *esophagus:* _____ / ____ / _____ *stomach:* _____ / ____ / _____

6-59 Common surgical suffixes that refer to cutting are summarized below. Review and use them to complete subsequent frames related to operative procedures.

Surgical Suffix	Meaning
-ectomy	excision, removal
-tome	instrument to cut
-tomy	incision

esophagus ē-SŎF-ă-gŭs	**6-60** Whenever you see a suffix or word with **tom** in it, relate it to an incision. *Esophag/o/tomy* is an incision through the wall of the _____.
esophag/o/tome ē-SŎF-ă-gō-tōm	**6-61** When *esophag/eal* surgery necessitates an incision, the physician will ask for an instrument called an _____ / ____ / _____.
gastr/ectomy găs-TRĔK-tō-mē	**6-62** A surgical procedure to remove all or, more commonly, part of the stomach is called a _____ / _____.
gastr **-ectomy**	**6-63** Partial or total *gastr/ectomy* is commonly performed to treat stomach cancer. From *gastr/ectomy*, identify the element that means *stomach:* _____ *excision or removal:* _____

gastr/ectomy găs-TRĔK-tō-mē	**6-64** A perforated (punctured) stomach ulcer may require a partial _____ / _____.
stomach	**6-65** A *gastr/o/tome* is an instrument to cut or incise the _____.
gastr/o/tome GĂS-trō-tōm	**6-66** When the stomach is incised, the physician uses an instrument called a _____ / _____ / _____.
esophag/us ē-SŎF-ă-gŭs	**6-67** *Esophag/o/tomy* is an incision of the _____ / _____.
gastr/o/tomy găs-TRŎT-ō-mē	**6-68** Develop a word that means *incision of the stomach.* _____ / _____ / _____
carcin/oma kăr-sĭ-NŌ-mă	**6-69** *Cancer* (CA) is a general term used to indicate various types of malignant neoplasms. Most cancers invade surrounding tissues and metastasize (spread) to other sites in the body. The CF for cancer is **carcin/o**. Combine **carcin/o** + *-oma* to build a word that means *cancerous tumor.* _____ / _____
cancer	**6-70** CA, especially sarc/oma, can recur even though the tumor is excised. Ultimately, it may cause death. Whenever you see *CA* in a medical report, you will know it means _____.
-ous	**6-71** *Cancer/ous* means *pertaining to cancer.* Identify the adjective element that means *pertaining to.* _____
cancerous *or* malignant	**6-72** A carcin/oma is a tumor that is _____.
cancer; tumor	**6-73** The largest group of carcin/omas are solid tumors derived from epithelial tissue. This is the tissue that lines the surfaces of the body. It includes the skin and the tissues that line the internal organs, including the digestive organs. Analyze *carcin/oma* by defining the elements **carcin:** _____; *-oma:* _____
gastr/itis găs-TRĪ-tĭs **epi/gastr/ic** ĕp-ĭ-GĂS-trĭk	**6-74** *Epi-* means *above, upon.* Epi/gastr/ic pain may result from an acute form of gastr/itis. Identify words in this frame that mean *inflammation of the stomach:* _____ / _____ *pertaining to above or upon the stomach:* _____ / _____ / _____

hyper/emesis hī-pĕr-ĔM-ĕ-sĭs	**6-75** *Emesis* is a term that means *vomiting;* however, it may also be used as a suffix. A symptomatic term that means *excessive vomiting* is *hyper /* _____.
hyper- **-emesis**	**6-76** *Hyper/emesis* is characterized by excessive vomiting. Unless treated, it can lead to malnutrition. Determine elements in this frame that mean *excessive, above normal:* _____ *vomiting:* _____
hemat/emesis hĕm-ăt-ĔM-ĕ-sĭs	**6-77** *Hemat/o* refers to *blood.* A patient with acute gastr/itis or a peptic ulcer may vomit blood. Build a word that means *vomiting blood.* _____ / _____
hemat/emesis hĕm-ăt-ĔM-ĕ-sĭs	**6-78** Bleeding in the stomach may be due to a gastr/ic ulcer and may cause vomiting of blood. A Dx of vomiting blood is entered in the medical record as _____ / _____.
epi/gastr/ic ĕp-ĭ-GĂS-trĭk	**6-79** A common symptom of gastr/ic disease is pain. When pain occurs in the region above the stomach, it is called *epi/gastr/ic pain.* Form a word that means *pertaining to above or on the stomach.* _____ / _____ / _____
-pepsia **dys-**	**6-80** *Dys/pepsia* literally means *painful or difficult digestion* and is a form of gastric indigestion. It is not a disease in itself but may be symptomatic of other diseases. Determine word elements in this frame that mean *digestion:* _____ *bad, painful, difficult:* _____
dys/pepsia dĭs-PĔP-sē-ă	**6-81** Over-the-counter antacids (agents that neutralize acidity) usually provide prompt relief of pain from _____ / _____.
dys/phagia dĭs-FĀ-jē-ă **bad, painful, difficult** **swallowing, eating**	**6-82** The suffix *-phagia* means *swallowing, eating.* Use *dys-* and *-phagia* to form a word that means *difficult or painful swallowing.* _____ / _____ Analyze *dys/phagia* by defining its elements: *dys-:* _____, _____, _____ *-phagia:* _____, _____

aer/o	**6-83** Swallowing air, usually followed by belching and gastric distention, is a condition known as *aer/o/phagia.* The CF for *air* is _____ / _____.
aer/o/phagia ĕr-ō-FĀ-jē-ă	**6-84** Infants have a tendency to swallow air as they suck milk from a bottle, a condition charted as _____ / _____ / _____.

SECTION REVIEW 6-2

Using the following table, write the CF, suffix, or prefix that matches its definition in the space provided to the left of the definition. There may be more than one word element that matches a definition.

Combining Forms		Suffixes		Prefixes
dent/o	odont/o	-al	-oma	an-
gastr/o	or/o	-ary	-orexia	dia-
gingiv/o	orth/o	-algia	-pepsia	dys-
gloss/o	pylor/o	-dynia	-phagia	hyper-
lingu/o	sial/o	-ic	-rrhea	hypo-
myc/o	stomat/o	-ist	-scope	peri-
			-tomy	

1. _____ tumor
2. _____ pertaining to
3. _____ around
4. _____ under, below, deficient
5. _____ discharge, flow
6. _____ fungus
7. _____ gum(s)
8. _____ pylorus
9. _____ bad; painful; difficult
10. _____ excessive, above normal
11. _____ saliva, salivary gland
12. _____ stomach
13. _____ specialist

14. _____ straight
15. _____ teeth
16. _____ through, across
17. _____ tongue
18. _____ instrument for examining
19. _____ incision
20. _____ appetite
21. _____ mouth
22. _____ pain
23. _____ swallowing, eating
24. _____ without, not
25. _____ digestion

Competency Verification: Check your answers in Appendix B, Answer Key, page 565. If you are not satisfied with your level of comprehension, go back to Frame 6–1 and rework the frames.

Correct Answers _____ × 4 = _____ % Score

WORD ELEMENTS

This section introduces CFs related to the small intestine and colon. Key suffixes are defined in the right-hand column as needed. Review the following table, and pronounce each word in the word analysis column aloud before you begin to work the frames.

Word Element	Meaning	Word Analysis
Combining Forms		

SMALL INTESTINE

duoden/o	duodenum (first part of small intestine)	**duoden**/o/scopy (dū-ŏd-ĕ-NŎS-kō-pē): visual examination of the duodenum *-scopy:* visual examination
enter/o	intestine (usually small intestine)	**enter**/o/pathy (ĕn-tĕr-ŎP-ă-thē): any intestinal disease *-pathy:* disease
jejun/o	jejunum (second part of small intestine)	**jejun**/o/rrhaphy (jĕ-joo-NOR-ă-fē): suture of the jejunum *-rrhaphy:* suture
ile/o	ileum (third part of small intestine)	**ile**/o/stomy (ĭl-ē-ŎS-tō-mē): incision of the ileum (ileotomy) and creation of a permanent opening *-stomy*:* forming an opening (mouth) *Ileostomy is performed following a total colectomy. The ileum is pulled out through the abdominal wall. The edges of the wall of the colon are rolled to make a mouth (stoma) that is then sutured to the abdominal wall. The patient wears a plastic pouch on the abdomen to collect feces.*

LARGE INTESTINE

append/o	appendix	**append**/ectomy (ăp-ĕn-DĔK-tō-mē): removal of the appendix *-ectomy:* excision, removal *Appendectomy is performed to remove a diseased appendix that is in danger of rupturing.*
appendic/o	appendix	**appendic**/itis (ă-pĕn-dĭ-SĪ-tĭs): inflammation of the appendix *-itis:* inflammation

*When the suffix *-stomy* is used with a combining form that denotes an organ, it refers to a surgical opening to the outside of the body.

(continued)

Word Element	Meaning	Word Analysis
col/o	colon	**col/o**/stomy (kō-LŎS-tō-mē): creation of an opening between the colon and the abdominal wall *-stomy:* forming an opening (mouth) *A colostomy creates a place for fecal matter to exit the body other than through the anus. It may be temporary or permanent.*
colon/o		**colon/o**/scopy (kō-lŏn-ŎS-kō-pē): visual examination of the inner surface of the colon using a long, flexible endoscope *-scopy:* visual examination
proct/o	anus, rectum	**proct/o**/logist (prŏk-TŎL-ō-jĭst): physician who specializes in treating disorders of the colon, rectum, and anus *-logist:* specialist in study of
rect/o	rectum	**rect/o**/cele (RĔK-tō-sēl): herniation or protrusion of the rectum; also called *proctocele* *-cele:* hernia, swelling
sigmoid/o	sigmoid colon	**sigmoid/o**/tomy (sĭg-moyd-ŎT-ō-mē): incision of sigmoid colon *-tomy:* incision

Listen and Learn, the audio CD-ROM included in this book, will help you master pronunciation of selected medical words. Use it to practice pronunciations of the above-listed medical terms and for instructions to complete the *Listen and Learn* exercise for this section.

SECTION REVIEW 6-3

For the following medical terms, first write the suffix and its meaning. Then translate the meaning of the remaining elements starting with the first part of the word. The first word is completed for you.

Term	Meaning
1. duoden/o/scopy	*-scopy: visual examination; duodenum (first part of small intestine)*
2. appendic/itis	_____
3. enter/o/pathy	_____
4. col/o/stomy	_____
5. rect/o/cele	_____
6. sigmoid/o/tomy	_____
7. proct/o/logist	_____
8. jejun/o/rrhaphy	_____
9. append/ectomy	_____
10. ile/o/stomy	_____

Competency Verification: Check your answers in Appendix B, Answer Key, page 565. If you are not satisfied with your level of comprehension, review the vocabulary and retake the review.

Correct Answers _____ × 10 = _____ % Score

Lower GI Tract

The lower GI tract consists of the small and large intestine as well as the anus and rectum.

Small and Large Intestine

6-85 The small intestine is a continuation of the GI tract. It is where digestion of food is completed as nutrients are absorbed into the bloodstream through tiny, fingerlike projections called *villi.* Any unabsorbed material is passed on to the large intestine to be excreted from the body. There are three parts of the small intestine: the (1) **duodenum,** the (2) **jejunum,** and the (3) **ileum.** Label these parts in Figure 6–3.

duodenum dū-ŎD-ĕ-nŭm **jejunum** jē-JŪ-nŭm **ileum** ĬL-ē-ŭm	**6–86** Here is a review of the small intestine. The CF *duoden/o* refers to the first part of the small intestine, called the _____. The CF *jejun/o* refers to the second part of the small intestine, called the _____. The CF *ile/o* refers to the third part of the small intestine, called the _____.
duoden/ectomy dū-ŏd-ĕ-NĔK-tō-mē **jejun/ectomy** jē-jū-NĔK-tō-mē **ile/ectomy** ĭl-ē-ĔK-tō-mē	**6–87** *Duoden/ectomy, jejun/ectomy,* and *ile/ectomy* are total or partial excisions of different sections of the small intestine. Build a word that means *excision of the* *duodenum:* _____ / _____ *jejunum:* _____ / _____ *ileum:* _____ / _____
duodenum, duoden/o dū-ŎD-ĕ-nŭm **jejunum, jejun/o** jē-JŪ-nŭm **ileum, ile/o** ĬL-ē-ŭm	**6–88** Name the three parts of the small intestine and their CFs. **Part** **Combining Form** 1. _____ _____ / _____ 2. _____ _____ / _____ 3. _____ _____ / _____
duodenum dū-ŎD-ĕ-nŭm	**6–89** Duoden/o/stomy is performed to form an opening (mouth) into the _____.
-stomy	**6–90** Identify the element in Frame 6–89 that means *forming an opening* *(mouth):* _____.
opening, jejunum jē-JŪ-nŭm	**6–91** Jejun/o/stomy is a surgical procedure meaning forming an _____ into the _____.
opening, ileum ĬL-ē-ŭm	**6–92** When the colon is removed because of colon CA, an ile/o/stomy is performed. The patient must wear an ile/o/stomy bag to collect fecal material from the ile/um. The surgical procedure *ile/o/stomy* means *forming an* _____ into the _____.

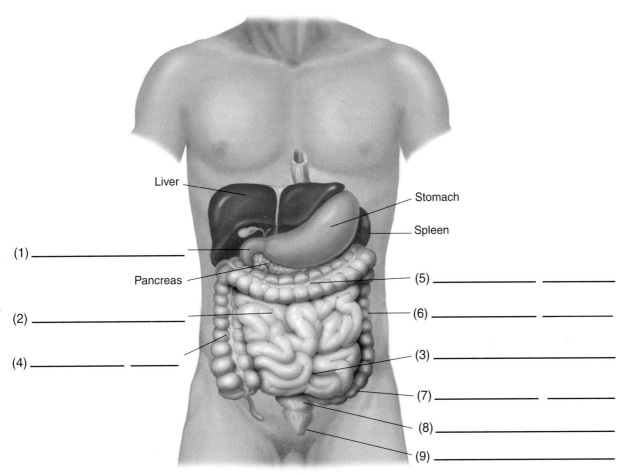

Liver

Stomach

Spleen

(1) _____

Pancreas

(5) _____ _____

(2) _____

(6) _____ _____

(4) _____ _____

(3) _____

(7) _____ _____

(8) _____

(9) _____

Figure 6-3 The small intestine and colon.

-stomy	**6–93** The medical term *stoma* refers to an opening shaped like a mouth. The suffix that means *forming an opening (mouth)* is _____.
-tomy **jejun/o/tomy** jē-jū-NŎT-ō-mē	**6–94** For patients who cannot eat by mouth, a jejun/al (pertaining to the jejunum) feeding tube is commonly placed through a jejun/o/tomy incision. The surgical suffix that means *incision* is _____. An incision of the jejunum is called _____ / _____ / _____.
duoden/o/tomy dū-ŏd-ĕ-NŎT-ō-mē	**6–95** Incision of the duodenum is called _____ / _____ / _____.
ile/o/tomy ĭl-ē-ŎT-ō-mē	**6–96** Incision of the ileum is called _____ / _____ / _____.

ileum
ĬL-ē-ŭm

suture

6–97 The suffix -rrhaphy refers to *suture* (sew). *Ile/o/rrhaphy* is performed to surgically repair the ile/um.
Analyze *ile/o/rrhaphy* by defining the elements.

ile/o: _____

-rrhaphy: _____

---

duoden/ectomy
dū-ŏd-ĕ-NĔK-tō-mē
duoden/o/rrhaphy
dū-ŏ-dĕ-NOR-ă-fē

6–98 In a bleeding duoden/al ulcer, a suture over the bleeding portion can prevent performing duoden/ectomy. Develop surgical words that mean

excision of duodenum: _____ / _____

suture of duodenum: _____ / _____ / _____

---

jejun/o/rrhaphy
jĕ-joo-NOR-ă-fē
ile/o/rrhaphy
ĭl-ē-OR-ă-fē

6–99 Form surgical words that mean *suture of*

jejunum: _____ / _____ / _____

ileum: _____ / _____ / _____

**opening
(mouth)**

6–100 The suffix -stomy means *forming an*

_____ (_____).

---

stomach, duodenum
dū-ŎD-ĕ-nŭm

6–101 Gastr/o/duoden/o/stomy is the formation of an opening

between the _____ and _____.

---

stomach, ileum
ĬL-ē-ŭm

6–102 Gastr/o/ile/o/stomy is the formation of an opening between the

_____ and _____.

---

stomach, small intestine

6–103 Anastomosis (connection between two vessels, bowel segments, or ducts) is performed to provide a connecton from one structure to another.
Gastr/o/enter/o/anastomosis is a surgical connection between the

_____ and _____ _____.

**gastr/o/enter/o/
anastomosis, gastr/o/
enter/o/stomy**
găs-trō-ĕn-tĕr-ō-
ă-năs-tō-MŌ-sĭs, găs-trō-ĕn-
tĕr-ŎS-tō-mē

6–104 Gastr/o/enter/o/anastomosis, also called *gastr/o/enter/o/stomy*, may be performed when there is a malignant or benign gastr/o/duoden/al disease.
Terms in this frame that mean *creation of a passage between the stomach and some part of the small intestine* are

_____ / _____ / _____ / _____ / _____ and

_____ / _____ / _____ / _____ / _____

-stomy	**6–105** Another type of anastomosis, *gastr/o/duoden/o/stomy* (see Figure 2-7), is a procedure in which the lower part of the stomach is excised, and the remainder is anastomosed to the duodenum. The element in this frame that means *forming an opening (mouth)* is _____.
ileum ĬL-ē-ŭm	**6–106** Most absorption of food takes place in the third part of the small intestine, which is the _____.
inflammation, ileum ĬL-ē-ŭm	**6–107** *Crohn disease*, a chronic inflammation of the ile/um, may affect any part of the intestinal tract. It is distinguished from closely related bowel disorders by its inflammatory pattern; it is also called *regional ile/itis.* *Ile/itis* is a(n) _____ of the _____.
enter/o	**6–108** Enter/al means pertaining to the intestine (usually the small intestine). From *enter/al,* construct the CF for *intestine.* _____ / _____
enter/ectomy ĕn-tĕr-ĔK-tō-mē **enter/o/rrhaphy** ĕn-tĕr-OR-ă-fē	**6–109** Build medical terms that mean *excision of intestine (usually small):* _____ / _____ *suture of intestine (such as an intestinal wound):* _____ / _____ / _____
inflammation, intestine	**6–110** *Enter/itis* is an _____ of the _____ (usually small).
enter/itis ĕn-tĕr-Ī-tĭs	**6–111** Crohn disease is distinguished from closely related bowel disorders by its inflammatory pattern. It is also known as *regional enter/itis.* Form a word that means *inflammation of the intestine.* _____ / _____
	6–112 Continue labeling Figure 6–3 as you read the following: The large intestine, also called the colon, extends from the ileum of the small intestine to the anus. The colon consists of four segments: (4) **ascending colon**, (5) **transverse colon**, (6) **descending colon**, and (7) **sigmoid colon**.
col/ectomy kō-LĔK-tō-mē **col/itis** kō-LĪ-tĭs **col/o/tomy** kō-LŎT-ō-mē	**6–113** The CF *col/o* refers to the *colon.* Form medical words that mean *excision of colon:* _____ / _____ *inflammation of colon:* _____ / _____ *incision into colon:* _____ / _____ / _____

col/o/stomy
kō-LŎS-tō-mē

col/o/rrhaphy
kō-LOR-ă-fē

6–114 *Col/o/stomy* is the surgical creation of an opening into the colon (through the surface of the abdomen). It may be temporary or permanent and may be performed as treatment for CA or diverticul/itis. Col/o/stomy allows elimination of feces into a bag attached to the skin. (See Figure 6–4.) Build medical terms that mean

forming an opening (mouth) into the colon: _____ / _____ / _____

suture of the colon: _____ / _____ / _____

6–115 Absorption of water by the colon changes intestin/al contents from a fluid to a more solid consistency known as *feces* or *stool.* Use your medical dictionary to define *feces.*

_____

_____

liver

spleen

6–116 The ascending colon is located superior to the cecum. (See Figure 6–1.) It curves horizontally at the hepatic flexure and descends at the splenic flexure.

Name the organ that is in close proximity to the

hepat/ic flexure: _____

splen/ic flexure: _____

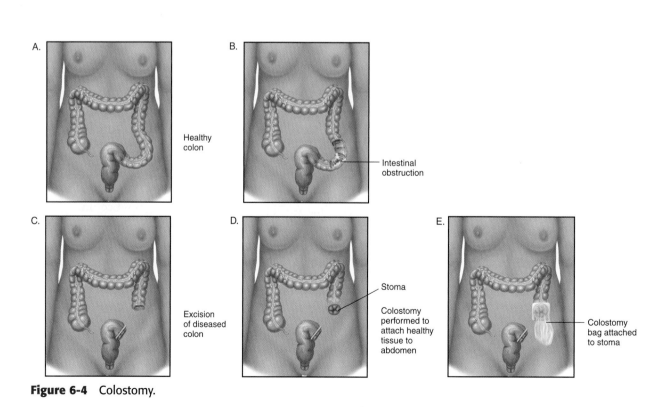

A.

Healthy colon

B.

Intestinal obstruction

C.

Excision of diseased colon

D.

Stoma

Colostomy performed to attach healthy tissue to abdomen

E.

Colostomy bag attached to stoma

Figure 6-4 Colostomy.

6-117 The sigmoid colon is *S*-shaped and extends from the descending colon into the (8) **rectum**. The rectum terminates in the lower opening of the gastrointestinal tract, the (9) **anus**. Label Figure 6–3 to identify and locate the rectum and anus.

---

sigmoid/o	**6-118** Sigmoid/ectomy, an excision of all or part of the sigmoid colon, is most commonly performed to remove a malignant tumor. A large percentage of lower bowel cancers occur in the sigmoid colon. From *sigmoid/ectomy*, construct the CF for *sigmoid colon*. _____ / _____
sigmoid/itis sĭg-moyd-Ī-tĭs	**6-119** Form a term that means *inflammation of the sigmoid colon*. _____ / _____

Competency Verification: Check your labeling of Figure 6–3 with the answers in Appendix B, Answer Key, page 566.

Rectum and Anus

inflammation, rectum RĔK-tŭm	**6-120** The CF **rect/o** refers to the *rectum*. *Rect/itis* is a(n) _____ of the _____.
inflammation, rectum, colon RĔK-tŭm, KŌ-lŏn	**6-121** *Rect/o/col/itis* is a(n) _____ of the _____ and _____.
pain	**6-122** *Proct/algia* refers to a neur/o/logic/al pain in or around the anus or lower rectum, which is also called *rect/algia*. Whenever you see *-algia* in a term, you will know it means _____.
surgical repair, rectum RĔK-tŭm	**6-123** *Rect/o/plasty* is a _____ _____ of the _____.
pertaining to, rectum RĔK-tŭm	**6-124** *Rect/o/vagin/al* means _____ _____ the _____ and vagina.
through, across **discharge, flow**	**6-125** *Dia-* is a prefix that means *through, across*. *Dia/rrhea* refers to frequent passage of watery bowel movements. Analyze *dia/rrhea* by defining the elements. *dia-:* _____, _____ *-rrhea:* _____, _____

dia/rrhea dī-ă-RĒ-ă	**6-126** A patient with an irritable bowel (IB) may experience frequent passage of watery bowel movements or have symptoms of a condition called _____ / _____.
dia/rrhea dī-ă-RĒ-ă	**6-127** Some foods, such as prunes, are likely to cause _____ / _____.
stenosis stĕ-NŌ-sĭs	**6-128** *Stenosis* refers to a narrowing or stricture of a passageway or orifice. This condition may result in an obstruction. *Stenosis* may also be used as a suffix. A narrowing or stricture of the pylorus is called pyloric _____.
rect/o **-stenosis**	**6-129** *Rect/o/stenosis* is a narrowing or stricture of the rectum. Determine elements in this frame that mean *rectum:* _____ / _____ *narrowing, stricture:* _____
proct/itis prŏk-TĪ-tĭs	**6-130** The CF **proct/o** refers to the *anus* and *rectum*. Locate the anus and rectum in Figure 6–1. Inflammation of the anus and rectum is known as _____ / _____.
rectum, anus RĔK-tŭm, Ā-nŭs	**6-131** *Proct/o/dynia* is a pain in the _____ and _____.
proct/algia prŏk-TĂL-jē-ă	**6-132** Use *-algia* to form another word that means *pain in the rectum and anus.* _____ / _____
rectum RĔK-tŭm **rectum, anus** RĔK-tŭm, Ā-nŭs	**6-133** The word *spasm* refers to an involuntary contraction or twitching. It is also used in medical words as a suffix. *Rect/o/spasm* is an involuntary contraction of the _____. *Proct/o/spasm* is an involuntary contraction of the _____ and _____.
path/o/log/ical păth-ō-LŎJ-ĭ-kăl	**6-134** *Endo/scopy* is an important tool in establishing or confirming a Dx or detecting a path/o/log/ical condition. A video recorder is commonly used during an endo/scop/ic procedure to guide the endo/scope and document abnormalities. Determine the word in this frame that means *study of disease.* _____ / _____ / _____ / _____

colon/o/scopy kō-lŏn-ŎS-kō-pē **proct/o/scopy** prŏk-TŎS-kō-pē	**6-135** The organ being examined dictates the name of the endoscopic procedure. Visual examination of colon is called *col/o/scopy* or _____ / _____ / _____. Visual examination of anus and rectum is called _____ / _____ / _____.
sigmoid colon SĬG-moyd KŌ-lŏn **visual examination**	**6-136** Sigmoid/o/scopy is used to screen for colon cancer. (See Figure 6–5.) The American Cancer Society recommends a first sigmoid/o/scopy after age 50. It is done sooner if there is a family history (FH) of colon cancer. Analyze *sigmoid/o/scopy* by defining its elements. The CF **sigmoid/o** means _____ _____. The suffix *-scopy* means _____ _____.
sigmoid/o/scopy sĭg-moy-DŎS-kō-pē	**6-137** To examine an abnormality in the colon, the physician performs a visual examination of the sigmoid colon called a _____ / _____ / _____.

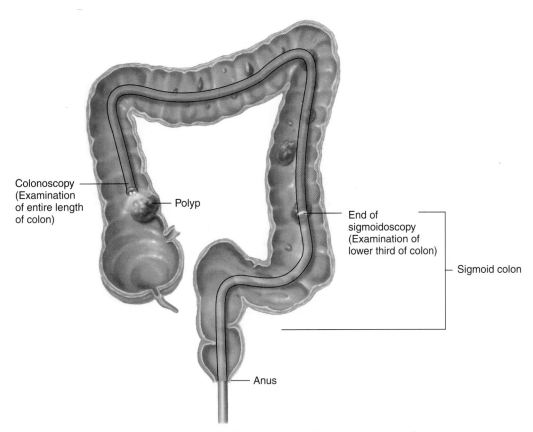

Figure 6-5 Sigmoidoscopy and colonoscopy. A colonoscopy involves examination of the entire length of the colon; a sigmoidoscopy involves examination of only the lower third of the colon.

sigmoid/o/scope
sĭg-MOY-dō-skōp

6-138 A sigmoid/o/scope, a flexible fiberoptic tube that permits transmission of light to visualize images around curves and corners, is placed through the anus to visualize part of the gastro/intestin/al tract.

To examine the colon, the physician uses a flexible fiberoptic instrument called a _____ / _____ / _____.

sigmoid/ectomy
sĭg-moyd-ĔK-tō-mē
carcin/oma
kăr-sĭ-NŌ-mă

6-139 The sigmoid colon is *S*-shaped and is the last part of the colon. (See Figure 6–5.) Sigmoid/ectomy is most commonly performed for carcin/oma of the sigmoid colon.

Identify words in this frame that mean

excision of sigmoid colon: _____ / _____

cancerous tumor: _____ / _____

examination, colon
KŌ-lŏn

6-140 A col/o/scopy is commonly referred to as a *colon/o/scopy*. Both terms mean *visual* _____ *of the* _____.

colon/itis
kō-lŏn-ī-tĭs
colon/o/scope
kō-LŎN-ō-skōp
colon/o/scopy
kō-lŏn-ŎS-kō-pē

6-141 Use *colon/o* to form medical words that mean

inflammation of colon: _____ / _____

instrument to examine colon: _____ / _____ / _____

visual examination of colon: _____ / _____ / _____

enter/o/scopy
ĕn-tĕr-ŎS-kō-pē

6-142 Enter/o/scopy is used to examine the small intestine. A visual examination of the intestines is known as a(n) _____ / _____ / _____.

enter/o/scope
ĔN-tĕr-ō-skōp

6-143 When there is a need to examine the intestine, the physician uses a(n) _____ / _____ / _____.

duoden/o/scopy
dū-ŏd-ĕ-NŎS-kō-pē
sigmoid/o/scopy
sĭg-moy-DŎS-kō-pē
gastr/o/scopy
găs-TRŎS-kō-pē

6-144 Use *-scopy* to form medical words that mean *visual examination of the*

duodenum: _____ / _____ / _____

sigmoid colon: _____ / _____ / _____

stomach: _____ / _____ / _____

S E C T I O N   R E V I E W   6-4

Using the following table, write the CF or suffix that matches its definition in the space provided to the left of the definition. There may be more than one word element that matches a definition.

Combining Forms		Suffixes	
col/o	jejun/o	-rrhaphy	-stomy
colon/o	proct/o	-scopy	-tome
duoden/o	rect/o	-spasm	-tomy
enter/o	sigmoid/o	-stenosis	
ile/o			

1. _____ intestine (usually small intestine)
2. _____ instrument to cut
3. _____ rectum
4. _____ involuntary contraction, twitching
5. _____ ileum (third part of small intestine)
6. _____ visual examination
7. _____ jejunum (second part of small intestine)
8. _____ colon
9. _____ duodenum (first part of small intestine)
10. _____ forming an opening (mouth)
11. _____ anus, rectum
12. _____ narrowing, stricture
13. _____ suture
14. _____ incision
15. _____ sigmoid colon

Competency Verification: Check your answers in Appendix B, Answer Key, page 566. If you are not satisfied with your level of comprehension, go back to Frame 6–85 and rework the frames.

   Correct Answers _____ × 6.67 = _____ % Score

WORD ELEMENTS

This section introduces CFs related to the accessory organs of digestion. Included are key suffixes; prefixes are defined in the right-hand column as needed. Review the following table and pronounce each word in the word analysis column aloud before you begin to work the frames.

Word Elements	Meaning	Word Analysis
Combining Forms		
cholangi/o	bile vessel	**cholangi**/ole (kō-LĂN-jē-ōl): small terminal portion of the bile duct *-ole:* small, minute
chol/e*	bile, gall	**chol**/e/lith (kō-lē-LĬTH): gallstone *-lith:* stone, calculus
cholecyst/o	gallbladder	**cholecyst**/ectomy (kō-lē-sĭs-TĔK-tō-mē): removal of gallbladder by laparoscopic or open surgery *-ectomy:* excision, removal *Cholecystectomy can be performed by open surgery or laparoscopically (placing a tube into the abdomen).*
choledoch/o	bile duct	**choledoch**/o/tomy (kō-lĕd-ō-KŎT-ō-mē): incision of the common bile duct *-tomy:* incision
hepat/o	liver	**hepat**/itis (hĕp-ă-TĪ-tĭs): inflammation of the liver *-itis:* inflammation
pancreat/o	pancreas	**pancreat**/o/lysis (păn-krē-ă-TŎL-ĭ-sĭs): destruction of pancreas by pancreatic enzymes *-lysis:* separation; destruction; loosening
Suffixes		
-iasis	abnormal condition (produced by something specified)	chol/e/lith/**iasis** (kō-lē-lĭ-THĪ-ă-sĭs): presence or formation of gallstones *chol/e:* bile, gall *lith/o:* stone, calculus
-megaly	enlargement	hepat/o/**megaly** (hĕp-ă-tō-MĔG-ă-lē): enlargement of the liver *hepat/o:* liver *Hepatomegaly may be caused by infection; fatty infiltration, as in alcoholism; biliary obstruction; or malignancy.*

*Using the combining vowel *e* instead of *o* is an exception to the rule.

Word Elements	Meaning	Word Analysis
-osis	abnormal condition; increase (used primarily with blood cells)	cirrh/**osis** (sĭr-RŌ-sĭs):abnormal condition of yellowness *Cirrhosis is a chronic liver disease characterized by destruction of liver cells. It eventually leads to impaired liver function and jaundice.*
-prandial	meal	post/**prandial** (pōst-PRĂN-dē-ăl): following a meal *post-:* after, behind

Listen and Learn, the audio CD-ROM included in this book, will help you master pronunciation of selected medical words. Use it to practice pronunciations of the above-listed medical terms and for instructions to complete the *Listen and Learn* exercise for this section.

S E C T I O N   R E V I E W   6 - 5

For the following medical terms, first write the suffix and its meaning. Then translate the meaning of the remaining elements starting with the first part of the word. The first word is completed for you.

Term	Meaning
1. hepat/itis	*-itis: inflammation; liver*
2. hepat/o/megaly	
3. chol/e/lith	
4. cholangi/ole	
5. cholecyst/ectomy	
6. post/prandial	
7. chol/e/lith/iasis	
8. choledoch/o/tomy	
9. pancreat/o/lith	
10. pancreat/o/lysis	

Competency Verification: Check your answers in Appendix B, Answer Key, page 566. If you are not satisfied with your level of comprehension, review the vocabulary and retake the review.

Correct Answers _____ × 10 = _____ % Score

Accessory Organs of Digestion

The accessory organs of digestion include the liver, gallbladder, and pancreas.

6-145 Label Figure 6–6 as you learn about the accessory organs of digestion.

Even though food does not pass through the (1) **liver,** (2) **gallbladder,** and (3) **pancreas,** these organs play a vital role in proper digestion and absorption of nutrients. The gallbladder serves as a storage site for bile, which is produced by the liver. When bile is needed for digestion, the gallbladder releases it through ducts into the (4) **duodenum** through the (5) **common bile duct.**

The three accessory organs of digestion are the _____, _____ and _____.

liver, gallbladder, pancreas

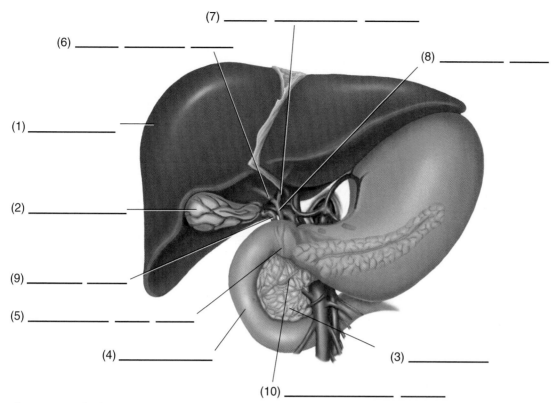

(7) _____ _____ _____
(6) _____ _____ _____
(8) _____ _____
(1) _____
(2) _____
(9) _____ _____
(5) _____ _____ _____
(4) _____
(3) _____
(10) _____ _____

Figure 6-6   The liver, gallbladder, pancreas, and duodenum with associated ducts and blood vessels.

hepat/o **cholecyst/o** **pancreat/o**	**6–146** Construct CFs for *liver:* _____ / _____ *gallbladder:* _____ / _____ *pancreas:* _____ / _____

Liver

hepat/itis hĕp-ă-TĪ-tĭs	**6–147** Hepat/itis, an inflammatory condition of the liver, may be caused by bacteri/al or viral infection, parasitic infestation, alcohol, drugs, toxins, or transfusion of incompatible blood. It may be mild and brief or severe and life-threatening. When a person has inflammation of the liver caused by a virus, the Dx is most likely _____ / _____.
hepat/o/megaly hĕp-ă-tō-MĔG-ă-lē	**6–148** Hepat/itis may be characterized by an enlarged liver. The medical term for enlarged liver is _____ / _____ / _____.
hepat/oma hĕp-ă-TŌ-mă	**6–149** Hepat/o/megaly may be a symptom of a rare malignant tumor of the liver called *hepat/oma*. The tumor occurs most commonly in association with hepat/itis or liver cirrh/osis. The Dx of a liver tumor is charted _____ / _____.

hepat/itis
hĕp-ă-TĪ-tĭs

6-150 Hepatitis B, the most common infectious hepatitis seen in hospitals, is transferred by blood and body secretions. As a preventive measure, hospital personnel are usually required to be vaccinated.

The medical term for inflammation of the liver is

_____ / _____.

hepat/o/dynia, hepat/algia
hĕp-ă-tō-DĬN-ē-ă, hĕp-ă-TĂL-jē-ă

hepat/o/rrhaphy
hĕp-ă -TŎR-ă-fē

hepat/ectomy
hĕp-ă-TĔK-tō-mē

6-151 Form medical words that mean

pain in the liver: _____ / _____ / _____ or

_____ / _____

suture of the liver: _____ / _____ / _____

excision of (a portion) of the liver: _____ / _____

hepat/o/cyte
HĔP-ă-tō-sīt

6-152 Combine *hepat/o* and *-cyte* to form a word that means *liver cell.*

_____ / _____ / _____

6-153 Identify and label the following structures in Figure 6–6 as you read about the accessory organs of digestion. Bile is released from the gallbladder and also drained directly from the liver through the (6) **right hepatic duct** and the (7) **left hepatic duct.** These two ducts eventually form the (8) **hepatic duct.** The (9) **cystic duct** merges with the hepatic duct to form the common bile duct and the (10) **pancreatic duct.** These ducts carry their digestive juices into the duodenum.

hepat/ic
hĕ-PĂT-ĭk

cyst/ic
SĬS-tĭk

pancreat/ic
păn-krē-ĂT-ĭk

6-154 Use *-ic* to form medical words that mean *pertaining to the*

liver: _____ / _____

bladder: _____ / _____

pancreas: _____ / _____

hepat/ic, cyst/ic, pancreat/ic
hĕ-PĂT-ĭk, SĬS-tĭk, păn-krē-ĂT-ĭk

6-155 Refer to Frame 6–154 to write the names of the ducts responsible for transporting digestive juices: _____ / _____,

_____ / _____, _____ / _____, and the

common bile duct.

Competency Verification: Check your labeling of Figure 6–6 in Appendix B, Answer Key, page 566.

Gallbladder

vomiting	**6-156** The CF *chol/e* means *bile, gall. Chol/emesis* means _____ bile.
cholecyst/o	**6-157** Bile, also called *gall,* is a yellow-green bitter secretion produced by the liver and stored in the gallbladder. It receives its color from the presence of bile pigments such as bilirubin. Bile passes from the gallbladder through the common bile duct into the small intestine. Bile emulsifies (breaks down) fats and prepares them for further digestion and absorption in the small intestine. Combine *chol/e* and *cyst/o* to develop the CF _____ / ____.
gallbladder	**6-158** *Cholecyst/itis* is an inflammation of the _____.
o	**6-159** The vowel *e* in *chol/e* is an exception to the rule of using an _____ as a connecting vowel.
bile, gall **vomiting**	**6-160** When a patient vomits bile, the condition is called *chol/emesis.* Analyze *chol/emesis* by defining the elements. The CF *chol/e* refers to _____ or _____. The suffix *-emesis* refers to _____.
liver	**6-161** The suffix *-lith* is used in words to mean stone or calculus. A *hepat/o/lith* is a stone or calculus in the _____.
pancreat/o/lith păn-krē-ĂT-ō-lĭth **cholecyst/o/lith** kō-lē-SĬS-tō-lĭth **hepat/o/lith** hĕp-Ă-tō-lĭth	**6-162** Form medical words that mean *stone or calculus in the* *pancreas:* _____ / ____ / _____ *gallbladder:* _____ / ____ / _____ *liver:* _____ / ____ / _____
chol/e	**6-163** *Chol/e/liths* are gallstones. Unless they obstruct a biliary duct, the stones may or may not cause symptoms. Exact causes of gallstones are unknown; however, they occur more commonly in women, elderly people, and obese persons. Figure 6–7 illustrates sites of gallstones. From *chol/e/lith,* determine the CF that means *bile, gall.* _____ / ____

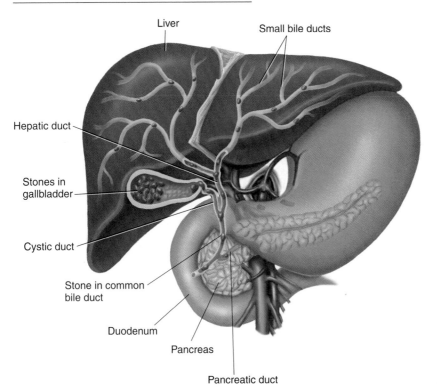

Liver

Small bile ducts

Hepatic duct

Stones in gallbladder

Cystic duct

Stone in common bile duct

Duodenum

Pancreas

Pancreatic duct

Figure 6-7   Cholelithiasis and choledocholithiasis.

chol/e/lith kō-lĕ-LĬTH **right upper quadrant**	**6-164** The most common type of gallstone contains cholesterol. These calculi are formed in the gallbladder or bile ducts. Calculi may cause jaund/ice, RUQ pain, obstruction, and inflammation of the gallbladder. The medical name for *gallstone* is _____ / _____ / _____. *RUQ* means _____ _____ _____.
cholang/oma kō-lăn-jē-Ō-mă	**6-165** A bil/i/ary duct, also called a *bile duct*, may become inflamed from a chol/e/lith. The CF *cholangi/o* refers to a bile vessel. *A tumor of the bile vessel* is called _____ / _____.
cholangi/o/graphy kō-lăn-jē-ŎG-ră-fē	**6-166** The Dx of *cholang/itis* is determined by ultrasound evaluation and cholangi/o/graphy. The radiographic procedure in this frame for outlining the major bile vessel is _____ / _____ / _____.
bile duct	**6-167** The CF *choledoch/o* means *bile duct*. A *choledoch/o/lith* is a stone in the _____ _____.
choledoch/o	**6-168** *Choledoch/o/lith/iasis* refers to the formation of a stone in the common bile duct, as illustrated in Figure 6–7. The CF for *bile duct* is _____ / _____.

choledoch/itis kō-lĕ-dō-KĪ-tĭs **choledoch/o/rrhaphy** kō-lĕd-ō-KŌR-ă-fē **choledoch/o/plasty** kō-LĔD-ō-kō-plăs-tē	**6-169** Use *choledoch/o* (bile duct) to develop medical words that mean *inflammation of the bile duct:* _____ / _____ *suture of the bile duct:* _____ / ____ / _____ *surgical repair of the bile duct:* _____ / ____ / _____
stone, calculus, bile duct	**6-170** *Choledoch/o/lith* is a _____ or _____ in the common _____ _____.
choledoch/o/lith kō-LĔD-ō-kō-līth **choledoch/o/rrhaphy** kō-lĕd-ō-KŌR-ă-fē **choledoch/o/tomy** kō-lĕd-ō-KŎT-ō-mē	**6-171** When a stone is trapped in the common bile duct, the duct may require an incision to remove the stone. Once the stone is removed, the duct is sutured. Form medical words that mean *stone in the bile duct:* _____ / ____ / _____ *suture of the bile duct:* _____ / ____ / _____ *incision of the bile duct:* _____ / ____ / _____
gallbladder	**6-172** Locate the gallbladder, also known as *cholecyst,* in Figure 6–6. This pouchlike structure is used to store bile, which is produced by the liver. *Cholecyst* is the medical name for _____.
cholecyst/itis kō-lē-sĭs-TĪ-tĭs	**6-173** Inflammation of the gallbladder may be caused by the presence of gallstones. The Dx *inflammation of gallbladder* is charted as _____ / _____.
gallstone	**6-174** A *chole/lith* is a _____.
stone, calculus KĂL-kū-lŭs	**6-175** The pancreat/ic duct transports pancreatic juices to the duodenum to help the digestive process. A *pancreat/o/lith* is a _____ or _____ within the pancreas.
pancreat/o **-lith**	**6-176** From *pancreat/o/lith,* identify the CF for *pancreas:* _____ / ____ Element that means *stone or calculus:* _____

stone, calculus KĂL-kū-lŭs	**6–177** *Lith/o* is also used in words as a CF that means *stone*, or *calculus*. Whenever you see *-lith* or **lith/o,** you will know that both elements mean _____ or _____.
stone, calculus KĂL-kū-lŭs	**6–178** The suffixes *-osis* and *-iasis* are used to indicate an abnormal or diseased condition. The difference between the two is that *-osis* is used to denote a disorder but does not indicate the specific cause of the abnormality. In contrast, *-iasis* is attached to a word root to identify an abnormal condition produced by something that is specified.* For example, *lith/iasis* is an abnormal condition produced by a _____ or _____.
liver	**6–179** *Hepat/osis* is an abnormal or diseased condition of the _____. The cause of the abnormality is not specified and could be the result of any number of liver diseases.
lith/iasis lĭth-Ī-ă-sĭs **pancreat/o/lith/iasis** păn-krē-ă-tō-lĭ-THĪ-ă-sĭs	**6–180** When forming a word that means *abnormal condition of stones, or calculi,* use *-iasis* because the abnormal condition is produced by something specified.* In this case, it is produced by the stones. Use *-iasis* to construct medical words that mean *abnormal condition of stones:* _____ / _____ *pancreat/ic stones:* _____ / _____ / _____ / _____
chol/e/lith/iasis kō-lē-lĭ-THĪ-ă-sĭs	**6–181** Chol/e/lith/iasis is common in obese women who are older than age 40. (See Figure 6–7.) A person who has an abnormal or diseased condition of gallstones suffers from _____ / _____ / _____ / _____.

> In some instances, you will find that *-osis* and *-iasis* are interchangeable. Whenever you are in doubt about which suffix to use, refer to your medical dictionary.

inflammation **gallbladder**	**6–182** Acute cholecyst/itis commonly leads to infection of the gallbladder and duct. Analyze *cholecyst/itis* by defining the elements. The suffix *-itis* refers to _____. The CF **cholecyst/o** refers to the _____.

*There are a few exceptions to this rule.

cholecyst/itis kō-lē-sĭs-TĬ-tĭs	**6-183** *Cholecyst/itis* is an inflammation of the gallbadder, usually caused by obstruction of gallstones in the bil/i/ary ducts. The disease is marked by pain in the RUQ of the abdomen. Usually, pain develops shortly after a meal and radiates to the shoulder and back. Use ***cholecyst/o*** to form medical words that mean *inflammation of the gallbladder:* _____ / _____
cholecyst/o/dynia, **cholecyst/algia** kō-lē-sĭs-tō-DĬN-ē-ă, kō-lē- sĭs-TĂL-jē-ă	*pain in the gallbladder:* _____ / ____ / _____ or _____ / _____
cholecyst/o/lith/iasis kŏ-lē-sĭs-tō-lĭ-THĬ-ă-sĭs	*abnormal condition of gallbladder stone(s):* _____ / ____ / _____ / _____

	6-184 *Chol/e/cyst/ectomy* is performed by *lapar/o/scop/ic* or open surgery. If bile ducts are obstructed, a classic "gallbladder attack," more properly referred to as *bili/ary colic*, results in pain in the RUQ. Nausea and vomiting may accompany the attack. Form medical terms that mean
cholecyst/ectomy kō-lē-sĭs-TĔK-tō-mē	*excision of the gallbladder:* _____ / _____
bil/i/ary BĬL-ē-ār-ē	*pertaining to bile or gall:* _____ / _____ / _____
lapar/o/scop/ic lăp-ă-rō-SKŎP-ĭk	*pertaining to visual examination of the abdomen:* _____ / ____ / _____ / _____

Pancreas

pancreat/ectomy păn-krē-ă-TĔK-tō-mē	**6-185** Because of its critical function of producing insulin and digestive enzymes, a complete excision of the pancreas is not usually performed. When excision of the pancreas is indicated, the surgeon performs a _____ / _____.

pancreat/ectomy păn-krē-ă-TĔK-tō-mē	**6-186** *Pancreat/ic CA* is an extremely lethal disease. Surgery is performed for relief, but it is not a cure for the CA. When part or all of the pancreas is removed, the surgeon performs a _____ / _____.

cholecyst/ectomy kō-lē-sĭs-TĔK-tō-mē	**6-187** Because the gallbladder performs no function except storage, it is not essential for life. When the gallbladder is excised, the surgical procedure is called _____ / _____.

esophag/o/plasty
ē-SŎF-ă-gō-plăs-tē

choledoch/o/plasty
kō-LĚD-ō-kō-plăs-tē

6-188 Plastic surgery is the specialty for restoration, repair, or reconstruction of body structures.

Develop operative terms that mean *repair of the*

esophagus: _____ / _____ / _____

bile duct: _____ / _____ / _____

---

discharge, flow

6-189 The suffix *-rrhea* refers to a _____ *or* _____.

---

dia/rrhea
dī-ă-RĒ-ă

6-190 Dia/rrhea is an abnormally frequent discharge of semisolid or fluid fecal matter from the intestine. Continuous passage of loose, watery stools most likely would be diagnosed as _____ / _____.

---

dia/rrhea
dī-ă-RĒ-ă

6-191 Frequent passage of watery bowel movements results in a condition known as _____ / _____.

---

dia/rrhea
dī-ă-RĒ-ă

6-192 Dia/rrhea is usually a symptom of an underlying disorder. *Irritable bowel syndrome*, GI tumors, or an inflammatory bowel disease may also cause _____ / _____.

---

therm/o/meter
thĕr-MŎM-ĕ-tĕr

6-193 A *therm/o/meter* is an instrument for measuring degrees of heat or cold. Normal temperature taken orally ranges from about 97.6° F to 99.6° F. Infection, malignancy, severe trauma, and drugs may cause fever. However, other conditions may also cause an elevated temperature. The CF *therm/o* refers to *heat*. The instrument used to determine body temperature is called a _____ / _____ / _____.

---

poison

6-194 *Poison* is any substance taken into the body by ingestion, inhalation, injection, or absorption that interferes with normal physiological function. Common elements used to refer to poison are *tox/o, toxic/o,* and *-toxic.* Whenever you see any of these elements in a word, you will know that the element refers to _____.

---

toxic/o/logy
tŏks-ĭ-KŎL-ō-jē

6-195 Virtually any substance can be poisonous if consumed in sufficient quantity. The term *poison* usually implies an excessive degree of a tox/ic dosage, rather than a specific group of substances. Aspirin is not usually thought of as a poison, but overdoses of this drug can result in the accidental death of a child.

Form a word that means *study of poisons.*

_____ / _____ / _____

abnormal condition, poison **toxic/o, tox/o**	**6–196** *Toxic/osis* literally means _____ _____ of _____. The CF for *poison* is _____ / _____ or _____ / _____.
toxic/o/logy tŏks-ĭ-KŎL-ō-jē	**6–197** Substances that impair health or destroy life when ingested, inhaled, or absorbed by the body in relatively small amounts are considered *tox/ic* substances. Identifying the tox/ic substance is critical to expeditious treatment. Scientific study of poisons is known as _____ / _____ / _____.
ultra/son/o/graphy ūl-tră-sŏn-ŎG-ră-fē	**6–198** The suffix *-gram* is used in words to mean *record, writing*. The suffix *-graphy* is used in words to mean *process of recording*. *Ultra/son/o/graphy* (US) is the process of imaging deep structures of the body by recording reflection of high-frequency sound waves (ultrasound) and displaying the reflected echoes on a monitor. US is also called *ultrasound* and *echo*. When confirmation of a suspected disease or tumor is needed, the physician may order the radi/o/graph/ic imaging procedure called *ultrasound*, also known as _____ / _____ / _____ / _____ (US).

	6–199 Adjective and noun suffixes are attached to roots to indicate a part of speech. Some adjective suffixes that mean *pertaining to* (such as *-ile, -ior,* and *-ous*) were previously introduced. Noun suffixes that mean *condition* (such as *-ia, -ism,* and *-ist*) were also introduced. See if you can identify the part of speech for the following terms. The first one is completed for you.	
adjective	pen/ile	*adjective* _____
adjective	cutane/ous	_____
noun	gastr/o/log/ist	_____
noun	thyroid/ism	_____
noun	pneumon/ia	_____
adjective	poster/ior	_____

gastr/o/megaly găs-trō-MĔG-ă-lē	**6–200** Use *-megaly* to build a word that means *enlargement of the stomach*. _____ / _____ / _____
hepat/o/megaly hĕp-ă-tō-MĔG-ă-lē	**6–201** Hepat/o/megaly may be caused by hepat/itis or another condition, such as fatty infiltration caused by alcoholism; bil/i/ary obstruction; or malignancy. The term used in the Dx of an enlargement of the liver is _____ / _____ / _____.

S E C T I O N   R E V I E W   6-6

Using the following table, write the combining form or suffix that matches its definition in the space provided to the left of the definition. There may be more than one word element that matches a definition.

Combining Forms		Suffixes		
chol/e	pancreat/o	-algia	-graphy	-plasty
cholecyst/o	therm/o	-dynia	-iasis	-rrhaphy
choledoch/o	toxic/o	-ectomy	-lith	-stomy
cyst/o	tox/o	-emesis	-megaly	-toxic
hepat/o		-gram	-osis	

1. _____ abnormal condition; increase (used primarily with blood cells)
2. _____ abnormal condition (produced by something specified)
3. _____ bile duct
4. _____ bile, gall
5. _____ bladder
6. _____ enlargement
7. _____ excision, removal
8. _____ forming an opening (mouth)
9. _____ gallbladder
10. _____ heat
11. _____ liver
12. _____ pain
13. _____ pancreas
14. _____ poison
15. _____ process of recording
16. _____ record, writing
17. _____ stone, calculus
18. _____ surgical repair
19. _____ suture
20. _____ vomiting

Competency Verification: Check your answers in Appendix B, Answer Key, page 567. If you are not satisfied with your level of comprehension, go back to Frame 6–145 and rework the frames.

Correct Answers _____ × 5 = _____ % Score

Abbreviations

This section introduces digestive system-related abbreviations and their meanings. Included are abbreviations contained in the medical record activities that follow.

Abbreviation	Meaning	Abbreviation	Meaning
Ba	barium	GTT	glucose tolerance test
BE	barium enema; below the elbow	HAV	hepatitis A virus
BM	bowel movement	HBV	hepatitis B virus
CA	cancer; chronological age; cardiac arrest	HF	heart failure
Ca	calcium; cancer	IBD	inflammatory bowel disease
cm	centimeter (1/100 of a meter)	IBS	irritable bowel syndrome
CT	computed tomography	IVC	intravenous cholangiogram; intravenous cholangiography
Dx	diagnosis	LES	lower esophageal sphincter
EGD	esophagogastroduodenoscopy	MRI	magnetic resonance imaging
ERCP	endoscopic retrograde cholangiopancreatography	OR	operating room
ESWL	extracorporeal shock-wave lithotripsy	RGB	Roux-en-Y gastric bypass
FBS	fasting blood sugar	RUQ	right upper quadrant
FH	family history	UGI	upper gastrointestinal
GERD	gastroesophageal reflux disease	UGIS	upper gastrointestinal series
GI	gastrointestinal	US	ultrasound; ultrasonography,

Additional Medical Terms

The following are additional medical terms related to the digestive system. Recognizing and learning these terms will help you understand the connection between common signs, symptoms, and diseases and their diagnoses as well as the rationale behind the method of treatment selected for a particular disorder.

Signs, Symptoms, and Diseases

appendicitis ă-pĕn-dĭ-SĪ-tĭs *appendic:* appendix *-itis:* inflammation	Inflammation of the appendix, which is usually acute and caused by blockage of the appendix followed by infection *Treatment for acute appendicitis is appendectomy within 48 hours of the first symptom. When left untreated, appendicitis rapidly leads to perforation and peritonitis as fecal matter is released into the peritoneal cavity. (See Figure 6–8.)*
ascites ă-SĪ-tēz	Abnormal accumulation of serous fluid in the peritoneal cavity *Ascites may be a symptom of inflammatory disorders in the abdomen, venous hypertension caused by liver disease, or heart failure (HF).*
borborygmus bŏr-bō-RĬG-mŭs	Gurgling or rumbling sound heard over the large intestine that is caused by gas moving through the intestines
cirrhosis sĭ-RŌ-sĭs *cirrh:* yellow *-osis:* abnormal condition; increase (used primarily with blood cells)	Chronic liver disease characterized by destruction of liver cells that eventually leads to ineffective liver function and jaundice
diverticular disease dī-vĕr-TĬK-ū-lăr	Condition in which bulging pouches (diverticula) in the gastrointestinal (GI) tract push the mucosal lining through the surrounding muscle *When feces become trapped inside a diverticular sac, it causes inflammation, infection, abdominal pain, and fever, a condition known as diverticulitis. (See Figure 6–9.)*

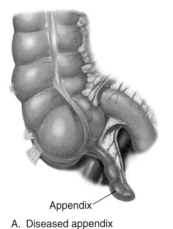

Appendix

A. Diseased appendix

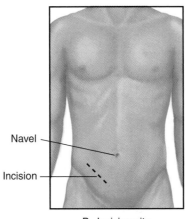

Navel

Incision

B. Incision site

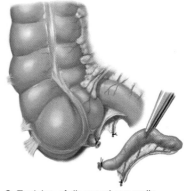

C. Excision of diseased appendix

Figure 6-8 Appendectomy.

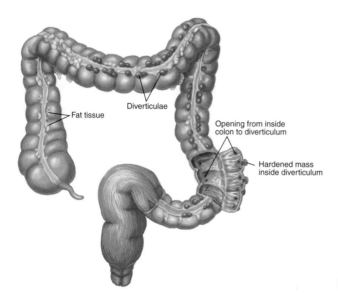

Figure 6-9   Diverticular disease.

dysentery
DĬS-ĕn-tĕr-ē
 	
dys-: bad; painful;
       difficult
enter: intestine (usually
       small intestine)
-y: condition; process
	Inflammation of the intestine, especially of the colon, which may be caused by chemical irritants, bacteria, protozoa, or parasites
	
	Dysentery is common in underdeveloped areas of the world and in times of disaster and social disorganization when sanitary living conditions, clean food, and safe water are not available. It is characterized by diarrhea, colitis, and abdominal cramps.

fistula FĬS-tū-lă	Abnormal passage from one organ to another, or from a hollow organ to the surface *An anal fistula is located near the anus and may open into the rectum.*
gastroesophageal reflux disease (GERD) găs-trō-ē-sŏf-ă-JĒ-ăl RĒ-flŭks dĭ-ZĒZ *gastr/o:* stomach *esophag:* esophagus *-eal:* pertaining to	Backflow (reflux) of gastric contents into the esophagus due to malfunction of the lower esophageal sphincter (LES) *Symptoms of GERD include heartburn (burning sensation caused by regurgitation of hydrochloric acid from the stomach to the esophagus), belching, and regurgitation of food. Treatment includes elevating the head of the bed while sleeping, avoiding alcohol and foods that stimulate acid secretion, and administering drugs to decrease production of acid.*
hematochezia hĕm-ă-tō-KĒ-zē-ă	Passage of stools containing bright red blood
hemorrhoid HĔM-ō-royd	Mass of enlarged, twisted varicose veins in the mucous membrane inside (internal) or just outside (external) the rectum; also known as *piles*
hernia HĔR-nē-ă	Protrusion or projection of an organ or a part of an organ through the wall of the cavity that normally contains it (See Figure 6–10.)

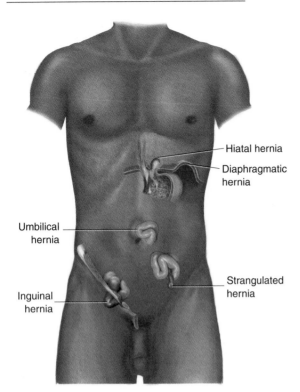

Hiatal hernia

Diaphragmatic hernia

Umbilical hernia

Inguinal hernia

Strangulated hernia

Figure 6-10 Common locations of hernias.

inflammatory bowel disease (IBD) ĭn-FLĂM-ă-tŏr-ē BŎ-wăl	Ulceration of the colon mucosa *Crohn disease and ulcerative colitis are forms of IBD.*
Crohn disease KRŌN	Chronic IBD that usually affects the ileum but may affect any portion of the intestinal tract *Crohn disease is distinguished from closely related bowel disorders by its inflammatory pattern, which tends to be patchy or segmented; also called regional colitis.*
ulcerative colitis ŬL-sĕr-ā-tĭv kō-LĪ-tĭs *col:* colon *-itis:* inflammation	Chronic IBD of the colon characterized by episodes of diarrhea, rectal bleeding, and pain
irritable bowel syndrome (IBS) ĬR-ĭ-tă-bl BŎ-wăl SĬN-drōm	Condition characterized by gastrointestinal signs and symptoms, including constipation, diarrhea, gas, and bloating, all in the absence of organic pathology; also called *spastic colon* *Contributing factors of IBS include stress and tension. Treatment consists of dietary modifications, such as avoiding irritating foods or adding a high-fiber diet and laxatives if constipation is a symptom. It also includes antidiarrheal and antispasmodic drugs as well as alleviating anxiety and stress.*
jaundice JAWN-dĭs *jaund:* yellow *-ice:* noun ending	Yellow discoloration of the skin, mucous membranes, and the outer white layer of the eyeballs (sclera). This condition is caused by excessive levels of bilirubin in the blood (hyperbilirubinemia)

obesity	Condition in which a person accumulates an amount of fat that exceeds the body's skeletal and physical standards, usually an increase of 20 percent or more above ideal body weight
morbid obesity	More severe obesity in which a person has a body mass index (BMI) of 40 or greater, which is generally 100 or more pounds over ideal body weight
	Morbid obesity is a disease with serious medical, psychological, and social ramifications.

polyp PŎL-ĭp	Small, tumorlike, benign growth that projects from a mucous membrane surface
	Polyps have potential of becoming cancerous, so they are checked frequently or removed to detect any abnormalities at an early stage. Colonic polyps have a high likelihood of becoming colorectal cancer.
colonic polyposis kō-LŎN-ĭk pŏl-ē-PŌ-sĭs *colon:* colon *-ic:* pertaining to *polyp:* small growth *-osis:* abnormal condition; increase (used primarily with blood cells)	Condition in which polyps project from the mucous membrane of the colon
polyposis pŏl-ē-PŌ-sĭs *polyp:* small growth *-osis:* abnormal condition; increase (used primarily with blood cells)	Condition in which polyps develop in the intestinal tract

ulcer UL-sĕr	Open sore or lesion of the skin or mucous membrane accompanied by sloughing of inflamed necrotic tissue
	An ulcer may be shallow, involving only the epidermis, or it may be deep, involving multiple layers of the skin. Examples of ulcers are peptic ulcer, duodenal ulcer, and pressure ulcer (decubitus ulcer).

volvulus VŎL-vū-lŭs	Twisting of the bowel on itself, causing obstruction
	Volvulus usually requires surgery to untwist the loop of bowel.

Diagnostic Procedures

barium enema (BE) BĂ-rē-ŭm ĔN-ĕ-mă	Radiographic examination of the rectum and colon after administration of barium sulfate (radiopaque contrast medium) into the rectum
	BE is used for diagnosis of obstructions, tumors, or other abnormalities, such as ulcerative colitis.

barium swallow BĂ-rē-ŭm	Radiographic examination of the esophagus, stomach, and small intestine after oral administration of barium sulfate (radiopaque contrast medium); also called *upper GI series* *Structural abnormalities of the esophagus and vessels, such as esophageal varices, may be diagnosed using this technique.*
computed tomography (CT) kŏm-PŪ-tĕd tō-MŎG-ră-fē *tom/o:* to cut *-graphy:* process of recording	Radiographic technique that uses a narrow beam of x-rays that rotates in a full arc around the patient to acquire multiple views of the body that a computer interprets to produce cross-sectional images of that body part *CT scans are used to view the gallbladder, liver, bile ducts, and pancreas and diagnose tumors, cysts, inflammation, abscesses, perforation, bleeding, and obstructions. A contrast material may be used to enhance the structures.*
endoscopy ĕn-DŎS-kō-pē *endo-:* in, within *-scopy:* visual examination **upper GI** **lower GI**	Visual examination of a cavity or canal using a specialized lighted instrument called an *endoscope* *The organ, cavity, or canal being examined dictates the name of the endoscopic procedure. A camera and video recorder are commonly used during the procedure to provide a permanent record.* Endoscopy of the esophagus (esophagoscopy), stomach (gastroscopy), and duodenum (duodenoscopy) *Endoscopy of the upper GI tract is performed to identify tumors, esophagitis, gastroesophageal varices, peptic ulcers, and the source of upper GI bleeding. It is also used to confirm the presence and extent of varices in the lower esophagus and stomach in patients with liver disease.* Endoscopy of colon (colonoscopy), sigmoid colon (sigmoidoscopy), and rectum and anal canal (proctoscopy) (See Figure 6–5.) *Endoscopy of the lower GI tract is used to identify pathological conditions in the colon. It may also be used to remove polyps. When polyps are discovered in the colon, they are removed and tested for cancer.*
magnetic resonance imaging (MRI) măg-NĔT-ĭc RĔZ-ĕn-ăns ĬM-ĭj-ĭng	Radiographic technique that uses electromagnetic energy to produce multiplanar cross-sectional images of the body *In the digestive system, MRI is particularly useful in detecting abdominal masses and viewing images of abdominal structures.*
stool guaiac GWĪ-ăk	Test performed on feces to detect presence of blood in the stool (bowel movement) that is not apparent on visual inspection; also called *hemoccult test*
ultrasonography (US) ŭl-tră-sŏn-ŎG-ră-fē *ultra-:* excess, beyond *son/o:* sound *-graphy:* process of recording	Imaging technique that uses high-frequency sound waves (ultrasound) that bounce off body tissues and are recorded to produce an image of an internal organ or tissue *Ultrasound is used to view the liver, gallbladder, bile ducts, and pancreas, among other structures. It is also used to diagnose digestive disorders, locate cysts and tumors, and guide insertion of instruments during surgical procedures.*

Medical and Surgical Procedures

bariatric surgery BĂR-ē-ă-trĭk	Group of procedures that treat morbid obesity *Commonly employed bariatric surgeries include vertical banded gastroplasty and Roux-en-Y gastric bypass. (See Figure 6–11.)*
vertical banded gastroplasty găs-trō-PLĂS-tē *gastr/o:* stomach *-plasty:* surgical repair	Bariatric surgery in which the upper stomach near the esophagus is stapled vertically to reduce it to a small pouch and a band is inserted that restricts and delays food from leaving the pouch, causing a feeling of fullness (See Figure 6–11A.)
Roux-en-Y gastric bypass (RGB) rū-ĕn-WĪ GĂS-trĭk	Bariatric surgery in which the stomach is first stapled to decrease it to a small pouch and then the jejunum is shortened and connected to the small stomach pouch, causing the base of the duodenum leading from the nonfunctioning portion of the stomach to form a Y configuration, which decreases the pathway of food through the intestine, thus reducing absorption of calories and fats *RGB is performed laparoscopically using instruments inserted through small incisions in the abdomen. When laparoscopy is not possible, gastric bypass can be performed as an open procedure (laparotomy) and involves a large incision in the middle of the abdomen. RGB is the most commonly performed weight loss surgery today. (See Figure 6–11B.)*
lithotripsy LĬTH-ō-trĭp-sē *lith/o:* stone, calculus *-tripsy:* crushing	Procedure for eliminating a stone within the gallbladder or urinary system by crushing the stone surgically or using a noninvasive method, such as ultrasonic shock waves, to shatter it *The crushed fragments may be expelled or washed out.*
extracorporeal shock-wave lithotripsy (ESWL) ĕks-tră-kor-POR-ē-ăl LĬTH-ō-trĭp-sē *extra-:* outside *corpor:* body *-eal:* pertaining to *lith/o:* stone, calculus *-tripsy:* crushing	Use of shock waves as a noninvasive method to destroy stones in the gallbladder and biliary ducts *In ESWL, ultrasound is used to locate the stone or stones and monitor their destruction. The patient usually undergoes a course of oral dissolution drugs to ensure complete removal of all stones and stone fragments.*

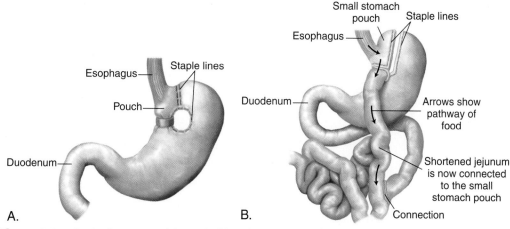

Figure 6-11   Bariatric surgery. (A) Vertical banded gastroplasty. (B) Roux-en-Y gastric bypass.

nasogastric intubation nā-zō-GĂS-trĭk ĭn-tū-BĀ-shŭn *nas/o:* nose *gastr:* stomach *-ic:* pertaining to	Insertion of a nasogastric tube through the nose into the stomach *Nasogastric intubation is used to relieve gastric distention by removing gas, gastric secretions, or food. It is also used to instill medication, food, or fluids or obtain a specimen for laboratory analysis.*

Pharmacology

antacids ănt-ĂS-ĭds	Agents that neutralize acids in the stomach

antidiarrheals ăn-tĭ-dī-ă-RĒ-ăls	Agents that control loose stools and relieve diarrhea by absorbing excess water in the bowel or slowing peristalsis in the intestinal tract

antiemetics ăn-tĭ-ē-MĔT-ĭks	Agents that control nausea and vomiting by blocking nerve impulses to the vomiting center of the brain

laxatives LĂK-să-tĭvz	Agents that relieve constipation and facilitate passage of feces through the lower GI tract

Pronunciation Help	**Long Sound**	ā in rāte	ē in rēbirth	ī in īsle	ō in ōver	ū in ūnite
	Short Sound	ă in ălone	ĕ in ĕver	ĭ in ĭt	ŏ in nŏt	ŭ in cŭt

Additional Medical Terms Review

Match the medical term(s) below with the definitions in the numbered list.

ascites	fistula	jaundice
barium enema	hematochezia	lithotripsy
barium swallow	hemoccult	nasogastric intubation
cirrhosis	IBD	polyp
Crohn disease	IBS	volvulus

1. _____ is a test performed on feces that detects the presence of blood that is not apparent on visual inspection; also called stool guiac.

2. _____ refers to insertion of a tube through the nose into the stomach for therapeutic and diagnostic purposes.

3. _____ is a small benign growth that projects from a mucous membrane.

4. _____ is an abnormal accumulation of serous fluid in the peritoneal cavity.

5. _____ refers to chronic inflammatory bowel disease, which usually affects the ileum.

6. _____ refers to surgically crushing a stone.

7. _____ is an abnormal tubelike passage from one organ to another or from one organ to the surface.

8. _____ is a yellow discoloration of the skin caused by hyperbilirubinemia.

9. _____ is a radiographic examination of the rectum and colon after administration of barium sulfate.

10. _____ refers to ulceration of the mucosa of the colon, as seen in *Crohn disease*.

11. _____ refers to passage of stools containing red blood.

12. _____ means twisting of the bowel on itself, causing obstruction.

13. _____ refers to a chronic liver disease characterized pathologically by destruction of liver cells and jaundice.

14. _____ is a radiographic examination of the esophagus, stomach, and small intestine after oral administration of barium sulfate.

15. _____ is a condition characterized by constipation, diarrhea, gas, and bloating without organic pathology and is also called *spastic colon*.

Competency Verification: Check your answers in Appendix B, Answer Key, page 567. If you are not satisfied with your level of comprehension, review the pathological, diagnostic, and therapeutic terms and retake the review.

Correct Answers _____ × 6.67 = _____ % Score

Medical Record Activities

Medical reports included in the following activities reflect common, real-life clinical scenarios to show how medical terminology is used to document patient care.

MEDICAL RECORD ACTIVITY 6-1

Rectal Bleeding

Terminology

Terms listed in the table below come from the medical report *Rectal Bleeding* that follows. Use a medical dictionary such as *Taber's Cyclopedic Medical Dictionary,* the appendices of this book, or other resources to define each term. Then practice reading the pronunciations aloud for each term.

Term	Definition
angulation ăng-ū-LĀ-shŭn	_____
anorectal ā-nō-RĔK-tăl	_____
carcinoma kăr-sĭ-NŌ-mă	_____
cm	_____
diarrhea dī-ă-RĒ-ă	_____
diverticulum dī-věr-TĬK-ū-lŭm (See Figure 6–9.)	_____
dysphagia dĭs-FĀ-jē-ă	_____
emesis ĔM-ĕ-sĭs	_____
enteritis ĕn-těr-Ī-tĭs	_____
hematemesis hĕm-ăt-ĔM-ĕ-sĭs	_____
ileostomy ĭl-ē-ŌS-tō-mē	_____
nausea NAW-sē-ă	_____

Term	Definition
polyp PŎL-ĭp	
postprandial pōst-PRĂN-dē-ăl	
sigmoidoscopy sĭg-moy-DŎS-kō-pē	

 Listen and Learn Online! will help you master pronunciations of selected medical words from this medical report activity. Visit *http://davisplus.fadavis.com/gylys/simplified* to find instructions on completing the *Listen and Learn Online!* exercise for this section and to practice pronunciations.

Reading

Practice pronunciation of medical terms by reading the following medical report aloud.

Rectal Bleeding

This 50-year-old white man has lost approximately 40 pounds since his last examination. The patient says he has had no dysphagia or postprandial distress, and there is no report of diarrhea, nausea, emesis, hematemesis, or constipation. The patient has had a history of regional enteritis, appendicitis, and colonic bleeding.

The regional enteritis resulted in an ileostomy with appendectomy about 6 months ago. On 5/30/xx, a sigmoidoscopy using a 10-cm scope showed no evidence of bleeding at the anorectal area. A 35-cm scope was then inserted to a level of 13 cm. At this point, angulation prevented further passage of the scope. No abnormalities had been encountered, but there was dark blood noted at that level.

My impression is that the rectal bleeding could be due to a polyp, bleeding diverticulum, or rectal carcinoma.

Evaluation

Review the medical report above to answer the following questions. Use a medical dictionary such as *Taber's Cyclopedic Medical Dictionary* and other resources if needed.

1. What is the patient's symptom that made him seek medical help?

_____

2. What surgical procedures were performed on the patient for regional enteritis?

_____

3. What abnormality was found with the sigmoidoscopy?

_____

_____

4. What is causing the rectal bleeding?

_____

_____

5. Write the plural form of diverticulum.

_____

_____

MEDICAL RECORD ACTIVITY 6-2

Carcinosarcoma of the Esophagus

Terminology

Terms listed in the table below come from the medical report *Carcinosarcoma of the Esophagus* that follows. Use a medical dictionary such as *Taber's Cyclopedic Medical Dictionary,* the appendices of this book, or other resources to define each term. Then practice reading the pronunciations aloud for each term.

Term	Definition
aortic arch ā-OR-tĭk	_____
carcinosarcoma kăr-sĭ-nō-săr-KŌ-mă	_____
esophagoscopy ē-sŏf-ă-GŎS-kō-pē	_____
friable FRĪ-ă-bl	_____
intraluminal ĭn-tră-LŪ-mĭ-năl	_____
malignant mă-LĬG-nănt	_____
mediastinal mē-dē-ăs-TĪ-năl	_____
OR	_____
polypoid PŎL-ē-poyd	_____
reanastomosis rē-ăn-ăs-tō-MŌ-sĭs (See Figure 2-7.)	_____

Listen and Learn Online! will help you master pronunciations of selected medical words from this medical report activity. Visit *http://davisplus.fadavis.com/gylys/simplified* to find instructions on completing the *Listen and Learn Online!* exercise for this section and to practice pronunciations.

Reading

Practice pronunciation of medical terms by reading the following medical report aloud.

Carcinosarcoma of the Esophagus

ADMITTING DIAGNOSIS: Carcinosarcoma of the esophagus.

DISCHARGE DIAGNOSIS: Carcinosarcoma of the esophagus.

HISTORY OF PRESENT ILLNESS: Patient had been complaining of dysphagia over the last 4 months with a worsening recently in symptoms.

SURGERY: Esophagoscopy was performed, and a small friable biopsy specimen was obtained. Pathology tests confirmed it to be malignant. A barium x-ray study revealed polypoid, intraluminal, esophageal obstruction. Surgical findings revealed an infiltrating tumor of the middle third of the esophagus with intraluminal, friable, polypoid masses, each 3 cm in diameter. A resection of the esophagus was performed with reanastomosis of the stomach at the aortic arch. An adjacent mediastinal lymph node was excised. There were no complications during the procedure. Patient left the OR in stable condition.

Evaluation

Review the medical report above to answer the following questions. Use a medical dictionary such as *Taber's Cyclopedic Medical Dictionary* and other resources if needed.

1. What surgery was performed on this patient?

_____

_____

2. What diagnostic testing confirmed malignancy?

_____

_____

3. Where was the carcinosarcoma located?

_____

_____

4. Why was the adjacent lymph node excised?

_____

_____

Chapter Review

Word Elements Summary

The following table summarizes CFs, suffixes, and prefixes related to the digestive system.

Word Element	Meaning	Word Element	Meaning
Combining Forms			
appendic/o	appendix	**gloss/o, lingu/o**	tongue
chol/e	bile, gall	**hepat/o**	liver
cholecyst/o	gallbladder	**ile/o**	ileum (third part of small intestine)
choledoch/o	bile duct	**jejun/o**	jejunum (second part of small intestine)
col/o, colon/o	colon	**or/o, stomat/o**	mouth
dent/o, odont/o	teeth	**pancreat/o**	pancreas
duoden/o	duodenum (first part of small intestine)	**proct/o**	anus, rectum
enter/o	intestine (usually small intestine)	**ptyal/o, sial/o**	saliva, salivary gland
esophag/o	esophagus	**rect/o**	rectum
gastr/o	stomach	**sigmoid/o**	sigmoid colon
gingiv/o	gum(s)		
OTHER COMBINING FORMS			
aer/o	air	**nas/o**	nose
carcin/o	cancer	**orth/o**	straight
cirrh/o, jaund/o	yellow	**polyp/o**	small growth
corpor/o	body	**son/o**	sound
hemat/o, hem/o	blood	**therm/o**	heat
lith/o	stone, calculus	**tom/o**	to cut
myc/o	fungus	**tox/o, toxic/o**	poison
Suffixes			
SURGICAL			
-ectomy	excision, removal	**-stomy**	forming an opening (mouth)
-plasty	surgical repair	**-tome**	instrument to cut
-rrhaphy	suture	**-tomy**	incision

Word Element	Meaning	Word Element	Meaning
DIAGNOSTIC, SYMPTOMATIC, AND RELATED			
-algia, -dynia	pain	**-oma**	tumor
-emesis	vomiting	**-osis**	abnormal condition; increase (used primarily with blood cells)
-gram	record, writing	**-pepsia**	digestion
-graphy	process of recording	**-phagia**	swallowing, eating
-iasis	abnormal condition (produced by something specified)	**-rrhea**	discharge, flow
-itis	inflammation	**-scope**	instrument for examining
-lith	stone, calculus	**-scopy**	visual examination
-logist	specialist in study of	**-spasm**	involuntary contraction, twitching
-logy	study of	**-stenosis**	narrowing, stricture
-megaly	enlargement	**-tripsy**	crushing
-oid	resembling		
ADJECTIVE			
-al, -ar, -ary, -eal, -ic	pertaining to		
NOUN			
-ia, -ice	condition	**-y**	condition, process
-ist	specialist		
Prefixes			
ab-	from, away from	**hyper-**	excessive, above normal
dia-	through, across	**hypo-**	under, below, deficient
dys-	bad; painful; difficult	**peri-**	around
endo-	in, within	**sub-**	under, below
epi-	above, upon	**ultra-**	excess, beyond
extra-	outside		

 Enhance your study and reinforcement of word elements with the power of *Davis Plus.* Visit *http://davisplus.fadavis.com/gylys/simplified* for this chapter's flash-card activity. We recommend you complete the flash-card activity before completing the word elements review below.

Word Elements Review

After you review the Word Elements Summary, complete this activity by writing the meaning of each element in the space provided.

Word Element	Meaning	Word Element	Meaning
Combining Forms			

DIGESTIVE SYSTEM STRUCTURES

Word Element	Meaning	Word Element	Meaning
1. appendic/o	_____	13. hepat/o	_____
2. chol/e	_____	14. ile/o	_____
3. cholecyst/o	_____	15. jejun/o	_____
4. choledoch/o	_____	16. or/o, stomat/o	_____
5. col/o, colon/o	_____	17. pancreat/o	_____
6. dent/o, odont/o	_____	18. pharyng/o	_____
7. duoden/o	_____	19. proct/o	_____
8. enter/o	_____	20. ptyal/o	_____
9. esophag/o	_____	21. rect/o	_____
10. gastr/o	_____	22. sial/o	_____
11. gingiv/o	_____	23. sigmoid/o	_____
12. gloss/o, lingu/o	_____		

OTHER COMBINING FORMS

Word Element	Meaning	Word Element	Meaning
24. aer/o	_____	28. myc/o	_____
25. carcin/o	_____	29. polyp/o	_____
26. cirrh/o, jaund/o	_____	30. tom/o	_____
27. lith/o	_____	31. tox/o, toxic/o	_____

Suffixes			

SURGICAL

Word Element	Meaning	Word Element	Meaning
32. -plasty	_____	34. -stomy	_____
33. -rrhaphy	_____	35. -tome	_____

DIAGNOSTIC, SYMPTOMATIC, AND RELATED

Word Element	Meaning	Word Element	Meaning
36. -emesis	_____	44. -phagia	_____
37. -gram	_____	45. -rrhea	_____
38. -lith	_____	46. -scope	_____
39. -megaly	_____	47. -scopy	_____
40. -oid	_____	48. -spasm	_____
41. -oma	_____	49. -stenosis	_____
42. -osis	_____	50. -tripsy	_____
43. -pepsia	_____		

Word Element	Meaning	Word Element	Meaning
ADJECTIVE			
51. -al, -ar, -ary, -eal, -ic	_____		
NOUN			
52. -ia, -ice	_____	**54.** -y	_____
53. -ist	_____		
PREFIXES			
55. ab-	_____	**61.** hyper-	_____
56. dia-	_____	**62.** hypo-	_____
57. dys-	_____	**63.** peri-	_____
58. endo-	_____	**64.** sub-	_____
59. epi-	_____	**65.** ultra-	_____
60. extra-	_____		

Competency Verification: Check your answers in Appendix A, Glossary of Medical Word Elements, page 538. If you are not satisfied with your level of comprehension, review the word elements and retake the review.

Correct Answers _____ × 1.5 = _____ % Score

Vocabulary Review

Match the medical word(s) below with the definitions in the numbered list.

alimentary canal	cholelithiasis	gastroscopy	rectoplasty
anastomosis	duodenotomy	GERD	salivary glands
bariatric	dyspepsia	hematemesis	sigmoidotomy
cholecystectomy	dysphagia	hepatomegaly	stomatalgia
choledochal	friable	ileostomy	ultrasound

1. _____ refers to visual examination of the stomach.
2. _____ means bad, painful, difficult digestion.
3. _____ means vomiting blood.
4. _____ refers to high-frequency sound waves that produce internal images of the body.
5. _____ are glands that secrete saliva.
6. _____ is another term for GI tract.
7. _____ means pain in the mouth.
8. _____ is an incision of the duodenum.
9. _____ means enlargement of the liver.
10. _____ refers to painful swallowing.
11. _____ means removal of the gallbladder.
12. _____ is a surgical connection between two vessels
13. _____ is an incision of the sigmoid colon.
14. _____ refers to surgical repair of the rectum.
15. _____ is reflux of gastric contents into the esophagus with heartburn.
16. _____ refers to formation of an opening (mouth) into the ileum.
17. _____ refers to the presence or formation of gallstones.
18. _____ means easily broken or pulverized.
19. _____ means pertaining to the bile duct.
20. _____ surgery that treats morbid obesity by altering digestive structures to limit food intake.

Competency Verification: Check your answers in Appendix B, Answer Key, page 568. If you are not satisfied with your level of comprehension, review the chapter vocabulary and retake the review.

Correct Answers _____ × 5 = _____ % Score

7 Urinary System

OBJECTIVES

Upon completion of this chapter, you will be able to:

- Describe the type of medical treatment urologists and nephrologists provide.
- Identify urinary structures by labeling them on anatomical illustrations.
- Describe the primary functions of the urinary system.
- Describe common diseases related to the urinary system.
- Describe common diagnostic, medical, and surgical procedures related to the urinary system.
- Apply your word-building skills by constructing medical terms related to the urinary system.
- Describe common abbreviations and symbols related to the urinary system.
- Reinforce word elements by completing flash card activities.
- Recognize, define, pronounce, and spell terms correctly.
- Demonstrate your knowledge of this chapter by successfully completing the frames, reviews, and medical report evaluations.

Medical Specialties

Urology

The urinary system is associated with the medical specialty of **urology**. Physicians who specialize in clinical treatment of disorders of the female and the male urinary systems are called *urologists*. Because some urinary structures in the male perform a dual role, performing urinary functions and reproductive functions, the urologist also treats male reproductive disorders. These disorders include but are not limited to treatment of bladder cancer, infertility, and sexual dysfunctions. Urologists also perform various surgical procedures, such as transurethral resection of the prostate, cystoscopy, and various other procedures to treat numerous disorders of the urinary system.

Nephrology

Nephrologists specialize in the diagnosis and management of kidney disease, kidney transplantation, and dialysis therapies. The medical specialty of **nephrology** is a subspecialty of internal medicine. After completing a residency, the internist must complete additional training, or a fellowship, as a nephrologist.

Anatomy and Physiology Overview

The urinary system is composed of the kidneys, ureters, bladder, and urethra. Its purpose is to regulate the volume and composition of fluids in the body and remove waste substances and excess fluid from the blood. Waste substances are filtered from the blood by the kidneys and excreted in the urine, which exit via the ureters into the urinary bladder. Urine is stored in the bladder until the urge to urinate occurs, at which point the muscles at the bladder outlet relax, allowing the urine to be expelled through the urethra.

The main functions of the kidneys are to regulate the amount of water in the body and keep the body fluids at a constant concentration and acid-base level. They achieve these functions by filtering blood and excreting waste substances and excess water as urine. Other essential substances are reabsorbed into the bloodstream by the process called *reabsorption.*

The filtering-reabsorption process is necessary to maintain the balance of substances required for a relatively stable internal body environment. This stable internal environment, known as *homeostasis*, is necessary for the cells of the body to survive and carry out their functions effectively. If kidneys fail, waste substances cannot be eliminated from the body. Thus, the substances accumulate in the blood to toxic levels and the cells can no longer function. Death ultimately results unless impurities are filtered out of the blood by means of an artificial kidney known as *kidney dialysis* or the nonfunctioning kidneys are replaced with a healthy kidney through kidney transplantation. (See Figure 7–1.)

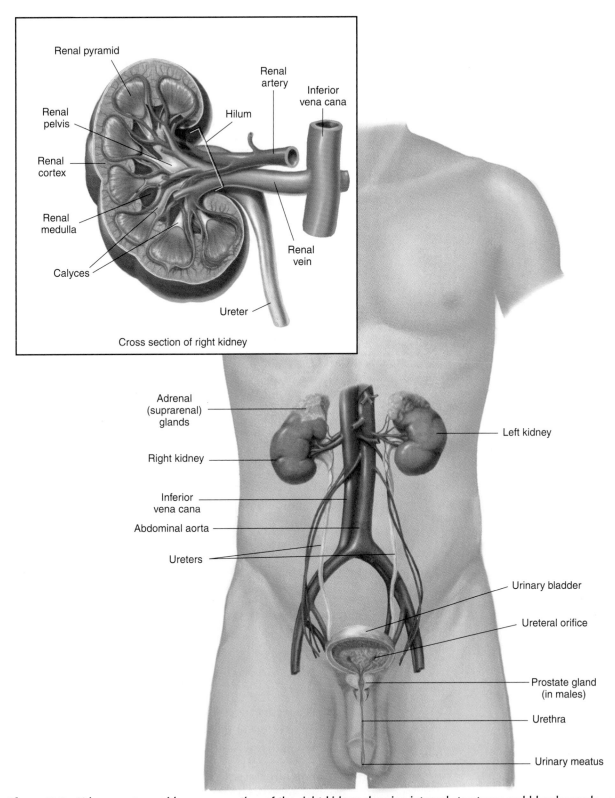

Figure 7-1 Urinary system with a cross-section of the right kidney showing internal structures and blood vessels.

WORD ELEMENTS

This section introduces combining forms (CFs) related to the urinary system. Included are key suffixes; prefixes are defined in the right-hand column as needed. Review the following table, and pronounce each word in the word analysis column aloud before you begin to work the frames.

Word Element	Meaning	Word Analysis
Combining Forms		
cyst/o	bladder	**cyst/o/scopy** (sĭs-TŎS-kō-pē): visual examination of the urinary tract using a cystoscope inserted through the urethra *-scopy:* visual examination *Cystoscopy is used to diagnose urinary tract disorders, obtain tissue and urine samples, excise tumors, or inject a contrast medium into the bladder.*
vesic/o		**vesic/o/cele** (VĔS-ĭ-kō-sēl): hernial protrusion of urinary bladder; also called *cystocele* *-cele:* hernia, swelling
glomerul/o	glomerulus	**glomerul/ar** (glō-MĔR-ū-lăr): pertaining to the glomerulus *-ar:* pertaining to *The glomerulus is a cluster of capillaries forming the structural and functional unit of the kidney known as the nephron. Glomerular capillaries filter fluid, the first step in urine formation.*
meat/o	opening, meatus	**meat/us** (mē-Ā-tŭs): opening or tunnel through any part of the body, such as the external opening of the urethra *-us:* condition, structure
nephr/o	kidney	**nephr/oma** (nĕ-FRŌ-mă): tumor of the kidney *oma:* tumor
ren/o		**ren/al** (RĒ-năl): pertaining to the kidney *-al:* pertaining to
pyel/o	renal pelvis	**pyel/o/plasty** (PĪ-ĕ-lō-plăs-tē): surgical repair of renal pelvis *-plasty:* surgical repair
ur/o	urine, urinary tract	**ur/emia** (ū-RĒ-mē-ă): excessive urea and other nitrogenous waste products in blood; also called *azotemia* *-emia:* blood condition *Healthy kidneys excrete waste products normally. Uremia occurs in renal failure.*
urin/o		**urin/ary** (Ū-rĭ-nār-ē): pertains to urine or formation of urine; also refers to the urinary tract *-ary:* pertaining to
ureter/o	ureter	**ureter/o/stenosis** (ū-rē-tĕr-ō-stĕ-NŌ-sĭs): narrowing or stricture of a ureter *-stenosis:* narrowing, stricture

Word Element	Meaning	Word Analysis
urethr/o	urethra	**urethr/o/cele** (ū-RĒ-thrō-sēl): hernial protrusion of the urethra *-cele:* hernia, swelling *Urethrocele may be congenital or acquired and secondary to obesity, childbirth, and poor muscle tone.*

Suffixes

Word Element	Meaning	Word Analysis
-emia	blood condition	azot/**emia** (ăz-ō-TĒ-mē-ă): excessive amounts of nitrogenous compounds in the blood *azot:* nitrogenous compounds *Azotemia is a toxic condition caused by the kidneys' failure to remove urea from the blood.*
-iasis	abnormal condition (produced by something specified)	lith/**iasis** (lĭth-Ī-ă-sĭs): abnormal condition of stones or calculi *lith:* stone, calculus *The calculi occur most commonly in the kidney, lower urinary tract, and gallbladder.*
-lysis	separation; destruction; loosening	dia/**lysis** (dī-ĂL-ĭ-sĭs): process of removing toxic wastes from blood when kidneys are unable to do so *dia-:* through, across
-pathy	disease	nephr/o/**pathy** (nĕ-FRŎP-ă-thē): disease of the kidneys *nephr:* kidney
-pexy	fixation (of an organ)	nephr/o/**pexy** (NĔF-rō-pĕks-ē): surgical procedure to affix a displaced kidney *nephr/o:* kidney
-ptosis	prolapse, downward displacement	nephr/o/**ptosis** (nĕf-rŏp-TŌ-sĭs): downward displacement or dropping of a kidney *nephr/o:* kidney
-tripsy	crushing	lith/o/**tripsy** (LĬTH-ō-trĭp-sē): crushing of a stone *lith/o:* stone, calculus *Lithotripsy is a surgical procedure that employs sound waves to crush a stone in the kidney, ureter, bladder, or gallbladder. The fragments may then be expelled or washed out.*
-uria	urine	poly/**uria** (pōl-ē-Ū-rē-ă): excessive urination *poly-:* many, much

 Listen and Learn, the audio CD-ROM included in this book, will help you master pronunciation of selected medical words. Use it to practice pronunciations of the above-listed medical terms and for instructions to complete the *Listen and Learn* exercise for this section.

SECTION REVIEW 7-1

For the following medical terms, first write the suffix and its meaning. Then translate the meaning of the remaining elements starting with the first part of the word. The first word is completed for you.

Term	Meaning
1. glomerul/o/scler/osis	*-osis: abnormal condition, increase (used primarily with blood cells); glomerulus; hardening, sclera (white of eye)*
2. cyst/o/scopy	
3. poly/uria	
4. lith/o/tripsy	
5. dia/lysis	
6. ureter/o/stenosis	
7. meat/us	
8. ur/emia	
9. nephr/oma	
10. ureter/o/cele	

Competency Verification: Check your answers in Appendix B, Answer Key, page 568. If you are not satisfied with your level of comprehension, review the vocabulary and retake the review.

Correct Answers _____ × 10 = _____ % Score

Kidneys

7-1 Label urinary structures in Figure 7–2 as you read the following material. The urinary system is composed of a (1) **right kidney** and a left kidney. These are the primary structural units responsible for urine formation. Each kidney is composed of an outer layer, called the (2) *renal cortex,* and an inner region, called the (3) *renal medulla.* Blood enters the kidneys through the (4) **renal artery** and leaves through the (5) **renal vein.** Inside the kidney, the renal artery branches into smaller arteries called *arterioles* that lead into microscopic filtering units called *nephrons.* Each (6) **nephron** is designed to filter urea and other waste products effectively from the blood.

7-2 The CFs *nephr/o* and *ren/o* refer to the kidneys. Whenever you see terms such as *nephr/itis* and *ren/al,* you will know they refer to the

kidney(s)

_____.

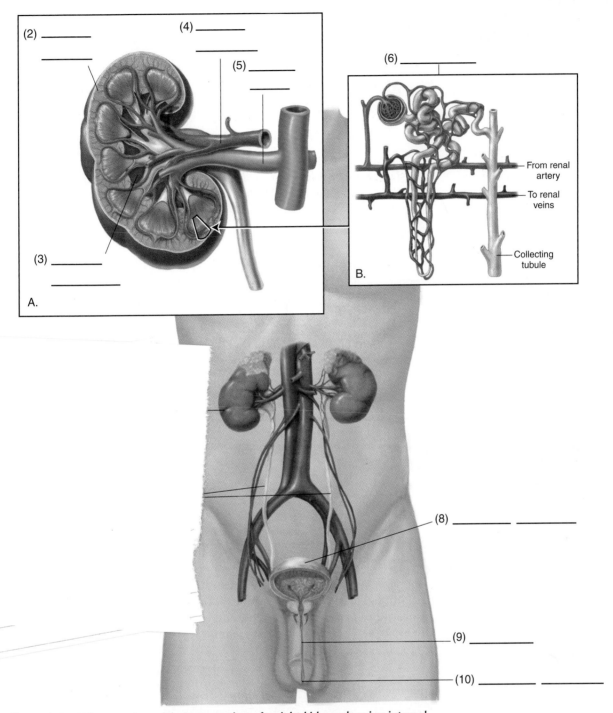

Figure 7-2 Urinary system. (A) Cross-section of a right kidney showing internal structures and blood vessels. (B) Single nephron with a collecting duct and associated blood vessels.

kidney(s)	**7-3** The term *ren/al* is commonly used as an adjective used to modify a noun. Some examples are *ren/al dialysis* and *ren/al biopsy*. Both of these terms mean *pertaining to* the _____.

nephr/ectomy nĕ-FRĔK-tō-mē	**7-4** A diseased kidney, or *renal cancer,* may necessitate its removal. Use ***nephr/o*** to form a word that means *excision of a kidney.* _____ / _____
nephr/ectomy nĕ-FRĔK-tō-mē	**7-5** When ren/al cancer occurs, the diseased kidney must be removed. The surgical procedure to remove a kidney is known as a _____ / _____ .
nephr/o/megaly nĕf-rō-MĔG-ă-lē	**7-6** When nephr/ectomy is performed, the remaining kidney most likely will become enlarged. Build a word that means *enlargement of a kidney.* _____ / _____ / _____

> If you had difficulty deciding whether to use ***nephr/o*** or ***ren/o*** in the previous frames, refer to your medical dictionary. Until you master the language of medicine, the dictionary will help you identify commonly used terms in medicine.

lith/iasis lĭth-Ī-ă-sĭs	**7-7** The suffix *-iasis* is used to describe an abnormal condition (produced by something specified). An abnormal condition of stones is called _____ / _____ .
nephr/o/lith NĔF-rō-lĭth **nephr/o/lith/iasis** nĕf-rō-lĭth-Ī-ă-sĭs	**7-8** Use ***nephr/o*** to construct medical words that mean *stone (in the) kidney:* _____ / _____ / _____ *abnormal condition of kidney stone(s):* _____ / _____ / _____ / _____
nephr/algia nĕ-FRĂL-jē-ă **nephr/itis** nĕf-RĪ-tĭs	**7-9** Formation of a kidney stone, or *ren/al calculus,* can vary in size from micro/scop/ic (commonly referrred to as *sand* or *gravel*) to a stone large enough to block the ureter or fill the ren/al pelvis. The stone commonly causes nephr/itis and nephr/algia. (See Figure 7–3.) Use ***nephr/o*** to build a word that means *pain in the kidney:* _____ / _____ *inflammation of the kidney:* _____ / _____
stone	**7-10** *Nephr/o/lith* and *ren/al calculus* mean the patient suffers from a kidney _____ .
nephr/o/lith/iasis nĕf-rō-lĭth-Ī-ă-sĭs	**7-11** A disorder that literally means *abnormal condition of a kidney stone* is: _____ / _____ / _____ / _____ .

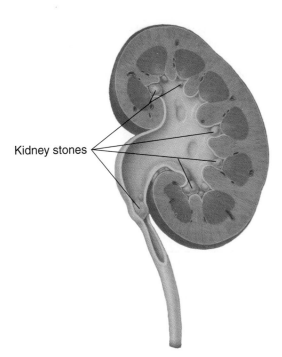

Kidney stones

Figure 7-3 Kidney stones shown in the calices and ureter.

7-12 Surgical suffixes *-ectomy, -tomy,* and *-tome* are commonly confusing to beginning medical terminology students. To reinforce your understanding of their meanings, review them in the following chart.

Surgical Suffix	Meaning
-ectomy	excision, removal
-tomy	incision
-tome	instrument to cut

---

incision, stone *or* **calculus**	**7-13** Stones trapped in the kidney or ureter may be removed surgically. *Nephr/o/lith/o/tomy* is an _____ to remove a ren/al _____.

	7-14 Ren/al hyper/tension produced by kidney disease is the most common type of hyper/tension caused by glomerul/o/nephr/itis or ren/al artery stenosis. Identify terms in this frame that mean
ren/al RĒ-năl	*pertaining to the kidney(s):* _____ / _____
stenosis stĕ-NŌ-sĭs	*narrowing, stricture:* _____
glomerul/o/nephr/itis glō-mĕr-ū-lō-nĕ-FRĪ-tĭs	*inflammation of the glomerulus of the kidney:* _____ / _____ / _____ / _____
hyper/tension hī-pĕr-TĔN-shŭn	*high blood pressure:* _____ / _____

protein/uria prō-tē-ĭn-Ū-rē-ă	**7–15** Nephr/o/tic syndrome, a group of symptoms characterized by chronic loss of protein in the urine (protein/uria), leads to depletion of body protein, especially albumin. Normally, albumin and other serum proteins maintain fluid within the vascular space. When levels of these proteins are low, fluid leaks from blood vessels into tissues, resulting in edema. The syndrome may also occur as a result of other disease processes. A chronic loss of protein in the urine is called _____ / _____.
swelling	**7–16** Although many disorders manifest fluid retention (excess fluid in tissues), a characteristic of nephr/o/tic syndrome is edema (swelling), especially around the ankles, feet, and eyes. The term *edema* indicates _____.
edema ĕ-DĒ-mă	**7–17** When body tissues contain excessive amounts of fluid that cause swelling, the term designated in a medical report for this condition would be noted as _____.
diuretic dī-ū-RĔT-ĭc	**7–18** Diuretics are agents or drugs prescribed to control edema and also to stimulate the flow of urine. Edema around the ankles and feet may also be due to a diet high in sodium. When this condition occurs, the physician may recommend a low-sodium diet and prescribe an agent known as a _____.
diuretic dī-ū-RĔT-ĭc	**7–19** Coffee increases production of urine, which means that coffee is a _____ agent.
supra- **ren** **-al**	**7–20** *Supra/ren/al* is a directional term that means *above the kidney.* Identify elements in this frame that mean *above, excessive, superior:* _____ *kidney:* _____ *pertaining to:* _____
scler/o	**7–21** The CF *scler/o* is used in words to indicate hardening of a body part. It also refers to the sclera (white of eye). To indicate a hardening, use the CF _____ / ____.
hardening	**7–22** Scler/osis is an abnormal condition of _____.

	7–23 Hyper/tension damages kidneys by causing scler/o/tic changes, such as arteri/o/scler/osis with thickening and hardening of ren/al blood vessels (nephr/o/scler/osis). Recall that *-iasis* is used to denote an abnormal condition (produced by something specified). Use ***nephr/o*** to form medical words that mean
nephr/osis něf-RŌ-sĭs	*abnormal condition of a kidney:* _____ / _____
nephr/o/scler/osis něf-rō-sklě-RŌ-sĭs	*abnormal condition of kidney hardening:* _____ / _____ / _____ / _____
nephr/o/lith NĚF-rō-lĭth	*calculus in a kidney:* _____ / _____ / _____
nephr/o/lith/iasis něf-rō-lĭth-Ī-ă-sĭs	*abnormal condition of kidney stone(s):* _____ / _____ / _____ / _____

-megaly	**7–24** The suffix for *enlargement* is _____.

	7–25 When kidneys become diseased, an enlargement of one or both kidneys may result. Use ***nephr/o*** to create a word that means *enlargement of a kidney*.
nephr/o/megaly něf-rō-MĚG-ă-lē	_____ / _____ / _____

kidney, stone *or* calculus KĂL-kū-lŭs	**7–26** *Lith/o/tomy* is an incision to remove a stone or calculus. A *nephr/o/lith/o/tomy* is an incision of the _____ to remove a _____.

	7–27 Many kidney disorders can be treated surgically. Learn these procedures by building surgical terms with ***nephr/o*** that mean
nephr/ectomy ně-FRĚK-tō-mē	*excision of a kidney:* _____ / _____
nephr/o/rrhaphy něf-ROR-ă-fē	*suture of a kidney:* _____ / _____ / _____
nephr/o/tomy ně-FRŎT-ō-mē	*incision of the kidney:* _____ / _____ / _____
nephr/o/lith/o/tomy něf-rō-lĭth-ŎT-ō-mē	*incision (to remove a) kidney stone:* _____ / _____ / _____ / _____ / _____

	7–28 A kidney may prolapse from its normal position because of a birth defect or injury. The downward displacement may occur because the kidney supports are weakened due to a sudden strain or blow. This condition is called *nephr/o/ptosis*, or *floating kidney*. A prolapsed kidney is noted in a medical chart as
nephr/o/ptosis něf-rŏp-TŌ-sĭs	_____ / _____ / _____.

-ptosis **nephr/o**	**7-29** Determine the element in *nephr/o/ptosis* that means *prolapse, downward displacement:* _____ *kidney:* _____ / _____
nephr/o/ptosis nĕf-rŏp-TŌ-sĭs	**7-30** Downward displacement of a kidney that results from a congenital defect or an injury is called _____ / _____ / _____.
nephr/o/pexy NĔF-rō-pĕks-ē	**7-31** Nephr/o/ptosis can be treated surgically. Use *-pexy* to build a surgical term that means *fixation of the kidney:* _____ / _____ / _____.

SECTION REVIEW 7-2

Using the following table, write the combining form, suffix, or prefix that matches its definition in the space provided to the left of the definition. There may be more than one word element that matches a definition.

Combining Forms	Suffixes		Prefixes
lith/o	-iasis	-ptosis	dia-
nephr/o	-megaly	-rrhaphy	poly-
ren/o	-osis	-tome	supra-
scler/o	-pathy	-tomy	
	-pexy		

1. _____ abnormal condition; increase (used primarily with blood cells)
2. _____ abnormal condition (produced by something specified)
3. _____ above; excessive; superior
4. _____ disease
5. _____ enlargement
6. _____ through, across
7. _____ fixation (of an organ)
8. _____ hardening; sclera (white of eye)
9. _____ instrument to cut
10. _____ incision
11. _____ kidney
12. _____ prolapse, downward displacement
13. _____ stone, calculus
14. _____ suture
15. _____ many, much

Competency Verification: Check your answers in Appendix B, Answer Key, page 568. If you are not satisfied with your level of comprehension, go back to Frame 7–1 and rework the frames.

Correct Answers _____ × 6.67 = _____ % Score

Ureters, Bladder, Urethra

	7-32 When urine is formed, it is conveyed from each kidney through the (7) **ureters** and stored in the (8) **urinary bladder** until it is expelled from the body through the (9) **urethra** and (10) **urinary meatus.** Label Figure 7–2 to locate the urinary structures.
ureters Ū-rĕ-tĕrs	**7-33** Locate the two pencil-like tubes in Figure 7–2 that transport urine from the kidneys to the urinary bladder. These structures are the _____.
enlargement, ureter(s) Ū-rĕ-tĕr	**7-34** The CF *ureter/o* means *ureter.* Ureter/o/megaly is an _____ of the _____.
ureter/o **-ectasis**	**7-35** *Ureter/ectasis* is a dilation of the ureter. The CF for *ureter* is _____ / _____. The element that denotes *dilation or expansion* is _____.
calculi KĂL-kū-lī	**7-36** A ren/al calculus (see Figure 7–3) is a concretion in the kidney. If the stone blocks the ureter and prevents flow of urine from the kidney, it must be removed. When there is one stone, it is referred to as a *calculus,* but multiple stones are referred to as _____.
calculus KĂL-kū-lŭs	**7-37** When stones form in the kidneys, the condition is called *nephr/o/lith/iasis.* Lith/o/tripsy may be used to crush the stones into small particles so they can be removed or expelled in the urine. The term *lith/o/tripsy* means *crushing of a stone, or* _____.
ureter/o/lith ū-RĒ-tĕr-ō-lĭth **ureter/o/lith/iasis** ū-rĕ-tĕr-ō-lĭth-Ī-ă-sĭs	**7-38** Ureter/itis may be caused by infection or by mechanical irritation of a stone. Develop some applicable terms related to ureter stones by building words that mean *stone or calculus in the ureter:* _____ / _____ / _____ *abnormal condition (produced by something specified) of a ureter(al) stone:* _____ / _____ / _____ / _____
incision, ureter, stone *or* **calculus** Ū-rĕ-tĕr, KĂL-kū-lŭs	**7-39** Ureter/o/lith/o/tomy is an _____ of a _____ to remove a _____.

dilation, ureter DĪ-lā-shŭn, Ū-rĕ-tĕr	**7-40** *Ureter/ectasis* is an expansion or _____ of a _____.

ureter/ectasis ū-rē-tĕr-ĔK-tă-sĭs	**7-41** When ren/al calculi get trapped in the ureter, urine is blocked, causing pressure on the walls of the ureter. This blockage results in an expansion or dilation of the ureter, which is called _____ / _____.

Competency Verification: Check your labeling of Figure 7–2 with Appendix B, Answer Key, page 568.

     cyst/o/lith SĬS-tō-lĭth **cyst/o/lith/iasis** sĭs-tō-lĭ-THĪ-ă-sĭs **cyst/o/lith/o/tomy** sĭs-tō-lĭth-ŎT-ō-mē	**7-42** The urinary bladder, which is a muscular sac, stores urine until it is voided. The CFs *cyst/o* and *vesic/o* are used in words to refer to the *bladder.* Use *cyst/o* to form words that mean *stone in the bladder:* _____ / _____ / _____ *abnormal condition of a bladder stone:* _____ / _____ / _____ / _____ *incision of the bladder to remove a stone:* _____ / _____ / _____ / _____ / _____

instrument, ureter ū-rē-tĕr	**7-43** A *ureter/o/cyst/o/scope* is a special _____ for examining the _____ and bladder.

ureter/algia ū-rē-tĕr-ĂL-jē-ă	**7-44** When *ureter/o/liths* become trapped in the ureter, a person may experience *ureter/o/dynia* or _____ / _____.

 ureter/o/liths ū-RĒ-tĕr-ō-lĭths **ureter/o/cyst/o/scope** ū-rē-tĕr-ō-SĬS-tō-skōp **ureter/o/cyst/o/scopy** ū-rē-tĕr-ō-sĭs-TŎS-kō-pē	**7-45** Form medical words that mean *stones in the ureter:* _____ / _____ / _____ *instrument to view the ureter and bladder:* _____ / _____ / _____ / _____ / _____ *visual examination of the ureter and bladder:* _____ / _____ / _____ / _____ / _____

suture SŪ-chūr	**7-46** The surgical suffix *-rrhaphy* is used in words to mean _____.

ureter/o/rrhaphy ū-rē-tĕr-OR-ră-fē **cyst/o/rrhaphy** sĭs-TOR-ă-fē	**7–47** Construct surgical words that mean *suture of the ureter:* _____ / _____ / _____ *suture of the bladder:* _____ / _____ / _____
vesic/o, cyst/o	**7–48** The CFs for *bladder* are _____ / _____ and _____ / _____.
bladder, intestine	**7–49** *Vesic/o/enter/ic* means *pertaining to the* _____ *and* _____.
        bladder **hernia, swelling** **rectum** RĔK-tŭm	**7–50** A *hernia* is a protrusion of an anatomical structure through the wall that normally contains it. Hernias may develop in several parts of the body. Two examples of hernias are cyst/o/cele and rect/o/cele. (See Figure 7–4.) A cyst/o/cele is herniation of part of the urin/ary bladder through the vagin/al wall caused by weakened pelv/ic muscles. A rect/o/cele is herniation of a portion of the rectum toward the vagina through weakened vagin/al muscles. Define the following word elements in this frame: *cyst/o:* _____ *-cele:* _____, _____ *rect/o:* _____
      cyst/o/cele SĬS-tō-sēl	**7–51** *Cyst/o/cele* develops over years as vaginal muscles weaken and can no longer support the weight of urine in the urinary bladder. This condition usually occurs after a woman has delivered several infants. It also occurs in elderly people because of weakened pelvic muscles resulting from the aging process. When the physician's diagnosis is a herniation of the bladder, you know the Dx will be stated as a _____ / _____ / _____.
rect/o/cele RĔK-tō-sēl	**7–52** Can you determine the Dx of herniation of the rectum into the vagina? _____ / _____ / _____
nephr/o/ptosis nĕf-rŏp-TŌ-sĭs **nephr/o/pexy** NĔF-rō-pĕks-ē	**7–53** Build medical words that mean *prolapse or downward displacement of a kidney:* _____ / _____ / _____ *surgical fixation of kidney:* _____ / _____ / _____

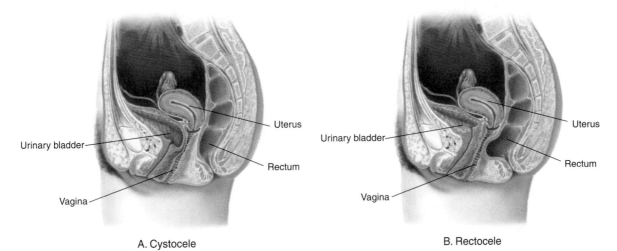

A. Cystocele   B. Rectocele

Figure 7-4   Herniations. (A) Cystocele. (B) Rectocele.

cyst/o/scope SĬST-ō-skōp **cyst/o/scopy** sĭs-TŎS-kō-pē	**7–54** Cyst/o/scopy is a procedure that uses a rigid or flexible cyst/o/scope inserted through the urethra to examine the urinary bladder. (See Figure 7–5.) The endo/scope used to perform cyst/o/scopy is called a _____ / _____ / _____. The cyst/o/scope is used to perform the diagnostic procedure called _____ / _____ / _____.
cyst/o/scope SĬST-ō-skōp	**7–55** The cyst/o/scope has an optical lighting system, special lenses and mirrors. It also contains a hollow channel for inserting operative devices to obtain biopsy specimens and remove tumors and small stones. A video attachment can be used to create a permanent visual record. (See Figure 7–5.) To excise polyps from the bladder, the ur/o/logist uses the special instrument called a _____ / _____ / _____.
cyst/o **-scope** **radi/o** **-graphy**	**7–56** In addition to inserting operative devices through a cyst/o/scope, catheters may be placed through the cyst/o/scope to obtain urine samples and to inject a contrast medium into the bladder during radi/o/graphy. Determine elements in this frame that mean *bladder:* _____ / _____ *instrument for examining:* _____ *radiation, x-ray; radius (lower arm bone on thumb side):* _____ / _____ *process of recording:* _____

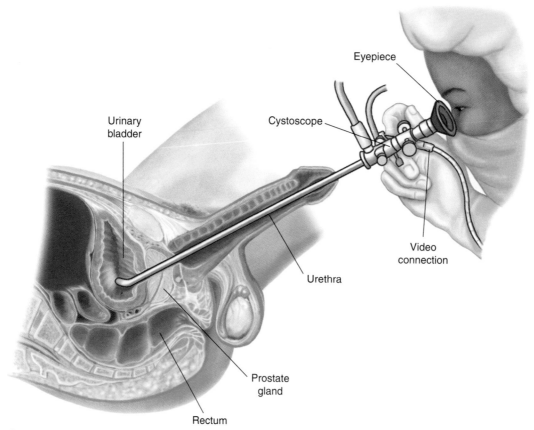

Figure 7-5 Cystoscopy.

cyst/ectomy sĭs-TĔK-tō-mē **cyst/o/plasty** SĬS-tō-plăs-tē **cyst/o/scope** SĬST-ō-skōp	**7-57** Construct surgical terms that mean *excision of the bladder:* _____ / _____ *surgical repair of the bladder:* _____ / _____ / _____ *instrument to view the bladder:* _____ / _____ / _____

urethr/o	**7-58** The urethra differs in men and women. In men, it serves a dual purpose of conveying sperm and discharging urine from the bladder. The female urethra performs only the latter function. Regardless of the sex, the CF for *urethra* is _____ / _____.

urethr/itis ū-rē-THRĪ-tĭs **urethr/ectomy** ū-rē-THRĔK-tō-mē **urethr/o/pexy** ū-RĒ-thrō-pĕks-ē **urethr/o/plasty** ū-RĒ-thrō-plăs-tē	**7-59** Form medical words that mean *inflammation of the urethra:* _____ / _____ *excision of the urethra:* _____ / _____ *surgical fixation of the urethra:* _____ / ____ / _____ *surgical repair of the urethra:* _____ / ____ / _____.
pain, urethra ū-RĒ-thră	**7-60** Urethr/o/dynia is a _____ in the _____.
urethr/algia ū-rē-THRĂL-jē-ă	**7-61** Besides urethr/o/dynia, construct another word that means *pain in the urethra:* _____ / _____.
cyst/itis sĭs-TĪ-tĭs **urethr/itis** ū-rē-THRĪ-tĭs **UTI**	**7-62** Cyst/itis and urethr/itis are two common lower urinary tract infections (UTIs) that frequently occur in women. Write terms that mean *inflammation of the* *bladder:* _____ / _____ *urethra:* _____ / _____ Write the abbreviation for *urinary tract infection.* _____
urethr/al ū-RĒ-thrăl **lumen** LŪ-mĕn	**7-63** Urethr/al stricture is a narrowing of the lumen (a tubular space within a structure) caused by scar tissue. Urethr/al stricture commonly results when catheters or surgical instruments are inserted into the urethra. Other causes are untreated gonorrhea and congenital abnormalities. Urethr/al stricture results in diminished urinary stream and causes UTIs because of urinary flow obstruction. Review terminology in this frame by identifying terms that mean *pertaining to the urethra:* _____ / _____ *tubular space within a structure:* _____
urethra, rectum ū-RĒ-thră, RĔK-tŭm	**7-64** *Urethr/o/rect/al* means *pertaining to the* _____ *and* _____.
urethr/o/cyst/itis ū-rē-thrō-sĭs-TĪ-tĭs	**7-65** Construct a medical word that means *inflammation of urethra and bladder.* _____ / ____ / _____ / _____

urethr/o/scope ū-RĒ-thrō-skōp **urethr/o/scopy** ū-rē-THRŎS-kō-pē	**7–66** Form diagnostic terms that mean *instrument for examining the urethra:* _____ / _____ / _____ *visual examination of the urethra:* _____ / _____ / _____
cyst/o/urethr/o/scope sĭs-tō-ū-RĒ-thrō-skōp	**7–67** Cyst/o/urethr/o/scopy is a visual examination of the urethra and bladder. The instrument used to perform a cyst/o/urethr/o/scopy is a _____ / ____ / _____ / ____ / _____.
-ia	**7–68** Identify the element in *-algia, -dynia, -pepsia,* and *-phagia* that means *condition.* _____
malignant mă-LĬG-nănt **benign** bĕ-NĪN	**7–69** Malignant tumors are cancerous; benign tumors are noncancerous. Use *malignant* or *benign* to complete the following statements. Cancerous tumors are _____ tumors. Noncancerous tumors are _____ tumors.
noncancerous	**7–70** Benign tumors do not invade surrounding tissue and are contained within a capsule. They become harmful only when they start placing pressure on adjacent structures. For example, a benign tumor of the uterus may place pressure on the urinary bladder and cause frequent urination. Benign tumors are (cancerous, noncancerous) _____ growths.
cancerous	**7–71** Malignant tumors spread rapidly and are invasive and life-threatening. Malignant tumors are (cancerous, noncancerous) _____.
pain, gland	**7–72** The CF **aden/o** is used in words to denote a *gland.* *Aden/o/dynia* is _____ in a _____.
gland **cancer** **tumor**	**7–73** Urin/ary tract tumors may be benign or malignant. The most common malignant ren/al tumor is an aden/o/carcin/oma. See if you can define the following elements: *aden/o:* _____ *carcin:* _____ *-oma:* _____

aden/oma ăd-ĕ-NŌ-mă **aden/o/carcin/oma** ăd-ĕ-nō-kăr-sĭn-Ō-mă	**7-74** An aden/oma is a benign glandular tumor composed of tissue from which it is developing; an aden/o/carcin/oma is a malignant glandular tumor. Determine words in this frame that mean *benign glandular tumor:* _____ / _____ *malignant glandular tumor:* _____ / _____ / _____ / _____
aden/itis ăd-ĕ-NĪ-tĭs **aden/oma** ăd-ĕ-NŌ-mă **aden/o/pathy** ăd-ĕ-NŎP-ă-thē	**7-75** Form medical words that mean *inflammation of a gland:* _____ / _____ *tumor of a gland:* _____ / _____ *disease of a gland:* _____ / _____ / _____
urinary tract infections	**7-76** Urinary tract infections (UTIs) account for most office visits by patients experiencing urinary tract problems. What does the abbreviation *UTIs* stand for? _____ _____ _____
nephrons NĔF-rŏnz	**7-77** *Nephrons* are micro/scop/ic filtering units of the kidneys (see Figure 7–2, structure 6). They are designed to filter urea and other waste products from blood. Nephrons are also responsible for maintaining home/o/stasis (keeping body fluids in balance). Complex structures designed to efficiently filter waste materials from blood are known as _____.
	7-78 Urine is collected in funnel-shaped extensions called **calyces** (singular, *calyx*) and empties into the **renal pelvis** and through the ureters. Both ureters convey the urine to the bladder for storage until it is expelled through the urethra during the process of urination (micturition). Locate the two structures in Figure 7–1 to see the path of urine as it is expelled through the ureters.
inflammation	**7-79** The CF **pyel/o** means *renal pelvis*. *Pelvis* is a word denoting any bowl-shaped structure. The symptomatic term *pyel/itis* refers to an _____ of the renal pelvis.

pyel/o/pathy
pī-ĕ-LŎP-ă-thē

pyel/o/tomy
pī-ĕ-LŎT-ō-mē

pyel/o/stomy
pī-ĕ-LŎS-tō-mē

7–80 Construct medical words that mean

disease of the renal pelvis: _____ / _____ / _____

incision of the renal pelvis: _____ / _____ / _____

forming an opening (mouth) into the renal pelvis:

_____ / _____ / _____

S E C T I O N   R E V I E W   7 - 3

Using the following table, write the CF or suffix that matches its definition in the space provided to the left of the definition. There may be more than one word element that matches a definition.

Combining Forms		Suffixes	
aden/o	ureter/o	-ectomy	-oma
carcin/o	urethr/o	-ectasis	-pathy
cyst/o	vesic/o	-iasis	-plasty
enter/o		-itis	-rrhaphy
pyel/o		-lith	-scope
rect/o		-megaly	-tomy

1. _____ abnormal condition (produced by something specified)
2. _____ bladder
3. _____ cancer
4. _____ disease
5. _____ enlargement
6. _____ excision, removal
7. _____ dilation, expansion
8. _____ gland
9. _____ incision
10. _____ inflammation
11. _____ instrument for examining
12. _____ intestine (usually small intestine)
13. _____ renal pelvis
14. _____ rectum
15. _____ stone, calculus
16. _____ surgical repair
17. _____ suture
18. _____ tumor
19. _____ ureter
20. _____ urethra

Competency Verification: Check your answers in Appendix B, Answer Key, page 569. If you are not satisfied with your level of comprehension, go back to Frame 7–1 and rework the frames.

Correct Answers _____ × 5 = _____ % Score

Nephron Structure

7-81 Label Figure 7–6 as you read the following information. The kidney is composed of an outer layer, called the (1) **renal cortex**, and an inner region, called the (2) **renal medulla.**

7-82 Nephrons, more than 1 million microscopic filtering units in each kidney, are designed to form urine in the process of filtration, reabsorption, and secretion.

In addition to numerous other structures, each nephron contains a (3) **glomerulus** (plural, *glomeruli*), which is a tiny ball of coiled, intertwined capillaries, and a (4) **collecting tubule.** The collecting tubule conveys newly formed urine to the renal pelvis where it is excreted by the kidneys. Nephrons maintain homeostasis in the body by selectively removing waste products from blood by forming urine, which is expelled from the body. The capsule that surrounds and encloses the glomerulus is called (5) **Bowman capsule.**

Label the urinary structures in Figure 7–6.

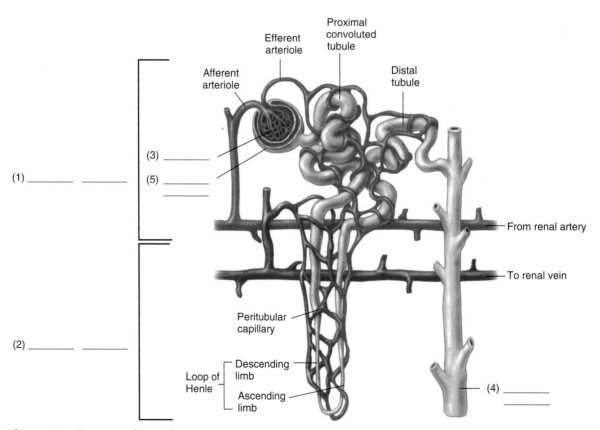

Figure 7-6 Structure of a nephron.

7-83 Glomerul/o/nephr/itis is an inflammatory disease of the kidney that primarily involves the glomerulus. It is characterized by hyper/tension, olig/uria, electrolyte imbalances, and edema. The CF *olig/o* means *scanty*. Identify terms in this frame that mean

hyper/tension
hī-pĕr-TĚN-shŭn

high blood pressure: _____ / _____

olig/uria
ŏl-ĭg-Ū-rē-ă

diminished capacity to pass urine: _____ / _____

edema
ĕ-DĒ-mă

swelling (of a body part): _____

glomerul/o/nephr/itis
glō-mĕr-ū-lō-nĕ-FRĪ-tĭs

inflammation of the glomerulus:

_____ / _____ / _____ / _____

7-84 Use *glomerul/o* to form medical words that mean

glomerul/itis
glō-mĕr-ū-LĪ-tĭs

inflammation of a glomerulus: _____ / _____

glomerul/o/pathy
glō-mĕr-ū-LŎP-ă-thē

disease of a glomerulus: _____ / _____ / _____

---

glomerulus *or* **glomeruli, hardening**
glō-MĚR-ū-lŭs, glō-MĚR-ū-lī

7-85 *Glomerul/o/scler/osis* literally means *an abnormal condition of*

_____ _____.

Competency Verification: Check your labeling of Figure 7–6 with Appendix B, Answer Key, page 569.

pyel/itis
pī-ĕ-LĪ-tĭs

7-86 The renal pelvis (see Figure 7–1) is a funnel-shaped dilation that drains urine from the kidney into the ureter. Inflammation of the renal pelvis is called _____ / _____.

KUB

7-87 To determine urinary tract abnormalities, such as tumors, swollen kidneys, and calculi, the physician may order a radi/o/graph/ic examination called *KUB (kidney, ureter, bladder)*. The radi/o/graph identifies location, size, shape, and malformation of the kidneys, ureters, and bladder. Stones and calcified areas may also be detected.
The diagnostic test of the kidneys, ureters, and bladder is recorded in the medical chart with the abbreviation _____.

IVP

7-88 Intra/ven/ous pyel/o/graphy (IVP) provides multiple radi/o/graph/ic images of the ren/al pelvis and urin/ary tract after injection of a contrast medium. IVP provides detailed information about the structure and function of the kidneys, ureters, bladder, and urethra.
To confirm a Dx of ren/al calculi or other urin/ary disorders, a radi/o/graph involving IV injection of a contrast dye may be ordered. The abbreviation for this type of radiograph is _____.

7–89 An intra/ven/ous pyel/o/gram (IVP) provides visualization of urinary structures. It is used to assess the urinary tract and identify nephr/o/liths and ureter/o/liths.
Determine words in this frame that mean

intra/ven/ous
ĭn-tră-VĒ-nŭs

within a vein: _____ / _____ / _____

pyel/o/gram
PĪ-ĕ-lō-grăm

record (x-ray) of renal pelvis: _____ / _____ / _____

nephr/o/liths
NĔF-rō-lĭths

stones in kidney: _____ / _____ / _____

ureter/o/liths
ū-RĔ-tĕr-ō-lĭths

stones in the ureter: _____ / _____ / _____

7–90 The prefix *retro-* means *backward, behind.* The suffix *-grade* means *to go.* The term *retro/grade* is used to describe a specific type of pyel/o/graphy. Retro/grade pyel/o/graphy (RP) consists of radi/o/graph/ic images taken after a contrast medium is injected through a urin/ary catheter directly into the urethra, bladder, and ureters.
Identify two types of pyel/o/graphy.

intra/ven/ous pyel/o/graphy (IVP)
ĭn-tră-VĒ-nŭs pī-ĕ-LŎG-ră-fē

Pyel/o/graphy in which a contrast medium is injected within a vein is called _____ / _____ / _____ _____ / _____ / _____ (_____).

retro/grade pyel/o/graphy (RP)
RĔT-rō-grād pī-ĕ-LŎG-ră-fē

Pyel/o/graphy in which a contrast medium is injected into the urethra is called _____ / _____ _____ / _____ / _____ (_____).

7–91 Build medical terms that mean

pyel/itis
pī-ĕ-LĪ-tĭs

inflammation of renal pelvis: _____ / _____

pyel/o/plasty
PĪ-ĕ-lō-plăs-tē

surgical repair of renal pelvis: _____ / _____ / _____

ureter/o/pyel/o/plasty
ū-rē-tĕr-ō-PĪ-ĕl-ō-plăs-tē

surgical repair of ureter and renal pelvis:
_____ / _____ / _____ / _____ / _____

7–92 The nephr/o/scope, a fiberoptic instrument, is used for visualization of the kidney and to disintegrate and remove ren/al calculi.
Use **nephr/o** to construct medical terms that mean

nephr/o/scope
NĔF-rō-skōp

instrument for examining the kidney: _____ / _____ / _____

nephr/o/scopy
nĕ-FRŎ-skŏ-pē

visual examination of the kidney: _____ / _____ / _____

nephr/o/scopy ně-FRŎ-skŏ-pē	**7-93** Incision of the renal pelvis is performed to insert a nephr/o/scope, usually to assess the kidney's interior. A visual examination of the kidney is known as _____ / _____ / _____.
pyel/itis pī-ě-LĪ-tĭs **pyel/o/nephr/itis** pī-ě-lō-ně-FRĪ-tĭs	**7-94** Pyel/o/nephr/itis is a bacterial infection of the ren/al pelvis and kidney caused by bacterial invasion from the middle and lower urinary tract or bloodstream. Bacteria may gain access to the bladder via the urethra and ascend to the kidney. Form medical words that mean *inflammation of the* *renal pelvis:* _____ / _____ *renal pelvis and kidney:* _____ / _____ / _____ / _____
pyel/o/nephr/itis pī-ě-lō-ně-FRĪ-tĭs	**7-95** Pyel/o/nephr/itis is an extremely dangerous condition, especially in pregnant women, because it can cause premature labor. The medical term for bacterial infection of the renal pelvis and kidneys is _____ / _____ / _____ / _____.
bladder **urethra** ū-RĒ-thră **rectum** RĔK-tŭm **intestine** ĭn-TĔS-tĭn	**7-96** Four common types of hernias that occur as downward displacements are *cyst/o/cele,* herniation of the _____ *urethr/o/cele,* herniation of the _____ *rect/o/cele,* herniation of the _____ *enter/o/cele,* herniation of the _____
cyst/o/cele SĬS-tō-sēl **urethr/o/cele** ū-RĒ-thrō-sēl **rect/o/cele** RĔK-tō-sēl	**7-97** Cyst/o/cele is a hernia in which the bladder bulges through a weakness in the muscular wall of the vagina or rectum. This causes urinary retention in the part of the bladder that pouches into the vagina or rectum. In the female, herniation of the bladder into the vagina may be caused by childbirth or age. Practice building medical terms that mean *herniation of the* *bladder:* _____ / _____ / _____ *urethra:* _____ / _____ / _____ *rectum:* _____ / _____ / _____

*For an illustration of a cystocele and a rectocele, see Figure 7–4.

white **red**	**7-98** The CF *erythr/o* denotes the color *red;* **leuk/o** denotes the color *white.* *Leuk/o/rrhea* is a discharge that is _____ . *Erythr/uria* is urine that is _____ .
cell **cell**	**7-99** The CF for *cell* is **cyt/o.** The suffix *-cyte* also means *cell.* *Erythr/o/cyte* is a red blood _____ . *Leuk/o/cyte* is a white blood _____ .
urine Ū-rĭn	**7-100** *Ur/o/toxin* is a poisonous substance in _____ .
toxin TŎKS-ĭn	**7-101** From *ur/o/toxin,* determine the element that means *poisonous.* _____
poison	**7-102** A toxic substance in the body is a substance that resembles or is caused by _____ .
ur/o/logy ū-RŎL-ō-jē **ur/o/logist** ū-RŎL-ō-jĭst	**7-103** Use **ur/o** to form words that mean *study of the urinary tract:* _____ / _____ / _____ *specialist in study of the urinary tract:* _____ / _____ / _____

Two combining forms that sound alike but have different meanings are **pyel/o** and **py/o**. Here is a useful clarification:

Combining Form	Meaning	Example
pyel/o	renal pelvis	pyel/o/pathy
py/o	pus	py/o/rrhea

pyel/o/plasty PĪ-ĕ-lō-plăs-tē **pyel/o/gram** PĪ-ĕ-lō-grăm	**7-104** Form medical words that mean *surgical repair of renal pelvis:* _____ / _____ / _____ *record (x-ray) of renal pelvis:* _____ / _____ / _____
py/o/rrhea pī-ō-RĒ-ă **py/o/nephr/osis** pī-ō-nĕf-RŌ-sĭs	**7-105** Use **py/o** *(pus)* to build words that mean *discharge or flow of pus:* _____ / _____ / _____ *abnormal condition of pus from the kidney:* _____ / _____ / _____ / _____

Note: Remember not to use *-iasis* because the pus is not produced by something specified; the term just denotes that there is pus in the kidneys.

---

py/uria
pī-Ū-rē-ă

7-106 An important diagnostic test that provides early detection of ren/al disease is urinalysis. Urine samples are analyzed for abnormalities, such as blood or pus in urine and other physical and chemical properties. *Hemat/uria* is a condition of blood in the urine. Form a word meaning pus in the urine.

_____ / _____

---

an/uria
ăn-Ū-rē-ă

7-107 The prefixes *a-* and *an-* are used in words to mean *without* or *not*. The *a-* is usually used before a consonant; the *an-* is usually used before a vowel.
Construct a word that literally means *without urine*.

_____ / _____

---

proxim/al

dist/al

7-108 *Hydr/o/nephr/osis* is an enlargement of the kidney due to constant pressure from backed-up urine in the ureter. It may be caused by a stricture, tumor, or a stone in the proxim/al part of a ureter that obstructs urine flow. When obstruction occurs in the dist/al part of the ureter, the condition is called *hydr/o/ureter with hydr/o/nephr/osis*. (See Figure 7–7.)
Identify the terms in this frame that mean

nearest the point of attachment: _____ / _____

farthest from the point of attachment: _____ / _____

---

hydr/o/nephr/osis
hī-drō-nĕf-RŌ-sĭs

7-109 Although partial obstruction in hydr/o/nephr/osis may not produce symptoms initially, the built-up pressure behind the area of obstruction eventually results in symptoms of ren/al dysfunction.
When calculi obstruction causes cessation of urine flow, it may result in a

condition called _____ / _____ / _____ / _____.

---

hydr/o/nephr/osis
hī-drō-nĕf-RŌ-sĭs

7-110 Presence of ren/al calculi increases the risk of urinary tract infections (UTIs) because they obstruct the free flow of urine. Untreated obstruction of a stone in any of the urin/ary structures can also result in retention of urine and damage to the kidney. (See Figure 7–7.)
Build a word that means *abnormal condition of water (urine) in*

the kidney _____ / _____ / _____ / _____.

---

py/uria
pī-Ū-rē-ă

hemat/uria
hĕm-ă-TŪ-rē-ă

7-111 A person who suffers from hydr/o/nephr/osis may experience pain, hemat/uria, and py/uria. Blood or pus may be present in the urine. Build medical words that mean

pus in the urine: _____ / _____

blood in the urine: _____ / _____

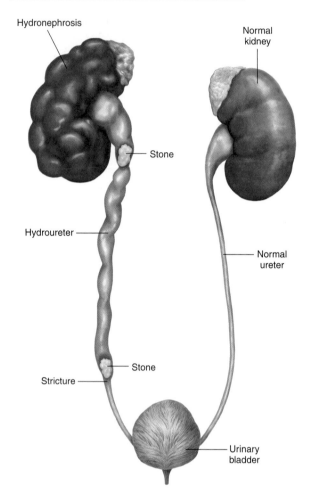

Hydronephrosis

Stone

Hydroureter

Stone

Stricture

Normal kidney

Normal ureter

Urinary bladder

Figure 7-7   Hydronephrosis.

olig/uria ŏl-ĭg-Ū-rē-ă	**7-112** The CF *olig/o* means *scanty*. Combine *olig/o* and *-uria* to form a word that means *scanty urination*. _____ / _____
olig/uria ŏl-ĭg-Ū-rē-ă	**7-113** Diminished or scanty amount of urine formation is known as _____ / _____.
py/uria pī-Ū-rē-ă	**7-114** Py/uria is the presence of an excessive number of white blood cells in urine. It is generally a sign of a urinary tract infection. A viral infection of the bladder and urethra may result in the condition called _____ / _____.
poly/uria pŏl-ē-Ū-rē-ă	**7-115** The prefix *poly-* means *many, much*. Combine *poly-* and *-uria* to build a word that means *excessive urination*. _____ / _____

poly/cyst/ic pŏl-ē-SĬS-tĭk **ur/emia** ū-RĒ-mē-ă	**7–116** Poly/cyst/ic kidney disease (PKD) is an abnormal condition in which the kidneys are enlarged and contain many cysts. Kidney failure commonly develops over time, requiring dialysis or kidney transplantation. Identify terms in this frame that mean *pertaining to many cysts:* _____ / _____ / _____ *increase in concentration of urea and other nitrogenous wastes in the blood:* _____ / _____
azot/uria ăz-ō-TŪ-rē-ă	**7–117** Azot/emia also means an increase in concentration of urea and other nitrogenous wastes in blood. Use **azot/o** to form a word meaning increase of nitrogenous wastes in urine. _____ / _____.
noct/uria nŏk-TŪ-rē-ă	**7–118** Noct/uria refers to urination at night. If a child has a tendency to urinate at night, the condition is known as _____ / _____.
urination *or* **urine** ū-rĭ-NĀ-shŭn	**7–119** Continence is the ability to control urination and defecation. A person who has urinary continence is able to control urination. A person with urinary in/continence is not able to control _____.
in/continence ĭn-KON-tĭ-nēns	**7–120** Elderly patients in nursing homes may experience uncontrolled loss of urine from the bladder. They may suffer from the condition known as *urinary* _____ / _____.
ur/o/logist ū-RŎL-ō-jĭst **nephr/o/logist** nĕ-FRŎL-ō-jĭst	**7–121** Ur/o/logists specialize in treating urin/ary tract disorders; Nephr/o/logists specialize in management of kidney disease, kidney transplantation, and dia/lysis therapies. Persons with urin/ary disorders see the medical specialist called a _____ / _____ / _____. Persons with kidney disorders, including transplantations and dia/lysis see the medical specialist called a _____ / _____ / _____.
hemat/uria hĕm-ă-TŪ-rē-ă	**7–122** Cyst/itis, an inflammatory condition of the urin/ary bladder, is commonly caused by bacterial infection and is characterized by pain, frequency of urination, urgency and, sometimes, hemat/uria. If cyst/itis results in traces of blood in urine, the medical term for this condition is _____ / _____.
cyst/itis sĭs-TĪ-tĭs	**7–123** When a patient has inflammation of the bladder, the condition is diagnosed as _____ / _____.

7-124 Cyst/itis is more common in women, due to their shorter urethra and the closeness of the urethr/al orifice to the anus. Symptoms of cyst/itis include dys/uria, urgency, and urinary frequency. Urinalysis reveals bacteri/uria, and py/uria.
Identify words in this frame that mean

py/uria
pī-Ū-rē-ă

pus in urine: _____ / _____

dys/uria
dĭs-Ū-rē-ă

painful urination: _____ / _____

bacteri/uria
băk-tē-rē-Ū-rē-ă

bacteria in urine: _____ / _____

cyst/itis
sĭs-TĪ-tĭs

inflammation of bladder: _____ / _____

7-125 Pyel/o/nephr/itis, an inflammation of the renal pelvis and the kidney, is a common type of kidney disease and a frequent complication of cystitis.
Build a medical term that means *inflammation of the*

nephr/itis
nĕf-RĪ-tĭs

kidney: _____ / _____

pyel/o/nephr/itis
pī-ĕ-lō-nĕ-FRĪ-tĭs

renal pelvis and kidney: _____ / ____ / _____ / _____

7-126 Glomerul/o/nephr/itis, a form of nephr/itis in which lesions involve primarily the glomeruli, may result in protein/uria and hemat/uria. Determine medical words in this frame that mean

hemat/uria
hĕm-ă-TŪ-rē-ă

blood in urine: _____ / _____

protein/uria
prō-tē-ĭn-Ū-rē-ă

protein in urine: _____ / _____

nephr/itis
nĕf-RĪ-tĭs

inflammation of the kidney: _____ / _____

glomerul/o/nephr/itis
glō-mĕr-Ū-lō-nĕ-FRĪ-tĭs

7-127 A form of nephr/itis that involves the glomeruli is called
_____ / ____ / _____ / _____ .

7-128 Any condition that impairs flow of blood to the kidneys, such as shock, injury, or exposure to toxins, may result in acute renal failure (ARF).

acute renal failure

The abbreviation *ARF* refers to

_____ _____ _____ .

7-129 Nephr/o/lith/iasis occurs when salts in the urine precipitate (settle out of solution and grow in size). Elimination of the stone(s) may occur spontaneously, but crushing the stone(s) by means of lith/o/tripsy may sometimes be necessary.
Build medical terms that mean

lith/ectomy
lĭ-THĔK-tō-mē

excision of a stone: _____ / _____

lith/o/tripsy
LĬTH-ō-trĭp-sē

crushing a stone: _____ / _____ / _____

nephr/o/lith/iasis
nĕf-rō-lĭth-Ī-ă-sĭs

abnormal condition (produced by something specified) of kidney stone(s):

_____ / _____ / _____ / _____

7-130 *Extracorporeal shock-wave lithotripsy (ESWL)* uses powerful sound wave vibrations to break up calculi in the urin/ary tract or gallbladder. (See Figure 7–8.) Ultrasound (US) is used to locate and monitor stones as they are being destroyed. Complete removal of stones and their fragments during urination is ensured by administration of an oral dissolution drug. Identify abbreviations for

US

ultrasound: _____

ESWL

extracorporeal shock-wave lithotripsy: _____

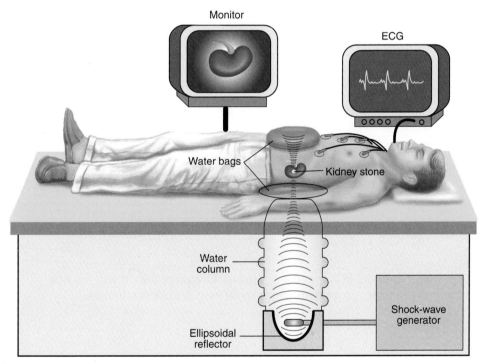

Figure 7-8 Extracorporeal shock-wave lithotripsy.

SECTION REVIEW 7-4

Using the following table, write the CF, suffix, or prefix that matches its definition in the space provided to the left of the definition. There may be more than one word element that matches a definition.

Combining Forms		Suffixes	Prefixes
cyst/o	pyel/o	-cele	a-
cyt/o	py/o	-cyte	an-
erythr/o	ren/o	-ist	intra-
glomerul/o	scler/o	-ptosis	poly-
hemat/o	ureter/o		
leuk/o	urethr/o		
nephr/o	ur/o		
olig/o	vesic/o		

1. _____ bladder
2. _____ blood
3. _____ cell
4. _____ glomerulus
5. _____ hardening; sclera (white of eye)
6. _____ specialist
7. _____ kidney
8. _____ pus
9. _____ red
10. _____ renal pelvis

11. _____ scanty
12. _____ ureter
13. _____ urethra
14. _____ urine; urinary tract
15. _____ white
16. _____ hernia, swelling
17. _____ many, much
18. _____ prolapse, downward displacement
19. _____ in, within
20. _____ without, not

Competency Verification: Check your answers in Appendix B, Answer Key, page 569. If you are not satisfied with your level of comprehension, go back to Frame 7–81 and rework the frames.

Correct Answers _____ × 5 = _____ % Score

Abbreviations

This section introduces urinary system-related abbreviations and their meanings. Included are abbreviations contained in the medical record activities that follow.

Abbreviation	Meaning	Abbreviation	Meaning
ARF	acute renal failure	EU	excretory urography
		IVP	intravenous pyelogram; intravenous pyelography
BNO	bladder neck obstruction	IVU	intravenous urogram; intravenous urography
BPH	benign prostatic hyperplasia; benign prostatic hypertrophy	KUB	kidney, ureter, bladder
BUN	blood urea nitrogen	PKD	polycystic kidney disease
CRF	chronic renal failure	PSA	prostate-specific antigen
CT	computed tomography	RP	retrograde pyelography
cysto	cystoscopy	TURP	transurethral resection of the prostate
DRE	digital rectal examination	UA	urinalysis
ED	erectile dysfuntion; emergency department	US	ultrasonography, ultrasound
ESRD	end-stage renal disease	UTI	urinary tract infection
ESWL	extracorporeal shock-wave lithotripsy	VCUG	voiding cystourethrogram; voiding cystourethrography

Additional Medical Terms

The following are additional terms related to the urinary system. Recognizing and learning these terms will help you understand the connection between a pathological condition, its diagnosis, and the rationale behind the method of treatment selected for a particular disorder.

Signs, Symptoms, and Diseases

azoturia ăz-ō-TŪ-rē-ă *azot:* nitrogenous compounds *-uria:* urine	Increase of nitrogenous substances, especially urea, in urine
diuresis dī-ū-RĒ-sĭs *di-:* double *ur:* urine *-esis:* condition	Increased formation and secretion of urine
dysuria dĭs-Ū-rē-ă *dys-:* bad; painful; difficult *-uria:* urine	Painful or difficult urination, symptomatic of cystitis and other urinary tract conditions
end-stage renal disease (ESRD) RĒ-năl	Kidney disease that has advanced to the point that the kidneys can no longer adequately filter the blood and, ultimately, requires dialysis or renal transplantation for survival; also called *chronic renal failure* (CRF) (See Figure 7–9.) *Common diseases leading to ESRD include malignant hypertension, infections, diabetes mellitus, and glomerulonephritis. Diabetes is the most common cause of kidney transplantation.*
enuresis ĕn-ū-RĒ-sĭs *en-:* in, within *ur:* urine *-esis:* condition	Involuntary discharge of urine after the age at which bladder control should be established; also called *bed-wetting at night* or *nocturnal enuresis* *In children, voluntary control of urination is usually present by age 5.*
hypospadias hī-pō-SPĀ-dē-ăs *hypo-:* under, below, deficient *-spadias:* slit, fissure	Abnormal congenital opening of the male urethra on the undersurface of the penis
interstitial nephritis ĭn-tĕr-STĬSH-ăl nĕf-RĪ-tĭs *nephr:* kidney *-itis:* inflammation	Condition associated with pathological changes in the renal interstitial tissue that may be primary or due to a toxic agent, such as a drug or chemical, which results in destruction of nephrons and severe impairment in renal function

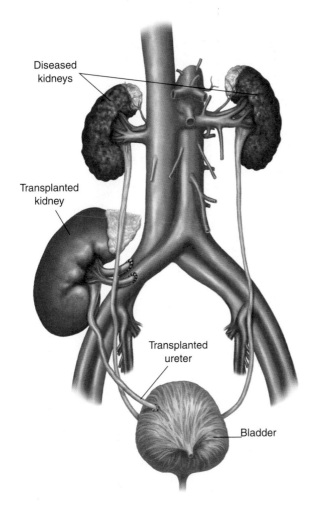

- Diseased kidneys
- Transplanted kidney
- Transplanted ureter
- Bladder

Figure 7-9   Renal transplantation.

renal hypertension RĒ-năl hī-pĕr-TĔN-shŭn *ren:* kidney *-al:* pertaining to *hyper-:* excessive, above normal *-tension:* to stretch	High blood pressure that results from kidney disease
uremia ū-RĒ-mē-ă *ur:* urine *-emia:* blood	Elevated level of urea and other nitrogenous waste products in the blood, as occurs in renal failure; also called *azotemia*
Wilms tumor VĬLMZ TOO-mor	Malignant neoplasm of the kidney that occurs in young children, usually before age 5 *The most common early signs of Wilms tumor are hypertension, a palpable mass, pain, and hematuria.*

Diagnostic Procedures

blood urea nitrogen (BUN) ū-RĒ-ă NĪ-trō-jĕn	Laboratory test that measures the amount of urea (nitrogenous waste product) in the blood and demonstrates the kidneys' ability to filter urea from the blood for excretion in urine *An increase in BUN level may indicate impaired kidney function.*
computed tomography (CT) kŏm-PŪ-tĕd tō-MŎG-ră-fē *tom/o:* to cut *-graphy:* process of recording	Radiographic technique that uses a narrow beam of x-rays that rotates in a full arc around the patient to acquire multiple views of the body that a computer interprets to produce cross-sectional images of that body part *CT scanning is used to diagnose kidney, ureter, and bladder tumors, cysts; inflammation; abscesses; perforation; bleeding; and obstructions. It may be administered with or without a contrast medium.*
kidney, ureter, bladder (KUB)	Radiographic examination to determine the location, size, shape, and malformation of the kidneys, ureters, and bladder *KUB radiography may also detect stones and calcified areas.*
pyelography pī-ĕ-LŎG-ră-fē *pyel/o:* renal pelvis *-graphy:* process of recording	Radiographic study of the kidney, ureters, and usually the bladder after injection of a contrast agent *A contrast medium is injected into a vein (intravenous pyelography) or through a catheter placed through the urethra, bladder, or ureter and into the renal pelvis (retrograde pyelography).*
intravenous pyelography (IVP) ĭn-tră-VĒ-nŭs pī-ĕ-LŎG-ră-fē *intra:* in, within *ven:* vein *-ous:* pertaining to *pyel/o:* renal pelvis *-graphy:* process of recording	Radiographic imaging in which a contrast medium is injected intravenously and serial x-ray films are taken to provide visualization of the entire urinary tract; also called *intravenous urography* (IVU) or *excretory urography* (EU) *In IVP, the x-ray image produced is known as a pyelogram or urogram.*
retrograde pyelography (RP) RĔT-rō-grād pī-ĕ-LŎG-ră-fē *retro-:* backward, behind *-grade:* to go *pyel/o:* renal pelvis *-graphy:* process of recording	Radiographic imaging in which a contrast medium is introduced through a cystoscope directly into the bladder and ureters using small-caliber catheters *RP provides detailed visualization of the urinary collecting system (pelvis and calices of the kidney as well as the ureters). It is useful in locating urinary tract obstruction. It may also be used as a substitute for IVP when a patient is allergic to the contrast medium.*

renal scan RĒ-năl *ren:* kidney *-al:* pertaining to	Nuclear medicine imaging procedure that determines renal function and shape through measurement of a radioactive substance that is injected intravenously and concentrates in the kidney
urinalysis ū-rĭ-NĂL-ĭ-sĭs	Physical, chemical, and microscopic evaluation of urine
voiding cystourethrography (VCUG) sĭs-tō-ū-rē-THRŎG-ră-fē *cyst/o:* bladder *urethr/o:* urethra *-graphy:* process of recording	Radiography of the bladder and urethra after filling the bladder with a contrast medium and during the process of voiding urine

Medical and Surgical Procedures

catheterization kăth-ĕ-tĕr-ĭ-ZĀ-shŭn	Insertion of a catheter (hollow flexible tube) into a body cavity or organ to instill a substance or remove fluid, most commonly. through the urethra into the bladder to withdraw urine (See Figure 7–10.) *Catheters are available in two basic types: straight and indweeling, with many variations in shape, coatings, and so forth.*

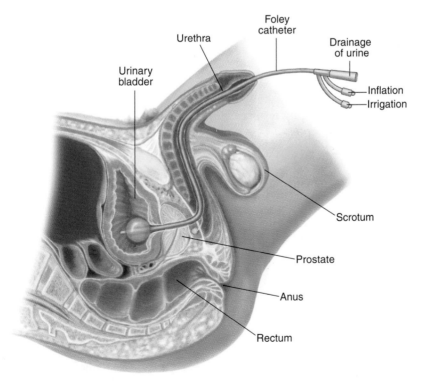

Figure 7-10 Catheterization.

dialysis dī-ĂL-ĭ-sĭs *dia-:* through, across *-lysis:* separation; destruction; loosening	Mechanical filtering process used to cleanse blood of high concentrations of metabolic waste products, draw off excess fluids, and regulate body chemistry when kidneys fail to function properly *Two primary methods are used to dialyze the blood: hemodialysis and peritoneal dialysis.*
hemodialysis hē-mō-dī-ĂL-ĭ-sĭs	Process of removing excess fluids and toxins from the blood by continually shunting (diverting) the patient's blood from the body into a dialysis machine for filtering, and then returning the clean blood to the patient's body via tubes connected to the circulatory system (See Figure 7–11.)
peritoneal dialysis pĕr-ĭ-tō-NĒ-ăl dī-ĂL-ĭ-sĭs	Dialysis in which the patient's own peritoneum is used as the dialyzing membrane (See Figure 7–12.) *In peritoneal dialysis, dialyzing fluid passes through a tube into the peritoneal cavity and remains there for a prescribed period. During this time, wastes diffuse across the peritoneal membrane into the fluid. Contaminated fluid then drains out and is replaced with fresh solution. This process is repeated as often as required and may be continuous or intermittent.*
renal transplantation RĒ-năl trăns-plăn-TĀ-shŭn *ren:* kidney *-al:* pertaining to	Transplant of a kidney in a patient with end-stage renal disease; also called *kidney transplantation* (See Figure 7–9.)

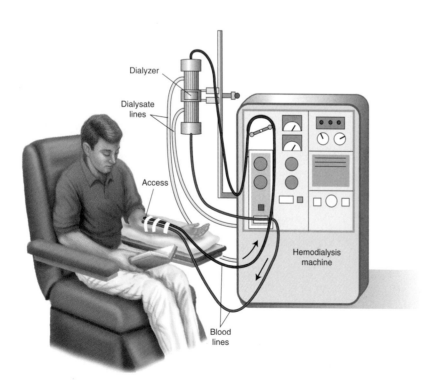

Figure 7-11 Hemodialysis.

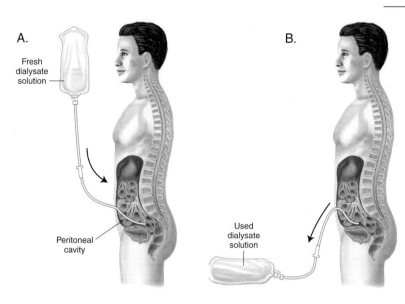

A.

Fresh
dialysate
solution

Peritoneal
cavity

B.

Used
dialysate
solution

Figure 7-12 Peritoneal dialysis.
(A) Introducing dialysis fluid into the
peritoneal cavity. (B) Draining dialysate
with waste products from peritoneal
cavity.

Pharmacology

antibiotics ăn-tĭ-bī-ŎT-ĭks	Agents that treat bacterial infections of the urinary tract by acting on the bacterial membrane or one of its metabolic processes
antispasmodics ăn-tĭ-spăz-MŌT-ĭks	Agents that decrease spasms in the urethra and bladder (caused by UTIs and catheterization) by relaxing the smooth muscles lining their walls, thus allowing normal emptying of the bladder
diuretics dī-ū-RĔT-ĭks	Agents that block reabsorption of sodium by the kidneys, thereby increasing the amount of salt and water excreted in the urine (causes reduction of fluid retained in the body and prevents edema)

Additional Medical Terms Review

Match the medical term(s) below with the definitions in the numbered list.

azoturia	diuresis	interstitial nephritis	urinalysis
BUN	dysuria	renal hypertension	VCUG
catheterization	enuresis	retrograde pyelography	Wilms tumor
dialysis	hypospadias	uremia	

1. _____ refers to physical, chemical, and microscopic examination of urine.

2. _____ is a malignant neoplasm in the kidney that occurs in young children.

3. _____ is an increase in nitrogenous compounds in urine.

4. _____ means painful or difficult urination, symptomatic of numerous conditions.

5. _____ means increased formation and secretion of urine.

6. _____ is a radiologic technique in which a contrast medium is introduced through a cystoscope to provide detailed visualization of urinary collecting system.

7. _____ is an abnormal congenital opening of the male urethra on the undersurface of the penis.

8. _____ is nephritis associated with pathological changes in the renal interstitial tissue, which may be primary or due to a toxic agent.

9. _____ is a test that measures the amount of urea excreted by kidneys into the blood.

10. _____ means urinary incontinence, including bed-wetting.

11. _____ refers to insertion of a hollow, flexible tube into a body cavity or organ to instill a substance or remove fluid.

12. _____ is radiography of the bladder and urethra after introduction of a contrast medium and during the process of urination.

13. _____ refers to an elevated level of urea and other nitrogenous waste products in blood.

14. _____ refers to high blood pressure that results from kidney disease.

15. _____ is the mechanical filtering process used to cleanse blood of high concentrations of metabolic waste products.

Competency Verification: Check your answers in Appendix B, Answer Key, page 569. If you are not satisfied with your level of comprehension, review the pathological, diagnostic, and therapeutic terms and retake the review.

Correct Answers _____ × 6.67 = _____ % Score

Medical Record Activities

Medical reports included in the following activities reflect common, real-life clinical scenarios using medical terminology to document patient care.

MEDICAL RECORD ACTIVITY 7-1

Cystitis

Terminology

Terms listed in the table below come from the medical report *Cystitis* that follows. Use a medical dictionary such as *Taber's Cyclopedic Medical Dictionary*, the appendices of this book, or other resources to define each term. Then practice reading the pronunciations aloud for each term.

Term	Definition
cholecystectomy kō-lē-sĭs-TĔK-tō-mē	_____
cholecystitis kō-lē-sĭs-TĪ-tĭs	_____
choledocholithiasis kō-lĕd-ō-kō-lĭ-THĪ-ă-sĭs	_____
choledocholithotomy kō-lĕd-ō-kō-lĭth-ŎT-ō-mē	_____
cholelithiasis kō-lē-lĭ-THĪ-ă-sĭs	_____
cystitis sĭs-TĪ-tĭs	_____
cystoscopy sĭs-TŎS-kō-pē	_____
epigastric ĕp-ĭ-GĂS-trĭk	_____
hematuria hĕm-ă-TŪ-rē-ă	_____
nocturia nŏk-TŪ-rē-ă	_____
polyuria pŏl-ē-Ū-rē-ă	_____
urinary incontinence Ū-rĭ-nār-ē ĭn-KŎNT-ĭn-ĕns	_____

Listen and Learn Online! will help you master pronunciations of selected medical words from this medical record activity. Visit *http://davisplus.fadavis.com/gylys/simplified* to find instructions on completing the *Listen and Learn Online!* exercise for this section and to practice pronunciations.

Reading

Practice pronunciation of medical terms by reading the following medical report aloud.

Cystitis

This 50-year-old white woman has been complaining of diffuse pelvic pain with urinary bladder spasm since cystoscopy 10 days ago, at which time marked cystitis was noted. She reports nocturia 3–4 times, urinary frequency, urgency, and epigastric discomfort. The patient has a history of polyuria, hematuria, and urinary incontinence. There is a history of numerous stones, large and small, in the gallbladder. In 20xx she was admitted to the hospital with cholecystitis, chronic and acute; cholelithiasis; and choledocholithiasis. Subsequently, cholecystectomy, choledocholithotomy, and incidental appendectomy were performed. My impression is that the urinary incontinence is due to cystitis and is temporary in nature.

Evaluation

Review the medical report above to answer the following questions. Use a medical dictionary such as *Taber's Cyclopedic Medical Dictionary* and other resources if needed.

1. What was found when the patient had a cystoscopy?

_____

_____

2. What are the symptoms of cystitis?

_____

_____

3. What is the patient's past surgical history?

_____

_____

4. What is the treatment for cystitis?

_____

_____

5. What are the dangers of untreated cystitis?

_____

_____

6. What instrument is used to perform a cystoscopy?

_____

_____

Dysuria with Benign Prostatic Hypertrophy

Terminology

Terms listed in the table below come from the medical report *Dysuria with Benign Prostatic Hypertrophy* that follows. Use a medical dictionary such as *Taber's Cyclopedic Medical Dictionary,* the appendices of this book, or other resources to define each term. Then practice reading the pronunciations aloud for each term.

Term	Definition
asymptomatic ā-sĭmp-tō-MĂT-ĭk	
auscultation aws-kŭl-TĀ-shŭn	
basal cell carcinoma BĀ-săl SĔL kăr-sĭ-NŌ-mă	
benign prostatic hypertrophy bē-NĪN prŏs-TĂT-ĭk hī-PĔR-trō-fē	
bilateral bī-LĂT-ĕr-ăl	
bruits brwēz	
catheterization kăth-ĕ-tĕr-ĭ-ZĀ-shŭn	
colectomy kō-LĔK-tō-mē	
distended dĭs-TĔND-ĕd	
dysuria dĭs-Ū-rē-ă	
frequency FRĒ-kwĕn-sē	
hemorrhoid HĔM-ō-royd	
hydrocele HĪ-drō-sēl	
impotence ĬM-pō-tĕns	

(continued)

Term	Definition
inguinal hernia ĬNG-gwĭ-năl HĔR-nē-ă	
normocephalic nor-mō-sĕ-FĂL-ĭk	
palpable PĂL-pă-bl	
percussion pĕr-KŬSH-ŭn	
pneumothorax nū-mō-THŌ-răks	
transurethral trăns-ū-RĔ-thrăl	

Listen and Learn Online! will help you master pronunciations of selected medical words from this medical record activity. Visit *http://davisplus.fadavis.com/gylys/simplified* to find instructions on completing the *Listen and Learn Online!* exercise for this section and to practice pronunciations.

Reading

Practice pronunciation of medical terms by reading the following medical report aloud.

Dysuria with Benign Prostatic Hypertrophy

HISTORY OF PRESENT ILLNESS: Patient is a 72-year-old white man with symptoms of dysuria and frequency before this admission. He recently was found to have colon cancer and is being admitted for colectomy. Preoperative catheterization was not possible, and consultation with Dr. Moriarty was obtained.

PAST HISTORY: Negative for transurethral resection of the prostate or any urological trauma or venereal disease. Past medical history includes hemorrhoid symptoms, bilateral inguinal hernia repair, high cholesterol, retinal surgery, spontaneous pneumothorax ×2 requiring chest tube insertion. He also had a basal cell carcinoma.

PHYSICAL EXAMINATION: Head: Normocephalic. **Eyes, Ears, Nose, and Throat:** Within normal limits. **Neck:** No nodes. No bruits over carotids. **Chest:** Clear to auscultation and percussion. **Heart:** Normal heart sounds. No murmur. **Abdomen:** Soft and nontender. No masses are palpable. It is very distended. **Penis:** Normal. There is a right hydrocele. **Rectal:** Examination reveals benign prostatic hypertrophy.

ASSESSMENT: 1. Mild to moderate benign prostatic hypertrophy.
2. Status post colon resection for carcinoma of the colon.
3. Right hydrocele, asymptomatic.

Evaluation

Review the medical report to answer the following questions. Use a medical dictionary such as *Taber's Cyclopedic Medical Dictionary* and other resources if needed.

1. What prompted the consultation with the urologist, Dr. Moriarty?

_____

_____

2. What abnormality did the urologist discover?

_____

_____

3. Did the patient have any previous surgery on his prostate?

_____

_____

4. Where was the patient's hernia?

_____

_____

5. What in the patient's past medical history contributed to his present urological problem?

_____

_____

Chapter Review

Word Elements Summary

The following table summarizes CFs, suffixes, and prefixes related to the urinary system.

Word Element	Meaning	Word Element	Meaning
Combining Forms			
URINARY STRUCTURES			
cyst/o, vesic/o	bladder	**pyel/o**	renal pelvis
glomerul/o	glomerulus	**ureter/o**	ureter
nephr/o, ren/o	kidney	**urethr/o**	urethra
OTHER COMBINING FORMS			
aden/o	gland	**noct/o**	night
carcin/o	cancer	**olig/o**	scanty
enter/o	intestine (usually small intestine)	**py/o**	pus
erythr/o	red	**rect/o**	rectum
gastr/o	stomach	**scler/o**	hardening; sclera (white of eye)
hemat/o	blood	**ur/o, urin/o**	urine
hepat/o	liver	**ven/o**	vein
lith/o	stone, calculus		
Suffixes			
SURGICAL			
-ectomy	excision, removal	**-stomy**	forming an opening (mouth)
-pexy	fixation (of an organ)	**-tome**	instrument to cut
-plasty	surgical repair	**-tomy**	incision
-rrhaphy	suture	**-tripsy**	crushing
DIAGNOSTIC, SYMPTOMATIC, AND RELATED			
-algia, -dynia	pain	**-logy**	study of
-cele	hernia, swelling	**-megaly**	enlargement
-cyte	cell	**-oma**	tumor

Word Element	Meaning	Word Element	Meaning
-ectasis	dilation, expansion	-osis	abnormal condition; increase (used primarily with blood cells)
-edema	swelling	-pathy	disease
-emesis	vomiting	-pepsia	digestion
-grade	to go	-phagia	swallowing, eating
-gram	record, writing	-phobia	fear
-graphy	process of recording	-ptosis	prolapse, downward displacement
-iasis	abnormal condition (produced by something specified)	-rrhea	discharge, flow
-itis	inflammation	-scope	instrument for examining
-lith	stone, calculus	-scopy	visual examination
-logist	specialist in study of	-uria	urine

ADJECTIVE

-al, -ic, -ous	pertaining to		

NOUN

-ia	condition	-ist	specialist

Prefixes			
a-, an-	without, not	poly-	many, much
dys-	bad; painful; difficult	retro-	backward, behind
in-	in, not	supra-	above; excessive; superior
Intra-	in, within		

Enhance your study and reinforcement of word elements with the power of *Davis Plus*. Visit *http://davisplus.fadavis.com/gylys/simplified* for this chapter's flash-card activity. We recommend you complete the flash-card activity before completing the word elements review below.

Word Elements Review

After you review the Word Elements Summary, complete this activity by writing the meaning of each element in the space provided.

Word Element	Meaning	Word Element	Meaning
Combining Forms			
URINARY STRUCTURES			
1. cyst/o, vesic/o	_____	5. ureter/o	_____
2. glomerul/o	_____	6. urethr/o	_____
3. nephr/o, ren/o	_____	7. ur/o	_____
4. pyel/o	_____		
OTHER COMBINING FORMS			
8. aden/o	_____	14. noct/o	_____
9. carcin/o	_____	15. olig/o	_____
10. erythr/o	_____	16. py/o	_____
11. gastr/o	_____	17. rect/o	_____
12. hemat/o	_____	18. scler/o	_____
13. lith/o	_____		
Suffixes			
SURGICAL			
19. -ectomy	_____	23. -stomy	_____
20. -pexy	_____	24. -tome	_____
21. -plasty	_____	25. -tomy	_____
22. -rrhaphy	_____	26. -tripsy	_____
DIAGNOSTIC, SYMPTOMATIC, AND RELATED			
27. -algia, dynia	_____	36. -megaly	_____
28. -cele	_____	37. -oma	_____
29. -cyte	_____	38. -osis	_____
30. -ectasis	_____	39. -pathy	_____
31. -edema	_____	40. -ptosis	_____
32. -gram	_____	41. -scope	_____
33. -graphy	_____	42. -scopy	_____
34. -iasis	_____	43. -uria	_____
35. -lith	_____		

Word Element	Meaning	Word Element	Meaning
Prefixes			
44. a-, an-	_____	**48.** poly-	_____
45. dys-	_____	**49.** retro-	_____
46. in-	_____	**50.** supra-	_____
47. intra-	_____		

Competency Verification: Check your answers in Appendix A, Glossary of Medical Word Elements, page 538. If you are not satisfied with your level of comprehension, review the word elements and retake the review.

Correct Answers _____ × 2 = _____ % Score

Vocabulary Review

Match the medical term(s) with the definitions in the numbered list.

acute renal failure	cystocele	malignant	oliguria
anuria	diuretics	nephrolithotomy	polyuria
benign	edema	nephrons	renal pelvis
bilateral	hematuria	nephroptosis	ureteropyeloplasty
cholelithiasis	IVP	nocturia	urinary incontinence

1. _____ means tending or threatening to produce death; refers to cancerous growths.

2. _____ are microscopic filtering units in the kidney that are responsible for keeping body fluids in balance.

3. _____ refers to formation of gallstones.

4. _____ is a funnel-shaped reservoir that is the basin of the kidney.

5. _____ is an x-ray film of the kidneys after injection of dye.

6. _____ are drugs that stimulate flow of urine.

7. _____ means swelling (of body tissues).

8. _____ means noncancerous.

9. _____ is an incision into a kidney to remove a stone.

10. _____ is a condition that results from lack of blood flow to the kidneys.

11. _____ is downward displacement of a kidney.

12. _____ is surgical repair of a ureter and renal pelvis.

13. _____ means pertaining to two sides.

14. _____ means excessive urination at night.

15. _____ refers to inability to hold urine.

16. _____ refers to presence of blood cells in urine.

17. _____ means excessive discharge of urine.

18. _____ is a diminished amount of urine formation.

19. _____ is absence of urine formation.

20. _____ is herniation of the urinary bladder.

Competency Verification: Check your answers in Appendix B, Answer Key, page 570. If you are not satisfied with your level of comprehension, review the chapter vocabulary and retake the review.

Correct Answers _____ × 5 = _____ % Score

8 Reproductive Systems

OBJECTIVES

Upon completion of this chapter, you will be able to:

■ Describe the type of medical treatment gynecologists and obstetricians provide.

■ Identify female and male reproductive structures by labeling them on the anatomical illustrations.

■ Describe primary functions of the female and male reproductive systems.

■ Describe common diseases related to the female and male reproductive systems.

■ Describe common diagnostic, medical, and surgical procedures related to the female and male reproductive systems.

■ Apply your word-building skills by constructing medical terms related to the female and male reproductive systems.

■ Describe common abbreviations and symbols related to the female and male reproductive systems.

■ Reinforce word elements by completing flash card activities.

■ Recognize, define, pronounce, and spell terms correctly.

■ Demonstrate your knowledge of this chapter by successfully completing the frames, reviews, and medical report evaluations.

Medical Specialties

Gynecology and Obstetrics

Gynecology is the medical specialty concerned with diagnosis and treatment of female reproductive disorders, including the breasts. Unlike most medical specialties, gynecology encompasses surgical and nonsurgical expertise of the physician. The gynecologist is a physician who specializes in gynecology. Because obstetrics is studied in conjunction with gynecology, the physician's medical practice commonly includes both areas of expertise. This branch of medicine is called *obstetrics and gynecology (OB-GYN)*. The obstetrician and gynecologist possess knowledge of endocrinology because hormones play an important role in the functions of the female reproductive system, especially the process of secondary sex characteristics, menstruation, pregnancy, and menopause. Therefore infertility, birth control, and hormone imbalance are all part of the treatment provided by an OB-GYN physician.

 Obstetrics is the branch of medicine concerned with pregnancy and childbirth, including the study of the physiological and pathological functions of the female reproductive tract. It also involves the care of the mother and fetus throughout pregnancy, childbirth, and the immediate **postpartum** (after birth) period. An **obstetrician** is a physician who specializes in obstetrics. The branch of medicine that concentrates on the care of the neonate (newborn) and in the diagnosis and treatment of disorders of the neonate is known as *neonatology*. Once the infant is born, physicians called *neonatologists* specialize in providing their medical care.

Urology

Urology is the branch of medicine concerned with disorders and care of the urinary tract in men and women and of the male reproductive system. **Urologists** diagnose and treat disorders of the male reproductive system, such as sexual dysfunction and infertility. Their scope of practice includes various surgeries, such as transurethral resection of the prostate and cystoscopy. In addition, urologists treat genitourinary tract diseases that affect the urinary system of men and women.

Anatomy and Physiology Overview

Although structures of the female and male reproductive systems differ, both have a common purpose. They are specialized to produce and unite *gametes* (reproductive cells) and transport them to sites of fertilization. Reproductive systems of both sexes are designed specifically to perpetuate the species and pass genetic material from generation to generation. In addition, both sexes produce hormones, which are vital in the development and maintenance of sexual characteristics and regulation of reproductive physiology. In women, the reproductive system includes the ovaries, fallopian tubes, uterus, vagina, clitoris, and vulva. (See Figure 8–1.) In men, the reproductive system includes the testes, epididymis, vas deferens, seminal vesicles, ejaculatory duct, prostate, and penis.

Female Reproductive System

The female reproductive system is composed of internal organs of reproduction and external genitalia. The internal organs are the ovaries, fallopian tubes (oviducts, uterine tubes), uterus, and vagina. External organs, also called the *genitalia,* are known collectively as the *vulva.* Included in the vulva are the mons pubis, labia majora, labia minora, clitoris, and Bartholin glands. (See Figure 8–1.) The combined organs of the female reproductive system are designed to produce and transport ova (female sex cells), discharge ova from the body if fertilization does not occur, and nourish and provide a place for the developing fetus throughout pregnancy if fertilization occurs. The female reproductive system also produces the female sex hormones estrogen and progesterone, which are responsible for development of secondary sex characteristics, such as breast development and regulation of the menstrual cycle.

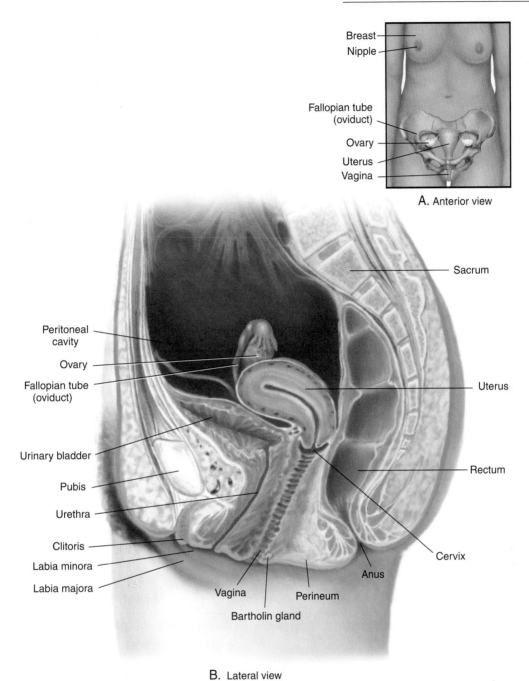

Breast
Nipple

Fallopian tube
(oviduct)
Ovary
Uterus
Vagina

A. Anterior view

Peritoneal
cavity
Ovary
Fallopian tube
(oviduct)

Urinary bladder

Pubis

Urethra

Clitoris
Labia minora
Labia majora

Vagina
Bartholin gland
Perineum
Anus
Cervix
Rectum
Uterus
Sacrum

B. Lateral view

Figure 8-1   Female reproductive system. (A) Anterior view. (B) Lateral view.

WORD ELEMENTS

This section introduces combining forms (CFs) related to the female reproductive system. Included are key suffixes; prefixes are defined in the right-hand column as needed. Review the following table and pronounce each word in the word analysis column aloud before you begin to work the frames.

Word Element	Meaning	Word Analysis
Combining Forms		
amni/o	amnion (amniotic sac)	**amni/o**/centesis (ăm-nē-ō-sĕn-TĒ-sĭs): surgical puncture of the amniotic sac *-centesis:* surgical puncture *The sample of amniotic fluid obtained in amniocentesis is studied chemically and cytologically to detect genetic abnormalities, biochemical disorders, and maternal-fetal blood incompatibility.*
cervic/o	neck; cervix uteri (neck of uterus)	**cervic**/itis (sĕr-vĭ-SĪ-tĭs): inflammation of cervix uteri *-itis:* inflammation
colp/o	vagina	**colp/o**/scopy (kŏl-PŎS-kō-pē): examination of the vagina and cervix with an optical magnifying instrument (colposcope) *-scopy:* visual examination *Colposcopy is commonly performed after a Papanicolaou (Pap) test for treatment of cervical dysplasia and to obtain biopsy specimens of the cervix.*
vagin/o		**vagin/o**/cele (VĂJ-ĭn-ō-sēl): herniation into the vagina; also called a *colpocele* *-cele:* hernia, swelling
galact/o	milk	**galact/o**/rrhea (gă-lăk-tō-RĒ-ă): discharge or flow of milk *-rrhea:* discharge, flow
lact/o		**lact/o**/gen (LĂK-tō-jĕn): production and secretion of milk *-gen:* forming, producing, origin
gynec/o	woman, female	**gynec/o**/logist (gī-nĕ-KŎL-ō-jĭst): physician specializing in treating disorders of the female reproductive system *-logist:* specialist in study of
hyster/o	uterus (womb)	**hyster**/ectomy (hĭs-tĕr-ĔK-tō-mē): excision of uterus *-ectomy:* excision, removal
uter/o		**uter/o**/vagin/al (ū-tĕr-ō-VĂJ-ĭ-năl): pertaining to the uterus and vagina *vagin:* vagina *-al:* pertaining to

Word Element	Meaning	Word Analysis
mamm/o	breast	**mamm**/o/gram (MĂM-ō-grăm): radiograph of the breast *-gram:* record, writing
mast/o		**mast**/o/pexy (MĂS-tō-pĕks-ē): surgical fixation of the breast(s) *-pexy:* fixation (of an organ) *Mastopexy is performed to affix sagging breasts in a more elevated position, commonly improving their shape.*
men/o	menses, menstruation	**men**/o/rrhagia (mĕn-ō-RĀ-jē-ă): excessive amount of menstrual flow over a longer duration than normal *-rrhagia:* bursting forth (of)
metr/o	uterus (womb); measure	endo/**metr**/itis (ĕn-dō-mē-TRĪ-tĭs): inflammation of the endometrium *endo-:* in, within *-itis:* inflammation
nat/o	birth	pre/**nat**/al (prē-NĀ-tl): pertaining to (the period) before birth *pre-:* before, in front of *-al:* pertaining to
oophor/o	ovary	**oophor**/oma (ō-ŏf-ōr-Ō-mă): ovarian tumor *-oma:* tumor
ovari/o		**ovari**/o/rrhexis (ō-văr-rē-ō-RĔK-sĭs): rupture of an ovary *-rrhexis:* rupture
perine/o	perineum	**perine**/o/rrhaphy (pĕr-ĭ-nē-OR-ă-fē): suture of the perineum *-rrhaphy:* suture *Perineorrhaphy is performed to repair a laceration that occurs spontaneously or is made surgically during the delivery of the fetus.*
salping/o	tube (usually fallopian or eustachian [auditory] tubes)	**salping**/ectomy (săl-pĭn-JĔK-tō-mē): excision of a fallopian tube *-ectomy:* excision, removal
vulv/o	vulva	**vulv**/o/pathy (vŭl-VŎP-ă-thē): disease of the vulva *-pathy:* disease
episi/o		**episi**/o/tomy (ĕ-pēs-ē-ŎT-ō-mē): incision of the perineum *Episiotomy is performed to enlarge the vaginal opening for delivery of the fetus.* *-tomy:* incision

(continued)

Word Element	Meaning	Word Analysis
Suffixes		
-arche	beginning	men/**arche** (měn-ĂR-kē): initial menstrual period *men:* menses, menstruation *Menarche usually occurs between ages 9 and 17.*
-cyesis	pregnancy	pseudo/**cyesis** (soo-dō-sī-Ē-sĭs): false pregnancy *In pseudocyesis, a woman believes she is pregnant when she is not.* *pseudo-:* false
-gravida	pregnant woman	primi/**gravida** (prī-mĭ-GRĂV-ĭ-dă): woman during her first pregnancy *primi-:* first
-para	to bear (offspring)	multi/**para** (mŭl-TĬP-ă-ră): woman who has delivered more than one viable infant *multi-:* many, much
-salpinx	tube (usually fallopian or eustachian [auditory] tubes)	hemat/o/**salpinx** (hěm-ă-tō-SĂL-pinks): collection of blood in a fallopian tube; also called *hemosalpinx.* *hemat/o:* blood *Hematosalpinx is commonly associated with a tubal pregnancy.*
-tocia	childbirth, labor	dys/**tocia** (dĭs-TŌ-sē-ă): childbirth that is painful and difficult *dys-:* bad; painful; difficult *Dystocia may be caused by an obstruction or constriction of the birth passage or abnormal size, shape, position, or condition of the fetus.*
-version	turning	retro/**version** (rět-rō-VĚR-shŭn): tipping back of an organ *retro-:* backward, behind *Uterine retroversion is measured as first, second, or third degree, depending on the angle of tilt in relationship to the vagina.*

Pronunciation Help	Long Sound Short Sound	ā in rāte ă in ălone	ē in rēbirth ĕ in ĕver	ī in īsle ĭ in ĭt	ō in ōver ŏ in nŏt	ū in ūnite ŭ in cŭt

 Listen and Learn, the audio CD-ROM included in this book, will help you master pronunciation of selected medical words. Use it to practice pronunciations of the above-listed medical terms and for instructions to complete the *Listen and Learn* exercise for this section.

SECTION REVIEW 8-1

For the following medical terms, first write the suffix and its meaning. Then translate the meaning of the remaining elements starting with the first part of the word. The first word is completed for you.

Term	Definition
1. primi/gravida	*-gravida: pregnant woman; first*
2. colp/o/scopy	
3. gynec/o/logist	
4. perine/o/rrhaphy	
5. hyster/ectomy	
6. oophor/oma	
7. dys/tocia	
8. endo/metr/itis	
9. mamm/o/gram	
10. amni/o/centesis	

Competency Verification: Check your answers in Appendix B, Answer Key, page 570. If you are not satisfied with your level of comprehension, review the vocabulary and retake the review.

Correct Answers _____ × 10 = _____ % Score

Internal Structures

8-1 The female reproductive system is composed of internal and external organs of reproduction. The internal reproductive organs are the (1) **ovaries**, (2) **fallopian tubes**, (3) **uterus**, and (4) **vagina**. Label these organs in Figures 8–2 and 8–3 as you learn the names of the internal reproductive organs.

---

tumor
TOO-mŏr

8-2 An *oophor/oma* is an ovarian _____. Pronounce the initial *o* and the second *o* in words with *oophor/o*.

---

oophor/o

8-3 The main purpose of the ovaries is to produce ovum, the female reproductive cell. This process is called *ovulation*. Another important function of the ovaries is to produce the hormones estrogen and progesterone. From *oophor/oma*, construct the CF for *ovary*.

_____ / _____

oophor/o/pathy
ō-ŏf-ŏr-ŎP-ă-thē

oophor/o/plasty
ō-ŎF-ŏr-ō-plăs-tē

oophor/o/pexy
ō-ŏf-ō-rō-PĔK-sē

8-4 Use *oophor/o* to build medical words that mean

disease of the ovaries: _____ / _____ / _____

surgical repair of an ovary:

_____ / _____ / _____

fixation of a displaced ovary: _____ / _____ / _____

8-5 The CF *salping/o* means *tube (usually fallopian or eustachian [auditory] tube)* and is related to the female reproductive system. Eustachian (auditory) tubes are related to the sense of hearing and are discussed in Chapter 11.

salping/o/plasty
săl-PĬNG-gō-plăs-tē

Surgical repair of a fallopian tube (also known as *oviduct*) is called

_____ / _____ / _____.

---

salping/o

8-6 Approximately once a month, maturation of the ovum, or *ovulation,* occurs when the egg leaves the ovary and slowly travels down the fallopian tube to the uterus. (See Figure 8–3.) If union of the ovum with sperm takes place during this time, fertilization (pregnancy) results.
To form words for the fallopian tube(s), uterine tube(s), or oviduct(s), use the CF _____ / _____.

---

salping/ectomy
săl-pĭn-JĔK-tō-mē

8-7 If the fertilized egg attaches to the wall of the fallopian tube (instead of the uterus), the tube must be removed to prevent serious bleeding in or possible death of the mother.
When a fallopian tube is removed, the surgical procedure is called

_____ / _____.

---

instrument

8-8 A salping/o/scope is an _____ for viewing the fallopian tube(s).

---

salping/o/scopy
săl-pĭng-GŎS-kō-pē

8-9 Visual examination of the fallopian tube(s) is called
_____ / _____ / _____.

---

salping/o/cele
săl-PĬNG-ō-sēl

8-10 Herniation of a fallopian tube(s) is known as
_____ / _____ / _____.

---

oviducts
Ŏ-vĭ-dŭkts

8-11 Locate the two small tubes leading to each ovary that are called
fallopian tubes, uterine tubes, or _____. (See Figure 8–3.)

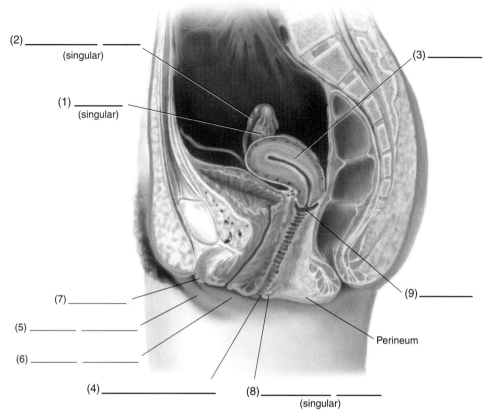

(2) _____ _____
(singular)

(1) _____
(singular)

(3) _____

(7) _____

(5) _____ _____

(6) _____ _____

(4) _____

(9) _____

Perineum

(8) _____ _____
(singular)

Figure 8-2 Lateral view of the female reproductive system.

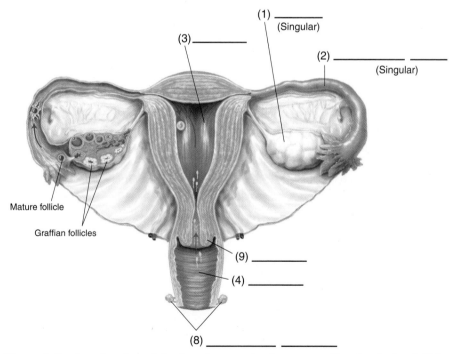

(1) _____
(Singular)

(3) _____

(2) _____ _____
(Singular)

Mature follicle

Graffian follicles

(9) _____

(4) _____

(8) _____ _____

Figure 8-3 Anterior view of the female reproductive system. The developing follicles are shown in the sectioned left ovary, fertilization in the sectioned left fallopian tube, and internal structures of the vagina and uterus. The red arrow indicates the movement of the ovum toward the uterus; the blue arrow indicates the movement of the sperm toward the fallopian tube.

hernia *or* **herniation,** **uterus** HĔR-nē-ă *or* hĕr-nē-Ā-shŭn, Ū-tĕr-ŭs	**8-12** The uterus, also called the *womb,* is the organ that contains and nourishes the embryo and fetus from the time the fertilized egg is implanted to the time of birth. The CF *hyster/o* is used to form words about the uterus as an organ. A *hyster/ o/cele* is a _____ of the _____.
hyster/o/pathy hĭs-tēr-ŎP-ă-thē **hyster/algia, hyster/o/ dynia** hĭs-tĕr-ĂL-jē-ā, hĭs-tĕr-ō-DĬN-ē-ă **hyster/o/spasm** HĬS-tĕr-ō-spăzm	**8-13** Use *hyster/o* to construct medical words that mean *disease of the uterus:* _____ / _____ / _____ *pain in the uterus:* _____ / _____ or _____ / _____ / _____ *involuntary contraction, twitching of uterus:* _____ / _____ / _____
hyster/ectomy hĭs-tĕr-ĔK-tō-mē **hyster/o/tomy** hĭs-tĕr-ŎT-ō-mē	**8-14** Presence of one or more tumors (either benign or malignant) in the uterus may necessitate its removal. (See Figure 8–4.) Use *hyster/o* to form surgical terms that mean *excision of uterus:* _____ / _____ *incision of uterus:* _____ / _____ / _____
dictionary	**8-15** Besides *hyster/o,* the CFs *metr/o* and *uter/o* are also used to denote the *uterus.* When in doubt about forming medical words with *hyster/o, uter/o,* or *metr/o,* refer to your medical _____.
hyster/o/scopy hĭs-tĕr-ŎS-kō-pē **uter/o/scopy** Ū-tĕr-ŏs-kō-pē	**8-16** The uterus is a muscular, hollow, pear-shaped structure located in the pelvic area between the bladder and rectum. (See Figure 8–1.) Use *hyster/o* to form a word that means *visual examination of the uterus.* _____ / _____ / _____ Use *uter/o* to form another word that means *visual examination of the uterus.* _____ / _____ / _____
hyster/o/ptosis hĭs-tĕr-ŏp-TŌ-sĭs	**8-17** The uterus is supported and held in place by ligaments. Weakening of these ligaments may cause a downward displacement, or *prolapse,* of the uterus. Combine *hyster/o* and *-ptosis* to form a word that means *a prolapse or downward displacement of the uterus.* _____ / _____ / _____

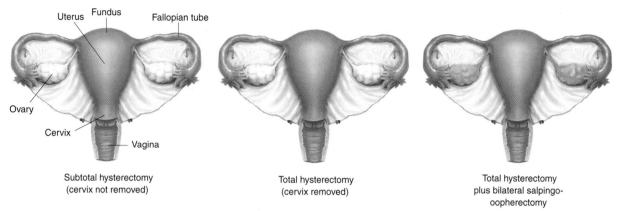

Figure 8-4   Hysterectomy showing the excised structure shaded in purple.

uterus Ū-tēr-ŭs **-ine**	**8-18** A diagnosis (Dx) of uter/ine hemorrhage denotes bleeding from the _____. The element in this frame that means *pertaining to* is _____.
hyster/o, uter/o **-pexy**	**8-19** A prolapsed uterus may be caused by heavy physical exertion, pregnancy, or an inherent weakness. The surgical procedure to correct a prolapsed uterus is known as *hyster/o/pexy* or *uter/o/pexy*. Write the elements in this frame that mean *uterus:* _____ / ____, _____ / ____ *fixation (of an organ):* _____
surgical repair, uterus Ū-tĕr-ŭs	**8-20** Surgical repair is denoted by the suffix *-plasty*. *Hyster/o/plasty, uter/o/plasty,* and *metr/o/plasty* all refer to _____ _____ of the _____.
hyster/o/cele HĬS-tĕr-ō-sēl	**8-21** Hyster/o/cele, a protrusion of uter/ine contents into a weakened area of the uterine wall, may occur as a result of pregnancy. A Dx of *herniation of the uterus* would be documented in the medical chart as _____ / ____ / _____.
estrogen, progesterone ĔS-trō-jĕn, prō-JĔS-tĕr-ōn	**8-22** Two important hormones, estrogen and progesterone, are secreted by the ovaries. These hormones play an important role in the processes of menstruation and pregnancy as well as the development of secondary sex characteristics. When ovaries are diseased and necessitate removal, the body becomes deficient in the hormones known as _____ and _____.

men/o/pause
MĔN-ō-pawz

trans/derm/al
trănz-DĔR-măl

8-23   Men/o/pause, a natural process, is the gradual ending of the menstrual cycle, which also results in an estrogen hormone deficiency. Hormone replacement therapy (HRT) given orally or as a trans/derm/al patch may be used to relieve uncomfortable symptoms of men/o/pause. Identify terms in this frame that mean

cessation of the menses: _____ / _____ / _____

through, across the skin: _____ / _____ / _____

---

post/men/o/pause
pōst-MĔN-ō-pawz

8-24   The term *pre/men/o/pause* refers to a time period before men/o/pause. Can you build a word that refers to a time period after men/o/pause?

_____ / _____ / _____ / _____

---

bursting forth

8-25   The suffixes *-rrhage* and *-rrhagia* are used in words to mean *bursting forth (of)*. Hem/o/rrhage denotes a _____ _____ *(of) blood.*

---

hem/o

8-26   The CF in *hem/o/rrhage* that denotes *blood* is _____ / _____.

---

blood

8-27   The elements **hemat/o, hem/o,** and *-emia* refer to _____.

---

blood

8-28   *Hemat/o/logy* is the study of _____.

---

blood
tumor
TOO-mŏr

8-29   A hemat/oma is a localized collection or swelling of blood, usually clotted, in an organ, space, or tissue, caused by a break in the wall of a blood vessel.
Analyze *hemat/oma* by defining the elements.

hemat/o: _____

-oma: _____

---

hemat/o/logist
hē-mă-TŎL-ō-jĭst

hemat/o/pathy
hē-mă-TŎP-ă-thē

hemat/emesis
hĕm-ăt-ĔM-ĕ-sĭs

8-30   Use **hemat/o** to build medical words that mean

specialist in the study of blood: _____ / _____ / _____

disease of the blood: _____ / _____ / _____

vomiting blood: _____ / _____

cervic/itis sĕr-vĭ-SĪ-tĭs	**8-31** The CF ***cervic/o*** means *neck; cervix uteri (neck of uterus).* In the female reproductive system ***cervic/o*** is used in reference to the cervix uteri. The medical term for *inflammation of the cervix uteri* is _____ / _____.
curet kū-RĔT	**8-32** Dilation and curettage (D&C) is a surgical procedure to widen (dilate) the cervic/al canal of the uterus and scrape (curet) the endo/metri/um of the uterus. The instrument used to scrape the endo/metri/um is known as a _____. (See Figure 8–5.)
uterine sound **serrated**	**8-33** Review Figure 8–5 to learn about the surgical procedure and instruments used to perform D&C. What type of instrument is used to measure the uterus? _____ _____ What type of curet is used to scrape the uterine lining? _____

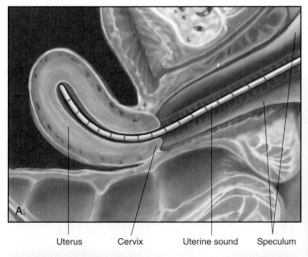

A.

Uterus   Cervix   Uterine sound   Speculum

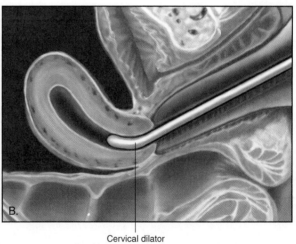

B.

Cervical dilator

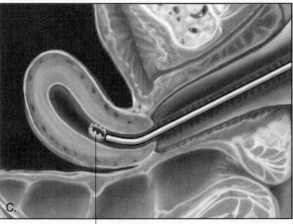

C.

Serrated curet

Figure 8-5 Dilation and curettage of the uterus. (A) Examination of the uterine cavity with a uterine sound, which measures the innermost part of the uterus to prevent perforation during dilation. (B) Dilation of the cervix with a series of dilators of increasing size to allow insertion of a curet into the uterus. (C) Scraping (curettage) of the uterine lining with a serrated uterine curet and collection of tissue samples for diagnostic purposes.

inflammation, vagina vă-JĪ-nă	**8-34** The vagina is a muscular tube that extends from the cervix (neck of the uterus) to the exterior of the body. (See Figure 8–3.) In addition to serving as the organ of sexual intercourse and the receptor of semen, the vagina discharges menstrual flow and acts as a passageway for the delivery of the fetus. The CFs *colp/o* and *vagin/o* refer to the vagina. *Colp/itis* is an _____ of the _____.
vagin/itis văj-ĭn-Ī-tĭs	**8-35** Form another word in addition to *colp/itis* that means *inflammation of the vagina.* _____ / _____
colp/algia kŏl-PĂL-jē-ā	**8-36** *Colp/o/dynia* is pain in the vagina. Use *colp/o* to build another term for *pain in the vagina.* _____ / _____
colp/o/spasm KŎL-pō-spăzm **colp/o/ptosis** kŏl-pŏp-TŌ-sĭs **colp/o/pexy** KŎL-pō-pĕk-sē	**8-37** Use *colp/o* to construct medical words that mean *spasm or twitching of the vagina:* _____ / _____ / _____ *prolapse or downward displacement of the vagina:* _____ / _____ / _____ *fixation of the vagina:* _____ / _____ / _____
vagin/o/plasty vă-JĪ-nō-plăs-tē **vagin/o/scope** VĂJ-ĭn-ō-skōp **vagin/o/tomy** văj-ĭ-NŎT-ō-mē	**8-38** Use *vagin/o* to form medical words that mean *surgical repair of the vagina:* _____ / _____ / _____ *instrument to view the vagina:* _____ / _____ / _____ *incision of the vagina:* _____ / _____ / _____
suture, vagina SŪ-chŭr, vă-JĪ-nă	**8-39** A prolapsed vagina usually is sutured to the abdominal wall. *Colp/o/rrhaphy* is a _____ of the _____.
vesic/o/vagin/al fistula vĕs-ĭ-kō-VĂJ-ĭ-năl, FĬS-tū-lă	**8-40** A vesic/o/vagin/al fistula is another type of path/o/logy that can develop in the female reproductive system. This is an an abnormal passage between the urinary bladder and the vagina. (See Figure 8–6.) An abnormal connection that develops between the bladder and vagina is known as a _____ / _____ / _____ / _____ _____.

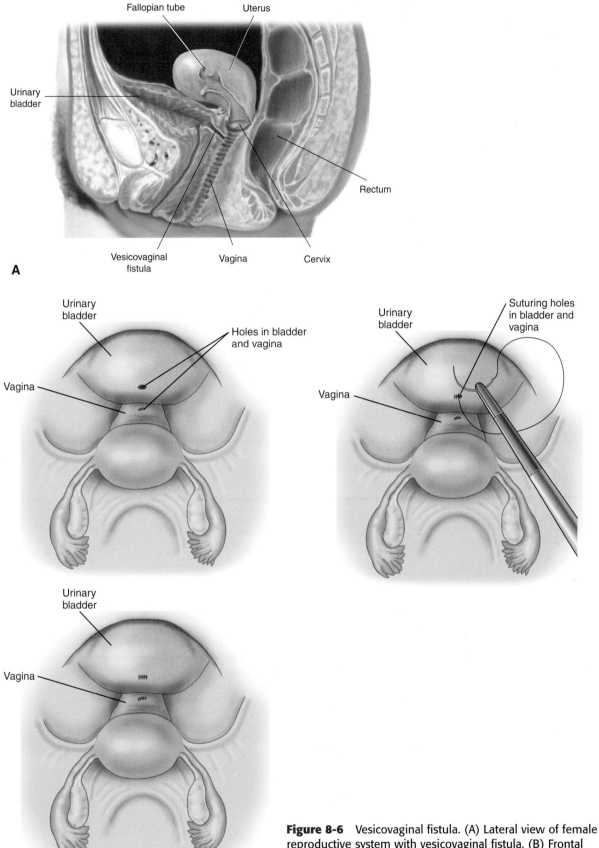

Fallopian tube

Uterus

Urinary
bladder

Rectum

Vesicovaginal
fistula

Vagina

Cervix

A

Urinary
bladder

Holes in bladder
and vagina

Vagina

Urinary
bladder

Suturing holes
in bladder and
vagina

Vagina

Urinary
bladder

Vagina

B

Vesicovaginal fistula repaired

Figure 8-6   Vesicovaginal fistula. (A) Lateral view of female
reproductive system with vesicovaginal fistula. (B) Frontal
view of the urinary bladder and vagina with vesicovaginal
fistula repair.

vagina vă-JĪ-nă	**8-41** The term *fistula* refers to an abnormal passage from one epithelial surface to another epithelial surface. It can occur in any body system. Thus, a vesic/o/vagin/al fistula is only one type of fistula. A ureter/o/vagin/al fistula occurs between the lower ureter and the _____.
vagina vă-JĪ-nă	**8-42** A rect/o/vagin/al fistula is one that develops between the rectum and the _____.
-rrhagia, -rrhage	**8-43** Colp/o/rrhagia is an excessive vagin/al discharge or a vagin/al hem/o/rrhage. The elements in these words that mean *bursting forth (of)* are _____ and _____.
hem/o/rrhage HĔM-ĕ-rĭj	**8-44** Form a word that means *bursting forth (of)* blood. _____ / ____ / _____
hernia, swelling HĔR-nē-ă	**8-45** Recall that *-cele* means _____ or _____.
vagina vă-JĪ-nă	**8-46** A colp/o/cyst/o/cele is swelling or herniation of the bladder into the _____.
vagina vă-JĪ-nă **bladder** **hernia, swelling** HĔR-nē-ă	**8-47** Women who have had several vagin/al childbirths may suffer from herniation of the bladder, or *colp/o/cyst/o/cele*. Identify the elements in *colp/o/cyst/o/cele*. *colp/o:* _____ *cyst/o:* _____ *-cele:* _____ or _____
vagin/al VĂJ-ĭn-ăl **hyster/ectomy** hĭs-tĕr-ĔK-tō-mē	**8-48** When the uterus is removed through the vagina, the surgical procedure is known as a *vagin/al hyster/ectomy* or a *colp/o/hyster/ectomy*. Identify words in this frame that mean *pertaining to the vagina:* _____ / _____ *excision of the uterus:* _____ / _____

muc/ous MŪ-kŭs	**8-49** The vagina is lubricated by mucus. ***Muc/o*** is the CF for mucus. Use the adjective ending *-ous* to form a word that means *pertaining to mucus*. _____ / _____
-oid	**8-50** The term *muc/oid* means *resembling mucus*. The adjective element that means *resembling* is _____.
resembling fat	**8-51** *Lip/oid* means _____ _____.
adip/oid ĂD-ĭ-poyd	**8-52** Use ***adip/o*** to form another term that means *resembling fat*. _____ / _____

SECTION REVIEW 8-2

Using the following table, write the CF and suffix that matches its definition in the space provided to the left of the definition. There may be more than one word element that matches a definition.

Combining Forms		Suffixes	
colp/o	muc/o	-arche	-ptosis
cyst/o	oophor/o	-cele	-rrhage
hemat/o	ovari/o	-logist	-rrhagia
hem/o	salping/o	-logy	-salpinx
hyster/o	uter/o	-oid	-scope
metr/o	vagin/o	-pexy	-tome
		-plasty	-tomy

1. _____ bladder

2. _____ blood

3. _____ bursting forth (of)

4. _____ uterus (womb)

5. _____ hernia, swelling

6. _____ incision

7. _____ instrument to cut

8. _____ instrument for examining

9. _____ tube (usually fallopian or eustachian [auditory] tubes)

10. _____ fixation (of an organ)

11. _____ mucus

12. _____ ovary

13. _____ beginning

14. _____ uterus (womb); measure

15. _____ prolapse, downward displacement

16. _____ resembling

17. _____ specialist in study of

18. _____ study of

19. _____ surgical repair

20. _____ vagina

Competency Verification: Check your answers in Appendix B, Answer Key, page 571. If you are not satisfied with your level of comprehension, go back to Frame 8–1 and rework the frames.

Correct Answers _____ × 5 = _____ % Score

External Structures

8-53 The external structures, or *genitalia*, include the (5) **labia majora** (the outer lips of the vagina), (6) **labia minora** (the smaller, inner lips of the vagina), (7) **clitoris**, and (8) **Bartholin glands**. Label Figures 8–2 and 8–3 to locate the structures of the genitalia.

---

vulva
VŬL-vă

8-54 The CF *vulv/o* refers to the vulva, the combined external structures of the female reproductive system. *Vulv/o/uter/ine* refers to the uterus and _____.

---

clitoris, Bartholin glands
KLĬT-ō-rĭs, BĂR-tō-lĭn

8-55 The external structures, or *genitalia* (also known as the *vulva*), include the labia majora, labia minora, _____ , and _____ _____.

---

muc/ous
MŪ-kŭs

8-56 Mucus secretions from Bartholin glands help keep the vagina moist and lubricated, facilitating intercourse.
Use *-ous* to build a word that means *pertaining to mucus*.
_____ / _____ (adjective ending)

---

vulv/itis
vŭl-VĪ-tĭs

vulv/o/pathy
vŭl-VŎP-ă-thē

8-57 Use *vulv/o* to construct words that mean

inflammation of the vulva: _____ / _____

disease of the vulva: _____ / _____ / _____

8-58 The (9) **cervix** is the neck of the uterus and extends into the upper portion of the vagina. Examine the position of the cervix in the lateral and anterior view as you label Figures 8–2 and 8–3.

---

cervic/itis
sĕr-vĭ-SĪ-tĭs

8-59 The CF *cervic/o* denotes the *cervix uteri* or the *neck*. Inflammation of the cervix uteri is called _____ / _____.

---

vagina, uteri
vă-JĪ-nă, Ū-tĕ-rī

8-60 When *cervic/o* is used in a word, you can determine whether it refers to the *neck* or the *cervix uteri* by reviewing the other parts of the word.
Colp/o/cervic/al refers to the _____ and cervix _____.

---

colp/o/scopy
kŏl-PŎS-kō-pē

8-61 A colp/o/scope, an instrument with a magnifying lens, is used to examine vagin/al and cervic/al tissue. Visual examination of vagin/al and cervic/al tissue using a colposcope is called
_____ / _____ / _____.

colp/o/scope
KŎL-pō-skōp

colp/o/scopy
kŏl-PŎS-kō-pē

vagin/al
VĂJ-ĭn-ăl

cervic/al
SĔR-vĭ-kăl

8–62 Determine the words in Frame 8–61 that mean

instrument for examining the vagina and cervix uteri:

_____ / ____ / _____

visual examination of the vagina and cervix uteri using a colp/o/scope:

_____ / ____ / _____

pertaining to the vagina: _____ / _____

pertaining to the cervix uteri: _____ / _____

---

uterus
Ū-tĕr-ŭs

8–63 Cervix uteri refers to the neck of the _____.

Competency Verification: Check your labeling of Figures 8–2 and 8–3 in Appendix B, Answer Key, page 571.

gynec/o/logist
gī-nĕ-KŎL-ō-jĭst

8–64 The term *gynec/o/logy* means *study of females or women* and is the medical specialty for treating female reproductive disorders. A specialist in study of female reproductive disorders is called a

_____ / ____ / _____.

---

gynec/o

8–65 The CF in *gynec/o/logy* that means *woman* or *female* is

_____ / ____.

---

gynec/o/pathy
gī-nĕ-KŎP-ă-thē

8–66 Use *-pathy* to form a word that means *disease of a female.*

_____ / ____ / _____

---

gynec/o/logy
gī-nĕ-KŎL-ō-jē

8–67 *GYN* is the abbreviation for *gynec/o/logy. OB-GYN* refers to *obstetrics*
and _____ / ____ / _____.

8–68 Use your medical dictionary to define *obstetrics.*

_____

---

menses, menstruation
MĔN-sēz, mĕn-stroo-Ā-shŭn

8–69 The CF **men/o** means *menses* or *menstruation*, which is the monthly flow of blood and tissue from the uterus.

Men/o/rrhea is a flow of _____ or _____.

dys/men/o/rrhea dĭs-mĕn-ō-RĒ-ă	**8-70** Use *dys-* and *men/o/rrhea* to develop a word that means *painful or difficult menstrual flow.* _____ / _____ / _____ / _____
dys/men/o/rrhea dĭs-mĕn-ō-RĒ-ă	**8-71** Dys/men/o/rrhea is pain associated with menstruation. Primary dys/men/o/rrhea is menstrual pain that results from factors intrinsic to the uterus and the process of menstruation. It is extremely common, occurring at least occasionally in almost all women. If the painful episode is mild and brief, it is considered functional and normal and requires no treatment. The symptomatic term that literally means *bad, painful, difficult menstruation* is _____ / _____ / _____ / _____ .
bursting forth, menses *or* menstruation MĔN-sēz, mĕn-stroo-Ā-shŭn	**8-72** Men/o/rrhagia is excessive bleeding at the time of a menstrual period. Literally, it means _____ _____ of _____ .
menstruation mĕn-stroo-Ā-shun	**8-73** Men/o/pause terminates the reproductive period of life and is a permanent cessation of menses or _____ .
menstruation mĕn-stroo-Ā-shun	**8-74** *A/men/o/rrhea* is absence or abnormal stoppage of menstruation. *Men/o/rrhea* is a flow of the menses or _____ .
-pause	**8-75** Identify the element in men/o/pause that means *cessation*. _____
after, before	**8-76** The terms *post/men/o/paus/al* and *pre/men/o/paus/al* refer to bleeding occurring at times other than during the normal menstrual flow. *Post-* means _____, or *behind*. *Pre-* means _____, or *in front of.*

Breasts

mamm/o, mast/o	**8-77** The breasts, also called *mamm/ary glands*, are present in both sexes but they normally function only in females. The biological role of the mammary glands is to secrete milk for the nourishment of the infant, a process called *lactation*. The CFs that refer to the breast are _____ / _____ and _____ / _____ .

excision *or* **removal** ĕk-SĬ-zhŭn	**8-78** *Mast/ectomy* is a(n) _____ of a breast.
mast/ectomy măs-TĔK-tō-mē	**8-79** To prevent spread of CA, a malignant breast tumor may be treated with a partial or complete excision. When a breast has to be removed, the patient has a _____ / _____.
	8-80 During puberty, the female's breasts develop as a result of periodic stimulation of the ovarian hormones estrogen and progesterone. Estrogen is responsible for the development of (1) **adipose tissue**, which enlarges the size of the breasts until they reach full maturity around age 16. Breast size is primarily determined by the amount of fat around the (2) **glandular tissue**, but is not a factor in the ability to produce and secrete milk. Label the adipose and glandular tissues in Figure 8–7.
	8-81 During pregnancy, high levels of estrogen and progesterone prepare the mammary glands for milk production. Each breast has approximately 20 lobes. Each (3) **lobe** is drained by a (4) **lactiferous duct** that opens on the tip of the raised (5) **nipple**. Circling the nipple is a border of slightly darker skin called the (6) **areola**. Label the structures of the mammary glands in Figure 8–7.
lactation lăk-TĀ-shŭn	**8-82** During pregnancy, the breasts enlarge and remain so until lactation ceases. At menopause, breast tissue begins to atrophy. The ability of mammary glands to secrete milk for the nourishment of the infant is a process called _____.
-graphy **mamm/o**	**8-83** Mamm/o/graphy, an x-ray examination of the breast, is used in the Dx of CA. Determine the elements in this frame that mean *process of recording:* _____ *breast:* _____ / _____
mamm/o/plasty MĂM-ō-plăs-tē	**8-84** Use *mamm/o* to construct a word that means *surgical reconstruction or surgical repair of a breast.* _____ / _____ / _____
mast/o/plasty MĂS-tō-plăs-tē **mast/o/pexy** MĂS-to-pĕk-sē	**8-85** Correction of pendulous breasts can be performed by reconstructive cosmetic surgery to lift the breasts. Use *mast/o* to develop surgical terms that mean *surgical repair of the breast:* _____ / _____ / _____ *fixation of the breast:* _____ / _____ / _____

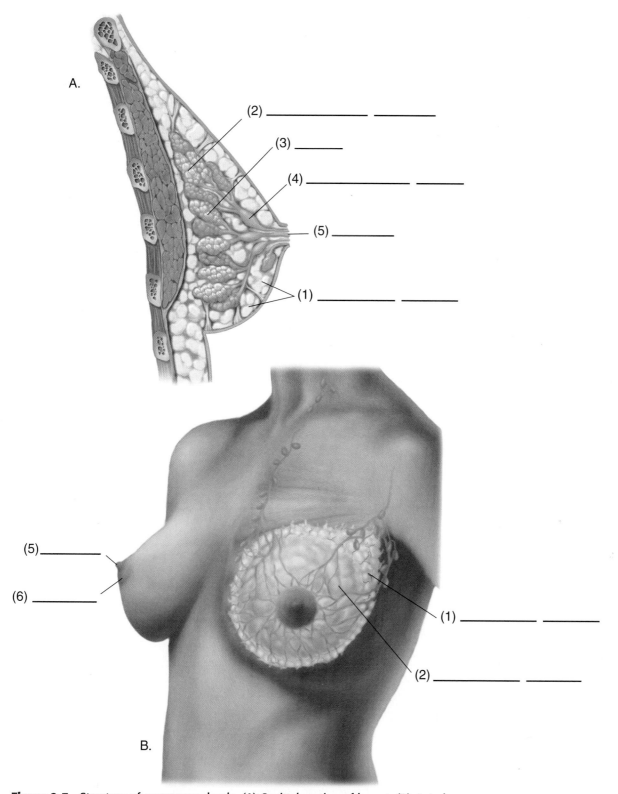

A.

(2) _____ _____

(3) _____

(4) _____ _____

(5) _____

(1) _____ _____

(5) _____

(6) _____

(1) _____ _____

(2) _____ _____

B.

Figure 8-7 Structure of mammary glands. (A) Sagittal section of breast. (B) Anterior view showing lymph nodes and structures of the breast.

8–86 When a small primary tumor is localized, the surgeon performs a lumpectomy. In these instances, the tumor and some of the normal tissue surrounding it are excised. All tissue removed from the breast is biopsied to determine if CA cells are present in the normal tissue surrounding the tumor. (See Figure 8–8.)

mast/o, mamm/o	**8–87** The CFs for *breast* are _____ / _____ and _____ / _____.
inflammation, breast(s)	**8–88** Breast-feeding may cause a blockage of the milk ducts and mast/itis, which is an _____ of the _____.
mast/o/dynia, mast/algia măst-ō-DĬN-ē-ă, măst-ĂL-jē-ă	**8–89** Use *mast/o* to form a word that means *pain in the breast.* _____ / _____ / _____ or _____ / _____

Competency Verification: Check your labeling of Figure 8–7 in Appendix B, Answer Key, page 571.

before, after	**8–90** The term *nat/al* means *pertaining to birth. Pre/nat/al* refers to the time period _____ birth; *post/nat/al* refers to the time period _____ birth.
neo- **nat/o** **-logy**	**8–91** Identify elements in *neo/nat/o/logy* that mean *new:* _____ *birth:* _____ / _____ *study of:* _____

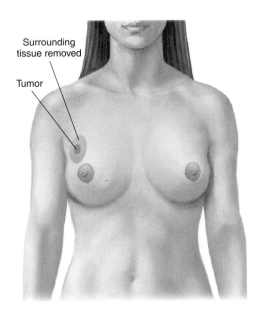

Surrounding tissue removed

Tumor

Figure 8-8 Lumpectomy, with the primary tumor in red and the surrounding tissue removed during lumpectomy highlighted pink.

neo/nat/o/logist nē-ō-nā-TŎL-ō-jĭst	**8-92** Neo/nat/o/logy is the study and treatment of the neonate (new-born infant). A physician who specializes in the care and treatment of the neonate is called a _____ / _____ / _____ / _____.
woman	**8-93** *Gravida* is used to describe a pregnant woman, as is the suffix *-gravida*. A *primi/gravida* is a woman pregnant for the first time; a *multi/gravida* is a woman who has been pregnant more than once. Whenever you see *gravida* in a word, you will know it denotes a pregnant _____.
fourth **second**	**8-94** *Gravida* may also be followed by numbers to denote the number of pregnancies, as in *gravida 1, 2, 3,* and *4* (or *I, II, III,* and *IV*). *Gravida 4* is a woman in her _____ pregnancy. *Gravida 2* is a woman in her _____ pregnancy.
gravida 3 GRĂV-ĭ-dă **gravida 5** GRĂV-ĭ-dă	**8-95** A woman in her third pregnancy is a _____ _____. A woman in her fifth pregnancy is a _____ _____.
two, five	**8-96** The word *para* refers to a woman who has given birth to an infant, regardless of whether or not the offspring was alive at birth. It also may be followed by numbers to indicate the number of deliveries, as in *para 1, 2, 3,* or *4* (or *I, II, III,* or *IV*). *Para 2* means _____ deliveries; *para 5* means _____ deliveries.
para 6 PĂR-ă	**8-97** A woman who has delivered three infants would be described as *para 3*. A woman who has delivered six infants would be described as _____ _____.
PID	**8-98** *Pelvic inflammatory disease* (PID) is a collective term for inflammation of the uterus, fallopian tubes, ovaries, and adjacent pelvic structures. This disease is usually caused by bacterial infection. The abbreviation for pelvic inflammatory disease is _____.
path/o/gen PĂTH-ō-jĕn	**8-99** In the female reproductive system, an infection may be confined to a single organ or it may involve all of the internal female reproductive organs. Path/o/gens generally enter through the vagina during coitus, induced abortion, childbirth, or the postpartum period. As an ascending infection, pathogens spread from the vagina and cervix to the upper structures of the female reproductive tract. A term in this frame that means *forming, producing, or origin of disease* is _____ / _____ / _____.

sexually transmitted disease

pelvic inflammatory disease

8-100 The two most common causes of PID are gonorrhea and chlamydia, both of which are sexually transmitted diseases (STDs). Unless treated promptly, PID may result in sterility because the fallopian tubes and ovaries become scarred. Widespread infection of reproductive structures may also lead to fatal septicemia.

The abbreviation *STD* refers to _____ _____ _____.

The abbreviation *PID* refers to _____ _____ _____.

---

pelvic inflammatory disease

8-101 Because regions of the fallopian tubes have an internal diameter as small as the width of a human hair, the scarring and closure of the tubes caused by PID is one of the major causes of female sterility (infertility). Chlamydia and gonorrhea are two main causes of PID. The abbreviation *PID* means _____ _____ _____.

---

ovary *or* **ovaries**
Ō-vă-rē, Ō-vă-rēz

8-102 A pelvic infection confined to the uterine or fallopian tubes is known as *salping/itis;* a pelvic infection confined to the ovaries is known as *oophor/itis.*

The CF *oophor/o* refers to the _____.

---

oophor/itis
ō-ŏf-ō-RĪ-tĭs

oophor/oma
ō-ŏf-ō-RŌ-mă

8-103 A pelvic infection that involves the ovaries is known as *oophor/itis.* Use *oophor/o* to build a term that means

inflammation of the ovaries: _____ / _____

tumor of the ovaries: _____ / _____

---

diagnosis

8-104 Dx of a cyst or tumor in a fallopian tube may necessitate the surgical procedure known as *salping/ectomy.* When the abbreviation *Dx* is used in a medical report, it means _____.

---

salping/ectomy
săl-pĭn-JĔK-tō-mē

8-105 Build a surgical term that means excision of one or both fallopian tubes.

_____ / _____

---

uterus
Ū-tĕr-ŭs

8-106 A hyster/o/tome is an instrument for incising the _____.

incision, uterus	**8-107** Abdominal incision of the uterus (hyster/o/tomy) is performed to remove the fetus during a cesarean section (CS), also called *C-section*. Hyster/o/tomy is an _____ into the _____.

CS, C-section	**8-108** Abbreviations for *cesarean section* are _____ and _____.

SECTION REVIEW 8-3

Using the following table, write the CF, suffix, or prefix that matches its definition in the space provided to the left of the definition. There may be more than one word element that matches a definition.

Combining Forms		Suffixes		Prefixes
cervic/o	men/o	-algia	-ous	dys-
colp/o	salping/o	-ary	-pathy	post-
episi/o	vagin/o	-dynia	-rrhea	pre-
gynec/o	vulv/o	-ectomy	-scope	
mamm/o		-itis	-scopy	
mast/o		-logist	-tome	

1. _____ after, behind

2. _____ woman, female

3. _____ before, in front of

4. _____ breast

5. _____ disease

6. _____ excision, removal

7. _____ discharge, flow

8. _____ inflammation

9. _____ instrument to cut

10. _____ instrument for examining

11. _____ visual examination

12. _____ menses, menstruation

13. _____ neck; cervix uteri (neck of uterus)

14. _____ pain

15. _____ pertaining to

16. _____ specialist in study of

17. _____ tube (usually fallopian or eustachian [auditory] tubes)

18. _____ vagina

19. _____ vulva

20. _____ bad; painful; difficult

Competency Verification: Check your answers in Appendix B, Answer Key, page 571. If you are not satisfied with your level of comprehension, go back to Frame 8–53 and rework the frames.

Correct Answers _____ × 5 = _____ % Score

Male Reproductive System

The primary sex organs of the male are called *gonads,* specifically the testes (singular, *testis*). Gonads produce gametes (sperm) and secrete sex hormones. The remaining accessory reproductive organs are the structures that are essential in caring for and transporting sperm. All of these organs and structures are designed to accomplish the male's reproductive role of producing and delivering sperm to the female reproductive tract, where fertilization can occur.

These structures can be divided into three categories:

- *sperm transporting ducts,* which include the *epididymis, ductus deferens* (also referred to as *vas deferens*), *ejaculatory duct,* and *urethra*

- accessory glands, which include the *seminal vesicles, prostate gland,* and *bulbourethral glands*

- copulatory organ, the *penis,* which contains *erectile tissue.* (See Figure 8–9.)

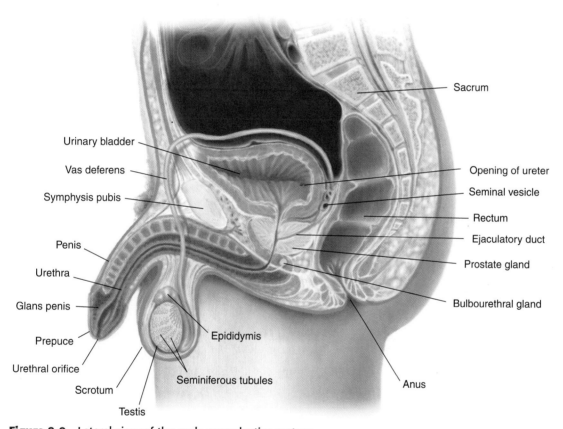

Figure 8-9 Lateral view of the male reproductive system.

WORD ELEMENTS

This section introduces combining forms related to the male reproductive system. Included are key suffixes; prefixes are defined in the right-hand column as needed. Review the following table and pronounce each word in the word analysis column aloud before you begin to work the frames.

Word Element	Meaning	Word Analysis
Combining Forms		
andr/o	male	**andr**/o/gen (ĂN-drō-jĕn): forming or producing male (hormones)
		-gen: forming, producing, origin
		Hormones such as testosterone and androsterone produce or stimulate the development of male characteristics (masculinization).
balan/o	glans penis	**balan**/itis (băl-ă-NĪ-tĭs): inflammation of the glans penis
		-itis: inflammation
gonad/o	gonads, sex glands	**gonad**/o/tropin (gŏn-ă-dō-TRŌ-pĭn): hormone that stimulates the gonads
		-tropin: stimulate
		Gonadotropin is a hormone that stimulates the function of the testes and ovaries (gonads).
orch/o	testis (plural, testes)	crypt/**orch**/ism (krĭpt-OR-kĭzm): condition of a hidden testicle
		crypt: hidden
		-ism: condition
		In cryptorchism, the testicles are retained in the abdomen or inguinal canal. If spontaneous descent does not occur by age 1, hormone therapy or surgery may be performed.
orchi/o		**orchi**/o/pexy (ŌR-kē-ō-pĕk-sē): surgical fixation of a testis
		-pexy: fixation (of an organ)
		An orchiopexy is performed to mobilize an undescended testis, bring it into the scrotum, and attach it so that it will not retract.
orchid/o		**orchid**/ectomy (or-kĭ-DĚK-tō-mē): excision of one or both testes
		-ectomy: excision, removal
test/o		**test**/algia (tĕs-TĂL-jē-ă): pain in the testes
		-algia: pain

Word Element	Meaning	Word Analysis
spermat/o	spermatozoa, sperm cells	**spermat/o/cyte** (spĕr-MĂT-ō-sīt) sperm cell *cyte:* cell
sperm/i		**sperm/i/cide** (SPĔR-mĭ-sīd): agent that kills spermatozoa *-cide:* killing
sperm/o		a/**sperm**/ia (ă-SPĔR-mē-ă): without semen *a-:* without, not *-ia:* condition *In aspermia, semen fail to form or ejaculate.*
varic/o	dilated vein	**varic/o/cele** (VĂR-ĭ-kō-sēl): dilated or enlarged vein of the spermatic cord *-cele:* hernia, swelling
vas/o	vessel; vas deferens; duct	**vas**/ectomy (văs-ĔK-tō-mē): removal of all or part of the vas deferens *-ectomy:* excision, removal
vesicul/o	seminal vesicle	**vesicul**/itis (vĕ-sĭk-ū-LĪ-tĭs): inflammation of the seminal vesicle *-itis:* inflammation

Listen and Learn, the audio CD-ROM included in this book, will help you master pronunciations of selected medical words. Use it to practice pronunciations of the above-listed medical terms and for instructions to complete the *Listen and Learn* exercise for this section.

SECTION REVIEW 8-4

For the following medical terms, first write the suffix and its meaning. Then translate the meaning of the remaining elements starting with the first part of the word. The first word is completed for you.

Term	Meaning
1. vas/ectomy	*-ectomy: excision, removal; vessel, vas deferens, duct*
2. balan/itis	
3. spermat/i/cide	
4. gonad/o/tropin	
5. orchi/o/pexy	
6. a/sperm/ia	
7. vesicul/itis	
8. orchid/ectomy	
9. andr/o/gen	
10. crypt/orch/ism	

Competency Verification: Check your answers in Appendix B, Answer Key, page 572. If you are not satisfied with your level of comprehension, review the vocabulary and retake the review.

Correct Answers _____ × 10 = _____ % Score

8–109 The (1) **testes** (singular, *testis*), also called *testicles* (singular, *testicle*), are paired oval glands that descend into the (2) **scrotum**. At the onset of puberty, the testes produce the hormone testosterone. Label Figure 8–10 as you learn about the organs of reproduction.

---

disease, testes *or* testicles
TĔS-tēs, TĔS-tĭ-klz

8–110 The CF *test/o* refers to the testis. *Test/o/pathy* is a _____ of the _____ (plural).

8–111 The male hormone testosterone stimulates and promotes the growth of secondary sex characteristics in the male. This hormone is produced by the testes (plural).

testis
TĔS-tēs

The singular form of *testes* is _____.

testicle
TĔS-tĭ-kl

The singular form of *testicles* is _____.

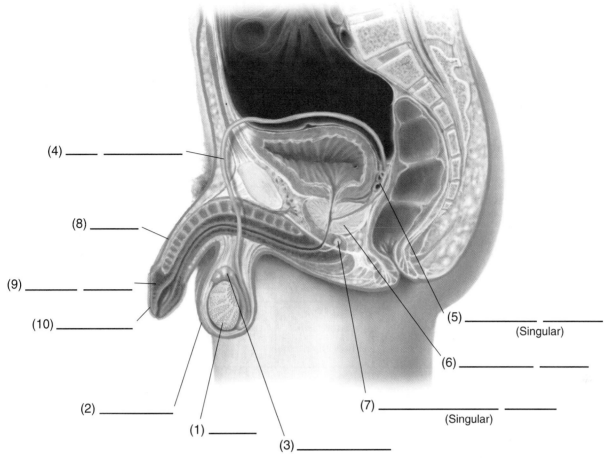

(4) _____ _____

(8) _____

(9) _____ _____

(10) _____

(5) _____ _____
(Singular)

(6) _____ _____

(7) _____ _____
(Singular)

(2) _____

(1) _____

(3) _____

Figure 8-10 Lateral view of the male reproductive system.

test/itis tĕs-TĪ-tĭs **test/ectomy** tĕs-TĔK-tō-mē **test/o/pathy** tĕs-TŎP-ă-thē	**8-112** Use *test/o* to form medical words that mean *inflammation of testis:* _____ / _____ *excision of testis:* _____ / _____ *disease of testis:* _____ / _____ / _____
spermatozoa spĕr-măt-ō-ZŌ-ă	**8-113** The CF *spermat/o* means *spermatozoa, sperm cells*. These are the male sex cell produced by the testes. Spermat/o/genesis is the beginning or formation of sperm cells, or _____.
stone, calculus KĂL-kū-lŭs	**8-114** A *spermat/o/lith* is a _____ or _____ in the spermatic duct.

spermat/o/genesis
spĕr-măt-ō-JĔN-ĕ-sĭs

8-115 The suffix *-genesis* is used in words to mean *forming, producing,* or *origin.*

Construct a word that means *producing or forming sperm.*

_____ / _____ / _____

---

spermat/o/cyte
spĕr-MĂT-ō-sīt

8-116 Use **spermat/o** to form a word that means *sperm cell.*

_____ / _____ / _____

---

spermat/oid
SPĔR-mă-toyd

8-117 Build a word that means *resembling spermatozoa.*

_____ / _____

---

spermat/uria
spĕr-mă-TŪ-rē-ă

8-118 Spermat/uria is a condition in which there is sperm in the urine. A discharge of semen in urine is also called

_____ / _____.

---

without

8-119 A/spermat/ism is a condition in which there is lack of male sperm. *A/spermat/ism* literally means _____ sperm.

---

scanty

8-120 A man who produces a scanty amount of sperm in the semen has a condition called *olig/o/sperm/ia.*

Olig/o means _____.

---

olig/o/sperm/ia
ŏl-ĭ-gō-SPĔR-mē-ă

8-121 When the physician detects an insufficient number of spermatozoa in the semen, the Dx is noted in the medical record as

_____ / _____ / _____ / _____.

8-122 A comma-shaped organ, the (3) **epididymis,** stores and propels sperm toward the urethra during ejaculation. The (4) **vas deferens,** also called *ductus deferens,* is a duct that transports sperm from the testes to the urethra. The sperm is excreted in the semen, or *seminal fluid.* Semen is a mixture of secretions from the (5) **seminal vesicles,** (6) **prostate gland,** and (7) **bulbourethral glands,** also known as *Cowper glands.* Label Figure 8–10 as you continue to learn about the male reproductive organs.

---

muc/o

8-123 Ducts of Cowper glands open into the urethra and secrete thick mucus that acts as a lubricant during sexual stimulation.
Write the CF that refers to mucus.

_____ / _____

---

adjective

8-124 *Muc/us* is a noun. *Muc/ous* is a (n) (noun, adjective)

_____.

muc/oid MŪ-koyd	**8-125** Use *-oid* to construct a medical term that means *resembling mucus.* _____ / _____
orchi/o/plasty OR-kē-ō-plăs-tē **orchi/o/rrhaphy** or-kē-OR-ă-fē **orchi/o/pexy** or-kē-ō-PĔK-sē	**8-126** In addition to ***test/o,*** two other CFs that refer to the testes are ***orchi/o*** and ***orchid/o.*** Use ***orchi/o*** to develop medical words that mean *surgical repair of the testicle:* _____ / _____ / _____ *suture of a testicle:* _____ / _____ / _____ *fixation of a testicle:* _____ / _____ / _____
enlargement	**8-127** The CF for *prostate gland* is ***prostat/o.*** The prostate gland secretes a thick fluid that, as part of the semen, helps the sperm to move spontaneously. *Prostat/o/megaly* is a(n) _____ of the prostate gland.
prostat/o/megaly prŏs-tă-tō-MĔG-ă-lē	**8-128** Benign prostatic hyperplasia (BPH), a gradual enlargement of the prostate gland, normally occurs as a man ages. It is a common disorder in men older than age 60. The enlarged prostate compresses the urethra and causes the bladder to retain urine. Symptoms include inability to empty the bladder completely and a weak urine stream. (See Figure 8–11.) Construct a medical word that means *enlargement of the prostate gland.* _____ / _____ / _____
growth; nourishment	**8-129** Benign prostat/ic hyper/plasia (BPH) is also known as *benign prostat/ic hyper/trophy* (BPH). The suffix *-plasia* means *formation,* _____. The suffix *-trophy* means *development,* _____.
trans/urethr/al trăns-ū-RĒ-thrăl	**8-130** Common symptoms of BPH include hesitancy and dribbling on urination and a weak urine stream. Treatment for BPH includes drugs to decrease prostate size or the surgical procedure known as *trans/urethr/al resection of the prostate* (TURP) in which the obstructing tissue is removed. TURP makes it possible to perform surgery on certain organs that lie near the urethra without having an abdominal incision. (See Figure 8–11.) Because this surgery is performed by passing a resect/o/scope through the urethra, it is called _____ / _____ / _____ resection of the prostate.
resect/o/scope rē-SĔK-tō-skōp	**8-131** The resect/o/scope (special type of endoscope) contains a light, valves for controlling irrigating fluid, and an electrical loop that cuts tissue and seals blood vessels. The wire loop is used to remove obstructing tissue piece-by-piece through the resectoscope. The chips of tissue are irrigated into the bladder and then flushed out at the end of the surgical procedure. The endo/scop/ic instrument used by the urologist to perform TURP is called a _____ / _____ / _____.

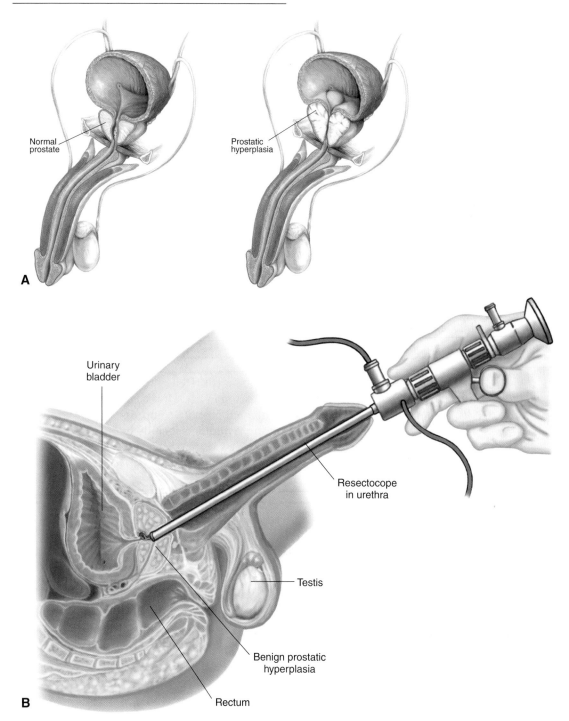

Normal prostate

Prostatic hyperplasia

A

Urinary bladder

Resectocope in urethra

Testis

Benign prostatic hyperplasia

B

Rectum

Figure 8-11 Benign prostatic hyperplasia (A) and transurethral resection of the prostate (B).

8-132 *PSA* refers to a blood test used to detect prostat/ic cancer and to monitor the patient's response to therapy. The abbreviation for *prostate-specific antigen* test is _____.

PSA

prostat/itis prŏs-tă-TĪ-tĭs **prostat/o/cyst/itis** prŏs-tă-tō-sĭs-TĪ-tĭs	**8–133** Build medical terms that mean *inflammation of the prostate gland:* _____ / _____ *inflammation of the prostate gland and bladder:* _____ / ____ / _____ / _____
prostate, bladder PRŎS-tāt	**8–134** Prostat/o/cyst/o/tomy is an incision of the _____ and _____.
	8–135 The (8) **penis** is the male sex organ that transports the sperm into the female vagina. A slightly enlarged region at the tip of the penis is the (9) **glans penis**. The tip of the penis is covered by a fold of skin called the (10) **foreskin** or prepuce. Label Figure 8–10 as you learn the names of organs of reproduction.
   water **hernia, swelling** HĔR-nē-ă	**8–136** Hydr/o/cele is a collection of fluid in a saclike cavity, specifically the testis. Analyze *hydr/o/cele* by defining the elements. *hydr/o:* _____ *-cele:* _____, _____

Competency Verification: Check your labeling of Figure 8–10 in Appendix B, Answer Key, page 572.

    prostat/ectomy prŏs-tă-TĔK-tō-mē	**8–137** Prostate CA is the third leading cause of cancer deaths in men (after lung and colon CA). Surgery may be performed to remove the prostate and adjacent affected tissues. Develop a surgical term that means *excision of the prostate gland.* _____ / _____
cancer	**8–138** Currently PSA is considered the most sensitive tumor marker for prostate _____.
  threatening	**8–139** Tumors may be benign or malignant. Benign tumors are not malignant (cancerous) and not life-threatening. A malignant tumor, however, is cancerous and life-_____.
benign bē-NĪN	**8–140** Tumors are also called *neo/plasms* (new growths or formations). Similar to tumors, neo/plasms can be malignant or _____.
cancer/ous KĂN-sĕr-ŭs	**8–141** A benign tumor is non/cancer/ous. A malignant tumor is _____ / _____.

neo/plasm NĒ-ō-plăzm	**8-142** Carcin/omas are also known as malignant neo/plasms. Form a word that means *formation or growth that is new.* _____ / _____
neo/plasm NĒ-ō-plăzm	**8-143** A new growth in any body system or organ is called a _____ / _____.
prostate PRŎS-tāt	**8-144** Prostate CA also is called *carcinoma of the* _____.
prostat/itis prŏs-tă-TĪ-tĭs	**8-145** Prostat/itis, an acute or chronic inflammation of the prostate gland, is usually the result of infection. The patient usually complains of burning, urinary frequency, and urgency. Build a symptomatic term that means *inflammation of the prostate gland.* _____ / _____
growth	**8-146** The suffixes *-plasm* and *-plasia* refer to *formation or* _____.
dys- **-plasia**	**8-147** Dys/plasia is an abnormal development of tissue. Identify the element in *dys/plasia* that means *bad, painful, or difficult:* _____ *formation, growth:* _____
without, not **formation, growth**	**8-148** A/plasia means *without formation,* and it is a condition that is due to failure of an organ to develop or form normally. Analyze *a/plasia* by defining the elements. *a-:* _____, _____ *-plasia:* _____ or _____
hyper- **-plasia**	**8-149** Hyper/plasia is an excessive increase in the number of cells in a tissue or organ. (See Figure 8–11.) Determine the element in *hyper/plasia* that means *excessive:* _____ *formation or growth:* _____
vas/o	**8-150** Vas/ectomy, a sterilization procedure, involves bi/later/al cutting and tying of the vas deferens to prevent the passage of sperm. (See Figure 8–12.) This sterilization procedure is most commonly performed at an outpatient surgery center using local an/esthesia. From the term vas/ectomy, construct the combining form that means *vessel, vas deferens, or duct.* _____ / ___

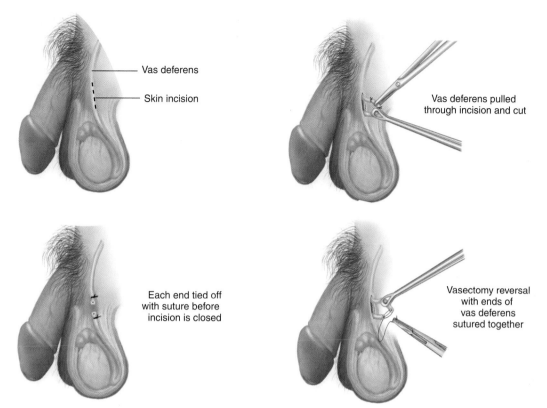

Vas deferens

Skin incision

Vas deferens pulled
through incision and cut

Each end tied off
with suture before
incision is closed

Vasectomy reversal
with ends of
vas deferens
sutured together

Figure 8-12   Vasectomy and its reversal.

---

an/esthesia ăn-ĕs-THĒ-zē-ă **bi/later/al** bī-LĂT-ĕr-ăl **vas/ectomy** văs-ĔK-tō-mē	**8–151** Identify the terms in Frame 8–150 that mean *without feeling:* _____ / _____ *pertaining to two sides:* _____ / _____ / _____ *excision of the vas deferens:* _____ / _____

prostat/itis prŏs-tă-TĪ-tĭs	**8–152** Vas/ectomy is also performed routinely before removal of the prostate gland to prevent inflammation of the testes and epididymides. Potency is not affected. Inflammation of the prostate gland is called _____ / _____.

vas/ectomy reversal văs-ĔK-tō-mē	**8–153** Vas/o/vas/o/stomy, also called *vas/ectomy reversal,* is a surgical procedure in which the function of the vas deferens on each side of the testes is restored, having been cut and ligated in a preceding vasectomy. (See Figure 8–12.) Another term for *vas/o/vas/o/stomy* is _____ / _____ _____.

ur/o/genit/al

ū-rō-JĔN-ĭ-tăl

vas/o/vas/o/stomy

văs-ō-vă-SŎS-tō-mē

8-154 Vas/ectomy reversal may be performed if a man wants to regain his fertility. In most cases, patency (opening up) of the canals is achieved. However, in many cases, fertility does not result, possibly due to circulating autoantibodies that disrupt normal sperm activity. The antibodies apparently develop after vas/ectomy because the developing sperm cannot be excreted through the ur/o/genit/al tract.

Identify the term in this frame that means *pertaining to urine and the organs of reproduction.*

_____ / ____ / _____ / ____

Identify the surgical term in Frame 8–153 that is synonymous with *vas/ectomy reversal.*

_____ / ____ / _____ / ____ / _____

S E C T I O N   R E V I E W   8 - 5

Using the following table, write the CF, suffix, or prefix that matches its definition in the space provided to the left of the definition. There may be more than one word element that matches a definition.

Combining Forms		Suffixes		Prefixes
carcin/o	prostat/o	-cele	-pexy	dys-
cyst/o	spermat/o	-cyte	-rrhaphy	hyper-
muc/o	sperm/o	-genesis	-tome	neo-
olig/o	test/o	-itis		
orchid/o	vas/o	-megaly		
orchi/o		-pathy		

1. _____ suture
2. _____ bad; painful; difficult
3. _____ bladder
4. _____ cancer
5. _____ cell
6. _____ disease
7. _____ enlargement
8. _____ hernia, swelling
9. _____ inflammation
10. _____ instrument to cut
11. _____ vessel; vas deferens; duct
12. _____ mucus
13. _____ new
14. _____ forming, producing, origin
15. _____ prostate gland
16. _____ testes
17. _____ scanty
18. _____ spermatozoa, sperm cells
19. _____ fixation (of an organ)
20. _____ excessive, above normal

Competency Verification: Check your answers in Appendix B, Answer Key, page 572. If you are not satisfied with your level of comprehension, go back to Frame 8–109 and rework the frames.

Correct Answers _____ × 5 = _____ % Score

Abbreviations

This section introduces reproductive system-related abbreviations and their meanings. Included are abbreviations contained in the medical record activities that follow.

Abbreviation	Meaning	Abbreviation	Meaning
Female Reproductive System			
CS, C-section	cesarean section	**Pap**	Papanicolaou (test)
D&C	dilatation (dilation) and curettage	**para 1, 2, 3**	unipara, bipara, tripara (number of viable births)
Dx	diagnosis	**PID**	pelvic inflammatory disease
G	gravida (pregnant)	**PIH**	pregnancy-induced hypertension
GYN	gynecology	**PMP**	previous menstrual period
HRT	hormone replacement therapy	**PSA**	prostate-specific antigen
IUD	intrauterine device	**TAH**	total abdominal hysterectomy
IVF	*in vitro* fertilization	**TRAM**	transverse rectus abdominis muscle
LMP	last menstrual period	**TSS**	toxic shock syndrome
OB-GYN	obstetrics and gynecology	**TVH**	total vaginal hysterectomy
OCPs	oral contraceptive pills		
Male Reproductive System			
BPH	benign prostatic hyperplasia, benign prostatic hypertrophy	**TURP, TUR**	transurethral resection of the prostate
DRE	digital rectal examination	**XY**	male sex chromosomes
GU	genitourinary		
Sexually Transmitted Diseases			
GC	gonorrhea	**STD**	sexually transmitted disease
HPV	human papillomavirus	**VD**	venereal disease
HSV	herpes simplex virus		

Additional Medical Terms

The following are additional terms related to the female and male reproductive systems. Recognizing and learning these terms will help you understand the connection between a pathological condition, its diagnosis, and the rationale behind the method of treatment selected for a particular disorder.

Signs, Symptoms, and Diseases

Female Reproductive System

candidiasis kăn-dĭ-DĪ-ă-sĭs	Vaginal fungal infection caused by *Candida albicans;* characterized by a curdy or cheeselike discharge and extreme itching

cervicitis
sĕr-vĭ-SĪ-tĭs
 	
cervic: neck; cervix uteri
     (neck of uterus)
  -itis: inflammation
	Inflammation of the uterine cervix
	
	Cervicitis is usually the result of infection or a sexually transmitted disease. It may also become chronic, because the cervical lining is not renewed each month as is the uterine lining during menstruation.

ectopic pregnancy ĕk-TŎP-ik	Implantation of the fertilized ovum outside of the uterine cavity (See Figure 8–13) *Ectopic pregnancy occurs in approximately 1% of pregnancies, most commonly in the oviducts (tubal pregnancy). Some types of ectopic pregnancies include ovarian, interstitial, and isthmic.*

endometriosis
ĕn-dō-mē-trē-Ō-sĭs
 	
endo: in, within
metri: uterus (womb)
  -osis: abnormal
     condition; increase
     (used primarily
     with blood cells)
	Presence of endometrial tissue outside (ectopic) the uterine cavity, such as the pelvis or abdomen (See Figure 8–14.)

fibroid FĪ-broyd *fibr:* fiber, fibrous tissue *-oids:* resembling	Benign neoplasm in the uterus that is composed largely of fibrous tissue; also called *leiomyoma* *Uterine fibroids are the most common tumors in women. If fibroids grow too large and cause symptoms such as pelvic pain or menorrhagia, hysterectomy may be indicated.*
leukorrhea loo-kō-RĒ-ă *leuk/o:* white *-rrhea:* discharge, flow	White discharge from the vagina *A greater than usual amount of leukorrhea is normal in pregnancy, and a decrease is to be expected after delivery, during lactation, and after menopause. Leukorrhea is the most common reason women seek gynecological care.*

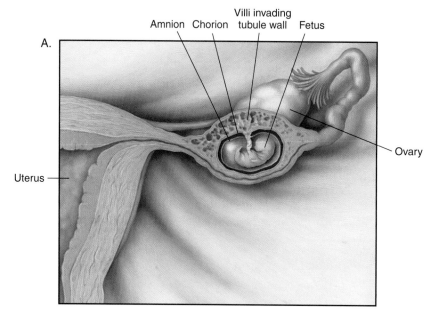

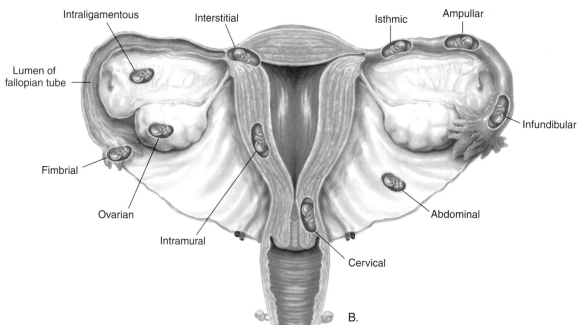

Figure 8-13 Ectopic pregnancy (A) and sites of ectopic pregnancy (B).

oligomenorrhea	Scanty or infrequent menstrual flow
ŏl-ĭ-gō-mĕn-ō-RĒ-ă	
olig/o: scanty	
men/o: menses, menstruation	
-rrhea: discharge, flow	

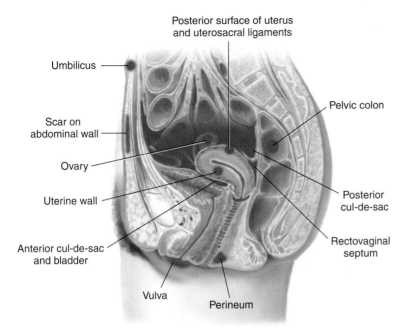

Posterior surface of uterus
and uterosacral ligaments

Umbilicus

Scar on
abdominal wall

Ovary

Uterine wall

Anterior cul-de-sac
and bladder

Vulva

Perineum

Pelvic colon

Posterior
cul-de-sac

Rectovaginal
septum

Figure 8-14 Endometriosis.

pregnancy-induced hypertension (PIH)	Potentially life-threatening disorder that usually develops after the 20th week of pregnancy and is characterized by edema and proteinuria
	PIH may occur in nonconvulsive or convulsive forms.
preeclampsia prē-ē-KLĂMP-sē-ă	Nonconvulsive form of PIH
	If left untreated, preeclampsia may progress to eclampsia. Treatment includes bed rest and blood pressure monitoring.
eclampsia ē-KLĂMP-sē-ă	Convulsive form of PIH
	Treatment for eclampsia includes bed rest, blood pressure monitoring, and antiseizure drugs.
pyosalpinx pī-ō-SĂL-pĭnks *py/o:* pus *-salpinx:* tube (usually fallopian or eustachian [auditory] tube)	Pus in the fallopian tube
retroversion rĕt-rō-VĔR-shŭn *retro-:* backward, behind *-version:* turning	Turning, or state of being turned back, especially an entire organ being tipped from its normal position (such as the uterus) *Uterine retroversion is measured as first-, second-, or third-degree, depending on the angle of tilt in relationship to the vagina.*
sterility stĕr-ĬL-ĭ-tē	Inability of a woman to become pregnant or for a man to impregnate a woman

| **toxic shock syndrome (TSS)** TŎK-sĭk SHŎK SĬN-drōm *tox:* poison *-ic:* pertaining to | Rare and sometimes fatal staphylococcus infection that generally occurs in menstruating women, most of whom use vaginal tampons for menstrual protection *In TSS, the normally harmless vaginal bacterium Staphylococcus aureus multiplies in the old blood in the tampon and releases toxins. The tampon itself creates small tears in the vaginal wall that allow the toxins to enter the blood.* |
| **trichomoniasis** trĭk-ō-mō-NĪ-ă-sĭs | Protozoal infestation of the vagina, urethra, or prostate |

Male Reproductive System

anorchism ăn-ŎR-kĭzm *an:* without, not *orch:* testis (plural, *testes*) *-ism:* condition	Congenital absence of one or both testes; also called *anorchia*
balanitis băl-ă-NĪ-tĭs *balan:* glans penis *-itis:* inflammation	Inflammation of the skin covering the glans penis *Balanitis is caused by irritation and invasion of microorganisms. It is commonly associated with inadequate hygiene of the prepuce and phimosis.*
cryptorchidism krĭpt-OR-kĭd-ĭzm *crypt:* hidden *orchid:* testis (plural, *testes*) *-ism:* condition	Failure of one or both testicles to descend into the scrotum *Cryptorchidism is associated with a high risk of sterility, causing a low sperm count and male infertility. If testes do not descend on their own at an early age, orchiopexy is performed to bring the testicles into the scrotum.*
epispadias ĕp-ĭ-SPĀ-dē-ăs *epi-:* above, upon *-spadias:* slit, fissure	Congenital defect in which the urethra opens on upper side of the penis near the glans penis instead of the tip
hypospadias hī-pō-SPĀ-dē-ăs *hypo:* under, below, deficient *-spadias:* slit, fissure	Congenital defect in which the male urethra opens on undersurface of the penis instead of the tip
impotence ĬM-pŏ-tĕns	Inability of a man to achieve or maintain a penile erection; commonly called *erectile dysfunction*

phimosis fī-MŌ-sĭs *phim:* muzzle *-osis:* abnormal condition; increase (used primarily with blood cells)	Stenosis or narrowness of the preputial orifice so that the foreskin cannot be pushed back over the glans penis
sexually transmitted disease (STD)	Any disease that may be acquired as a result of sexual intercourse or other intimate contact with an infected individual and affects the male and female reproductive systems; also called *venereal disease*
chlamydia klă-MĬD-ē-ă	STD caused by infection with the bacterium *Chlamydia trachomatis* *Chlamydia is the most common and among the most damaging of all STDs. In women, chlamydial infections cause cervicitis with a mucopurulent discharge and an alarming increase in pelvic infections. In men, chlamydial infections cause urethritis with a whitish discharge from the penis.*
genital warts JĔN-ĭ-tăl WORTZ *genit:* genitalia *-al:* pertaining to	Wart(s) in the genitalia caused by human papillomavirus (HPV) *In women, genital warts may be associated with cervical cancer.*
gonorrhea gŏn-ō-RĒ-ă *gon/o:* seed (ovum or spermatozoon) *-rrhea:* discharge, flow	Contagious bacterial infection that most commonly affects the genitourinary tract and, occasionally, the pharynx or rectum *Gonorrheal infection results from contact with an infected person or with secretions containing the causative organism Neisseria gonorrhoeae. In men, symptoms include dysuria and a greenish yellow discharge from the urethra. In women, the chief symptom is a vaginal greenish yellow discharge. Gonorrhea can be transmitted to the fetus during delivery.*
herpes genitalis HĔR-pēz jĕn-ĭ-TĂL-ĭs	Infection in females and males of the genital and anorectal skin and mucosa with herpes simplex virus type 2 *This viral infection may be transmitted to the fetus during delivery and may be fatal.*
syphilis SĬF-ĭ-lĭs	Infectious, chronic STD characterized by lesions that change to a chancre and may involve any organ or tissue *Syphilis usually exhibits cutaneous manifestations and relapses are common without treatment. It may exist without symptoms for years and can be transmitted from mother to fetus.*

Diagnostic Procedures

Female Reproductive System

amniocentesis ăm-nē-ō-sĕn-TĒ-sĭs *amni/o:* amnion (amniotic sac) *-centesis:* surgical puncture	Obstetric procedure that involves surgical puncture of the amniotic sac under ultrasound guidance to remove amniotic fluid *In amniocentesis, cells of the fetus found in the fluid are cultured and studied chemically and cytologically to detect genetic abnormalities, biochemical disorders, and maternal-fetal blood incompatibility. (See Figure 8–15.)*

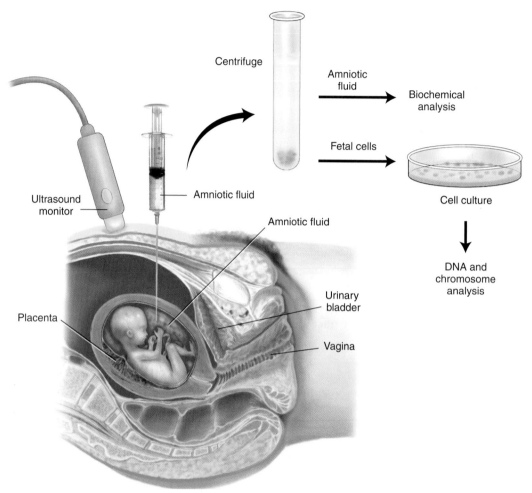

Figure 8-15 Amniocentesis using transabdominal puncture of the amniotic sac with ultrasound guidance to remove amniotic fluid for laboratory analysis.

colposcopy kŏl-PŎS-kō-pē *colp/o:* vagina *-scopy:* visual examination	Examination of the vagina and cervix with an optical magnifying instrument (colposcope) *Colposcopy is commonly performed after a Papanicolaou test to obtain biopsy specimens of the cervix.*

hysterosalpingography hĭs-tĕr-ō-săl-pĭn-GŎG-ră-fē *hyster/o:* uterus (womb) *salping/o:* tube (usually fallopian or eustachian [auditory] tube) *-graphy:* process of recording	Radiography of the uterus and oviducts after injection of a contrast medium

laparoscopy lăp-ăr-ŎS-kō-pē *lapar/o:* abdomen *-scopy:* visual examination	Visual examination of the abdominal cavity with a laparoscope through one or more small incisions in the abdominal wall, usually at the umbilicus (See Figure 8–16.) *Laparoscopy is used for inspection of the ovaries and fallopian tubes, diagnosis of endometriosis, destruction of uterine leiomyomas, myomectomy, and gynecologic sterilization.*

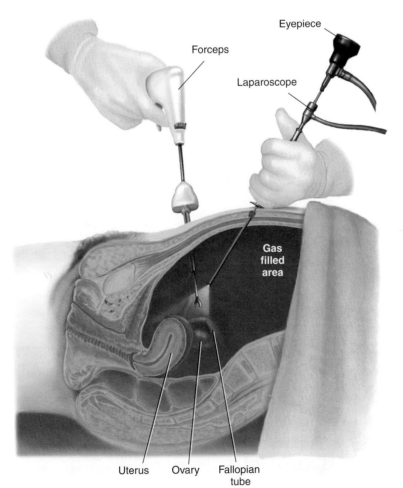

Eyepiece

Forceps

Laparoscope

Gas filled area

Uterus   Ovary   Fallopian tube

Figure 8-16   Laparoscopy.

mammography măm-ŎG-ră-fē *mamm/o:* breast *-graphy:* process of recording	Radiography of breast; used to diagnose benign and malignant tumors
Papanicolaou (Pap) test pă-pă-NĬ-kō-lŏw	Microscopic analysis of cells taken from the cervix and vagina to detect the presence of carcinoma Cells are obtained for a Pap test via insertion of a vaginal speculum and the use of a swab to scrape a small tissue sample from the cervix and vagina.
ultrasonography (US) ŭl-tră-sŏn-ŎG-ră-fē *ultra-:* excess, beyond *son/o:* sound *-graphy:* process of recording	Imaging technique that uses high-frequency sound waves (ultrasound) that bounce off body tissues and are recorded to produce an image of an internal organ or tissue *Pelvic US is used to evaluate the female reproductive organs and the fetus during pregnancy. Transvaginal US places the sound probe in the vagina instead of across the pelvis or abdomen, producing a sharper examination of normal and pathologic structures within the pelvis.*

Male Reproductive System

digital rectal examination (DRE) DĬJ-ĭ-tăl RĔK-tăl *rect:* rectum *-al:* pertaining to	Examination of the prostate gland by finger palpation through the anal canal and the rectum (See Figure 8–17.) *DRE is usually performed during physical examination to detect prostate enlargement. It is also used to check for problems with organs or other structures in the pelvis and lower abdomen.*
prostate-specific antigen (PSA) test ĂN-tĭ-jĕn	Blood test to screen for prostate cancer *Elevated levels of PSA are associated with prostate enlargement and cancer.*

Medical and Surgical Procedures

Female Reproductive System

cerclage sār-KLŎZH	Obstetric procedure in which a nonabsorbable suture is used for holding the cervix closed to prevent spontaneous abortion in a woman who has an incompetent cervix
dilation and curettage (D&C) DĬ-lā-shŭn, kū-rĕ-TĂZH	Surgical procedure that widens the cervical canal of the uterus (dilation) so that the endometrium of the uterus can be scraped (curettage) (See Figure 8–5.) *D&C is performed to stop prolonged or heavy uterine bleeding, diagnose uterine abnormalities, and obtain tissue for microscopic examination. It is also performed to remove tumors, rule out carcinoma of the uterus, remove retained placental fragments after delivery or after an incomplete abortion, and determine the cause of infertility.*

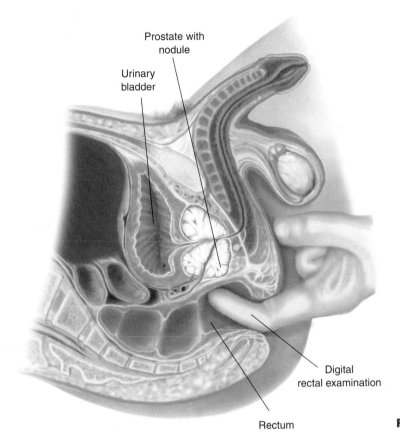

Prostate with nodule

Urinary bladder

Digital rectal examination

Rectum

Figure 8-17 Digital rectal examination.

hysterosalpingo-oophorectomy hĭs-tĕr-ō-săl-pĭng-gō-ō-ŏ-for-ĔK-tō-mē *hyster/o:* uterus (womb) *salping/o:* tube (usually fallopian or eustachian [auditory] tube) *oophor:* ovary *-ectomy:* excision	Surgical removal of a uterus, a fallopian tube, and an ovary
lumpectomy lŭm-PĔK-tō-mē	Excision of a small primary breast tumor ("lump") and some of the normal tissue that surrounds it (See Figure 8–8.) *In lumpectomy, lymph nodes may also be removed because they are located within the breast tissue taken during surgery. All tissue removed from the breast is biopsied to determine whether cancer cells are present in the normal tissue surrounding the tumor. Lumpectomy is the most common form of breast cancer surgery today.*

mastectomy
măs-TĔK-tō-mē
 	
  mast: breast
  -ectomy: excision,
       removal
	Complete or partial excision of one or both breasts, most commonly performed to remove a malignant tumor
	
	Mastectomy may be simple, radical, or modified depending on the extent of the malignancy and amount of breast tissue excised.

total	Excision of an entire breast, nipple, areola, and the involved overlying skin; also called *simple mastectomy* *In total mastectomy, lymph nodes are removed only if they are included in the breast tissue being removed.*
modified radical	Excision of an entire breast, including lymph nodes in the underarm (axillary dissection) (See Figure 8–18.) *Most women who have mastectomies today have modified radical mastectomies.*
radical	Excision of an entire breast, all underarm lymph nodes, and chest wall muscles under the breast

Entire breast and underarm lymph nodes removed, chest muscles left intact

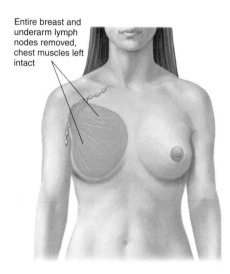

Figure 8-18 Modified radical mastectomy.

reconstructive breast surgery	Reconstruction of a breast that has been removed due to cancer or other disease *Reconstruction is commonly possible immediately following mastectomy so the patient awakens from anesthesia with a breast mound already in place.*
tissue (skin) expansion	Common breast reconstruction technique in which a balloon expander is inserted beneath the skin and chest muscle, saline solution is gradually injected to increase size, and the expander is then replaced with a more permanent implant (See Figure 8–19.)
transverse rectus abdominis muscle (TRAM) flap	Surgical creation of a skin flap (using skin and fat from the lower half of the abdomen), which is passed under the skin to the breast area, shaped into a natural-looking breast, and sutured into place (See Figure 8–20.) *The TRAM flap procedure is one of the most popular reconstruction options.*

tubal ligation TŪ-băl lī-GĀ-shŭn	Sterilization procedure that involves blocking both fallopian tubes by cutting or burning them and tying them off

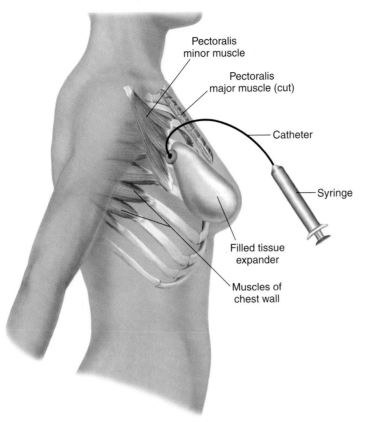

Pectoralis minor muscle

Pectoralis major muscle (cut)

Catheter

Syringe

Filled tissue expander

Muscles of chest wall

Figure 8-19   Tissue expander for breast reconstruction.

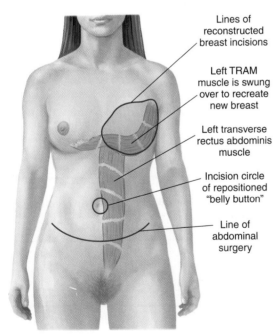

Lines of reconstructed breast incisions

Left TRAM muscle is swung over to recreate new breast

Left transverse rectus abdominis muscle

Incision circle of repositioned "belly button"

Line of abdominal surgery

Figure 8-20   TRAM flap.

Male Reproductive System

circumcision sĕr-kŭm-SĬ-zhŭn	Surgical removal of the foreskin or prepuce of the penis, usually performed on the male as an infant
transurethral resection of the prostate (TURP)	Surgical procedure to relieve obstruction caused by benign prostatic hyperplasia (excessive overgrowth of normal tissue) by insertion of a resectoscope into the penis and through the urethra to "chip away" at prostatic tissue and flush out chips (using an irrigating solution) *The pieces of prostatic tissue obtained through TURP are sent to the laboratory to be analyzed for possible evidence of CA. (See Figure 8–11.) Although TURP relieves the obstruction, overgrowth of tissue may recur over several years. Lasers may also be used to destroy prostatic tissue and relieve obstruction.*

Pharmacology

antifungals ăn-tĭ-FŬN-gălz	Agents used to treat vaginal fungal infection, such as *candidiasis*
estrogens ĔS-trō-jĕnz	Agents used to treat symptoms of menopause (hot flashes, vaginal dryness) through hormone replacement therapy (HRT)
gonadotropin gŏn-ă-dō-TRŌ-pĭn *gonad/o:* gonads, sex glands *-tropin:* stimulate	Agents used to increase sperm count in infertility cases
oral contraceptives (OCPs) kŏn-tră-SĔP-tĭvz	Agents that prevent ovulation in order to avoid pregnancy; also known as *birth control pills*
spermicides SPĔR-mĭ-sīdz	Agents used as a method of birth control that destroy sperm by creating a highly acidic environment in the uterus

Additional Medical Terms Review

Match the medical term(s) below with the definitions in the numbered list.

anorchism	cryptorchidism	impotence	pyosalpinx
candidiasis	D&C	leukorrhea	sterility
cerclage	endometriosis	mammography	syphilis
chlamydia	gonadotropins	oligomenorrhea	toxic shock
circumcision	gonorrhea	phimosis	trichomoniasis

1. _____ refers to failure of testicles to descend into scrotum.

2. _____ is pus in the fallopian tube.

3. _____ refers to inability of a woman to become pregnant or for a man to impregnate a woman.

4. _____ refers to congenital absence of one or both testes.

5. _____ is a vaginal fungal infection caused by *Candida albicans* and marked by a curdy discharge and extreme itching.

6. _____ is caused by infection with the bacterium *Chlamydia trachomatis* and occurs in both sexes.

7. _____ is surgical removal of foreskin or prepuce of the penis.

8. _____ is an obstetric procedure to prevent spontaneous abortion in a woman who has an incompetent cervix.

9. _____ is a discharge from the vagina; common reason for women to seek gynecological care.

10. _____ is a condition in which endometrial tissue is found in various abnormal sites throughout the pelvis or in the abdominal wall.

11. _____ refers to radiography of the breast and is used to diagnose benign and malignant tumors.

12. _____ is a sexually transmitted bacterial infection that most commonly affects the genitourinary tract and, occasionally, the pharynx or rectum.

13. _____ is a sexually transmitted disease that is characterized by lesions that change to a chancre, may involve any organ or tissue, and usually exhibits cutaneous manifestations.

14. _____ is a rare and sometimes fatal staphylococcal infection that occurs in menstruating women who use vaginal tampons.

15. _____ is a protozoal infestation of the vagina, urethra, or prostate.

16. _____ refers to widening of the uterine cervix so that the surface lining of the uterus can be scraped.

17. _____ means stenosis of the preputial orifice so that the foreskin does not retract over the glans penis.

18. _____ refers to the inability of a man to achieve a penile erection.

19. _____ refers to scanty or infrequent menstrual flow.

20. _____ are hormonal preparations used to increase the sperm count in cases of infertility.

Competency Verification: Check your answers in Appendix B, Answer Key, page 572. If you are not satisfied with your level of comprehension, review the pathological, diagnostic, and therapeutic terms and retake the review.

Correct Answers _____ × 5 = _____ % Score

Medical Record Activities

The following medical reports reflect common, real-life clinical scenarios using medical terminology to document patient care.

MEDICAL RECORD ACTIVITY 8-1

Postmenopausal Bleeding

Terminology

Terms listed in the table below come from the medical report *Postmenopausal Bleeding* that follows. Use a medical dictionary such as *Taber's Cyclopedic Medical Dictionary,* the appendices of this book, or other resources to define each term. Then practice reading the pronunciations aloud for each term.

Term	Definition
axilla ăk-SĬL-ă	
D&C	
gravida 4 GRĂV-ĭ-dă	
laparoscopy lăp-ăr-ŎS-kō-pē (See Figure 8–16.)	
lesion LĒ-zhŭn	
mastectomy măs-TĔK-tŏ-mē	
menstrual MĔN-stroo-ăl	
metastases mě-TĂS-tă-sēz	
neoplastic nē-ō-PLĂS-tĭk	
para 4 PĂR-ă	
postmenopausal pōst-měn-ō-PAW-zăl	

Term	Definition
Premarin PRĔM-ă-rĭn	_____
preulcerating prē-ŬL-sĕr-āt-ĭng	_____

 Listen and Learn Online! will help you master pronunciations of selected medical words from this medical record activity. Visit *http://davisplus.fadavis.com/gylys/simplified* to find instructions on completing the *Listen and Learn Online!* exercise for this section and practice pronunciations.

Reading

Practice pronunciation of medical terms by reading the following medical report aloud.

Postmenopausal Bleeding

A 52-year-old gravida 4, para 4 woman had her last menstrual period at age 48. She was in our office last month for an evaluation because of postmenopausal bleeding. She has been taking Premarin and has had vaginal bleeding. The patient is currently admitted for gynecological laparoscopy and diagnostic D&C to rule out the possibility of a neoplastic process.

Last year this patient was admitted to the hospital for a simple mastectomy. The patient had a large preulcerating lesion of the left breast with metastases to the axilla, liver, and bone. Further medical evaluation will be performed next week.

Evaluation

Review the medical record to answer the following questions. Use a medical dictionary such as *Taber's Cyclopedic Medical Dictionary* and other resources if needed.

1. How many times has the patient been pregnant? How many children has the patient given birth to?

_____

_____

2. Why is the patient being admitted to the hospital?

_____

_____

3. What is a D&C?

_____

_____

4. What is the patient's past surgical history?

_____

_____

5. At what sites did the patient have malignant growth?

_____

_____

MEDICAL RECORD ACTIVITY 8-2

Bilateral Vasectomy

Terminology

Terms listed in the table below come from the medical report _Bilateral Vasectomy_ that follows. Use a medical dictionary such as _Taber's Cyclopedic Medical Dictionary,_ the appendices of this book, or other resources to define each term. Then practice reading the pronunciations aloud for each term.

Term	Definition
bilateral bī-LĂT-ĕr-ăl	_____
cauterized KAW-tĕr-īzd	_____
Darvocet-N DĂHR-vō-sĕt	_____
hemostat HĒ-mō-stăt	_____
semen SĒ-mĕn	_____
supine sū-PĪN	_____
vas văs	_____
vasectomy văs-ĔK-tō-mē (See Figure 8–12.)	_____
Xylocaine ZĪ-lō-kān	_____

Listen and Learn Online! will help you master pronunciations of selected medical words from this medical record activity. Visit _http://davisplus.fadavis.com/gylys/simplified_ to find instructions on completing the _Listen and Learn Online!_ exercise for this section and practice pronunciations.

Reading

Practice pronunciation of medical terms by reading the following medical report aloud.

Bilateral Vasectomy

Patient was placed on the table in supine position and prepped, scrotum shaved, and draped in the usual fashion. The right testicle was grasped and brought to skin level. This area was injected with 1% Xylocaine anesthesia. After a few minutes, a small incision was made, and the right vas was located. A hemostat was used and clamped on the right and left vas. A segment of the right vas was removed, and both ends were cauterized and tied independently with 3-0 silk suture. The skin was closed with 2-0 chromic suture. The same procedure was performed on the left side. The hemostats were removed. There were no complications or bleeding. Patient was discharged to home in care of his wife. Postoperative care instruction sheet was given along with prescription of Darvocet-N 100 mg, 1 q4h as required for pain. Patient will be seen for follow-up semen analysis in 6 weeks.

Evaluation

Review the medical record to answer the following questions. Use a medical dictionary such as *Taber's Cyclopedic Medical Dictionary* and other resources if needed.

1. What is the end result of a bilateral vasectomy?

_____

_____

2. Was the patient awake during the surgery? What type of anesthesia was used?

_____

_____

3. What was used to prevent bleeding?

_____

_____

4. What type of suture material was used to close the incision?

_____

_____

5. What was the patient given for pain relief at home?

_____

_____

6. Why is it important for the patient to go for a follow-up visit?

_____

_____

Chapter Review

Word Elements Summary

The following table summarizes CFs, suffixes, and prefixes related to the reproductive system.

Word Element	Meaning	Word Element	Meaning
Combining Forms			
FEMALE REPRODUCTIVE SYSTEM			
amni/o	amnion (amniotic sac)	**metr/o**	uterus (womb); measure
cervic/o	neck; cervix uteri (neck of uterus)	**mamm/o, mast/o**	breast
colp/o, vagin/o	vagina	**men/o**	menses, menstruation
episi/o, vulv/o	vulva	**nat/o**	birth
galact/o, lact/o	milk	**oophor/o, ovari/o**	ovary
gynec/o	woman, female	**perine/o**	perineum
hyster/o, uter/o	uterus (womb)	**salping/o**	tube (usually fallopian or eustachian [auditory] tubes)
lapar/o	abdomen		
MALE REPRODUCTIVE SYSTEM			
andr/o	male	**prostat/o**	prostate gland
balan/o	glans penis	**spermat/o**	spermatozoa, sperm cells
orchid/o, orchi/o, orch/o, test/o	testis (plural, testes)	**vas/o**	vessel; vas deferens; duct
OTHER COMBINING FORMS			
adip/o, lip/o	fat	**hydr/o**	water
carcin/o	cancer	**muc/o**	mucus
cyst/o	bladder	**olig/o**	scanty
hemat/o, hem/o	blood		
Suffixes			
SURGICAL			
-ectomy	excision, removal	**-rrhaphy**	suture
-pexy	fixation (of an organ)	**-tome**	instrument to cut

Word Element	Meaning	Word Element	Meaning
-plasty	surgical repair	-tomy	incision

DIAGNOSTIC, SYMPTOMATIC, AND RELATED

Word Element	Meaning	Word Element	Meaning
-algia, -dynia	pain	-oma	tumor
-cele	hernia, swelling	-pathy	disease
-genesis	forming, producing, origin	-plasia, -plasm	formation, growth
-itis	inflammation	-ptosis	prolapse, downward displacement
-lith	stone, calculus	-rrhage, -rrhagia	bursting forth (of)
-logy	study of	-rrhea	discharge, flow
-logist	specialist in study of	-scope	instrument for examining
-megaly	enlargement	-spasm	involuntary contraction, twitching
-oid	resembling	-uria	urine

FEMALE REPRODUCTIVE SYSTEM

Word Element	Meaning	Word Element	Meaning
-arche	beginning	-salpinx	tube (usually fallopian or eustachian [auditory] tubes)
-cyesis	pregnancy	-tocia	childbirth, labor
-gravida	pregnant woman	-version	turning
-para	to bear (offspring)		

ADJECTIVE

Word Element	Meaning	Word Element	Meaning
-al, -ic, -ous	pertaining to, relating to		

NOUN

Word Element	Meaning	Word Element	Meaning
-ia	condition	-ist	specialist

Prefixes

Word Element	Meaning	Word Element	Meaning
a-, an-	without, not	neo-	new
dys-	bad; painful; difficult	post-	after, behind
hyper-	excessive, above normal	pre-	before, in front of

Enhance your study and reinforcement of word elements with the power of *Davis Plus.* Visit *http://davisplus.fadavis.com/gylys/simplified* for this chapter's flash-card activity. We recommend you complete the flash-card activity before completing the word elements review below.

Word Elements Review

After you review the Word Elements Summary, complete this activity by writing the meaning of each element in the space provided.

Word Element	Meaning	Word Element	Meaning
Combining Forms			
FEMALE REPRODUCTIVE SYSTEM			
1. amni/o		6. hyster/o, metr/o, uter/o	
2. colp/o, vagin/o		7. nat/o	
3. episi/o, vulv/o		8. oophor/o, ovari/o	
4. galact/o, lact/o		9. perine/o	
5. gynec/o			
MALE REPRODUCTIVE SYSTEM			
10. vas/o		12. andr/o	
11. orchid/o, orchi/o, orch/o, test/o		13. balan/o	
OTHER COMBINING FORMS			
14. adip/o, lip/o		17. hydr/o	
15. olig/o		18. muc/o	
16. hemat/o, hem/o			
Suffixes			
SURGICAL			
19. -ectomy		21. -pexy	
20. -plasty		22. -tomy	
DIAGNOSTIC, SYMPTOMATIC, AND RELATED			
23. -logist		26. -megaly	
24. -genesis		27. -cele	
25. -algia, -dynia			
FEMALE REPRODUCTIVE SYSTEM			
28. -para		32. -salpinx	
29. -tocia		33. -gravida	
30. -version		34. -arche	
31. -cyesis			

Word Element	Meaning	Word Element	Meaning
NOUN			
35. -ist	_____		
ADJECTIVE			
37. -al, -ic, -ous	_____		
Prefixes			
38. neo-	_____	**40.** a-, an-	_____
39. dys-	_____		

Competency Verification: Check your answers in Appendix A, Glossary of Medical Word Elements, page 538. If you are not satisfied with your level of comprehension, review the word elements and retake the review.

Correct Answers: _____ × 2.5 = _____ % Score

Vocabulary Review

Match the medical term(s) below with the definitions in the numbered list.

amenorrhea	estrogen	postmenopausal	uterus
aplasia	gravida 4	progesterone	vas deferens
aspermatism	hydrocele	prostatic cancer	vasectomy
cervix uteri	oophoritis	prostatomegaly	
dysmenorrhea	para 4	testopathy	
epididymis	PID	testosterone	

1. _____ means enlargement of prostate gland.

2. _____ refers to disease of the testes.

3. _____ is a male hormone produced by testes.

4. _____ is absence or abnormal stoppage of the menses.

5. _____ is a (are) female hormone(s) produced by the ovaries.

6. _____ is an inflamed condition of the ovaries.

7. _____ is a condition in which there is a lack of male sperm.

8. _____ refers to a woman in her fourth pregnancy.

9. _____ is an organ that nourishes the embryo.

10. _____ is a malignant neoplasm of the prostate.

11. _____ is a tube that temporarily stores sperm.

12. _____ is a collection of fluid in a saclike cavity.

13. _____ is a duct that transports sperm from the testes to the urethra.

14. _____ refers to a woman who has delivered four infants.

15. _____ means neck of the uterus.

16. _____ refers to painful menstruation.

17. _____ means occurring after menopause.

18. _____ is failure or lack of formation or growth.

19. _____ is a procedure to sterilize a man by cutting the vas deferens, preventing the release of sperm.

20. _____ is a collective term for any extensive bacterial infection of the pelvic organs, especially the uterus, uterine tubes, or ovaries.

Competency Verification: Check your answers in Appendix B, Answer Key, page 573. If you are not satisfied with your level of comprehension, review the chapter vocabulary and retake the review.

Correct Answers _____ × 5 = _____ % Score

9 Endocrine and Nervous Systems

OBJECTIVES

Upon completion of this chapter, you will be able to:

- Describe the type of medical treatment endocrinologists and neurologists provide.
- Identify endocrine and nervous systems structures by labeling them on the anatomical illustrations.
- Describe the primary functions of the endocrine and nervous systems.
- Describe common diseases related to the endocrine and nervous systems.
- Describe common diagnostic, medical,and surgical procedures related to the endocrine and nervous systems.
- Apply your word-building skills by constructing various medical terms related to the endocrine and nervous systems.
- Describe common abbreviations and symbols related to the endocrine and nervous systems.
- Reinforce word elements by completing flash card activities.
- Recognize, define, pronounce, and spell terms correctly.
- Demonstrate your knowledge of this chapter by successfully completing the frames, reviews, and medical report evaluations.

Medical Specialties

Endocrinology

Endocrinology is the branch of medicine concerned with treatment of disorders that affect glands that control metabolism, reproduction, and sexual growth and development. **Endocrinologists** evaluate the body's overall metabolic function and diagnose and treat hormone imbalances. They treat such conditions as diabetes mellitus, thyroid diseases, and osteoporosis and other disorders involving the underproduction or overproduction of hormones, control of overall fluid concentrations, and disorders of blood glucose metabolism. When surgery is required, the endocrinologist works closely with the surgeon to provide the most beneficial patient care. Endocrinologists also play important roles related to their field of expertise in university academic research and in the pharmaceutical industry.

Neurology

Neurology is the branch of medicine concerned with the diagnosis and treatment of diseases of the nervous system, which includes the brain, spinal cord, and peripheral nerves. **Neurologists** are physicians who provide evaluation, diagnosis, and treatment of conditions involving the nervous system. The nervous system controls voluntary and involuntary movements as well as some organ and gland functioning. It also controls all the processes of cognition, such as thinking, feeling, and remembering. The neurologist attempts to detect, diagnose, and treat symptoms and disorders that indicate an impairment of any of these functions. These disorders can include but are not limited to vascular problems that affect the brain, infections or inflammations of the brain or the spinal cord tissue, nervous tissue tumors, degenerative neuromuscular disorders, and traumatic brain or spinal cord injury. Neurologists use specialized examination procedures, laboratory tests, and brain imaging techniques to diagnose nervous disorders. Pharmacological, surgical, and rehabilitative techniques are used to treat neurological disorders. The branch of surgery involving the nervous system, including the brain and spinal cord, is called **neurosurgery**. The physician who specializes in neurosurgery is a **neurosurgeon**.

Anatomy and Physiology Overview

The endocrine and nervous systems work together like interlocking supersystems to control many intricate activities of the body. Together they monitor changes in the body and in the external environment, interpret these changes, and coordinate appropriate responses to reestablish and maintain a relative equilibrium in the internal environment of the body **(homeostasis)**.

The endocrine system is made up of a network of ductless glands, which have a rich blood supply that enables the hormones they produce to enter the bloodstream. (See Figure 9–1.) Hormone production occurs at one site, but their effects take place at various other sites in the body. The tissues or organs that respond to the effects of a hormone are called *target tissues* or *target organs*.

In contrast to the endocrine system, which slowly discharges hormones into the bloodstream, the nervous system is designed to act instantaneously by transmitting electrical impulses to specific body locations. The nervous system controls all critical body activities and reactions. It is one of the most complicated systems of the body. The nervous system coordinates voluntary (conscious) activities, such as walking, talking, and eating. It also coordinates involuntary (unconscious) functions, such as reflexes to pain, body changes related to stress, and thought and emotional processes.

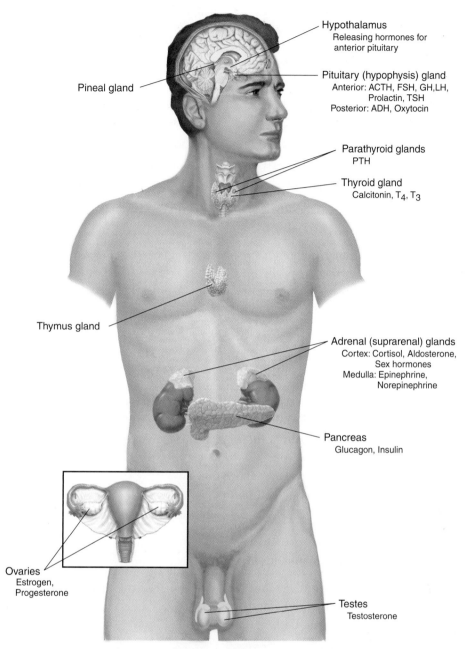

Hypothalamus
Releasing hormones for
anterior pituitary

Pituitary (hypophysis) gland
Anterior: ACTH, FSH, GH,LH,
Prolactin, TSH
Posterior: ADH, Oxytocin

Pineal gland

Parathyroid glands
PTH

Thyroid gland
Calcitonin, T$_4$, T$_3$

Thymus gland

Adrenal (suprarenal) glands
Cortex: Cortisol, Aldosterone,
Sex hormones
Medulla: Epinephrine,
Norepinephrine

Pancreas
Glucagon, Insulin

Ovaries
Estrogen,
Progesterone

Testes
Testosterone

Figure 9-1   Locations of major endocrine glands.

WORD ELEMENTS

This section introduces CFs related to the endocrine system. Included are key suffixes; prefixes are defined in the right-hand column as needed. Review the following table, and pronounce each word in the word analysis column aloud before you begin to work the frames.

Word Element	Meaning	Word Analysis
Combining Forms		
aden/o	gland	**aden**/oma (ăd-ĕ-NŌ-mă): tumor composed of glandular tissue *-oma:* tumor
adren/o		**adren**/al (ăd-RĒ-năl): pertaining to the adrenal glands *-al:* pertaining to
adrenal/o	adrenal glands	**adrenal**/ectomy (ăd-rē-năl-ĔK-tō-mē): excision of adrenal gland(s) *-ectomy:* excision, removal
calc/o	calcium	hypo/**calc**/emia (hī-pō-kăl-SĒ-mē-ă): deficiency of calcium in the blood *hypo-:* under, below, deficient *-emia:* blood condition
gluc/o	sugar, sweetness	**gluc**/o/genesis (gloo-kō-JĔN-ĕ-sĭs): formation of glucose *-genesis:* forming, producing, origin
glyc/o		hyper/**glyc**/emia (hī-pĕr-glī-SĒ-mē-ă): excessive glucose in the blood *hyper-:* excessive, above normal *-emia:* blood condition *Hyperglycemia is most commonly associated with diabetes mellitus.*
pancreat/o	pancreas	**pancreat**/itis (păn-krē-ă-TĪ-tĭs): inflammation of the pancreas *itis:* inflammation
parathyroid/o	parathyroid glands	**parathyroid**/ectomy (păr-ă-thī-royd-ĔK-tō-mē): excision of the parathyroid gland(s) *-ectomy:* excision, removal
pituitar/o	pituitary gland	hypo/**pituitar**/ism (hī-pō-pĭ-TŪ-ĭ-tă-rĭzm): condition of inadequate levels of the pituitary hormone in the body
thym/o	thymus gland	**thym**/oma (thī-MŌ-mă): tumor of the thymus gland *-oma:* tumor
thyr/o	thyroid gland	**thyr**/o/megaly (thī-rō-MĔG-ă-lē): enlargement of the thyroid gland *-megaly:* enlargement
thyroid/o		**thyroid**/ectomy (thī-royd-ĔK-tō-mē): excision of the thyroid gland *-ectomy:* excision, removal

Word Element	Meaning	Word Analysis
toxic/o	poison	**toxic/o**/logist (tŏks-ĭ-KŎL-ō-jĭst): specialist in the study of poisons or toxins *-logist:* specialist in study of

Suffixes

Word Element	Meaning	Word Analysis
-dipsia	thirst	poly/**dipsia** (pŏl-ē-DĬP-sē-ă): excessive thirst *poly-:* many, much *Polydipsia is a characteristic symptom of diabetes mellitus.*
-trophy	development, nourishment	hyper/**trophy** (hī-PĔR-trŏ-fē): increase in the size of an organ *hyper-:* excessive, above normal *Hypertrophy is due to an increase in the size of the cells of an organ, rather than an increase in the number of cells, as in carcinoma.*

Pronunciation Help	Long Sound	ā in rāte	ē in rēbirth	ī in īsle	ō in ōver	ū in ūnite
	Short Sound	ă in ălone	ĕ in ĕver	ĭ in ĭt	ŏ in nŏt	ŭ in cŭt

Listen and Learn, the audio CD-ROM included in this book, will help you master pronunciation of selected medical words. Use it to practice pronunciations of the above-listed medical terms and for instructions to complete the *Listen and Learn* exercise for this section.

SECTION REVIEW 9-1

For the following medical terms, first write the suffix and its meaning. Then translate the meaning of the remaining elements starting with the first part of the word. The first word is completed for you.

Term	Definition
1. toxic/o/logist	*-logist: specialist in study of; poison*
2. pancreat/itis	_____
3. thyr/o/megaly	_____
4. hyper/trophy	_____
5. gluc/o/genesis	_____
6. hypo/calc/emia	_____
7. adrenal/ectomy	_____
8. poly/dipsia	_____
9. aden/oma	_____
10. thyroid/ectomy	_____

Competency Verification: Check your answers in Appendix B, Answer Key, page 574. If you are not satisfied with your level of comprehension, review the vocabulary and retake the review.

Correct Answers _____ × 10 = _____ % Score

Endocrine System

Hormones

9-1 *Hormones* are chemical substances produced by specialized cells of the body. Because they travel in the blood, hormones reach all body tissues. However, only target organs contain receptors that recognize a particular hormone. The receptors maintain the tissue's responsiveness to hormonal stimulation.

Review Figure 9–2, which illustrates hormones of the pituitary gland and their target organs. The organs shown in Figure 9–2 are directly affected by the amounts of hormones released into the bloodstream by the pituitary gland. For example, underproduction of growth hormone (GH) in children results in dwarfism.

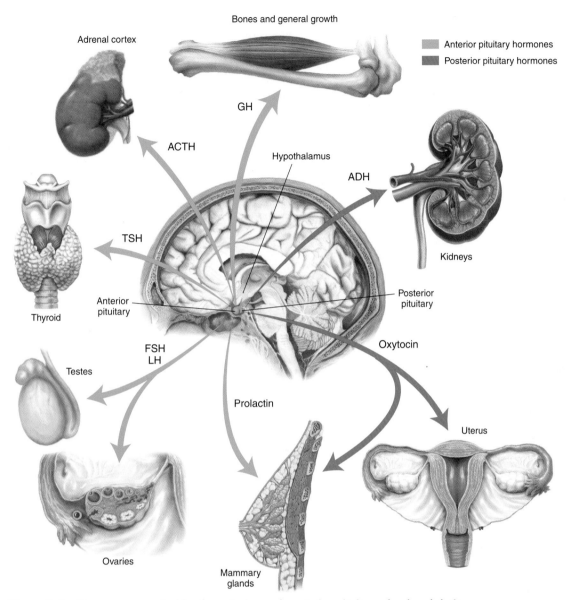

Figure 9-2 Hormones secreted by the anterior and posterior pituitary gland and their target organs.

9–2 Hormone secretion to a target organ is determined by the body's need for the hormone at any given time. Hormone secretion is regulated so that there is no overproduction (hyper/secretion) or underproduction (hypo/secretion). There are times when the body's regulating mechanism does not operate properly, and hormonal levels become excessive or deficient, causing various disorders.

List the term in this frame that is synonymous with

overproduction: _____ / _____

underproduction: _____ / _____

hyper/secretion
hī-pĕr-sē-KRĒ-shŭn

hypo/secretion
hī-pō-sē-KRĒ-shŭn

9–3 Although all major hormones circulate to virtually all tissues, each hormone exerts specific effects on its target organ. If a hormone has a specific effect on the stomach, that hormone's target organ is the stomach. If the hormone has a specific effect on the heart, the target organ is the

heart

_____.

9–4 Hormones have four key characteristics. They are:

- chemical substances produced by specialized cells of the body
- released slowly in minute amounts directly into the bloodstream
- produced primarily by the endocrine glands
- almost all inactivated or excreted by the liver and kidneys.

9–5 Refer to Frame 9–4 above to complete this frame.
List four common characteristics of hormones.

1. _____

_____

_____

2. _____

_____

_____

3. _____

_____

_____

To check answers, refer to Frame 9–4 above.

4. _____

_____

_____

9–6 Endo/crine gland dysfunction may result in hypo/secretion or hyper/secretion of its hormones. The prefix *hyper-* means *excessive, above normal*. The prefix *hypo-* means *under, below, deficient*.
Build medical terms that mean

hyper/secretion
hī-pĕr-sē-KRĒ-shŭn
hypo/secretion
hī-pō-sē-KRĒ-shŭn

excessive secretion: _____ / _____

deficient secretion: _____ / _____

Pituitary Gland

9–7 The (1) **pituitary gland** is one of the most important endocrine glands. Its hormone secretions influence the functions of many organs in the body, as illustrated in Figure 9–2. Located below the brain, it is no larger than a pea.
Label the pituitary gland in Figure 9–3.

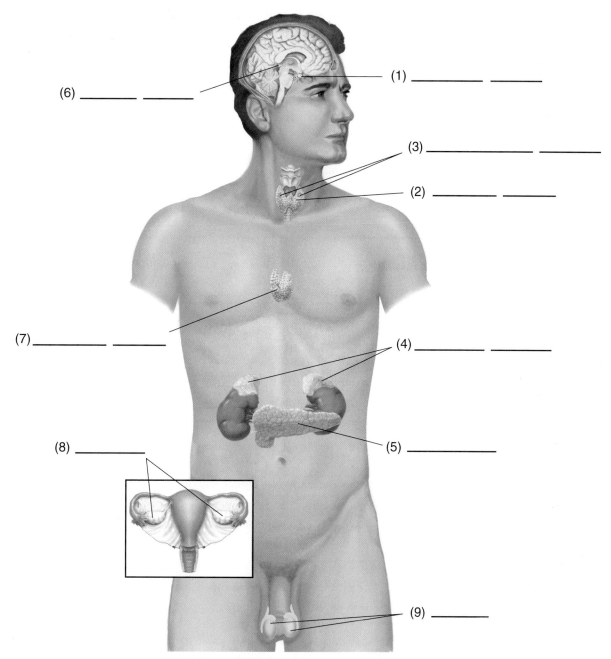

(6) _____ _____

(1) _____ _____

(3) _____ _____

(2) _____ _____

(7) _____ _____

(4) _____ _____

(5) _____

(8) _____

(9) _____

Figure 9-3 Locations of major endocrine glands.

anter/ior ăn-TĒ-rē-or **poster/ior** pŏs-TĒ-rē-or	**9–8** The pituitary gland consists of two distinct portions: an anter/ior lobe and a poster/ior lobe. The front lobe is called the _____ / _____ lobe. The back lobe back is called the _____ / _____ lobe.

anter/o **poster/o**	**9-9** Identify the CFs that mean *anterior, front:* _____ / _____ *back (of body), behind, posterior:* _____ / _____
radi/o	**9-10** The term *anter/o/poster/ior* (AP) is used in radi/o/logy to describe the direction or path of an x-ray beam. From *radi/o/logy*, determine the CF for *radiation, x-ray;radius (lower arm bone on thumb side).* _____ / _____
back	**9-11** AP is a directional abbreviation that means *passing from the front to* the _____ *(of the body).*
poster/ior pŏs-TĒ-rē-or	**9-12** An AP view of the abdomen is a view from the anter/ior to the _____ / _____ part of the abdomen.
AP **PA**	**9-13** The term *poster/o/anter/ior* (PA) means *directed from the back toward the front (of the body).* Write the abbreviations designating the path of an x-ray beam from the *anter/o/poster/ior (part of the body):* _____ *poster/o/anter/ior (part of the body):* _____
above **below** **behind, side**	**9-14** Use the terms *above, below, behind,* or *side* to define the following terms: *Poster/o/super/ior* means *located behind and* _____ *a structure.* *Poster/o/infer/ior* means *located behind and* _____ *a structure.* *Poster/o/later/al* means *located* _____ *and at the* _____ *of a structure.*
gland	**9-15** The pituitary gland is also called the *hypophysis.* The anterior lobe of the pituitary gland is called the *aden/o/hypophysis;* the poster/ior lobe is called the *neur/o/hypophysis.* The CF *neur/o* means *nerve.* The CF **aden/o** means _____.

9-16   The anter/ior lobe (aden/o/hypophysis) develops from an up-growth of the pharynx and is glandular in nature; the poster/ior lobe (neur/o/hypophysis) develops from a downgrowth from the base of the brain and consists of nervous tissue. Although both lobes secrete various hormones that regulate body functions, two hormones secreted by the neur/o/hypophysis are produced in the hypothalamus. The neur/o/hypophysis merely acts as a storage site until the hormones are released. (See Figure 9–2.)
Identify the words in this frame that mean

anter/ior
ăn-TĒ-rē-or

poster/ior
pŏs-TĒ-rē-or

neur/o/hypophysis
nū-rō-hī-PŎF-ĭs-ĭs

aden/o/hypophysis
ăd-ĕ-nō-hī-PŎF-ĭ-sĭs

in front of: _____ / _____

behind, back (of body): _____ / _____

hypophysis composed of nervous tissue: _____ / ____ / _____

hypophysis composed of glandular tissue: _____ / ____ / _____

---

neur/o/hypophysis
nū-rō-hī-PŎF-ĭs-ĭs

9-17   The poster/ior lobe of the pituitary gland, composed primarily of nervous tissue, is called the _____ / ____ / _____.

---

aden/o/hypophysis
ăd-ĕ-nō-hī-PŎF-ĭ-sĭs

9-18   The anter/ior lobe of the pituitary gland, composed primarily of glandular tissue, is called the _____ / ____ / _____.

9-19   Table 9–1 outlines pituitary hormones, along with their target organs and functions and selected associated disorders. Refer to Table 9–1 on page 399 to complete Frames 9–19 through 9–24.

The two hormones released by the neur/o/hypophysis are

_____ _____ and _____.

9-20   Define the following abbreviations related to the anterior pituitary (adenohypophysis) and posterior pituitary (neurohypophysis).

GH: _____

TSH: _____

ADH: _____ (vasopressin)

LH: _____

9-21   Briefly state the important function of ADH (posterior pituitary hormone) in the kidneys.

_____

_____

9–22 Write the abbreviation of the anterior pituitary hormone that initiates sperm production in men.

_____

9–23 What is the posterior pituitary hormone that causes contraction of the uterus during childbirth?

_____

To check answers for 9–19 through 9–24, refer to Table 9–1 on page 399.

9–24 Briefly state two functions of GH (anterior pituitary hormone).

_____

_____

_____

_____

dwarf/ism

gigant/ism

9–25 Overproduction of GH in children produces an exceptionally large person, a condition known as _gigant/ism._ Underproduction of GH in children is likely to produce an exceptionally small person, a condition called _dwarf/ism._

The clinical term for _condition of an abnormally_

short or undersized person is: _____ / _____

tall or oversized person is: _____ / _____

acr/o/megaly
ăk-rō-MĔG-ă-lē

9–26 The CF **acr/o** means _extremity._ Acr/o/megaly, a chronic metabolic condition, is characterized by a gradual, marked enlargement and thickening of the bones of the face and jaw. This condition, which afflicts middle-aged and older persons, is caused by overproduction of growth hormone and is treated by radiation, pharmacologic agents, or surgery, commonly involving partial resection of the pituitary gland.

A term that literally means _enlargement of the extremities_ is

_____ / _____ / _____.

Thyroid Gland

9–27 The (2) **thyroid gland** is located on the front and sides of the trachea just below the larynx. Its two lobes are separated by a strip of tissue called the isthmus. Label the thyroid gland in Figure 9–3.

thyroid/ectomy
thī-royd-ĔK-tō-mē

9–28 The CFs for _thyroid gland_ are **thyr/o** and **thyroid/o.**

Use **thyroid/o** to form a word that means _excision of the thyroid gland._

_____ / _____

table 9-1   PITUITARY HORMONES

This table identifies pituitary hormones, their target organs and functions, and associated disorders.

Hormone	Target Organ and Functions	Disorders
Anterior Pituitary Hormones (Adenohypophysis)		
Adrenocorticotropic hormone (ACTH)	• Adrenal cortex—promotes secretions of some hormones by adrenal cortex, especially cortisol	• Hyposecretion is rare. • Hypersecretion causes Cushing disease.
Follicle-stimulating hormone (FSH)	• Ovaries—in females, stimulates egg production; increases secretion of estrogen • Testes—in males, stimulates sperm production	• Hyposecretion causes failure of sexual maturation. • Hypersecretion has no known significant effects.
Growth hormone (GH), or somatotropin	• Bone, cartilage, liver, muscle, and other tissues—stimulates somatic growth; increases use of fats for energy	• Hyposecretion in children causes pituitary dwarfism. • Hypersecretion in children causes gigantism; hypersecretion in adults causes acromegaly.
Luteinizing hormone (LH)	• Ovaries—in females, promotes ovulation; stimulates production of estrogen and progesterone • Testes—in males, promotes secretion of testosterone	• Hyposecretion causes failure of sexual maturation. • Hypersecretion has no known significant effects.
Prolactin	• Breast—in conjunction with other hormones, promotes lactation	• Hyposecretion in nursing mothers causes poor lactation. • Hypersecretion in nursing mothers causes galactorrhea.
Thyroid-stimulating hormone (TSH)	• Thyroid gland—stimulates secretion of thyroid hormone	• Hyposecretion in infants causes cretinism; hyposecretion in adults causes myxedema. • Hypersecretion causes Graves disease, indicated by exophthalmos. (See Figure 9–4.)
Posterior Pituitary Hormones (Neurohypophysis)		
Antidiuretic hormone (ADH)	• Kidney—increases water reabsorption (water returns to the blood)	• Hyposecretion causes diabetes insipidus. • Hypersecretion causes syndrome of inappropriate antidiuretic hormone (SIADH).
Oxytocin	• Uterus—stimulates uterine contractions; initiates labor • Breast—promotes milk secretion from the mammary glands	• Unknown

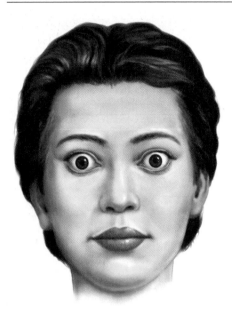

Figure 9-4   Exophthalmos caused by Graves disease.

thyr/o/megaly thī-rō-MĔG-ă-lē **thyr/o/pathy** thī-RŎP-ă-thē **thyr/o/tomy** thī-RŎT-ō-mē	**9–29** Use *thyr/o* to construct words that mean *enlargement of thyroid gland:* _____ / _____ / _____ *disease of thyroid gland:* _____ / _____ / _____ *incision of thyroid gland:* _____ / _____ / _____

9–30   Table 9–2 on page 402 outlines thyroid hormones along with their functions and selected associated disorders. Refer to the table to complete Frames 9–30 through 9–32.

The thyroid gland produces two hormones that regulate the body's metabolism (rate at which food is converted into heat and energy). These hormones are called _____ and _____.

9–31   In conjunction with PTH, calcium levels in the blood are regulated by secretion of the hormone called _____.

9–32   When does calcitonin exert its most important effects in the body?

To check answers for 9–30 through 9–32, refer to Table 9–2 on page 402.

_____

_____

_____

9-33 Hyper/thyroid/ism is caused by excessive secretion of the thyroid gland. The gland increases the body's metabolism and intensifies the demand for food.

Analyze *hyper/thyroid/ism* by defining the elements.

excessive, above normal

hyper-: _____, _____ _____

thyroid gland
THĪ-royd

thyroid/o: _____ _____

condition

-ism: _____

9-34 Hyper/thyroid/ism involves enlargement of the thyroid gland associated with hypersecretion of thyroxine. It is characterized by exophthalmos (bulging of the eyes), which develops because of edema in the tissues of the eye sockets and swelling of the extrinsic eye muscles. Hyper/thyroid/ism also is called *Graves disease, ex/ophthalm/ic goiter, thyr/o/toxic/osis,* and *tox/ic goiter.* (See Figure 9–5.)

Identify the terms in this frame that mean

ex/ophthalm/os *or*
ex/ophthalm/ic
ĕks-ŏf-THĂL-mŏs,
ĕks-ŏf-THĂL-mĭc

bulging of the eyes: _____ / _____ / _____

thyr/o/toxic/osis
thī-rō-tŏks-ĭ-KŌ-sĭs

abnormal condition of thyroid gland poisoning:

_____ / _____ / _____ / _____

9-35 Toxic/o/logy is the scientific study of poisons and treatment of conditions produced by them.

A specialist in the study of poisons is called a

toxic/o/logist
tŏks-ĭ-KŎL-ō-jĭst

_____ / _____ / _____.

---

poison

9-36 Toxic/o/pathy is any disease caused by _____.

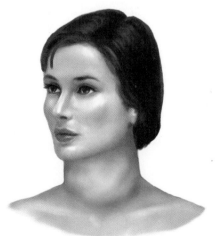

Figure 9-5 Enlargement of the thyroid gland in goiter.

thyroid/o/tomy thī-royd-ŎT-ō-mē **thyroid/o/tome** thī-ROYD-dō-tōm	**9-37** Use *thyroid/o* to form words that mean *incision of the thyroid gland:* _____ / ____ / _____ *instrument to incise the thyroid:* _____ / ____ / _____
blood	**9-38** The CF for *calcium* is **calc/o**. Calc/emia indicates an abnormal presence of calcium in the _____.
hyper/calc/emia hī-pěr-kăl-SĒ-mē-ă	**9-39** Hypo/calc/emia is a condition of abnormally low blood calcium. A person with excessively high blood calcium has a condition called _____ / _____ / _____

table 9-2   THYROID HORMONES

This table identifies thyroid hormones, their functions, and associated disorders.

Hormone	Functions	Disorders
Calcitonin	• Regulates calcium levels in the blood in conjunction with parathyroid hormone • Secreted when calcium levels in the blood are high in order to maintain homeostasis	• The most significant effects are exerted in childhood when bones are growing and changing dramatically in mass, size, and shape. • At best, calcitonin is a weak hypocalcemic agent in adults.
Thyroxine (T_4) and triiodothyronine (T_3)	• Increases energy production from all food types • Increases rate of protein synthesis	• Hyposecretion in infants causes cretinism; hyposecretion in adults causes myxedema. • Hypersecretion causes Graves disease, indicated by exophthalmos. (See Figure 9–4.)

SECTION REVIEW 9-2

Using the following table, write the CF, suffix, or prefix that matches its definition in the space provided to the left of the definition. There may be more than one word element that matches a definition.

Combining Forms		Suffixes		Prefixes
acr/o	poster/o	-emia	-tome	dys-
aden/o	radi/o	-logist	-tomy	hyper-
anter/o	thyr/o	-megaly		hypo-
calc/o	thyroid/o	-osis		poly-
neur/o	toxic/o	-pathy		

1. _____ abnormal condition; increase (used primarily with blood cells)
2. _____ excessive, above normal
3. _____ back (of body), behind, posterior
4. _____ bad; painful; difficult
5. _____ blood condition
6. _____ calcium
7. _____ disease
8. _____ enlargement
9. _____ extremity
10. _____ anterior, front
11. _____ gland
12. _____ incision
13. _____ instrument to cut
14. _____ nerve
15. _____ poison
16. _____ radiation, x-ray; radius (lower arm bone on thumb side)
17. _____ specialist in study of
18. _____ many, much
19. _____ thyroid gland
20. _____ under, below, deficient

Competency Verification: Check your answers in Appendix B, Answer Key, page 574. If you are not satisfied with your level of comprehension, go back to Frame 9–1 and rework the frames.

Correct Answers _____ × 5 = _____ % Score

Parathyroid Glands

9-40 The (3) **parathyroid glands** are located on the posterior surface of the thyroid gland. The parathyroid glands are so called because they are located around the thyroid gland. Label the parathyroid glands in Figure 9–3.

---

para/thyr/oid glands
păr-ă-THĪ-royd

9-41 Usually there are two pairs of para/thyr/oid glands associated with each of the thyroid's lobes, but the exact number varies. Nevertheless, as many as eight glands have been reported. The para/thyr/oid glands were detected accidentally. Surgeons observed that most patients who had either a partial or total thyroid/ectomy recovered uneventfully, whereas some experienced uncontrolled muscle spasms and severe pain and subsequently died. It was only after several such unexpected deaths that the parathyroid glands were discovered and their hormonal function, quite different from that of the thyroid gland hormones, became obvious. The parathyroid glands are responsible for controlling calcium levels in the blood.

When we discuss the two pairs of glands located in the posterior aspect of the thyroid glands, we are talking about the

_____ / _____ / _____ _____.

---

para-

9-42 Identify the element in the previous frame that means *located near, beside; beyond.*

_____

PTH

9-43 The hormone produced by the parathyroid glands is called *para/thormone* or *para/thyroid hormone* (PTH).

The abbreviation for *para/thormone* or *para/thyr/oid hormone* is _____.

To check answers, refer to Table 9–3 on page 405.

9-44 Table 9–3 on page 405 outlines parathyroid hormone along with its target organs and functions and associated disorders. Refer to the table to complete this frame.

The major function of PTH is to regulate levels of _____ and _____.

---

hyper/para/thyroid/ism
hī-pĕr-păr-ă-THĪ-roy-dĭzm

9-45 *Oste/itis fibrosa cystica* is an inflammatory degenerative condition in which normal bone is replaced by cysts and fibrous tissue. It is usually associated with hyper/para/thyroid/ism.

The term in this frame that means *abnormal endocrine condition characterized by hypersecretion of PTH* is

_____ / _____ / _____ / _____.

hyper/calc/emia hī-pĕr-kăl-SĒ-mē-ă **hypo/calc/emia** hī-pō-kăl-SĒ-mē-ă	**9–46** *Calc/emia* refers to calcium in the blood. Use *hypo-* and *hyper-* to form words that mean *excessive calcium in the blood:* _____ / _____ / _____ *deficiency of calcium in the blood:* _____ / _____ / _____

Adrenal Glands

	9–47 The (4) **adrenal glands,** also known as the *supra/ren/al glands,* are paired structures located super/ior to the kidneys. Label Figure 9–3 as you continue to learn about the endocrine system.

supra/ren/al soo-pră-RĒ-năl **super/ior**	**9–48** Indicate the words in Frame 9–46 that mean *above or superior to a kidney:* _____ / _____ / _____ *pertaining to upper or above:* _____ / _____

enlargement, adrenal **adrenal/ectomy** ăd-rē-năl-ĔK-tō-mē	**9–49** *Adren/o* and *adrenal/o* are CFs for the adrenal glands. *Adren/o/megaly* is an _____ of the _____ glands. Use **adrenal/o** to form a word that means *excision of an adrenal gland.* _____ / _____

kidneys	**9–50** Each adrenal gland is structurally and functionally differentiated into two sections: the outer adrenal cortex, which comprises the bulk of the gland, and the inner portion, the adrenal medulla. The hormones produced by each part have different functions. The adrenal glands are perched atop the _____.

table 9-3 PARATHYROID HORMONE

This table identifies parathyroid hormone along with its target organs and functions and associated disorders.

Hormone	Target Organ and Functions	Disorder
Parathyroid hormone (PTH)	• Bones—increases reabsorption of calcium and phosphate from bone to blood • Kidneys—increases calcium absorption and phosphate excretion • Small intestine—increases absorption of calcium and phosphate	• Hyposecretion causes tetany • Hypersecretion causes osteitis fibrosa cystica

9–51 Table 9–4 outlines adrenal hormones, along with their target organs and functions and selected associated disorders. Review the table to learn about hormones and their effects on target organs.

9–52 To complete Frames 9–52 through 9–57, refer to Table 9–4 on page 407.

Three hormones produced by the adrenal cortex are _____, _____ and _____.

To check answers, refer to Table 9–4 on page 407.

9–53 Identify two hormone(s) produced by the adrenal cortex that maintain(s) secondary sex characteristics.

_____ and _____

9–54 Epinephrine helps the body to cope with dangerous situations. Nerves transmit the message of fear to the glands, which react by rushing adrenaline to all parts of the system. Epinephrine is also called _____.

9–55 When a person is experiencing a stressful situation, the adrenal medulla produces adrenaline, which is also called _____.

9–56 Hormones produced by the adrenal medulla that increase blood pressure are _____ and _____.

9–57 The main glucocorticoid hormone secreted by the adrenal cortex is _____.

Pancreas (Islets of Langerhans)

9–58 The (5) **pancreas** is located posterior to the stomach. Hormone-producing cells of the pancreas are called *islets of Langerhans.* The islets produce two distinct hormones: alpha cells, which produce *glucagons,* and beta cells, which produce *insulin.* Both hormones play an important role in the proper metabolism of sugars and starches in the body. Label the pancreas in Figure 9–3.

table 9-4 ADRENAL HORMONES

This table identifies adrenal hormones, their target organs and functions, and associated disorders.

Hormone	Target Organ and Functions	Disorders
Adrenal Cortex Hormones		
Glucocorticoids (mainly cortisol)	• Body cells—promote gluconeogenesis; regulate metabolism of carbohydrates, proteins, and fats; and help depress inflammatory and immune responses	• Hyposecretion causes Addison disease. • Hypersecretion causes Cushing syndrome. (See Figure 9–6.)
Mineralocorticoids (mainly aldosterone)	• Kidneys—increase blood levels of sodium and decrease blood levels of potassium in the kidneys	• Hyposecretion causes Addison disease. • Hypersecretion causes aldosteronism.
Sex hormones (any of the androgens, estrogens, or related steroid hormones) produced by the ovaries, testes, and adrenal cortices	• In females, possibly responsible for female libido and source of estrogen after menopause (Otherwise, effects in adults are insignificant.)	• Hypersecretion of adrenal androgen in females leads to virilism (development of male characteristics). • Hypersecretion of adrenal estrogen and progestin secretion in males leads to feminization (development of feminine characteristics). • Hyposecretion has no known significant effects.
Adrenal Medullary Hormones		
Epinephrine (adrenaline) and norepinephrine	• Sympathetic nervous system target organs—hormone effects mimic sympathetic nervous system activation (sympathomimetic), increase metabolic rate and heart rate, and raise blood pressure by promoting vasoconstriction	• Hyposecretion has no known significant effects. • Hypersecretion causes prolonged "fight-or-flight" reaction and hypertension.

---

pancreat/oma
păn-krē-ă-TŌ-mă
pancreat/o/lith
păn-krē-ĂT-ō-lĭth
pancreat/o/lith/iasis
păn-krē-ă-tō-lĭ-THĪ-ă-sĭs
pancreat/o/pathy
păn-krē-ă-TŎP-ă-thē

9–59 Use *pancreat/o* (pancreas) to build medical words that mean

tumor of the pancreas: _____ / _____

calculus or stone in the pancreas: _____ / _____ / _____

abnormal condition of a pancreatic stone:
_____ / _____ / _____ / _____

disease of the pancreas: _____ / _____ / _____

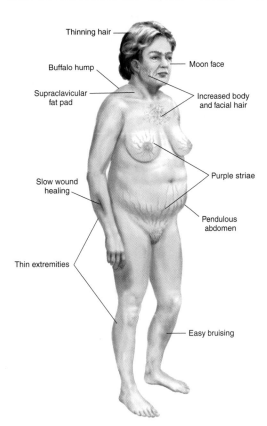

Thinning hair

Buffalo hump

Supraclavicular fat pad

Slow wound healing

Thin extremities

Moon face

Increased body and facial hair

Purple striae

Pendulous abdomen

Easy bruising

Figure 9-6 Physical manifestations seen in Cushing syndrome.

pancreas PĂN-krē-ăs	**9–60** The suffix *-lysis* is used in words to mean *separation, destruction, loosening.* Pancreat/o/lysis is a destruction of the _____.
To check answers, refer to Table 9–5 on page 411.	**9–61** Refer to Table 9–5 on page 411 to complete Frames 9–61 through 9–62. Two hormones produced by the pancreas are _____ and _____.
	9–62 Determine the pancreat/ic hormone that *lowers blood glucose:* _____ *increases blood glucose:* _____
To check answers, refer to Table 9–5 on page 411.	**9–63** Refer to Table 9–5 on page 411 to complete this frame. How does insulin lower blood glucose? _____ _____ _____

glyc/o/gen GLĪ-kō-jĕn	**9-64** Gluc/ose is the chief source of energy for living organisms. *Gluc/o* and *glyc/o* are CFs that mean *sugar, sweetness.* The suffixes *-gen* and *-genesis* mean *forming, producing, origin.* Combine **glyc/o** and *-gen* to form a word that means *forming or producing sugar.* _____ / _____ / _____
gluc/o/genesis gloo-kō-JĔN-ĕ-sĭs **glyc/o/genesis** glī-kō-JĔN-ĕ-sĭs	**9-65** Use *-genesis* to build words that mean *forming, producing, or origin of sugar.* _____ / _____ / _____ _____ / _____ / _____
gluc/o/meter gloo-KŎM-tĕr	**9-66** A gluc/o/meter is used to calculate blood glucose from one drop of blood. An instrument used by patients with diabetes to monitor their blood glucose levels is known as a _____ / _____ / _____ .
-emia **hyper-** **hypo-** **glyc**	**9-67** Hyper/glyc/emia is an excessive amount of glucose or sugar in the blood. Deficiency of glucose (sugar) in the blood is hypo/glyc/emia. Identify the elements in this frame that mean *blood condition:* _____ *excessive, above normal:* _____ *under, below, deficient:* _____ *sugar, sweetness:* _____
hypo/glyc/emia hī-pō-glī-SĒ-mē-ă **intravenous**	**9-68** A less than normal amount of gluc/ose in the blood, usually caused by excessive secretion of insulin by the pancreas, administration of too much insulin, or dietary deficiency, is called hypo/glyc/emia. Treatment is administration of gluc/ose by mouth if the person is conscious or an IV solution if the person is unconscious. Deficiency of blood glucose is called _____ / _____ / _____ The abbreviation *IV* means _____ .
-gen, -genesis	**9-69** In the terms glyc/o/gen and glyc/o/genesis, write the elements that mean *forming, producing, origin.* _____ , _____

insulin
ĬN-sū-lĭn

9–70 Insulin, an essential hormone for conversion of sugar, starches, and other food into energy, is required for normal daily living. Diabetes commonly results in hyper/glyc/emia. It occurs if the pancreas does not produce sufficient amounts of insulin or if the cells of the body become resistant to insulin and do not utilize insulin properly.

If hyper/glyc/emia occurs, the diabetic person can reduce the amount of gluc/ose in the blood by injecting himself or herself with the hormone called _____.

---

hyper/glyc/emia
hī-pĕr-glī-SĒ-mē-ă

hypo/glyc/emia
hī-pō-glī-SĒ-mē-ă

9–71 *Diabetes* is a general term that, when used alone, refers to *diabetes mellitus* (DM), a disease that occurs in two primary forms: *type 1 diabetes* and *type 2 diabetes*. When insulin is lacking, glucose does not enter cells but returns to the bloodstream with a subsequent rise in its concentration in the blood, a condition known as *hyper/glyc/emia*. Low blood glucose levels cause the opposite condition (*hypo/glyc/emia*).

Identify the terms in this frame that mean

excessive gluc/ose in the blood: _____ / _____ / _____

low or insufficient gluc/ose in the blood:

_____ / _____ / _____

---

hypo/glyc/emia
hī-pō-glī-SĒ-mē-ă

9–72 Diabetic patients whose bodies use excessive insulin have abnormally low glucose levels. The medical term for this condition is

_____ / _____ / _____.

---

hypo/glyc/emia
hī-pō-glī-SĒ-mē-ă

9–73 Hyper/glyc/emia can cause numerous complications, such as impairing wound healing, decreasing the body's ability to fight infection, and causing damage to the kidneys.

The opposite of *hyper/glyc/emia* is _____ / _____ / _____.

---

poly/dipsia
pŏl-ē-DĬP-sē-ă

poly/uria
pŏl-ē-Ū-rē-ă

poly/phagia
pŏl-ē-FĀ-jē-ă

9–74 The suffix *-dipsia* denotes a condition of thirst. Poly/dipsia, poly/uria, and poly/phagia are three cardinal signs of diabetes mellitus. Write the words in this frame that mean

excessive thirst: _____ / _____

excessive urination: _____ / _____

excessive eating: _____ / _____

---

poly/uria
pŏl-ē-Ū-rē-ă

9–75 When a person drinks too much water, he or she may experience a condition of excessive urine production (urination). The medical term for this condition is _____ / _____.

table 9-5	PANCREATIC HORMONES	

This table identifies pancreatic hormones, their target organs, functions, and associated disorders.

Hormone	Target Organ and Functions	Disorders
Glucagon	• Liver and blood—increases blood glucose level by accelerating conversion of glycogen into glucose in liver (glycogenolysis) and conversion of other nutrients into glucose in the liver (gluconeogenesis) and releasing glucose into blood; converts glycogen to glucose	• Persistently low blood sugar levels (hypoglycemia) may be caused by deficiency in glucagon.
Insulin	• Tissue cells—lowers blood glucose level by accelerating glucose transport into cells; converts glucose to glycogen	• Hyposecretion of insulin causes diabetes mellitus. • Hypersecretion of insulin causes hyperinsulinism.

Pineal and Thymus Glands

9–76 The (6) **pineal gland** and (7) **thymus gland** are classified as endocrine glands, but little is known about their endocrine function. Label these structures in Figure 9–3.

9–77 The CF *thym/o* means thymus gland. Build medical words that mean

thym/ectomy
thī-MĔK-tō-mē

excision of the thymus gland: _____ / _____

thym/oma
thī-MŌ-mă

tumor of the thymus gland: _____ / _____

thym/o/pathy
thī-MŎP-ă-thē

disease of the thymus gland: _____ / ____ / _____

thym/o/lysis
thī-MŎL-ĭ-sĭs

destruction of the thymus gland: _____ / ____ / _____

Ovaries and Testes

9–78 The (8) **ovaries** are a pair of small, almond-shaped glands positioned in the upper pelvic cavity, one on each side of the uterus. The (9) **testes** are paired oval glands surrounded by the scrotal sac. The functions of the ovaries and testes are covered in Chapter 8. Label the ovaries and testes in Figure 9–3.

oophor/o, ovari/o **orchid/o, orchi/o,** **orch/o, test/o**	**9–79** Recall the CFs for *ovaries:* _____ / _____ or _____ / _____ *testes:* _____ / _____ , _____ / _____ , _____ / _____ , or _____ / _____
oophor/o/pathy ō-ŏf-or-ŎP-ă-thē **oophor/o/tomy** ō-ŏf-or-ŎT-ō-mē	**9–80** Use *oophor/o* to construct medical words that mean *disease of an ovary:* _____ / _____ / _____ *incision of an ovary:* _____ / _____ / _____
orchid/o/pexy OR-kĭd-ō-pĕk-sē	**9–81** Use **orchid/o** to form a word that means *surgical fixation of a testis.* _____ / _____ / _____

Competency Verification: Check your labeling of Figure 9–3 in Appendix B, Answer Key, page 574.

SECTION REVIEW 9-3

Using the following table, write the CF, suffix, or prefix that matches its definition in the space provided to the left of the definition. There may be more than one word element that matches a definition.

Combining Forms		Suffixes		Prefixes
adrenal/o	orchid/o	-dipsia	-pathy	hypo-
adren/o	pancreat/o	-gen	-pexy	para-
gluc/o	thym/o	-genesis	-phagia	poly-
glyc/o	toxic/o	-iasis	-rrhea	supra-
orch/o		-lith	-uria	
orchi/o		-lysis		

1. _____ abnormal condition (produced by something specified)
2. _____ above; excessive; superior
3. _____ adrenal glands
4. _____ disease
5. _____ fixation (of an organ)
6. _____ discharge, flow
7. _____ many, much
8. _____ near, beside; beyond
9. _____ pancreas
10. _____ forming, producing, origin
11. _____ separation; destruction; loosening
12. _____ stone, calculus
13. _____ sugar, sweetness
14. _____ swallowing, eating
15. _____ testis (plural, testes)
16. _____ thirst
17. _____ thymus gland
18. _____ under, below, deficient
19. _____ urine
20. _____ poison

Competency Verification: Check your answers in Appendix B, Answer Key, page 574. If you are not satisfied with your level of comprehension, go back to Frame 9–40 and rework the frames.

Correct Answers _____ × 5 = _____ % Score

Nervous System

The nervous system is an extensive, intricate network of structures that activates, coordinates, and controls the functions of all other body systems. It can be grouped into two main divisions: the central nervous system (CNS) and the peripheral nervous system (PNS). The CNS consists of the brain and spinal cord and is the control center of the body. The PNS consists of the peripheral nerves, which include the cranial nerves (emerging from the base of the skull) and the spinal nerves (emerging from the spinal cord). The PNS connects the CNS to remote body parts to relay and receive messages, and its autonomic nerves regulate involuntary functions of the internal organs.

Despite the complex organization of the nervous system, it consists of only two principal types of cells, *neurons* and *neuroglia*. *Neurons* are the basic structural and functional units of the nervous system. (See Figure 9–7.) They are specialized to respond to physical and chemical stimuli, conduct electrochemical impulses, and release specific chemical regulators. Through these activities, neurons perform such functions as the perception of sensory stimuli, learning, memory, and control of muscles and glands. *Neuroglia* do not carry impulses, but perform the functions of support and protection. Many neuroglial, or *glial*, cells form a supporting network by twining around nerve cells or lining certain structures in the brain and spinal cord. Others bind nervous tissue to supporting structures and attach the neurons to their blood vessels. Certain small glial cells are phagocytic. In other words, they protect the CNS from disease by engulfing invading microbes and clearing away debris. *Neuroglia* are of clinical interest because they are a common source of tumors (gliomas) of the nervous system.

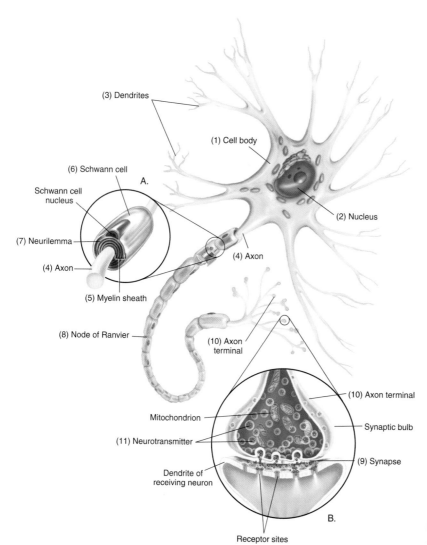

Figure 9-7   Neuron. (A) Schwann cell. (B) Axon terminal synapse.

WORD ELEMENTS

This section introduces CFs related to the nervous system. Included are key suffixes; prefixes are defined in the right-hand column as needed. Review the following table and pronounce each word in the word analysis column aloud before you begin to work the frames.

Word Element	Meaning	Word Analysis
Combining Forms		
cerebr/o	cerebrum	**cerebr/o**/spin/al (sĕr-ĕ-brō-SPĪ-năl): pertaining to the brain and spinal cord *spin:* spine *-al:* pertaining to
encephal/o	brain	**encephal**/itis (ĕn-sĕf-ă-LĪ-tĭs): inflammation of the brain (tissue) *-itis:* inflammation
gli/o	glue; neuroglial tissue	**gli**/oma (glī-Ō-mă): tumor composed of neuroglia tissue (supportive tissue of nervous system) *-oma:* tumor
mening/o	meninges (membranes covering brain and spinal cord)	**mening**/o/cele (mĕn-ĬN-gō-sēl): saclike protrusion of the meninges through the skull or vertebral column *-cele:* hernia, swelling *Meningocele is a congenital defect (occurs at birth) and can be repaired by surgery.*
meningi/o		**meningi**/oma (mĕn-ĭn-jē-Ō-mă): tumor composed of meninges *-oma:* tumor
myel/o	bone marrow; spinal cord	**myel**/algia (mī-ĕl-ĂL-jē-ă): pain of the spinal cord or its membranes *-algia:* pain
neur/o	nerve	**neur**/o/lysis (nū-RŎL-ĭs-ĭs): destruction of a nerve *-lysis:* separation; destruction; loosening
Suffixes		
-paresis	partial paralysis	hemi/**paresis** (hĕm-ē-păr-Ē-sĭs): paralysis of one half of the body (right half or left half) *hemi-:* one half
-phasia	speech	a/**phasia** (ă-FĀ-zē-ă): absence of speech *a-:* without, not *Aphasia is an abnormal neurologic condition in which language function is defective or absent because of an injury to certain areas of the cerebral cortex.*

(continued)

Word Element	Meaning	Word Analysis
-plegia	paralysis	quadri/**plegia** (kwŏd-rĭ-PLĒ-jē-ă): paralysis of all four extremities *quadri-:* four

Pronunciation Help	Long Sound Short Sound	ā in rāte ă in ălone	ē in rēbirth ĕ in ĕver	ī in īsle ĭ in ĭt	ō in ōver ŏ in nŏt	ū in ūnite ŭ in cŭt

 Listen and Learn, the audio CD-ROM included in this book, will help you master pronunciation of selected medical words. Use it to practice pronunciations of the above-listed medical terms and for instructions to complete the *Listen and Learn* exercise for this section.

SECTION REVIEW 9-4

For the following medical terms, first write the suffix and its meaning. Then translate the meaning of the remaining elements starting with the first part of the word. The first word is completed for you.

Term	Meaning
1. meningi/oma	*-oma: tumor; meninges*
2. neur/o/lysis	
3. hemi/paresis	
4. myel/algia	
5. cerebr/o/spin/al	
6. a/phasia	
7. mening/o/cele	
8. encephal/itis	
9. gli/oma	
10. quadri/plegia	

Competency Verification: Check your answers in Appendix B, Answer Key, page 575. If you are not satisfied with your level of comprehension, review the vocabulary and retake the review.

Correct Answers _____ × 10 = _____ % Score

Spinal Cord

The spinal cord is a long, narrow cable of nerve tissue within the spinal canal and is part of the CNS. It descends from the brain stem to the lumbar part of the back and contains about 100 million neurons. A slightly flattened cylinder, it is about as wide as a finger for most of its length, tapering to a threadlike tail. Thirty-one pairs of spinal nerves originate from the spinal cord. (See Figure 9–8.) Each pair of nerves serves a specific region on the right or left side of the body. The spinal nerves are mixed nerves that provide a two-way communication between the spinal cord and parts of the upper and lower limbs, neck, and trunk.

9–82 Spin/al nerves are named according to locations of their respective vertebrae. In Figure 9–8, there are 8 pairs of cervic/al nerves, identified as *C1–C8;* 12 pairs of thorac/ic nerves, identified as *T1–T12;* 5 pairs of lumb/ar nerves, identified as *L1–L5;* 5 pairs of sacr/al nerves, identified as *S1–S5;* and 1 pair of coccyg/eal nerves, identified as *Co1.*

Label the following nerves in Figure 9–8: (1) **cervical nerves**; (2) **thoracic nerves**; (3) **lumbar nerves**; (4) **sacral nerves**; and the (5) **coccygeal nerve**.

cervic/al nerves
SĔR-vĭ-kăl

thorac/ic nerves
thō-RĂS-ĭk

sacr/al nerves
SĀ-krăl

9–83 Build medical words that mean *pertaining to nerves*

of the neck: _____ / _____ _____

in back of the chest: _____ / _____ _____

of the sacrum: _____ / _____ _____

---

spin/al
SPĪ-năl

cerebr/o/spin/al
sĕr-ē-brō-SPĪ-năl

9–84 The spin/al cord, like the brain, is protected and nourished by the meninges, which consist of three layers: dura mater, the outermost membrane; arachnoid membrane, the second layer which surrounds the brain and spin/al cord; and pia mater, the third layer closest to the brain and spinal cord. Additional protection is provided by cerebr/o/spin/al fluid circulating in the subarachnoid space. (See Figure 9–8.)
Identify terms in this frame that mean *pertaining to*

the spine: _____ / _____

the cerebrum and the spine: _____ / ____ / _____ / _____

---

mening/itis
mĕn-ĭn-JĪ-tĭs

mening/o/cele
mĕn-ĬN-gō-sēl

meningi/oma
mĕn-ĭn-jē-Ō-mă

9–85 *Mening/o* and **meningi/o** both mean *meninges (membranes covering the brain and spinal cord).*
Use **mening/o** to construct a word that means *inflammation of the meninges.*
_____ / _____

Use **mening/o** to build a word that means *hernia or swelling of the meninges.*
_____ / ____ / _____

Use **meningi/o** to construct a word that means *tumor of the meninges.*
_____ / _____

---

mening/o/cele
mĕn-ĬN-gō-sēl

9–86 The outer layer of the spinal cord, the *dura mater,* is a tough, fibrous membrane that covers the entire length of the spinal cord and contains channels for blood to enter brain tissue. The middle layer, the *arachnoid,* runs across the space known as the *sub/dur/al space,* which contains cerebr/o/spin/al fluid. The innermost layer, the *pia mater,* is a thin membrane containing many blood vessels that nourish the spinal cord. Herniation of the meninges may occur through a defect in the skull or spinal cord. When herniation of the meninges occurs, the condition is called
_____ / ____ / _____.

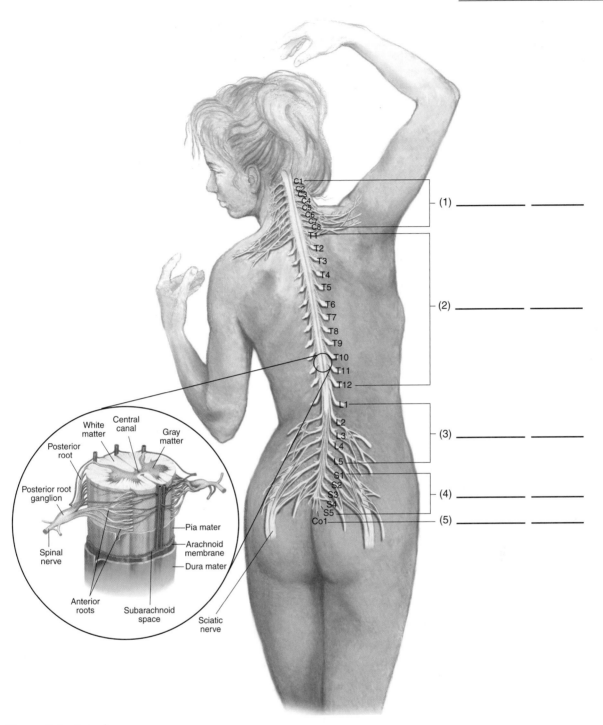

Figure 9-8 Spinal nerves.

The following labels appear in the figure:

C1, C2, C3, C4, C5, C6, C7, C8
T1, T2, T3, T4, T5, T6, T7, T8, T9, T10, T11, T12
L1, L2, L3, L4, L5
S1, S2, S3, S4, S5
Co1

(1) _____ _____
(2) _____ _____
(3) _____ _____
(4) _____ _____
(5) _____ _____

Enlarged inset labels:

White matter
Central canal
Gray matter
Posterior root
Posterior root ganglion
Spinal nerve
Anterior roots
Subarachnoid space
Pia mater
Arachnoid membrane
Dura mater
Sciatic nerve

epi-

dur

-al

9-87 The space between the *pia mater* and the bones of the spinal cord is called the *epi/dur/al space* and contains blood vessels and some fat. It is the space into which anesthetics may be injected to dull pain or contrast material may be injected for certain diagnostic procedures.
Identify the elements in this frame that mean

above, upon: _____

dura mater; hard: _____

pertaining to: _____

---

cerebr/o/spin/al
sĕr-ē-brō-SPĪ-năl

9-88 The fluid circulating in the subarachnoid space that protects the brain and spinal cord is known as

_____ / _____ / _____ / _____ fluid.

---

myel/itis
mī-ĕ-LĪ-tĭs

myel/o/pathy
mī-ĕ-LŎP-ă-thē

myel/o/tome
mī-ĔL-ō-tōm

9-89 The CF *myel/o* means *bone marrow; spinal cord.* Build medical words that mean

inflammation of the spinal cord: _____ / _____

any disease of the spinal cord: _____ / _____ / _____

instrument to cut or dissect the spinal cord: _____ / _____ / _____

---

spin/o

myel/o

neur/o

encephal/o

9-90 As discussed earlier, the nervous system consists of the brain, spin/al cord, and peripheral nerves. Together with the endo/crine system, the nervous system coordinates and controls many body activities.
Identify the CFs related to the nervous system that mean

pertaining to the spine: _____ / _____

bone marrow, spinal cord: _____ / _____

nerve: _____ / _____

brain: _____ / _____

---

encephal/itis
ĕn-sĕf-ă-LĪ-tĭs

encephal/oma
ĕn-sĕf-ă-LŌ-mă

9-91 *Encephal/itis,* an inflammatory condition of the brain, is usually caused by a viral infection transmitted by the bite of an infected mosquito. It may also be the result of lead or other poisoning.
Use *encephal/o* to build words that mean

inflammation of the brain: _____ / _____

tumor of the brain: _____ / _____

Competency Verification: Check your labeling of Figure 9-8 in Appendix B, Answer Key, page 575.

9-92 Each spin/al nerve has two roots, which are neurons entering or leaving the spinal cord. The dors/al root is made of sensory neurons that carry impulses into the spinal cord. The ventr/al root is the motor root. It is made of motor neurons carrying impulses from the spin/al cord to muscles or glands. The cell bodies of these motor neurons are in the gray matter of the spin/al cord. When the two nerve roots merge, the spin/al nerve thus formed is a mixed nerve.

Provide the meaning for the following CFs

back (of body)

dors/o: _____ (_____ _____)

nerve

neur/o: _____

belly, belly side

ventr/o: _____, _____ _____

9-93 Use *neur/o* to form medical terms that mean

neur/algia
nū-RĂL-jē-ă

pain in a nerve: _____ / _____

neur/itis
nū-RĪ-tĭs

inflammation of a nerve: _____ / _____

neur/oma
nū-RŌ-mă

tumor of nerve (tissue): _____ / _____

neur/o/pathy
nū-RŎP-ă-thē

any disease of nerves: _____ / _____ / _____

9-94 Use *myel/o* to form medical words that mean

myel/itis
mī-ĕ-LĪ-tĭs

inflammation of spinal cord: _____ / _____

myel/o/malacia
mī-ĕ-lō-mă-LĀ-shē-ă

softening of spinal cord: _____ / _____ / _____

myel/oma
mī-ĕ-LŌ-mă

tumor of bone marrow: _____ / _____

---

cell

thromb/o/cyte
THRŎM-bō-sīt

9-95 The CF *thromb/o* refers to a *blood clot*. A *thromb/o/cyte* is a blood-clotting _____.

A thromb/o/cyte (platelet) promotes the formation of clots and prevents bleeding. Another name for *platelet* is _____ / _____ / _____.

---

clot

9-96 Although the terms *embolus* and *thrombus* denote a disorder related to a clot, they both have different meanings. An **embolus** is a clot present in blood or lymphatic vessels and brought there by blood or lymph. A **thrombus** is a clot that adheres to the wall of a blood vessel or organ and may obstruct the vessel or organ in which it resides, preventing the flow of blood.

The term *thromb/o/lysis* refers to the destruction or loosening of a blood _____.

thromb/o/genesis thrŏm-bō-JĔN-ĕ-sĭs	**9-97** Use *-genesis* to form a word that means *producing, forming, or origin of a blood clot.* _____ / _____ / _____

hem/o/rrhage HĔM-ĕ-rĭj **cerebr/o/vascul/ar** sĕr-ĕ-brō-VĂS-kū-lăr **thrombus** THRŎM-bŭs	**9-98** Stroke, formerly called *cerebr/o/vascul/ar accident* (CVA), is a disruption of normal blood supply (ischemia) to the brain. It is characterized by occlusion from an embolus, thrombus, or hem/o/rrhage. The resulting neur/o/logic/al symptoms vary according to the site and degree of occlusion. Write the terms in this frame that mean *bursting forth (of) blood:* _____ / _____ / _____ *pertaining to the cerebrum and blood vessels:* _____ / _____ / _____ / _____ *stationary blood clot:* _____

aneurysm/ectomy ăn-ū-rĭz-MĔK-tō-mē	**9-99** Stroke caused by hem/o/rrhage from a cerebral artery is commonly fatal. This condition usually results from high blood pressure, atherosclerosis, or the bursting of an arterial aneurysm (localized dilation of the blood vessel wall). The CF **aneurysm/o** means *a widening or a widened blood vessel.* Use **aneurysm/o** to construct a medical word that means *excision of an aneurysm.* _____ / _____

cerebr/o/scler/osis sĕr-ĕ-brō-sklĕ-RŌ-sĭs	**9-100** Combine **cerebr/o** + **scler** + *-osis* to form a word that means *an abnormal condition of hardening of the cerebrum.* _____ / _____ / _____ / _____

cerebr/oid SĔR-ĕ-broyd	**9-101** Construct a medical term that means *resembling the cerebrum.* _____ / _____

-rrhagia, -rrhage	**9-102** Hem/o/rrhage occurs when there is a loss of large amounts of blood in a short period. Hem/o/rrhage may be arterial, venous, or capillary. The two suffixes that mean *bursting forth (of)* are _____ and _____ .

neur/o/glia nū-RŎG-lē-ă	**9-103** As discussed earlier, the entire nervous system is composed of two principal types of cells, *neurons* and *neuroglia.* The supporting cells in the CNS collectively are called neur/o/glia. A term that literally means *nerve glue* is _____ / _____ / _____ .

inflammation, nerves	**9-104** *Neur/itis* is an _____ of _____.
neur/algia nū-RĂL-jē-ă	**9-105** Another term in addition to *neur/o/dynia* that means *pain in a nerve* is _____ / _____.
inflammation, nerves	**9-106** *Neur/o/myel/itis* is an _____ of _____ and spinal cord.
neur/o/cyte NŪ-rō-sīt	**9-107** A *neur/o/cyte*, commonly called a *neuron*, is a nerve cell. A term that literally means *nerve cell* is _____ / _____ / _____.
carcin/o/phobia KĂR-sĭn-ō-fō-bē-ă	**9-108** The CF **neur/o** (nerve) is also used to form words that refer to mental disorders. For example, *neur/osis* is an emotional disorder that involves an ineffective way of coping with anxiety or inner conflict. *Neur/oses* are often named by combing the suffix *-phobia* (fear) with a root or prefix identifying the object feared, such as *hem/o/phobia* (fear of blood) and *necr/o/phobia* (fear of death or dead things). Whenever you see *-phobia* in a term, you will know it refers to "fear." Build a word that means *fear* of cancer: _____/____/_____
necr/o/phobia nĕk-rō-FŌ-bē-ă	**9-109** A person who has a fear of corpses or death suffers from the phobia known as _____/_____.
erot/o/mania ĕ-rŏt-ō-MĀ-nē-ă	**9-110** Another CF, **psych/o** (mind), is used to form words about a mental condition that represents a marked distortion of or sharp break from reality and is a serious personality disorder. Some psychoses are indicated by the suffix *–mania* (state of mental disorder, frenzy). Examples are *klept/o/mania* (urge to steal items you don't need and that usually have little value) and *pyr/o/mania* (craze for starting fires). Combine **erot/o** (sexual desire) + mania (state of mental disorder, frenzy) to form a word meaning *abnormally powerful sex drive*. _____/____/_____
psych/oses sī-KŌ-sēs	**9-111** Other types of psychoses include *schiz/o/phrenia* and paranoia. *Schiz/o/phrenia* is a *psych/osis* that involves delusions, such as believing that someone or something is controlling your thoughts. Another of its manifestations is hallucinations, most often "hearing" voices or other sounds. Paranoia is also a *psych/osis* but it is a type of personality disorder. It is characterized by unreasonable suspicion or jealousy, along with a tendency to interpret everything others do as hostile. *Schiz/o/phrenia* and *psych/osis* are two types of mental disorders known as _____/_____ (plural)

Pronunciation Help	**Long Sound** **Short Sound**	ā in rāte ă in ălone	ē in rēbirth ĕ in ĕver	ī in īsle ĭ in ĭt	ō in ōver ŏ in nŏt	ū in ūnite ŭ in cŭt

SECTION REVIEW 9-5

Using the following table, write the CF, suffix, or prefix that matches its definition in the space provided to the left of the definition. There may be more than one word element that matches a definition.

Combining Forms		Suffixes		Prefixes
cerebr/o	myel/o	-glia	-rrhagia	a-
encephal/o	neur/o	-malacia		dys-
gli/o	scler/o	-osis		
mening/o	thromb/o	-phasia		
meningi/o	vascul/o	-rrhage		

1. _____ abnormal condition; increase (used primarily with blood cells)
2. _____ bad; painful; difficult
3. _____ blood clot
4. _____ vessel
5. _____ brain
6. _____ bursting forth (of)
7. _____ glue; neuroglial tissue
8. _____ hardening; sclera (white of eye)
9. _____ meninges (membranes covering brain and spinal cord)
10. _____ nerve
11. _____ cerebrum
12. _____ softening
13. _____ speech
14. _____ bone marrow; spinal cord
15. _____ without, not

Competency Verification: Check your answers in Appendix B, Answer Key, page 575. If you are not satisfied with your level of comprehension, go back to Frame 9–82 and rework the frames.

Correct Answers _____ × 6.67 = _____ % Score

Abbreviations

This section introduces endocrine and nervous systems-related abbreviations and their meanings. Included are abbreviations contained in the medical record activities that follow.

Abbreviation	Meaning	Abbreviation	Meaning
Endocrine System			
ADH	antidiuretic hormone	**ICSH**	interstitial cell-stimulating hormone
BG	blood glucose	**LH**	luteinizing hormone
BS	blood sugar	**PGH**	pituitary growth hormone
DM	diabetes mellitus	**PTH**	parathyroid hormone
GH	growth hormone	**RAIU**	radioactive iodine uptake
HRT	hormone replacement therapy	**TSH**	thyroid-stimulating hormone
Nervous System			
C1, C2, and so on	first cervical vertebra, second cervical vertebra, and so on	**L1, L2, and so on**	first lumbar vertebra, second lumbar vertebra, and so on
CNS	central nervous system	**LP**	lumbar puncture
CO	cardiac output	**MS**	mitral stenosis; musculoskeletal; multiple sclerosis; mental status; magnesium sulfate
CSF	cerebrospinal fluid	**RBC, rbc**	red blood cell
CVA	cerebrovascular accident; costovertebral angle	**S1, S2**	first sacral vertebra, second sacral vertebra, and so on
CVD	cerebrovascular disease	**T1–T12**	first thoracic vertebra, second thoracic vertebra, and so on
EEG	electroencephalogram	**TIA**	transient ischemic attack
EMG	electromyography	**WBC, wbc**	white blood cell
Radiographic Procedures			
AP	anteroposterior	**CT**	computed tomography
PA	posteroanterior	**PET**	positron emission tomography
IV	intravenously	**MRI**	magnetic resonance imaging

Additional Medical Terms

The following are additional terms related to the endocrine and nervous systems. Recognizing and learning these terms will help you understand the connection between a pathological condition, its diagnosis, and the rationale behind the method of treatment selected for a particular disorder.

Signs, Symptoms, and Diseases

Endocrine System

Addison disease Ă-dĭ-sŭn	Relatively uncommon chronic disorder caused by deficiency of cortical hormones that results when the adrenal cortex is damaged or atrophied *Atrophy of adrenal glands is usually the result of an autoimmune process in which circulating adrenal antibodies slowly destroy the gland.*
Cushing syndrome KOOSH-ing	Cluster of symptoms caused by excessive amounts of cortisol or adrenocorticotropic hormone (ACTH) circulating in the blood *Most cases of Cushing syndrome are caused by administration of glucocorticoids in the treatment of immune disorders, such as asthma, rheumatoid arthritis, and lupus erythematosus.*
diabetes mellitus (DM) dī-ă-BĒ-tēz MĔ-lĭ-tŭs	Chronic metabolic disorder of impaired carbohydrate, protein, and fat metabolism due to insufficient production of insulin or the body's inability to utilize insulin properly *When used alone, the term* diabetes *refers to* diabetes mellitus. *Hyperglycemia and ketosis are responsible for its host of troubling and commonly life-threatening symptoms. Diabetes mellitus occurs in two primary forms:* type 1 diabetes *and* type 2 diabetes.
type 1 diabetes	Form of diabetes mellitus that is abrupt in onset and is due to the failure of the pancreas to produce insulin, making this type of disease difficult to regulate *Type 1 diabetes is usually diagnosed in children and young adults. Treatment includes insulin injections to maintain a normal level of glucose in the blood.*
type 2 diabetes	Form of diabetes mellitus that is gradual in onset and results from the body's deficiency in producing enough insulin or resistance to the action of insulin by the body's cells *Type 2 is the most common form of diabetes. It is usually diagnosed in adults older than age 40. Management of this disease is less problematic than that of type 1. Treatment includes diet, weight loss, and exercise. It may also include insulin or oral antidiabetic agents, which activate the release of pancreatic insulin and improve the body's sensitivity to insulin.*
exophthalmos ĕks-ŏf-THĂL-mŏs	Abnormal protrusion of the eyeball(s), possibly due to thyrotoxicosis, tumor of the orbit, orbital cellulitis, leukemia, or aneurysm

Graves disease GRĀVZ	Multisystem autoimmune disorder that involves growth of the thyroid (hyperthyroidism) associated with hypersecretion of thyroxine; also called *exophthalmic goiter, thyrotoxicosis,* or *toxic goiter* *Graves disease is characterized by an enlarged thyroid gland and exophthalmos (bulging of the eyes), which develops because of edema in the tissues of the eye sockets and swelling of the extrinsic eye muscles.*

insulinoma
ĭn-sū-lĭn-Ō-mă
  insulin: insulin
  -oma: tumor
	Tumor of the islets of Langerhans; also called a *pancreatic tumor*

myxedema
mĭks-ě-DĒ-mă
  myx: mucus
  -edema: swelling
	Advanced hypothyroidism in adults that results from hypofunction of the thyroid gland and affects body fluids, causing edema. This condition also increases blood volume and blood pressure

obesity ō-BĒ-sĭ-tē	Excessive accumulation of fat that exceeds the body's skeletal and physical standards, usually an increase of 20% or more above ideal body weight *Obesity may be due to excessive intake of food (exogenous) or metabolic or endocrine abnormalities (endogenous).*
morbid obesity	Body mass index (BMI) of 40 or greater, which is generally 100 lb or more over ideal body weight *Morbid obesity is a disease with serious psychological, social, and medical ramifications and one that threatens necessary body functions such as respiration.*

panhypopituitarism
păn-hī-pō-pĭ-TŪ-ĭ-tăr-ĭzm
  pan-: all
  hyp/o: under, below, deficient
  pituitar: pituitary gland
  -ism: condition
	Total pituitary impairment that brings about a progressive and general loss of hormone activity

pheochromocytoma fē-ō-krō-mō-sī-TŌ-mă	Small chromaffin cell tumor, usually located in the adrenal medulla

pituitarism
pĭ-TŪ-ĭ-tăr-ĭzm
  pituitar: pituitary gland
  -ism: condition
	Any disorder of the pituitary gland and its function

Nervous System

Alzheimer disease ĂLTS-hī-mĕr	Chronic, organic mental disorder that is a progressive form of presenile dementia caused by atrophy of the frontal and occipital lobes of the brain *The onset of Alzheimer disease is usually between ages 40 and 60. It involves progressive irreversible loss of memory, deterioration of intellectual functions, apathy, speech and gait disturbances, and disorientation. The course may take from a few months to 4 or 5 years to progress to complete loss of intellectual function.*
epilepsy ĔP-ĭ-lĕp-sē	Disorder affecting the central nervous system that is characterized by recurrent seizures
Huntington chorea HŬN-tĭng-tŭn kō-RĒ-ă	Hereditary nervous disorder caused by the progressive loss of brain cells, leading to bizarre, involuntary, dancelike movements

hydrocephalus
hī-drō-SĔF-ă-lŭs
 	
  hydro: water
  cephal: head
    -us: condition, structure
	Cranial enlargement caused by accumulation of fluid within the ventricles of the brain

multiple sclerosis
MŬL-tĭ-pl sklĕ-RŌ-sĭs
 	
  scler: hardening; sclera
    (white of eye)
  -osis: abnormal
    condition; increase
    (used primarily
    with blood cells)
	Progressive degenerative disease of the central nervous system characterized by inflammation, hardening, and loss of myelin throughout the spinal cord and brain, which produces weakness and other muscle symptoms

neuroblastoma
nū-rō-blăs-TŌ-mă
 	
  neur/o: nerve
    blast: embryonic cell
    -oma: tumor
	Malignant tumor composed principally of cells resembling neuroblasts
	Neuroblastoma occurs most commonly in infants and children.

palsy PAWL-zē	Partial or complete loss of motor function; also called *paralysis*
Bell palsy	Facial paralysis on one side of the face because of inflammation of a facial nerve (cranial nerve VII), most likely caused by a viral infection *Bell palsy commonly results in grotesque facial disfigurement and facial spasms. Treatment includes corticosteroid drugs to decrease nerve swelling. Ordinarily, the condition lasts a month and resolves by itself.*

cerebral palsy
  sĕr-ĕ-brăl
 	
  cerebr: cerebrum
    -al: pertaining to
	Bilateral, symmetrical, nonprogressive motor dysfunction and partial paralysis, which is usually caused by damage to the cerebrum during gestation or birth trauma but can also be hereditary

paralysis	Loss of muscle function, loss of sensation, or both
pă-RĂL-ĭ-sĭs	*Paralysis may be caused by a variety of problems, such as trauma, disease, and poisoning. Paralyses may be classified according to the cause, muscle tone, distribution, or body part affected. Common causes of paralysis are spinal cord injuries and strokes. (See Figure 9–9.)*

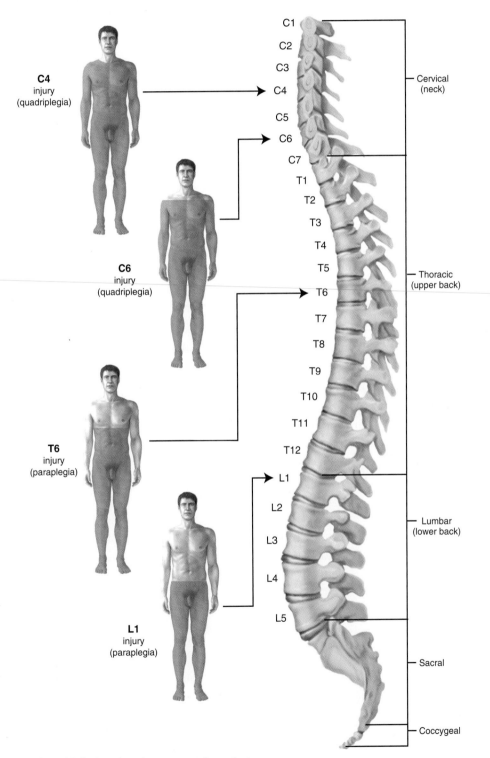

Figure 9-9 Spinal cord injuries showing extent of paralysis.

Parkinson disease PĂR-kĭn-sŭn	Progressive, degenerative neurological disorder affecting the portion of the brain responsible for controlling movement *The unnecessary skeletal muscle movements of Parkinson disease commonly interfere with voluntary movement, causing the hand to shake (called tremor), the most common symptom of Parkinson disease.*
poliomyelitis pō-lē-ō-mī-ĕl-Ī-tĭs *poli/o:* gray; gray matter (of brain or spinal cord) *myel:* bone marrow, spinal cord *-itis:* inflammation	Inflammation of the gray matter of the spinal cord caused by a virus, commonly resulting in spinal and muscle deformity and paralysis
sciatica sī-ĂT-ĭ-kă	Severe pain in the leg along the course of the sciatic nerve, which travels from the hip to the foot (See Figure 9–8.)
seizure SĒ-zhūr	Convulsion or other clinically detectable event caused by a sudden discharge of electrical activity in the brain that may be classified as partial or generalized *Seizure is a characteristic symptom of epilepsy.*
shingles SHĬNG-lz	Eruption of acute, inflammatory, herpetic vesicles caused by herpes zoster virus on the trunk of the body along a peripheral nerve
spina bifida SPĪ-nă BĬF-ĭ-dă	Congenital neural tube defect characterized by incomplete closure of the spinal canal through which the spinal cord and meninges may or may not protrude *Spina bifida usually occurs in the lumbosacral area and has several forms. (See Figure 9–10.)*
spina bifida occulta SPĪ-nă BĬF-ĭ-dă ŏ-KŬL-tă	Most common and least severe form of spina bifida without protrusion of the spinal cord or meninges
spina bifida cystica SPĪ-nă BĬF-ĭ-dă SĬS-tĭk-ă	More severe type of spina bifida that involves protrusion of the meninges (meningocele), spinal cord (myelocele), or both (meningomyelocele). *The severity of neurological dysfunction in spina bifida cystica depends directly on the degree of nerve involvement.*

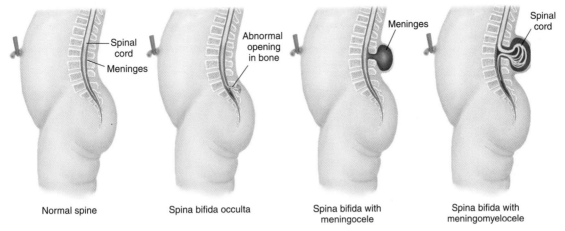

Normal spine | Spina bifida occulta | Spina bifida with meningocele | Spina bifida with meningomyelocele

Figure 9-10 Spina bifida.

spinal cord injuries	Severe injuries to the spinal cord, such as vertebral fractures and dislocations, resulting in impairment of spinal cord function below the level of the injury (See Figure 9–9) *Spinal cord injuries are commonly the result of trauma caused by motor vehicle accidents, falls, diving in shallow water, or accidents associated with contact sports. Such trauma may cause varying degrees of paraplegia and quadriplegia. These injuries are seen most commonly in the male adolescent and young adult population.*
paraplegia păr-ă-PLĒ-jē-ă *para:* near, beside; beyond *-plegia:* paralysis	Paralysis of the lower portion of the body and both legs *Paraplegia results in loss of sensory and motor control below the level of injury. Other common problems occurring with spinal cord injury to the lumbar and thoracic regions include loss of bladder, bowel, and sexual control.*
quadriplegia kwŏd-rĭ-PLĒ-jē-ă *quadri:* four *-plegia:* paralysis	Paralysis of all four extremities and, usually, the trunk *Quadriplegia generally results in loss of motor and sensory function below the level of injury. Paralysis includes the trunk, legs, and pelvic organs with partial or total paralysis in the upper extremities. The higher the trauma, the more debilitating the motor and sensory impairments will be.*
transient ischemic attack (TIA) TRĂN-zhĕnt ĭs-KĒ-mĭk *ischem:* to hold back; block *-ic:* pertaining to	Temporary interference with blood supply to the brain, lasting a few minutes to a few hours; also called *mini stroke*

Diagnostic Procedures

Endocrine System

computed tomography (CT) kŏm-PŪ-tĕd tō-MŎG-ră-fē *tom/o:* to cut *-graphy:* process of recording	Radiographic technique that uses a narrow beam of x-rays that rotates in a full arc around the patient to acquire multiple views of the body that a computer interprets to produce cross-sectional images of that body part *CT scans of endocrine organs are used to assist in the diagnosis of various pathologies and may involve the use of a contrast medium.*

magnetic resonance imaging (MRI) măg-NĔT-ĭc RĔZ-ĕn-ăns ĬM-ĭj-ĭng	Radiographic technique that uses electromagnetic energy to produce multiplanar cross-sectional images of the body *MRI scans of the endocrine system are used to identify abnormalities of pituitary, pancreatic, adrenal, and thyroid glands.*
radioactive iodine uptake (RAIU) test	Imaging procedure that measures levels of radioactivity in the thyroid after oral or IV administration of radioactive iodine *RAIU is used to determine thyroid function by monitoring the thyroid's ability to take up (uptake) iodine from the blood.*

Nervous System

cerebrospinal fluid (CSF) analysis sĕr-ĕ-brō-SPĪ-năl FLOO-ĭd *cerebr/o:* cerebrum *spin:* spine *-al:* pertaining to	Laboratory test in which CSF obtained from a lumbar puncture is evaluated macroscopically for clarity and color, microscopically for cells, and chemically for proteins and other substances *Normal CSF is clear and colorless. CSF has a pink or reddish tint when large numbers of red blood cells (RBCs) are present. RBCs indicate bleeding in the brain from trauma or a stroke. CSF appears cloudy when large numbers of white blood cells (WBCs) are present. WBCs indicate an infection such as meningitis or encephalitis. Elevated protein levels indicate infection or the presence of a tumor.*
computed tomography (CT) kŏm-PŪ-tĕd tō-MŎG-ră-fē *tom/o:* to cut *-graphy:* process of recording	Radiographic technique that uses a narrow beam of x-rays that rotates in a full arc around the patient to acquire multiple views of the body that a computer interprets to produce cross-sectional images of that body part *CT scans of the brain help in differentiating intracranial pathologies such as tumors, cysts, edema, hemorrhage, blood clots, and cerebral aneurysms. Contrast medium also may be injected intravenously.*
lumbar puncture LŬM-băr *lumb:* loins (lower back) *-ar:* pertaining to	Insertion of a needle into the subarachnoid space of the spinal column at the level of the fourth intervetebral space to withdraw cerebral spinal fluid (CSF) in order to perform various diagnostic and therapeutic procedures; also called *spinal tap* or *spinal puncture* *In lumbar puncture, CSF flows through the needle and is collected and sent to the laboratory for analysis. Therapeutic procedures include withdrawing CSF to reduce intracranial pressure, introducing a local anesthetic to induce spinal anesthesia, or to administer intrathecal medications. (See Figure 9–11.)*
magnetic resonance imaging (MRI) măg-NĔT-ĭc RĔZ-ĕn-ăns ĬM-ĭj-ĭng	Radiographic technique that uses electromagnetic energy to produce multiplanar cross-sectional images of the body *MRI of the brain produces cross-sectional, frontal, and sagittal plane views of the brain. It is regarded as superior to CT for most CNS abnormalities, particularly those of the brainstem and spinal cord. A contrast medium is not required but may be used to enhance internal structure visualization.*

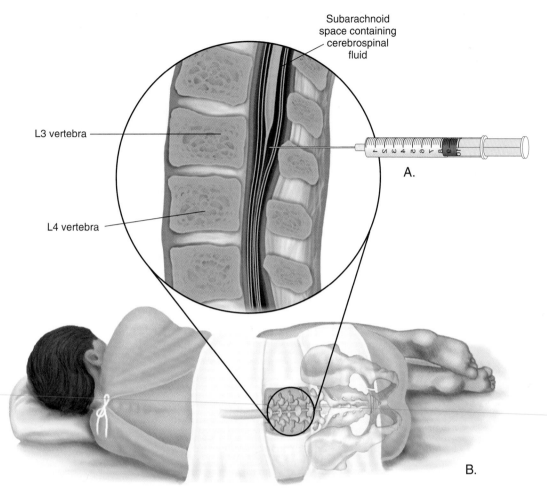

Figure 9-11 Lumbar puncture (spinal tap). (A) Collection of cerebrospinal fluid.
(B) Position for lumbar puncture.

positron emission tomography (PET) PŎZ-ĭ-trŏn ē-MĬSH-ŭn tō-MŎG-ră-fē *tom/o:* to cut *-graphy:* process of recording	Radiographic technique combining computed tomography with radiopharmaceuticals that produces a cross-sectional (transverse) image of the dispersement of radioactivity (through emission of positrons) in a section of the body to reveal the areas where the radiopharmaceutical is being metabolized and where there is a deficiency in metabolism *PET scanning aids in diagnosis of such neurologic disorders as brain tumors, epilepsy, stroke, Alzheimer disease, and abdominal and pulmonary disorders.*

Medical and Surgical Procedures

Endocrine System

adrenalectomy ăd-rē-năl-ĔK-tō-mē *adren/o:* adrenal glands *-ectomy:* excision, removal	Surgical removal of one or both adrenal glands to remove a benign or cancerous tumor, aid in correcting a hormone imbalance, prevent metastasis or, occasionally, prevent adrenal gland hormone excretion from exacerbating an existing condition such as breast cancer

thyroidectomy thī-royd-ĔK-tō-mē *thyroid:* thyroid gland *-ectomy:* excision, removal	Excision of one lobe (subtotal thyroidectomy) or the entire thyroid gland (thyroid lobectomy)

Nervous System

craniotomy **krā-nē-ŎT-ō-mē** *crani/o:* cranium (skull) *-tomy:* incision	Surgical procedure that creates an opening in the skull to gain access to the brain during neurosurgical procedures *A craniotomy is also performed to relieve intracranial pressure, control bleeding, or remove a tumor.*
thalamotomy thăl-ă-MŎT-ō-mē *thalam/o:* thalamus *-tomy:* incision	Partial destruction of the thalamus to treat psychosis or intractable pain

Pharmacology

Endocrine System

hormone replacement therapy (HRT)	Oral administration or injection of synthetic hormones to correct a deficiency in such hormones as of estrogen, testosterone, or thyroid hormone

Additional Medical Terms Review

Match the medical term(s) below with the definitions in the numbered list.

Alzheimer disease	insulinoma	poliomyelitis
Bell palsy	lumbar puncture	panhypopituitarism
CT	MRI	sciatica
epilepsy	myxedema	shingles
exophthalmos	Parkinson disease	spina bifida
Graves disease	PET	stroke
Huntington chorea	pheochromocytoma	thalamotomy
hydrocephalus	pituitarism	type 1 diabetes
neuroblastoma		

1. _____ is facial paralysis on one side of the face because of inflammation of a facial nerve.

2. _____ refers to brain tissue damage due to formation of a clot or a ruptured blood vessel.

3. _____ is a central nervous system disorder characterized by recurrent seizures.

4. _____ is abnormal protrusion of eyeball, possibly due to thyrotoxicosis.

5. _____ means hyperthyroidism, also called *toxic goiter*, which is characterized by exophthalmos.

6. _____ is a tumor of the pancreas.

7. _____ means advanced hypothyroidism in adults, resulting from hypofunction of the thyroid gland, causing edema and increasing blood pressure.

8. _____ is a small chromaffin cell tumor, usually located in the adrenal medulla.

9. _____ is a progressive degenerative neurological disorder that causes hand tremors.

10. _____ refers to inflammation of the gray matter caused by a virus, commonly resulting in spinal and muscle deformity and paralysis.

11. _____ refers to severe pain in the leg along the course of the sciatic nerve.

12. _____ is a congenital defect characterized by incomplete closure of the spinal canal through which the spinal cord and meninges may or may not protrude.

13. _____ is cranial enlargement caused by accumulation of fluid within the ventricles of the brain.

14. _____ is a malignant tumor composed principally of cells resembling neuroblasts; occurs chiefly in infants and children.

15. _____ is a brain disorder marked by deterioration of mental capacity (dementia), beginning in middle age, and leading to total disability and death.

16. _____ is a radiographic technique that uses electromagnetic energy to produce cross-sectional, frontal, and sagittal plane views of the brain.

17. _____ is a chronic disease due to insufficient production of insulin or the body's inability to utilize insulin properly.

18. _____ refers to eruption of acute, inflammatory, herpetic vesicles on the trunk of the body along a peripheral nerve.

19. _____ refers to any disorder of the pituitary gland and its function.

20. _____ refers to total pituitary impairment that brings about progressive and general loss of hormonal activity.

21. _____ is a hereditary nervous disorder caused by progressive loss of brain cells that leads to bizarre, involuntary, dancelike movements.

22. _____ withdrawal of spinal fluid for diagnostic or therapeutic purposes.

23. _____ is a radiographic technique that uses a narrow beam of x-rays that rotates in a full arc around the patient to acquire multiple views of the body that a computer interprets to produce cross-sectional images of that body part.

24. _____ refers to partial destruction of the thalamus to treat psychosis or intractable pain.

25. _____ produces cross-sectional image of radioactivity in a section of the body to reveal areas where the radiopharmaceutical is being metabolized and where there is a deficiency in metabolism.

Competency Verification: Check your answers in Appendix B, Answer Key, page 575. If you are not satisfied with your level of comprehension, review the additional medical terms and retake the review.

Correct Answers _____ × 4 = _____ % Score

Medical Record Activities

Medical reports included in the following activities reflect common, real-life clinical scenarios using medical terminology to document patient care.

MEDICAL RECORD ACTIVITY 9-1

Diabetes Mellitus

Terminology

Terms listed in the table below come from the medical report *Diabetes Mellitus* that follows. Use a medical dictionary such as *Taber's Cyclopedic Medical Dictionary,* the appendices of this book, or other resources to define each term. Then practice reading the pronunciations aloud for each term.

Term	Definition
acidosis ăs-ĭ-DŌ-sĭs	_____
ADA	_____
BS	_____
diabetes mellitus dī-ă-BĒ-tēz MĔ-lĭ-tŭs	_____
electrolytes ē-LĔK-trō-lītz	_____
glycemic glī-SĒ-mĭk	_____
glycosuria glī-kō-SŪ-rē-ă	_____
Humulin L HŪ-mū-lĭn	_____
Humulin R HŪ-mū-lĭn	_____
ketones KĒ-tōnz	_____
metabolically mĕt-ă-BŎL-ĭk-ă-lē	_____
polydipsia pŏl-ē-DĬP-sē-ă	_____

Term	Definition
polyuria pŏl-ē-Ū-rē-ă	
type 1 diabetes mellitus dī-ă-BĒ-tēz MĔ-lĭ-tŭs	
WNL	

 Listen and Learn Online! will help you master pronunciations of selected medical words from this medical record activity. Visit *http://davisplus.fadavis.com/gylys/simplified* to find instructions on completing the *Listen and Learn Online!* exercise for this section and to practice pronunciations.

Reading

Practice pronunciation of medical terms by reading the following medical report aloud.

Diabetes Mellitus

ADMITTING DIAGNOSIS: Diabetes mellitus, new onset.

DISCHARGE DIAGNOSIS: Type 1 diabetes mellitus, new onset.

HISTORY OF PRESENT ILLNESS: Patient is a 15-year-old white boy who presented in the office complaining of increased appetite, polydipsia, and polyuria and was found to have elevated blood glucose of 400 and glycosuria. He was sent to the hospital for further evaluation and treatment.

HOSPITAL COURSE: On admission, laboratory tests showed electrolytes, WNL, and ketones were negative. Urinalysis showed a trace of glucose, BG 380, and there was no evidence of acidosis. Metabolically the patient was stable. Patient was started on split-mixed insulin dosing. The patient and his family received full diabetic instruction during his hospitalization and seemed to understand this well. The patient picked up on all of this information quickly, asked appropriate questions, and appeared to be coping well with his new condition. By the 5th day, his polyuria and polydipsia resolved. When the patient was able to draw up and give his own insulin and perform his own fingersticks, he was discharged.

DISCHARGE INSTRUCTIONS: The patient was discharged to home with parents on a mixture of Humulin L 12 units and Humulin R 6 units each morning, with Humulin L 5 units and Humulin R 6 units each afternoon. He will continue with fingerstick BG 4 times daily at home until seen in the office for follow-up. I warned him of all glycemic symptoms to watch for, and he is to call the office with any problems that may occur. He is to follow an ADA 2,000-calorie diet.

DISCHARGE CONDITION: The patient's overall condition was much improved, and at the time of discharge BG levels were stabilized and he was doing well.

Evaluation

Review the medical record to answer the following questions. Use a medical dictionary such as *Taber's Cyclopedic Medical Dictionary* and other resources if needed.

1. What symptoms of DM did the patient experience before his office visit?

   _____

   _____

2. What confirmed the patient's new diagnosis of DM?

   _____

   _____

3. What conditions had to be met before the patient could be discharged from the hospital?

   _____

   _____

4. How many times a day does the patient have to take insulin?

   _____

   _____

5. Why does the patient have to perform fingersticks four times a day?

   _____

   _____

6. What is an ADA 2,000-calorie diet? Why is it important?

   _____

   _____

MEDICAL RECORD ACTIVITY 9-2

Stroke

Terminology

Terms listed in the table below come from the medical report *Stroke* that follows. Use a medical dictionary such as *Taber's Cyclopedic Medical Dictionary*, the appendices of this book, or other resources to define each term. Then practice reading the pronunciations aloud for each term.

Term	Definition
adenocarcinoma ăd-ĕ-nō-kăr-sĭn-Ō-mă	_____
anorexia ăn-ō-RĔK-sē-ă	_____
aphasia ă-FĀ-zē-ă	_____

Term	Definition
biliary BĬL-ē-ār-ē	_____
cardiovascular kăr-dē-ō-VĂS-kū-lăr	_____
cholecystojejunostomy kō-lē-sĭs-tō-jĕ-jū-NŎS-tō-mē	_____
deglutition dē-gloo-TĬSH-ŭn	_____
diplopia dĭp-LŌ-pē-ă	_____
jaundice JAWN-dĭs	_____
jejunojejunostomy jē-jū-nō-jĕ-jū-NŎS-tō-mē	_____
metastasis mĕ-TĂS-tă-sis	_____
pruritus proo-RĪ-tŭs	_____
vertigo VĔR-tĭ-gō	_____

Listen and Learn Online! will help you master pronunciations of selected medical words from this medical record activity. Visit *http://davisplus.fadavis.com/gylys/simplified* to find instructions on completing the *Listen and Learn Online!* exercise for this section and to practice pronunciations.

Reading

Practice pronunciation of medical terms by reading the following medical report aloud.

Stroke

The patient is a moderately obese white woman who was admitted to Riverside Hospital because of a sudden episode of stroke. She recalls an episode of vertigo 3 days ago. The patient is being nursed at home by her daughter because of terminal adenocarcinoma of the head of the pancreas with metastasis to the liver, which was diagnosed in December. The patient fell to the floor with paralysis of the right arm and right leg and aphasia. She has not noticed any difficulty with deglutition. Apparently with the onset of the stroke, she also experienced diplopia. She denies any difficulty with her cardiovascular system in the past. The patient was in the hospital 5 years ago because of generalized biliary-type disease with jaundice, pruritus, weight loss, and anorexia. Subsequently, she was seen in consultation, and cholecystojejunostomy and jejunojejunostomy were performed.

Diagnosis: 1. Stroke, probably secondary to metastatic lesion of the brain or cerebrovascular disease.
2. Evidence of the previously described deterioration secondary to carcinoma of the pancreas with metastases to the liver.

Evaluation

Review the medical record to answer the following questions. Use a medical dictionary such as *Taber's Cyclopedic Medical Dictionary* and other resources if needed.

1. Did the patient have a history of cardiovascular problems before her stroke?

_____

_____

2. What symptoms did the patient experience just before her stroke?

_____

_____

3. What is the primary site of this patient's cancer?

_____

_____

4. What is cerebrovascular disease?

_____

_____

5. What is the probable cause of the patient's stroke?

_____

_____

Chapter Review

Word Elements Summary

The following table summarizes CFs, suffixes, and prefixes related to the endocrine and nervous systems.

Word Element	Meaning	Word Element	Meaning
Combining Forms			
aden/o	gland	**mening/o, meningi/o**	meninges (membranes covering brain and spinal cord)
adren/o, adrenal/o	adrenal glands	**myel/o**	bone marrow; spinal cord
anter/o	anterior, front	**neur/o**	nerve
calc/o	calcium	**pancreat/o**	pancreas
cerebr/o	cerebrum	**thym/o**	thymus gland
encephal/o	brain	**thyroid/o**	thyroid gland
gli/o	glue; neuroglial tissue	**vascul/o**	blood vessel
gluc/o, glyc/o	sugar, sweetness		
Other Combining Forms			
acr/o	extremities	**hidr/o**	sweat
carcin/o	cancer	**nephr/o, ren/o**	kidney
cyst/o	bladder	**orchid/o, orchi/o, orch/o**	testis (plural, testes)
cyt/o	cell	**poster/o**	back (of body), behind, posterior
dermat/o	skin	**scler/o**	hardening; sclera (white of eye)
enter/o	intestine (usually small intestine)	**spin/o**	spine
gastr/o	stomach	**thromb/o**	blood clot
hem/o	blood	**toxic/o**	poison
hepat/o	liver		

(continued)

Word Element	Meaning	Word Element	Meaning
Suffixes			

SURGICAL

Word Element	Meaning	Word Element	Meaning
-ectomy	excision, removal	**-tome**	instrument to cut
-lysis	separation; destruction; loosening	**-tomy**	incision
-pexy	fixation (of an organ)		

DIAGNOSTIC, SYMPTOMATIC, AND RELATED

Word Element	Meaning	Word Element	Meaning
-algia, -dynia	pain	**-malacia**	softening
-dipsia	thirst	**-oid**	resembling
-emia	blood condition	**-oma**	tumor
-gen, -genesis	forming, producing, origin	**-osis**	abnormal condition; increase (used primarily with blood cells)
-glia	glue; neuroglial tissue	**-pathy**	disease
-iasis	abnormal condition (produced by something specified)	**-penia**	decrease, deficiency
-ism	condition	**-phagia**	swallowing, eating
-itis	inflammation	**-phasia**	speech
-lith	stone, calculus	**-plegia**	paralysis
-logist	specialist in study of	**-rrhagia**	bursting forth (of)
-logy	study of	**-rrhea**	discharge, flow
-megaly	enlargement	**-uria**	urine

Word Element	Meaning	Word Element	Meaning
Prefixes			
a-	without, not	**hyper-**	excessive, above normal
dys-	bad; painful; difficult	**hypo-**	under, below, deficient
endo-	within	**para-**	near, beside; beyond

 Enhance your study and reinforcement of word elements with the power of *Davis Plus.* Visit *http://davisplus.fadavis.com/gylys/simplified* for this chapter's flash-card activity. We recommend you complete the flash-card activity before completing the word elements review below.

Word Elements Review

After you review the word elements summary, complete this activity by writing the meaning of each element in the space provided.

Word Element	Meaning	Word Element	Meaning
Combining Forms			
1. aden/o	_____	8. mening/o, meningi/o	_____
2. adren/o, adrenal/o	_____	9. myel/o	_____
3. calc/o	_____	10. neur/o	_____
4. cerebr/o	_____	11. pancreat/o	_____
5. encephal/o	_____	12. thym/o	_____
6. gli/o	_____	13. thyroid/o	_____
7. gluc/o, glyc/o	_____		
OTHER COMBINING FORMS			
14. hem/o	_____	16. hidr/o	_____
15. hepat/o	_____	17. toxic/o	_____
Suffixes			
SURGICAL			
18. -ectomy	_____	21. -tome	_____
19. -lysis	_____	22. -tomy	_____
20. -pexy	_____		
DIAGNOSTIC, SYMPTOMATIC, AND RELATED			
23. -dipsia	_____	35. -oid	_____
24. -emia	_____	36. -oma	_____
25. -gen, -genesis	_____	37. -osis	_____
26. -glia	_____	38. -pathy	_____
27. -iasis	_____	39. -penia	_____
28. -ism	_____	40. -phagia	_____
29. -itis	_____	41. -phasia	_____
30. -lith	_____	42. -plegia	_____
31. -logist	_____	43. -rrhagia	_____
32. -logy	_____	44. -rrhea	_____
33. -megaly	_____	45. -uria	_____
34. -malacia	_____		
Prefixes			
46. a-	_____	49. hypo-	_____
47. endo-	_____	50. para-	_____
48. hyper-	_____		

Competency Verification: Check your answers in Appendix A, Glossary of Medical Word Elements, page 538. If you are not satisfied with your level of comprehension, review the word elements and retake the review.

Correct Answers _____ × 2 = _____ % Score

Vocabulary Review

Match the medical term(s) below with the definitions in the numbered list.

acromegaly	glycogenesis	metastasis	polyphagia
adenohypophysis	hormone	neurohypophysis	pruritus
adrenalectomy	hypercalcemia	neuromalacia	thyrotoxicosis
adrenaline	hyperglycemia	pancreatolith	vertigo
cerebral palsy	insulin	pancreatolysis	
deglutition	jaundice	pancreatopathy	
diabetes mellitus	meningocele	polydipsia	

1. _____ means enlargement of the extremities.

2. _____ means destruction of the pancreatic tissue due to a pathological condition.

3. _____ is the anterior lobe of the pituitary gland, composed of glandular tissue.

4. _____ refers to partial paralysis and lack of muscular coordination caused by damage to the cerebrum before or during the birth process.

5. _____ refers to excessive amounts of calcium in the blood.

6. _____ is a pancreatic hormone that decreases blood glucose level.

7. _____ is the posterior lobe of the pituitary, composed primarily of nerve tissue.

8. _____ means disease of the pancreas.

9. _____ refers to excessive consumption of food.

10. _____ is a chronic metabolic disorder marked by hyperglycemia; occurs in two primary forms.

11. _____ means increase of blood glucose, as in diabetes.

12. _____ is a calculus or stone in the pancreas.

13. _____ refers to excessive thirst.

14. _____ is a toxic condition due to hyperactivity of the thyroid gland.

15. _____ means excision of an adrenal gland.

16. _____ is a hormone secreted by the adrenal medulla that causes some of the physiological expressions of fear and anxiety; epinephrine.

17. _____ means production or formation of sugar.

18. _____ refers to protrusion of the membranes of the brain or spinal cord through a defect in the skull or spinal column.

19. _____ means softening of nerve tissue.

20. _____ refers to severe itching.

21. _____ refers to the act of swallowing.

22. _____ is an illusion of movement.

23. _____ is yellowish discoloration of the skin and eyes.

24. _____ refers to spread of a malignant tumor beyond its primary site to a secondary organ or location.

25. _____ is a chemical substance produced by specialized cells of the body and released slowly into the bloodstream.

Competency Verification: Check your answers in Appendix B, Answer Key, page 576. If you are not satisfied with your level of comprehension, review the chapter vocabulary and retake the review.

Correct Answers _____ × 4 = _____ % Score

10 Musculoskeletal System

OBJECTIVES

Upon completion of this chapter, you will be able to:

■ Describe the type of medical treatment orthopedists, rheumatologists, osteopathic physicians, and chiropractors provide.

■ Identify skeletal structures by labeling them on anatomical illustrations.

■ Describe the primary functions of the musculoskeletal system.

■ Describe common diseases related to the musculoskeletal system.

■ Describe common diagnostic, medical, and surgical procedures related to the musculoskeletal system.

■ Apply your word-building skills by constructing various medical terms related to the musculoskeletal system.

■ Describe common abbreviations and symbols related to the musculoskeletal system.

■ Reinforce word elements by completing flash card activities.

■ Recognize, define, pronounce, and spell terms correctly.

■ Demonstrate your knowledge of this chapter by successfully completing the frames, reviews, and medical report evaluations.

Medical Specialty

Orthopedics

Orthopedics is the branch of medicine concerned with prevention, diagnosis, care, and treatment of musculoskeletal disorders. These disorders include injury to or disease of the body's bones, joints, ligaments, muscles, and tendons. *Orthopedists* are surgeons who specialize in orthopedics. They employ medical, physical, and surgical methods to restore function that is lost as a result of injury or disease to the musculoskeletal system. Orthopedists coordinate their treatments with other health care providers, such as physical therapists, occupational therapists, and sports medicine physicians. In addition to the orthopedist who treats bone and joint diseases, the **rheumatologist** (also a medical doctor) specializes in treatment of arthritis and other diseases of joints, muscles, and bones.

Osteopathy

The *osteopathic physician* (**DO**) may also provide medical treatment for musculoskeletal disorders. The osteopathic philosophy maintains that good health requires a holistic approach that includes proper alignment of bones, muscles, ligaments, and nerves. Like a medical doctor (MD), osteopathic physicians provide state-of-the-art methods of medical treatment, including prescribing drugs and performing surgeries, and may specialize in such areas as orthopedics, cardiology, and pulmonology.

Chiropractic

Another health care provider who treats musculoskeletal disorders is the ***chiropractor***. Unlike medical doctors and osteopaths, chiropractors are not physicians. They do not employ drugs or surgery, the primary basis of treatment used by medical physicians. **Chiropractic medicine** is a system of therapy based on the theory that disease is caused by pressure on nerves. Nevertheless, chiropractors employ the use of radiographic images to diagnose pathological disorders and determine the most effective type of treatment. In most instances, chiropractic treatment involves physical manipulation of the spinal column.

Anatomy and Physiology Overview

The musculoskeletal system includes muscles, bones, joints, and related structures, such as tendons and connective tissue,that function in the movement of body parts and organs.

Muscles have four key functions: producing body movements, stabilizing body positions, storing and moving substances within the body, and generating heat. Through contraction, muscles cause motion and help maintain body posture. Less apparent motions that muscles are responsible for include the passage and elimination of food through the digestive system, propulsion of blood through the arteries, and contraction of the bladder to eliminate urine. In addition, muscles function in body movements in several different ways to allow a range of motion for the contraction and relaxation of muscle fibers. (See Figure 10–1.)

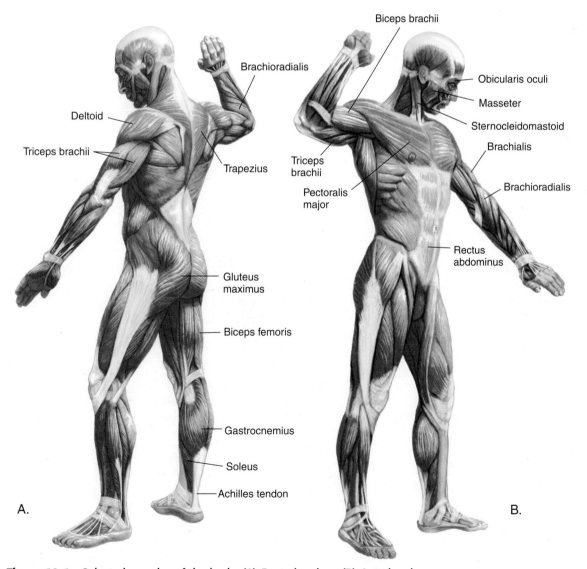

Figure 10-1   Selected muscles of the body. (A) Posterior view. (B) Anterior view.

The main function of bones is to form a skeleton to support and protect the body and serve as storage areas for mineral salts, especially calcium and phosphorus. Joints are the places where two bones articulate, or connect. Because bones cannot move without the help of muscles, contraction must be provided by muscle tissue.

WORD ELEMENTS

This section introduces combining forms (CFs) related to the muscles of the body. Included are key suffixes; prefixes are defined in the right-hand column as needed. Review the following table and pronounce each word in the word analysis column aloud before you begin to work the frames.

Word Element	Meaning	Word Analysis
Combining Forms		
MUSCLES AND RELATED STRUCTURES		
fasci/o	band, fascia (fibrous membrane supporting and separating muscles)	**fasci/o**/plasty (FĂSH-ē-ō-plăs-tē): surgical repair of fascia *-plasty:* surgical repair
fibr/o	fiber, fibrous tissue	**fibr**/oma (fī-BRŌ-mă): tumor of fibrous tissue *-oma:* tumor
leiomy/o	smooth muscle (visceral)	**leiomy**/oma (lī-ō-mī-Ō-mă): tumor of smooth muscle *-oma:* tumor
lumb/o	loins (lower back)	**lumb/o**/cost/al (lŭm-bō-KŎS-tăl): pertaining to the lumbar region and the ribs *cost:* ribs *-al:* pertaining to
muscul/o	muscle	**muscul**/ar (MŬS-kū-lăr): pertaining to muscles *-ar:* pertaining to
my/o		**my/o**/rrhexis (mī-or-ĔK-sĭs): rupture of a muscle *-rrhexis:* rupture
ten/o	tendon	**ten/o**/tomy (těn-ŎT-ō-mē): incision of a tendon *-tomy:* incision *Tenotomy is performed to correct muscle imbalance, such as in the correction of strabismus of the eye or clubfoot.*
tend/o		**tend/o**/plasty (TĔN-dō-plăs-tē): surgical repair of a tendon *-plasty:* surgical repair
tendin/o		**tendin**/itis (těn-dĭn-Ī-tĭs): inflammation of a tendon, usually resulting from strain; also called *tendonitis* *-itis:* inflammation *Tendinitis usually results from a strain.*

Word Element	Meaning	Word Analysis
Suffixes		
-algia	pain	my/**algia** (mī-ĂL-jē-ă): pain or tenderness in muscles *my:* muscle
-asthenia	weakness, debility	my/**asthenia** (mī-ăs-THĒ-nē-ă): weakness of muscle (and abnormal fatigue) *my:* muscle
-pathy	disease	my/o/**pathy** (mī-ŎP-ă-thē): disease of muscular tissue *my/o:* muscle *Myopathy is a disease that commonly indicates a skeletal muscle disorder.*
-plegia	paralysis	hemi/**plegia** (hĕm-ē-PLĒ-jē-ă): paralysis of one side of the body *hemi-:* one half *Types of hemiplegia include cerebral hemiplegia and facial hemiplegia.*
-rrhaphy	suture	my/o/**rrhaphy** (mī-OR-ă-fē): suture of muscle, usually due to a muscle wound *my/o:* muscle
-sarcoma	malignant tumor of connective tissue	my/o/**sarcoma** (mī-ō-sar-KŌ-mă): malignant tumor of muscle tissue *my/o:* muscle
-tomy	incision	chondr/o/**tomy** (kŏn-DRŎT-ō-mē): incision of cartilage *chondr/o:* cartilage

Pronunciation Help	Long Sound	ā in rāte	ē in rēbirth	ī in īsle	ō in ōver	ū in ūnite
	Short Sound	ă in ălone	ĕ in ĕver	ĭ in ĭt	ŏ in nŏt	ŭ in cŭt

 Listen and Learn, the audio CD-ROM included in this book, will help you master pronunciation of selected medical words. Use it to practice pronunciations of the above-listed medical terms and for instructions to complete the *Listen and Learn* exercise for this section.

S E C T I O N   R E V I E W   10-1

For the following medical terms, first write the suffix and its meaning. Then translate the meaning of the remaining elements starting with the first part of the word. The first word is completed for you.

Term	Meaning
1. my/o/sarcoma	*-sarcoma: malignant tumor of connective tissue; muscle*
2. my/o/rrhaphy	
3. hemi/plegia	
4. ten/o/tomy	
5. cost/o/chondr/itis	
6. tend/o/lysis	
7. my/o/pathy	
8. lumb/o/cost/al	
9. tendin/itis	
10. my/algia	

Competency Verification: Check your answers in Appendix B, Answer Key, page 577. If you are not satisfied with your level of comprehension, review the vocabulary and retake the review.

Correct Answers _____ × 10 = _____ % Score

Muscles

Types of Muscle Fibers

There are three types of muscular fibers or tissue:

- *Skeletal* muscle fibers are composed of striations that move bones of the skeleton and work mainly in a voluntary manner. Muscle fibers contract in response to stimulation and then relax when the stimulation ends. Their activity can be consciously controlled by neurons that are part of the somatic (voluntary) division of the nervous system. To some extent, skeletal muscles are also controlled subconsciously. For example, the diaphragm continues to alternately contract and relax without conscious control so that breathing does not stop.

- *Cardiac* muscle fibers, also composed of striations, are found only in the heart and form most of the heart wall. The alternating contraction and relaxation of the heart is involuntary and is not consciously controlled. Rather, the heart beats because it has a pacemaker that initiates each contraction. This built-in rhythm is called ***autorhythmicity.*** Several hormones and neurotransmitters can adjust heart rate by speeding or slowing the pacemaker.

- *Smooth* muscle fibers are shorter and lack the striations of skeletal and cardiac muscle tissue. For this reason, it has a smooth appearance, which gives it its name. The action of smooth muscle is usually involuntary and some smooth muscle tissue, such as the muscles that propel food through the gastrointestinal tract, has autorhythmicity. Smooth muscle and cardiac muscle are regulated by neurons that are part of the autonomic (involuntary) division of the nervous system and hormones released by endocrine glands.

muscle(s)	**10–1** Fibers within each muscle are characteristically arranged into specific patterns that provide specific functional capabilities. Most skeletal muscles lie between the skin and the skeleton. *My/o/genesis* is the embryonic formation of _____.
my/o/plasty MĪ-ō-plăs-tē **my/o/rrhaphy** mī-ŌR-ă-fē **my/o/tomy** mī-ŎT-ō-mē	**10–2** Practice building medical words that mean *surgical repair of muscle:* _____ / ____ / _____ *suture of muscle:* _____ / ____ / _____ *incision of muscle:* _____ / ____ / _____
my/o/rrhexis mī-or-ĔK-sĭs	**10–3** Sports-related injuries are commonly caused by the tremendous stress exerted on certain parts of musculoskeletal structures. In many instances, these types of athletic injuries may result in a torn muscle. Form a word that means *rupture (tear) of a muscle.* _____ / ____ / _____
hepat/o/rrhexis hĕp-ă-tō-RĔKS-ĭs **cyst/o/rrhexis** sĭs-tō-RĔKS-ĭs **enter/o/rrhexis** ĕn-tĕr-ō-RĔKS-ĭs	**10–4** Use *-rrhexis* to practice building words with the following organs. *rupture of the liver:* _____ / ____ / _____ *rupture of the bladder:* _____ / ____ / _____ *rupture of the intestine:* _____ / ____ / _____
my/algia mī-ĂL-jē-ă	**10–5** *My/o/dynia* refers to muscle pain. Form another word that means *muscle pain.* _____ / _____
my/o/pathy mī-ŎP-ă-thē	**10–6** The medical term that means *disease of muscle* is _____ / ____ / _____.
muscle	**10–7** *My/o/genesis* refers to forming, producing, or origin of _____.

hardening, sclera	**10-8** The CF *scler/o* refers to _____; _____ (white of eye).
scler/osis sklĕ-RŌ-sĭs **my/o/scler/osis** mī-ō-sklĕr-Ō-sĭs	**10-9** *Abnormal condition of hardening* is called _____ / _____. *Abnormal condition of muscle hardening* is called _____ / _____ / _____ / _____.
anterior **posterior**	**10-10** To become familiar with the names of the major muscles of the body, study Figure 10–1. Identify words in the caption for Figure 10–1 that mean *in front of:* _____ *back (of body), behind:* _____
tendon	**10-11** The CF *tend/o* means *tendon,* which is fibrous connective tissue that attaches muscles to bone. *Tend/o/plasty* is a surgical repair of a _____.
tend/o/tome TĔN-dō-tōm **tend/o/tomy** tĕn-DŎT-ō-mē **tend/o/plasty** TĔN-dō-plăs-tē	**10-12** Use *tend/o* to form words that mean *instrument to cut a tendon:* _____ / _____ / _____ *incision of a tendon:* _____ / _____ / _____ *surgical repair of a tendon:* _____ / _____ / _____
inferior	**10-13** The *Achilles tendon* is attached to a muscle in the lower leg. Locate the Achilles tendon in Figure 10–1A. It is located (superior, inferior) _____ to the gastrocnemius muscle.
paralysis pă-RĂL-ĭ-sĭs	**10-14** The prefix *quadri-* refers to *four. Quadri/plegia* is a _____ of all four extremities.
paralysis pă-RĂL-ĭ-sĭs	**10-15** The prefix *hemi-* means *one half. Hemi/plegia* is a _____ of half the body.
	10-16 With the exception of rotations of the body, other types of body movements occur in pairs as summarized in Table 10–1 on page 454 and illustrated in Figure 10–2.

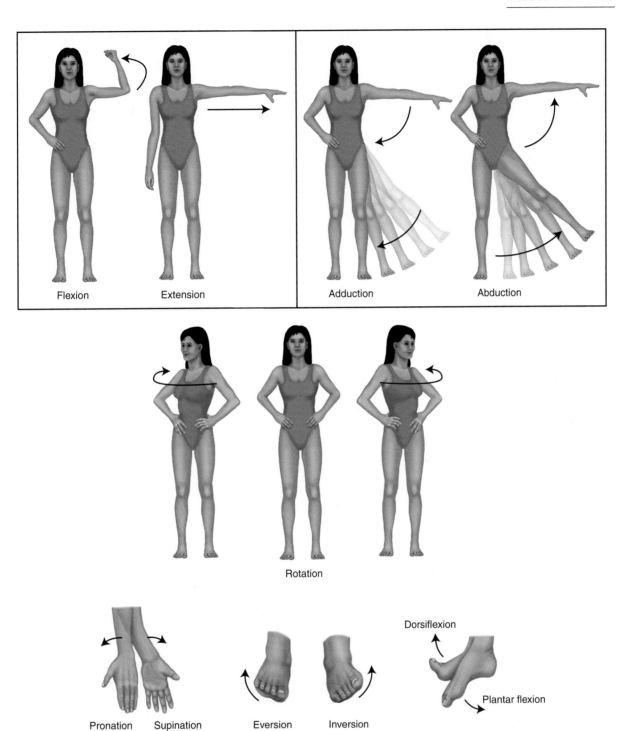

Flexion   Extension   Adduction   Abduction

Rotation

Pronation   Supination   Eversion   Inversion

Dorsiflexion

Plantar flexion

Figure 10-2 Body movements generated by muscles.

table 10-1 TYPES OF MOVEMENTS PRODUCED BY MUSCLES

This table examines movements and their actions, grouped in pairs of antagonistic (or opposite) functions.

Movement	Action
Flexion (FLĔK-shŭn) **Extension** (ĕks-TĔN-shŭn)	Bending and extension of a limb
Abduction (ăb-DŬK-shŭn) **Adduction** (ă-DŬK-shŭn)	Movement away from and toward the body
Rotation (rō-TĀ-shŭn)	Circular movement around an axis
Pronation (prō-NĀ-shŭn) **Supination** (sū-pĭn-Ā-shŭn)	Turning the hand to a palm down or palm up position
Dorsiflexion (dor-sĭ-FLĔK-shŭn) **Plantar flexion** (PLĂN-tăr FLĔK-shŭn)	Bending the foot or toes upward or downward
Eversion (ē-VĔR-zhŭn) **Inversion** (ĭn-VĔR-zhŭn)	Moving the sole of the foot outward or inward

S E C T I O N   R E V I E W   10-2

Using the table below, write the combining form, suffix, or prefix that matches its definition in the space provided to the left of the definition. There may be more than one word element that matches a definition.

Combining Forms		Suffixes		Prefixes
chondr/o	tendin/o	-cyte	-rrhaphy	hemi-
cyst/o	tend/o	-genesis	-rrhexis	quadri-
enter/o	ten/o	-lysis	-sarcoma	
hepat/o		-osis	-tome	
my/o		-plasty	-tomy	
scler/o		-plegia		

1. _____ abnormal condition; increase (used primarily with blood cells)
2. _____ bladder
3. _____ cell
4. _____ four
5. _____ one half
6. _____ hardening; sclera (white of eye)
7. _____ incision
8. _____ intestine (usually small intestine)
9. _____ liver
10. _____ muscle
11. _____ paralysis
12. _____ forming, producing, origin
13. _____ rupture
14. _____ surgical repair
15. _____ suture
16. _____ tendon
17. _____ instrument to cut
18. _____ cartilage
19. _____ malignant tumor of connective tissue
20. _____ separation; destruction; loosening

Competency Verification: Check your answers in Appendix B, Answer Key, page 577. If you are not satisfied with your level of comprehension, go back to Frame 10–1 to rework the frames.

Correct Answers _____ × 5 = _____ % Score

Skeletal System

The skeleton of a human adult consists of 206 individual bones, but this chapter covers only the major bones. For anatomical purposes, the human skeleton is divided into the axial skeleton (distinguished with bone color in Figure 10–3) and the appendicular skeleton (distinguished with blue color in Figure 10–3). The axial skeleton protects internal organs and provides central support of the body around which other parts move. It consists of the bones of the head, chest, and spine. The appendicular skeleton enables the body to move. It consists of the bones of the shoulders, arms, hips, and legs. The ability to walk, run, or catch a ball is possible due to the movable joints of the limbs.

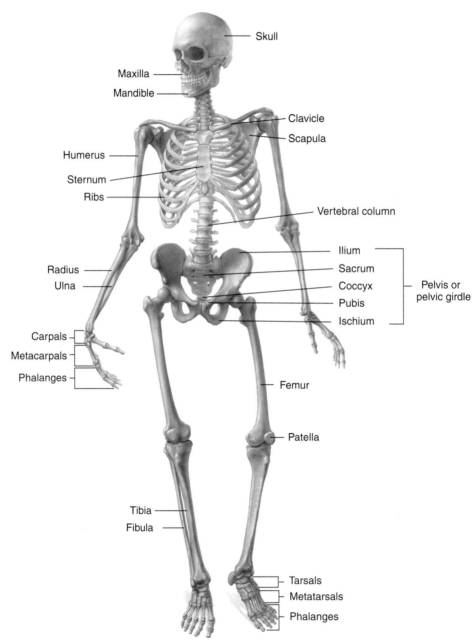

Figure 10-3 Anterior view of the skeleton.

WORD ELEMENTS

This section introduces CFs related to the bones. Included are key suffixes; prefixes are defined in the right-hand column as needed. Review the following table, and pronounce each word in the word analysis column aloud before you begin to work the frames.

Word Element	Meaning	Word Analysis
Combining Forms		

SPECIFIC BONES OF THE UPPER EXTREMITIES

Word Element	Meaning	Word Analysis
carp/o	carpus (wrist bones)	**carp/o/ptosis** (kăr-pŏp-TŌ-sĭs): downward displacement of the wrist; also called *dropped wrist* *-ptosis:* prolapse, downward displacement
cervic/o	neck; cervix uteri (neck of uterus)	**cervic/al** (SĔR-vĭ-kăl): pertaining to neck *-al:* pertaining to *The term cervical is also used to denote the region of the neck or a constricted area of a necklike structure, such as the neck of a tooth or the cervix uteri.*
cost/o	ribs	**sub/cost/al** (sŭb-KŎS-tăl): beneath the ribs *sub-:* under, below *-al:* pertaining to
crani/o	cranium (skull)	**crani/o/tomy** (krā-nē-ŎT-ō-mē): incision through the cranium, usually to gain access to the brain during neurosurgical procedures *-tomy:* incision *Craniotomy is performed to relieve intracranial pressure, control bleeding, or remove a tumor.*
humer/o	humerus (upper arm bone)	**humer/al** (HŪ-měr-ăl): pertaining to the humerus *-al:* pertaining to
metacarp/o	metacarpus (hand bones)	**metacarp/ectomy** (mĕt-ă-kăr-PĔK-tō-mē): excision of one or more metacarpal bones *-ectomy:* excision, removal
phalang/o	phalanges (bones of fingers and toes)	**phalang/itis** (făl-ăn-JĪ-tĭs): inflammation of one or more phalanges *-itis:* inflammation

(continued)

Word Element	Meaning	Word Analysis
spondyl/o*	vertebra (backbone)	**spondyl**/itis (spŏn-dĭl-Ī-tĭs): inflammation of any of the vertebrae (plural), usually characterized by stiffness and pain *-itis:* inflammation *Ankylosing spondylitis is a form of arthritis that may eventually cause the spine to fuse in a fixed, immobile position. Spondylitis may result from a traumatic injury to the spine, infection, or rheumatoid disease.*
vertebr/o*		**vertebr**/al (VĔR-tĕ-brăl): pertaining to a vertebra or the vertebral column *-al:* pertaining to
stern/o	sternum (breastbone)	**stern**/o/cost/al (stĕr-nō-KŎS-tăl): pertaining to the sternum and ribs *cost:* ribs *-al:* pertaining to

SPECIFIC BONES OF THE LOWER EXTREMITIES

Word Element	Meaning	Word Analysis
calcane/o	calcaneum (heel bone)	**calcane**/o/dynia (kăl-kăn-ē-ō-DĬN-ē-ă): painful condition of the heel *-dynia:* pain
femor/o	femur (thigh bone)	**femor**/al (FĔM-or-ăl): pertaining to the femur *-al:* pertaining to
fibul/o	fibula (smaller, outer bone of lower leg)	**fibul**/ar (FĬB-ū-lăr): pertaining to the fibula *-ar:* pertaining to
patell/o	patella (kneecap)	**patell**/ectomy (păt-ĕ-LĔK-tō-mē): excision of the patella *-ectomy:* excision, removal
pelv/i	pelvis	**pelv**/i/metry (pĕl-VĬM-ĕ-trē): measurement of the pelvic dimensions or proportions *-metry:* act of measuring *Pelvimetry helps determine whether or not it will be possible to deliver a fetus through the normal route.*
pelv/o		**pelv**/is (PĔL-vĭs): pertaining to the pelvis *-is:* noun ending *A woman's pelvis is usually less massive but wider and more circular than a man's pelvis.*
radi/o	radiation, x-ray; radius (lower arm bone, thumb side)	**radi**/o/graph (RĀ-dē-ō-grăf): x-ray image *-graph:* instrument for recording
tibi/o	tibia (larger bone of lower leg)	**tibi**/al (TĬB-ē-ăl): pertaining to the tibia (shin bone) *-al:* pertaining to

*The CF *spondyl/o* is used to form words about the condition of the structure. The CF *vertebr/o* is used to form words that describe the structure.

Word Element	Meaning	Word Analysis
OTHER RELATED STRUCTURES		
ankyl/o	stiffness; bent, crooked	**ankyl**/osis (ăng-kĭ-LŌ-sĭs): immobility of a joint *-osis:* abnormal condition; increase (used primarily with blood cells) *Ankylosis may be congenital or it may be due to disease, trauma, surgery, or contractures resulting from immobility.*
arthr/o	joint	**arthr**/itis (ăr-THRĪ-tĭs): inflammation of a joint *-itis:* inflammation *Arthritis is commonly accompanied by pain, swelling, stiffness, and deformity.*

chondr/o	cartilage	cost/o/**chondr**/itis (kŏs-tō-kŏn-DRĪ-tĭs): inflammation of cartilage of the anterior chest wall (ribs)
		  cost/o: ribs
		    -itis: inflammation
		Costochondritis is characterized by pain and tenderness that may radiate from the initial site of inflammation.

lamin/o	lamina (part of vertebral arch)	**lamin**/ectomy (lăm-ĭ-NĔK-tŏ-mē): excision of the lamina (bony arches of one or more vertebrae) *-ectomy:* excision, removal
myel/o	bone marrow; spinal cord	**myel**/o/cele (MĪ-ĕ-lō-sēl): herniation of the spinal cord *-cele:* hernia, swelling *Myelocele is a sacklike protrusion of the spinal cord through a congenital defect in the vertebral column.*

orth/o	straight	**orth**/o/ped/ics (or-thō-PĒ-dĭks): branch of medicine concerned with prevention and correction of musculoskeletal system disorders
		  ped: foot; child
		    -ics: pertaining to

oste/o	bone	**oste**/itis (ŏs-tē-Ī-tĭs): inflammation of bone *-itis:* inflammation
Suffixes		
-clasia	to break	arthr/o/**clasia** (ăr-thrō-KLĀ-zē-ă): forcible breaking of a joint *arthr/o:* joint
-clast	to break	oste/o/**clast** (ŎS-tē-ō-klăst): cell that breaks down bone *oste/o:* bone *Osteoclasts break down areas of old or damaged bone, while osteoblasts deposit new bone tissue in those areas*

(continued)

Word Element	Meaning	Word Analysis
-cyte	cell	oste/o/**cyte** (ŎS-tē-ō-sīt): bone cell *oste/o:* bone
-desis	binding, fixation (of a bone or joint)	arthr/o/**desis** (ăr-thrō-DĒ-sĭs): surgical immobilization of a joint *arthr/o:* joint
-malacia	softening	oste/o/**malacia** (ŏs-tē-ō-mă-LĀ-shē-ă): softening and bending of the bones *oste/o:* bone *Osteomalacia is caused by a deficiency in vitamin D that results in a shortage or loss of calcium salts, causing bones to become increasingly soft, flexible, brittle, and deformed.*
-physis	growth	dia/**physis** (dī-ĂF-ĭ-sĭs): shaft or middle region of a long bone *dia-:* through, across
-porosis	porous	oste/o/**porosis** (ŏs-tē-ō-por-Ō-sĭs): porous bones *oste/o:* bone *Osteoporosis is characterized by abnormal loss of bone density and deterioration of bone tissue with an increased risk of fracture.*

Pronunciation Help	**Long Sound** **Short Sound**	ā in rāte ă in ălone	ē in rēbirth ĕ in ĕver	ī in īsle ĭ in ĭt	ō in ōver ŏ in nŏt	ū in ūnite ŭ in cŭt

Listen and Learn, the audio CD-ROM included in this book, will help you master pronunciation of selected medical words. Use it to practice pronunciations of the above-listed medical terms and for instructions to complete the *Listen and Learn* exercise for this section.

SECTION REVIEW 10-3

For the following medical terms, first write the suffix and its meaning. Then translate the meaning of the remaining elements starting with the first part of the word. The first word is completed for you.

Term	Meaning
1. dia/physis	*-physis: growth; through, across*
2. sub/cost/al	
3. oste/o/malacia	
4. lamin/ectomy	
5. pelv/i/metry	
6. myel/o/cele	
7. oste/o/porosis	
8. ankyl/osis	
9. carp/o/ptosis	
10. crani/o/tomy	

Competency Verification: Check your answers in Appendix B, Answer Key, page 577. If you are not satisfied with your level of comprehension, review the vocabulary and retake the review.

Correct Answers _____ × 10 = _____ % Score

Structure and Function of Bones

	10-17 To understand the skeletal system, it is important to know the types and names of major bones, their functions, and where they are located. Regardless of the size or shape of a bone, the CF used to designate
oste/o	*bone* is _____ / _____.

10–18 There are four principal types of bones: *long, short, flat,* and *irregular.* The *long bones* of the extremities are the strongest bones of the arms and legs. The cube-shaped *short bones* include the bones of the ankles, wrists, and toes. *Flat bones* are the broad bones found in the skull, shoulder, and ribs. *Irregular bones* have varied shapes and sizes and are commonly clustered, such as the bones of the vertebrae and certain bones of the ears and face.

Identify the four types of bones described above.

short bones

flat bones

irregular bones

long bones

Cube-shaped bones of the wrists, ankles, and toes: _____ _____

Broad bones in the shoulders and ribs: _____ _____

Certain bones of the ears and the bones of the vertebrae:

_____ _____

Strongest bones of the arms and legs: _____ _____

10–19 Typically, long bones are found in the extremities of the body. The main elongated portion of such a bone, the (1) **diaphysis,** is composed of several tissue layers: the thin fibrous outer membrane, the (2) **periosteum;** the thick layer of hard (3) **compact bone;** and the inner (4) **medullary cavity.** Label the parts of the long bone in Figure 10–4.

10–20 The two ends of bones, the (5) **distal epiphysis** and (6) **proximal epiphysis,** have a bulbous shape to provide space for muscle and ligament attachments near the joints. Label these structures in Figure 10–4.

10–21 There are two kinds of bone tissue based on porosity, and most bones have both types. *Compact* (dense) bone tissue is the hard, outer layer; (7) **spongy** (cancellous) bone tissue is the porous, highly vascular inner portion. Compact bone tissue is covered by periosteum that serves as a place of attachment for muscles, provides protection, and gives durable strength to the bone. The spongy bone tissue makes the bone lighter and provides a space for bone marrow where blood cells are produced. Label the spongy bone in Figure 10–4, and note the position and structure of compact and spongy bone.

10–22 In Figure 10–4, observe how the diaphysis forms a cylinder that surrounds the medullary cavity. In adults, the medullary cavity contains fat yellow marrow, so named because of the large amounts of fat it contains.

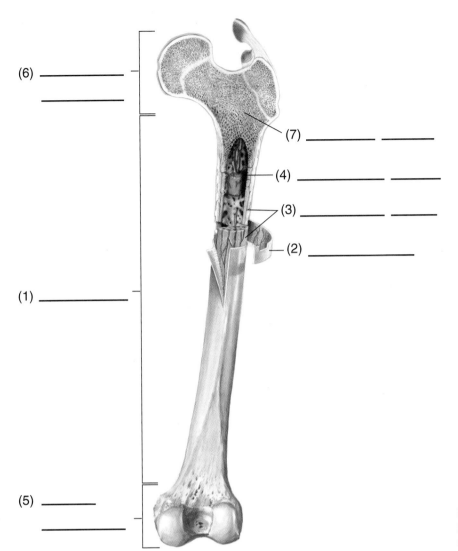

(6) _____ _____

(7) _____ _____

(4) _____ _____

(3) _____ _____

(2) _____

(1) _____

(5) _____

Figure 10-4 Longitudinal section of a long bone (femur) and interior bone structure.

10-23 The peri/oste/um, as illustrated in Figure 10–4, covers the entire surface of the bone. Its blood vessels supply nutrients, and its nerves signal pain. In growing bones, the inner layer contains bone-forming cells known as *oste/o/blasts*. Because blood vessels and oste/o/blasts are located here, the peri/oste/um provides a means for bone repair and general bone nutrition. Bones that lose peri/oste/um through injury or disease usually scale or die. As discussed earlier, the peri/oste/um also provides a point of attachment for muscles.

Identify terms in this frame that mean

embryonic cell (that develops into) bone:

_____ / _____ / _____

structure around bone: _____ / _____ / _____

oste/o/blasts
ŎS-tē-ō-blăstz

peri/oste/um
pĕr-ē-ŎS-tē-ŭm

-genesis

oste/o

oste/o/cytes
ŎS-tē-ō-sītz

10–24 *Oste/o/genesis* is the formation or development of bones. Identify elements in this frame that mean

forming, producing, origin: _____

bone: _____ / _____

When we are talking about bone cells, the medical term to use is

_____ / _____ / _____.

---

leuk/o/poiesis
loo-kō-poy-Ē-sĭs

erythr/o/poiesis
ĕ-rĭth-rō-poy-Ē-sĭs

10–25 In an adult, production of red blood cells *(erythr/o/poiesis)* occurs in red bone marrow. Red bone marrow is also responsible for formation of white blood cells *(leuk/o/poiesis)* and platelets.
Identify terms in this frame that mean

formation or production of white blood cells:

_____ / _____ / _____

formation or production of red blood cells:

_____ / _____ / _____

---

chondr/itis
kŏn-DRĪ-tĭs

chondr/oma
kŏn-DRŌ-mă

chondr/o/genesis
kŏn-drō-JĔN-ĕ-sĭs

10–26 Cartilage, which is more elastic than bone, composes parts of the skeleton. It is found chiefly in the joints, thorax, trachea, and nose.
Use **chondr/o** *(cartilage)* to form words that mean

inflammation of cartilage: _____ / _____

tumor composed of cartilage: _____ / _____

producing or forming cartilage:

_____ / _____ / _____

---

chondr/o/cyte
KŎN-drō-sīt

10–27 Use *-cyte* to build a word that means *cartilage cell.*

_____ / _____ / _____

Competency Verification: Check your labeling of Figure 10–4 in Appendix B, Answer Key, page 578.

---

oste/o/dynia
ŏs-tē-ō-DĬN-ē-ă

10–28 *Oste/algia* means pain in a bone. Form another term that means pain in a bone.

_____ / _____ / _____

---

oste/o/cytes
ŎS-tē-ō-sītz

10–29 Bone is living tissue composed of oste/o/cytes, blood vessels, and nerves.
Determine the medical term for *bone cells.*

_____ / _____ / _____

oste/itis ŏs-tē-Ī-tĭs **oste/o/pathy** ŏs-tē-ŎP-ă-thē **oste/o/tomy** ŏs-tē-ŎT-ō-mē **oste/o/rrhaphy** ŏs-tē-OR-ă-fē **oste/o/scler/osis** ŏs-tē-ō-sklĕ-RŌ-sĭs	**10–30** Practice developing medical words that mean *inflammation of bone:* _____ / _____ *disease of bone:* _____ / _____ / _____ *incision of bone:* _____ / _____ / _____ *suture of bone (wiring of bone fragments):* _____ / _____ / _____ *abnormal condition of bone hardening:* _____ / _____ / _____ / _____
dist/o	**10–31** *Dist/al* is a directional word that means *farthest from the point of attachment to the trunk,* or *far from the beginning of a structure.* From *dist/al,* build the CF that means *far* or *farthest.* _____ / _____
proxim/o	**10–32** *Proxim/al* is a directional word that means *near the point of attachment to the trunk,* or *near the beginning of a structure.* From *proxim/al,* build the CF that means *near or nearest.* _____ / _____
farthest from **nearest to**	**10–33** To complete this frame, use the words *farthest from* or *nearest to.* The dist/al epiphysis is located _____ _____ the trunk. The proxim/al epiphysis is located _____ _____ the trunk.
oste/o/malacia ŏs-tē-ō-mă-LĀ-shē-ă **oste/o/genesis** ŏs-tē-ō-JĔN-ĕ-sĭs	**10–34** Milk is a good source of vitamin D. Deficiency of this vitamin results in a softening and weakening of the skeleton, causing pain and bowing of the bones. Construct medical terms that mean *softening of bones:* _____ / _____ / _____ *producing or forming bone:* _____ / _____ / _____
oste/o/malacia ŏs-tē-ō-mă-LĀ-shē-ă	**10–35** Oste/o/malacia is the result of inadequate amounts of phosphorus and calcium in blood for mineralization of the bones. It may be caused by a diet lacking these minerals, deficiency in vitamin D, or a metabolic disorder that causes malabsorption of minerals. The medical term that means *softening of bones* is _____ / _____ / _____.

oste/o/malacia ŏs-tē-ō-mă-LĀ-shē-ă	**10-36** A form of oste/o/malacia known as *rickets* is seen in infants and children in many underdeveloped countries. It is a result of vitamin D deficiency. Symptoms of rickets include soft, pliable bones that cause such deformities as bowlegs and knock-knees. Rickets is another name for _____ / _____ / _____.
oste/o/malacia ŏs-tē-ō-mă-LĀ-shē-ă	**10-37** Rickets is marked by an abnormality in the shapes of bones and is a form of _____ / _____ / _____.
rickets RĬK-ĕts	**10-38** Calcium provides bone strength that is needed for its supportive functions. Many children in underdeveloped countries have rickets because of inadequate milk supply. When oste/o/malacia occurs in children, it is called _____.
calc/emia kăl-SĒ-mē-ă	**10-39** Combine **calc/o** and *-emia* to form a word that means *calcium in the blood*. _____ / _____
under, below, deficient	**10-40** Recall that *hypo-* means _____, _____, _____.
hyper/calc/emia hī-pĕr-kăl-SĒ-mē-ă	**10-41** Hypo/calc/emia is a deficiency of calcium in the blood. The term that means *excessive amount of calcium in the blood* is _____ / _____ / _____.
radi/o/logist rā-dē-ŎL-ō-jĭst	**10-42** Radi/o/logy, initially widely called *roentgen/o/logy,* was developed after discovery of an unknown ray in 1895 by Wilhelm Roentgen, who called his discovery a roentgen (x-ray). Occasionally you still may see words with **roentgen/o**, but **radi/o** is the preferred term used in the context of medical imaging today. *Radi/o/logy* is the branch of medicine concerned with radioactive substances. It is used to diagnose path/o/log/ical conditions of the skeletal system. A physician who specializes in the study of x-rays is called a _____ / _____ / _____.
radi/o/therapy rā-dē-ō-THĔR-ă-pē	**10-43** Radiation is used for diagnostic and therapeutic purposes. Radiation therapy, also called *radi/o/therapy,* is treatment of diseases using either an external source of high-energy rays or internally implanted radioactive substances. These rays and substances are effective in damaging cancer cells and halting their growth. Treatment of disease using radiation is called _____ / _____ / _____.

radi/o/logist rā-dē-ŎL-ō-jĭst	**10–44** Combine *radi/o* + *-logist* to build a word that means *specialist in the study of x-rays.* _____ / ____ / _____
muscle, bone marrow; spinal cord	**10–45** Although *my/o* and *myel/o* sound alike, they have different meanings. *My/o* refers to _____. *Myel/o* refers to _____ _____ or _____ _____.

10–46 Find three words that contain *myel/o* in your medical dictionary and write brief definitions in the spaces provided.

Term	Meaning
_____	_____
	_____
_____	_____
	_____
_____	_____

myel/o	**10–47** A myel/o/gram is a radi/o/graph of the spin/al cord after injection of a contrast medium. The CF for *bone marrow* and *spinal cord* is _____ / ____.
myel/o/genesis mī-ĕ-lō-JĔN-ĕ-sĭs	**10–48** Use *-genesis* to build a word that means *formation of bone marrow.* _____ / ____ / _____
myel/o/malacia mī-ĕl-ō-mă-LĀ-shē-ă **myel/o/gram** MĪ-ĕl-ō-grăm	**10–49** Develop medical words that mean *softening of the spinal cord:* _____ / ____ / _____ *record of the spinal cord:* _____ / ____ / _____
myel/o/gram MĪ-ĕl-ō-grăm	**10–50** A myel/o/gram, a radiograph of the spinal canal after injection of a contrast medium, is used to identify and study spinal lesions caused by trauma or disease. To identify any distortions of the spinal cord, the physician may order a radiograph called a _____ / ____ / _____.

SECTION REVIEW 10-4

Using the following table, write the CF, suffix, or prefix that matches its definition in the space provided to the left of the definition. There may be more than one word element that matches a definition.

Combining Forms		Suffixes		Prefixes
calc/o	radi/o	-algia	-graphy	hyper-
chondr/o	scler/o	-cele	-itis	hypo-
dist/o		-cyte	-logist	peri-
my/o		-dynia	-malacia	
myel/o		-emia	-oma	
oste/o		-genesis	-rrhaphy	
proxim/o		-gram	-tomy	

1. _____ excessive, above normal
2. _____ around
3. _____ blood condition
4. _____ bone
5. _____ cartilage
6. _____ calcium
7. _____ cell
8. _____ far, farthest
9. _____ hardening; sclera (white of eye)
10. _____ hernia, swelling
11. _____ incision
12. _____ inflammation
13. _____ near, nearest
14. _____ muscle

15. _____ pain
16. _____ process of recording
17. _____ forming, producing, origin
18. _____ record, writing
19. _____ softening
20. _____ specialist in study of
21. _____ bone marrow; spinal cord
22. _____ suture
23. _____ tumor
24. _____ under, below, deficient
25. _____ radiation, x-ray; radius (lower arm bone on thumb side)

Competency Verification: Check your answers in Appendix B, Answer Key, page 578. If you are not satisfied with your level of comprehension, go back to Frame 10–1 and rework the frames.

Correct Answers _____ × 4 = _____ % Score

Joints

synarthroses sĭn-ăhr-THRŌ-sēz **diarthroses** dī-ăhr-THRŌ-sēz **amphiarthroses** ăm-fē-ăr-THRŌ-sēz	**10–51** To allow for body movements, bones must have points where they meet *(articulate)*. These articulating points form joints that have various degrees of mobility. Some are freely movable *(diarthroses)*, others are only slightly movable *(amphiarthroses)*, and the remaining are totally immovable *(synarthroses)*. All three types are necessary for smooth, coordinated body movements. Use the information above to identify and pronounce the following types of joints. totally immovable joints: _____ freely movable joints: _____ slightly movable joints: _____
arthr/o/pathy ăr-THRŎP-ă-thē **arthr/itis** ăr-THRĪ-tĭs **arthr/o/centesis** ăr-thrō-sĕn-TĒ-sĭs	**10–52** Use *arthr/o* *(joint)* to develop medical words that mean *disease of a joint:* _____ / _____ / _____ *inflammation of a joint:* _____ / _____ *surgical puncture of a joint:* _____ / _____ / _____
arthr/o/scope ĂR-thrō-skōp	**10–53** Arthr/o/scopy is the visual examination of the interior of a joint performed by inserting an endo/scope through a small incision. Arthr/o/scopy is performed to repair and remove joint tissue, especially of the knee, ankle, and shoulder. (See Figure 10–5.) The endo/scope used to perform arthr/o/scopy is called an _____ / _____ / _____.
arthr/o/plasty ĂR-thrō-plăs-tē	**10–54** Total hip arthr/o/plasty is a surgical procedure to replace the femur and acetabulum with metal components. The acetabulum is plastic coated to avoid metal-to-metal articulating surfaces. (See Figure 10–6.) Surgical repair of a joint is known as _____ / _____ / _____.
joints	**10–55** Just as a piece of machinery is lubricated by oil, joints are lubricated by synovial fluid. The fluid is secreted within the synovial membranes. Synovial fluid allows free movement of the _____.
arthr/o/centesis ăr-thrō-sĕn-TĒ-sĭs	**10–56** To aspirate or remove accumulated fluid from a joint, a surgical puncture of a joint is performed. This surgical procedure is called _____ / _____ / _____.

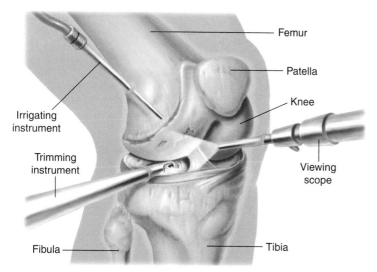

Irrigating instrument

Trimming instrument

Fibula

Femur

Patella

Knee

Viewing scope

Tibia

Figure 10-5 Arthroscopy.

---

arthr/o/dynia
ăr-thrō-DĬN-ē-ă

10–57 A person with arthr/itis suffers, not only from an inflammation of the joints, but also from arthr/algia.
Construct another medical word that means *pain in a joint*.

_____ / _____ / _____

---

arthr/itis
ăr-THRĪ-tĭs

oste/o/arthr/itis
ŏs-tē-ō-ăr-THRĪ-tĭs

10–58 Although there are various forms of arthr/itis, all of them result in an inflammation of the joints. This condition is accompanied by pain and swelling.
Form medical words that mean

inflammation of joints: _____ / _____

inflammation of bones and joints:

_____ / _____ / _____ / _____

---

oste/o/arthr/o/pathy
ŏs-tē-ō-ăr-THRŎP-ă-thē

10–59 A disease of the bones and joints is called

_____ / _____ / _____ / _____ / _____.

---

oste/o/arthr/o
sis
ŏs-tē-ō-ăr-THRŌ-sĭs

10–60 Select element(s) from oste/o/arthr/o/pathy to build a word that means *an abnormal condition of the bones and joints*.

_____ / _____ / _____ / _____

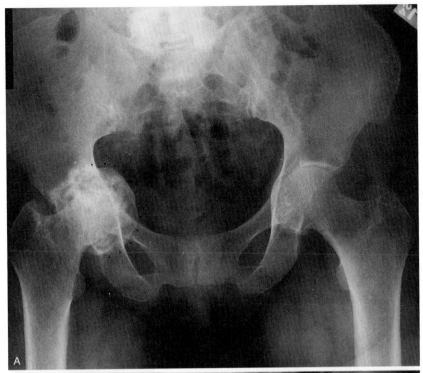

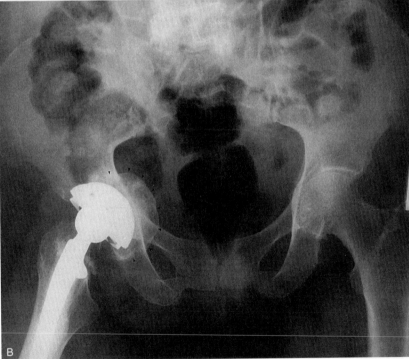

Figure 10-6 Total hip arthroplasty. (A) Arthritis of the right hip. (B) Total hip arthroplasty of arthritic hip. (From McKinnis, LN. *Fundamentals of Orthopedic Radiology.* Philadelphia: FA Davis, page 133, 1997, with permission.

Combining Forms Related to Specific Bones

The CF:

(1) *crani/o* refers to the cranium (skull).

(2) *stern/o* refers to the sternum (breastbone).

(3) *cost/o* refers to the ribs, which are attached to the sternum.

(4) *vertebr/o* refers to the vertebra (backbone). The vertebral column also is called the spinal column and is composed of 26 bones called vertebr/ae.

(5) *humer/o* refers to the humerus (upper arm bone). The humerus articulates with the scapula at the shoulder and with the radius and ulna at the elbow.

(6) *carp/o* refers to the carpus (wrist bones). There are eight wrist bones.

(7) *metacarp/o* refers to the metacarpus (hand bones). The metacarpals (plural) radiate from the wristlike spokes and form the palm of the hand.

(8) *phalang/o* refers to the phalanges (bones of fingers and toes).

(9) *pelv/i and pelv/o* refer to the pelvis. The pelvis, also called the pelvic girdle, is composed of three pairs of fused bones (the ilium, pubis, and ischium), the sacrum, and the coccyx. The pelvis provides attachment for the legs and supports the soft organs of the abdominal cavity (see Figure 10–3).

(10) *femor/o* refers to the femur (thigh bone). The femur is the longest and strongest bone in the body. It articulates with the hip bone and the bones of the lower leg.

(11) *patell/o* refers to the patella (kneecap). The patella articulates with the femur, but essentially is a floating bone. The main function of this bone is to protect the knee joint, but its exposed position makes it vulnerable to dislocation and fracture.

(12) *tibi/o* refers to the tibia (larger bone of lower leg). The tibia is the weight-bearing bone of the lower leg.

(13) *fibul/o* refers to the fibula (smaller bone of lower leg). The fibula is not a weight-bearing bone but is important because muscles are attached and anchored to it.

(14) *calcane/o* refers to the calcaneum (heel bone).

10–61 The word roots of bones are derived from the specific anatomical names of the bones. Learn the CFs for the bones as you label them in Figure 10–7.

Competency Verification: Check your labeling of Figure 10–7 with Appendix B, Answer Key, page 578.

 You are not expected to know the CFs and the names of bones from memory. If needed, you can always refer to Figure 10–7, Appendix A: Glossary of Medical Word Elements, or a medical dictionary to obtain information about a bone or its CF.

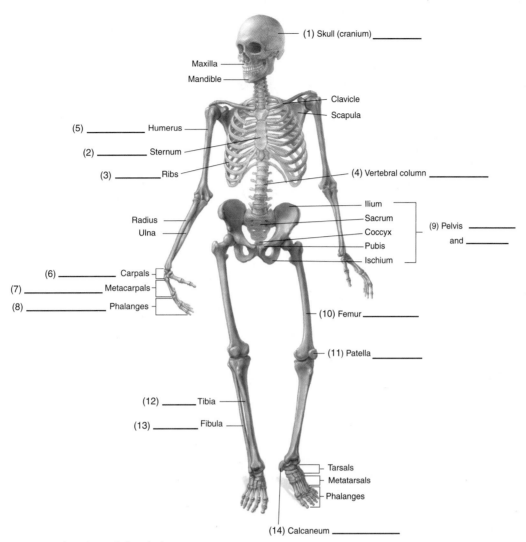

Figure 10-7 Anterior view of the skeleton.

pain, head	**10–62** Words that contain *cephal/o* refer to the *head*. *Cephal/o/dynia* is a _____ in the _____.
cephal/algia sĕf-ă-LĂL-gē-ă	**10–63** *Cephal/o/dynia* is the medical term for a headache. Construct another word that means *pain in the head*. _____ / _____
head **-meter**	**10–64** A meter is a metric unit of length equal to 39.37 inches. However, when used as a suffix *-meter* means *instrument for measuring*. Thus, a *cephal/o/meter* is an instrument for measuring the _____. In *cephal/o/meter,* the element that means *instrument for measuring* is _____.

encephal/o	**10-65** The prefix *en-* means *in, within*. Combine *en-* + **cephal/o** to create a new CF that refers to the brain. _____ / _____
encephal/oma ĕn-sĕf-ă-LŌ-mă **encephal/itis** ĕn-sĕf-ă-LĪ-tĭs **encephal/o/malacia** ĕn-sĕf-ă-lō-mă-LĀ-sē-ă	**10-66** Use *encephal/o* to build words that mean *tumor of the brain:* _____ / _____ *inflammation of the brain:* _____ / _____ *softening of the brain (tissue):* _____ / _____ / _____
encephal/itis ĕn-sĕf-ă-LĪ-tĭs	**10-67** Encephal/itis is usually caused by viruses (for example, *arborvirus, herpes virus*). Less commonly, it may occur as a component of rabies and acquired immune deficiency syndrome (AIDS). It may also occur as a result of systemic viral diseases, such as influenza, rubella, and chickenpox. The medical term for *an inflammatory condition of the brain* is _____ / _____.
disease, brain	**10-68** Encephal/o/pathy is a _____ of the _____.
brain	**10-69** An encephal/o/cele is a protrusion of _____ substance through an opening of the skull.
inter- **cost** **-al**	**10-70** Inter/cost/al muscles, located between the ribs, move the ribs during the breathing process. Write the elements in this frame that mean *between:* _____ *ribs:* _____ *pertaining to:* _____
under *or* below, ribs	**10-71** *Sub/cost/al* refers to the area _____ the _____.
pain, rib	**10-72** *Cost/algia* is a _____ in a _____.

Fractures and Repairs

10-73 A fracture is a break or crack in the bone. Fractures are defined according to the type and extent of the break. A (1) **closed fracture** means the bone is broken with no open wound, and surrounding tissue damage is minimal. An (2) **open fracture**, also called a *compound fracture*, means the broken end of a bone pierces the skin, creating an open wound. In such a fracture, there may be extensive damage to surrounding blood vessels, nerves, and muscles. Label the closed and open fractures in Figure 10–8.

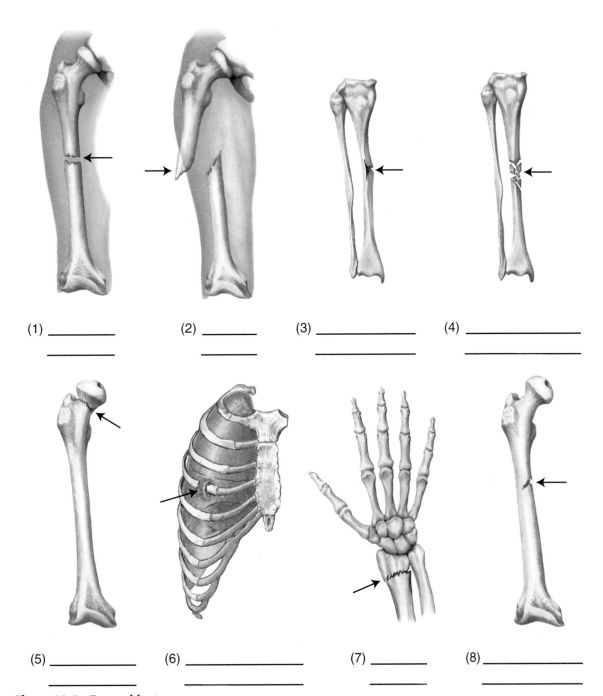

(1) _____
_____

(2) _____
_____

(3) _____
_____

(4) _____
_____

(5) _____
_____

(6) _____
_____

(7) _____
_____

(8) _____
_____

Figure 10-8   Types of fractures.

10-74 In addition to determining the extent of a break in a fracture, there are many different types of bone fractures, some of which are discussed here. A (3) **greenstick fracture** means there is an incomplete break of a soft bone, which means the bone is partially bent and partially broken. These fractures usually occur in children because their growing bones are soft and tend to splinter, rather than break completely. A (4) **comminuted fracture** occurs when the bone is broken into pieces. In an (5) **impacted fracture**, the broken ends of a bone are forced into one another; many bone fragments may be created by such a fracture. A (6) **complicated fracture** involves extensive soft tissue injury, such as when a broken rib pierces a lung. A (7) **Colles fracture** is a break of the lower end of the radius, which occurs just above the wrist. It causes displacement of the hand and usually occurs as a result of flexing a hand to cushion a fall. An (8) **incomplete fracture** is when the line of fracture does not include the whole bone. Label and study the different types of fractures in Figure 10–8.

Competency Verification: Check your labeling of Figure 10–8 in Appendix B, Answer Key, page 578.

open fracture, compound fracture **closed fracture**	**10-75** Refer to Figure 10–8 to identify the following fractures. A bone pierces the skin and causes extensive damage to surrounding blood vessels: _____ _____, also called _____ _____ A bone is broken with no external wound present: _____ _____
greenstick fracture **impacted fracture** ĭm-PĂK-tĕd	**10-76** Refer to Figure 10–8 to identify the following fractures. A bone is partially bent and partially broken (found more commonly in children): _____ _____ The broken ends of bone segments are wedged into one another: _____ _____

Vertebral Column

spin/al column SPĪ-năl **spin/o**	**10-77** The vertebr/al or spin/al column supports the body and provides a protective bony canal for the spinal cord. (See Figure 10–9.) Another name for the vertebr/al column is _____ / _____ _____. From the word *spin/al*, construct the CF for *spine*. _____ / _____
vertebra VĔR-tĕ-bră	**10-78** *Spondyl/o* and *vertebr/o* are CFs that refer to the vertebrae (backbone). The singular form of *vertebrae* is _____.
vertebra VĔR-tĕ-bră **vertebra** VĔR-tĕ-bră	**10-79** *Vertebr/ectomy* is an excision of a _____. *Spondyl/o/dynia* is a painful condition of a _____.

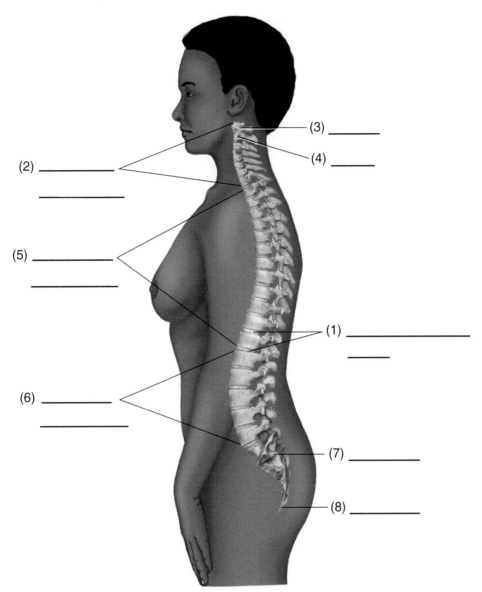

Figure 10-9 Vertebral column, lateral view, with regions of the spine shown with normal curves.

10–80 Change the following words from singular to plural form by retaining the *a* and adding an *e*.

Singular	**Plural**
vertebra	_____
bursa	_____
pleura	_____

vertebrae
VĔR-tĕ-brē
bursae
BĔR-sē
pleurae
PLOO-rē

spondyl/itis
spŏn-dĭl-Ī-tĭs

spondyl/o/pathy
spŏn-dĭl-ŎP-ă-thē

spondyl/o/malacia
spŏn-dĭl-ō-mă-LĀ-shē-ă

10–81 *Spondyl/o* is used to form words about the condition of a structure.
Build medical words that mean

inflammation of vertebrae: _____ / _____

disease of vertebrae: _____ / _____ / _____

softening of vertebrae: _____ / _____ / _____

---

vertebra, vertebra
VĔR-tĕ-bră

10–82 *Vertebr/o* is used to form words that describe the vertebral structure. For example, *vertebr/o/cost/al* means *pertaining to a* _____ *and a rib. Vertebr/o/stern/al* means *pertaining to a* _____ *and the sternum or chest plate.*

10–83 Vertebrae are separate and cushioned from each other by (1) **intervertebral disks** composed of cartilage. Label Figure 10–9 as you learn about the vertebr/al or spin/al column.

---

inter-

vertebr/o

-al

10–84 Determine the elements in *inter/vertebr/al* that mean

between: _____

vertebrae (backbone): _____ / _____

pertaining to: _____

10–85 The vertebr/al column, also called the *spin/al column* or *backbone,* is composed of 26 bones known as *vertebrae* (singular, *vertebra*). There are five regions of these bones in the vertebr/al column, each of which derives its name from its location along the length of the spin/al column. Seven (2) **cervical vertebrae** form the skeletal framework of the neck. The first cervic/al vertebra is called the (3) **atlas** and supports the skull. The second, the (4) **axis,** enables the skull to rotate on the neck. Label these structures in Figure 10–9.

---

neck

10–86 The CF *cervic/o* means *neck; cervix uteri (neck of the uterus). Cervic/o/facial* refers to the face and _____.

---

atlas
ĂT-lăs

cervic/al
SĔR-vi-kăl

10–87 The name of the first cervic/al vertebra is the _____.

A term that means *pertaining to the neck* is

_____ / _____.

C5 *or* **C₅**	**10-88** In medical reports, the first cervical vertebra is designated as *C1*, or C₁. The fifth cervical vertebra is designated as _____.
C5 *or* **C₅**	**10-89** A diagnosis of C4 to C5 herniation means the cervic/al disk between C4 and _____ is ruptured or herniated.
C2 *or* **C₂**	**10-90** The second vertebra is identified as _____.
seven	**10-91** There are a total of _____ cervic/al vertebrae.
	10-92 Twelve (5) **thoracic vertebrae** support the chest and serve as a point of articulation (joining together to allow motion between parts) for the ribs. The next five vertebrae are the (6) **lumbar vertebrae**. These are situated in the lower back and carry most of the weight of the torso. Label these structures in Figure 10-9.
articulation ăr-tĭk-ū-LĀ-shŭn **thorac/ic** thō-RĂS-ĭk	**10-93** Identify the terms in Frame 10-92 that mean *a place where two bones meet:* _____ *pertaining to the chest:* _____ / _____
pertaining to, back	**10-94** The CF *lumb/o* refers to the *loins (lower back)*. *Lumb/ar* means _____ _____ the loin or lower _____.
pain	**10-95** *Lumb/o/dynia* is a _____ in the lower back.
lumbar, five LŬM-băr	**10-96** Examine the position of the five lumbar vertebrae in Figure 10-9. These are designated as L1 to L5 in medical reports. An obese person with weak abdominal muscles tends to experience pain in the lower back area, or L1 to L5. *L5* refers to _____ vertebra _____.
	10-97 Below the lumbar vertebrae are five **sacral vertebrae** that are fused into a single bone in the adult. The single bone is known as the (7) *sacrum* and the tail of the vertebral column, the (8) *coccyx*. Label the sacrum and coccyx in Figure 10-9.

pain **sacr/um, spine** SĀ-krŭm	**10–98** The CF **sacr/o** means *sacr/um*. The suffix in the term *sacr/um* means *structure,thing*. *Sacr/o/dynia* is a _____ in the sacrum. *Sacr/o/spin/al* refers to the _____ / _____ and _____.
S5 *or* **S₅**	**10–99** To designate the exact position of abnormalities on the sacrum, the label *S1* to *S5* is used. The first vertebra of the sacrum is designated as *S1*. The fifth vertebra of the sacrum is designated as _____.
lumbar, sacrum LŬM-băr, SĀ-krŭm	**10–100** A ruptured disk can cause severe pain, muscle weakness, or numbness in either leg. The disk that most commonly ruptures is the L5 to S1 disk. *L5* refers to _____ five. *S1* refers to _____ one.

Competency Verification: Check your labeling of Figure 10–9 in Appendix B, Answer Key, page 578.

S E C T I O N   R E V I E W   10-5

Using the following table, write the CF or suffix that matches its definition in the space provided to the left of the definition. There may be more than one word element that matches a definition.

Combining Forms		Suffixes
arthr/o	oste/o	-centesis
cephal/o	sacr/o	-ectomy
cervic/o	spondyl/o	-osis
cost/o	thorac/o	-pathy
encephal/o	vertebr/o	-um
lumb/o		

1. _____ abnormal condition; increase (used primarily with blood cells)
2. _____ bone
3. _____ brain
4. _____ chest
5. _____ disease
6. _____ excision, removal
7. _____ head
8. _____ joint
9. _____ loins (lower back)
10. _____ neck; cervix uteri (neck of uterus)
11. _____ structure, thing
12. _____ ribs
13. _____ sacrum
14. _____ surgical puncture
15. _____ vertebra (backbone)

Competency Verification: Check your answers in Appendix B, Answer Key, page 578. If you are not satisfied with your level of comprehension, go back to Frame 10–51 and rework the frames.

Correct Answers _____ × 6.67 = _____ % Score

Abbreviations

This section introduces musculoskeletal system-related abbreviations and their meanings. Included are abbreviations contained in the medical record activities.

Abbreviation	Meaning	Abbreviation	Meaning
AE	above the elbow	HNP	herniated nucleus pulposus (herniated disk)
AIDS	acquired immune deficiency syndrome	IM	intramuscular
AK	above the knee	L1, L2, to L5	first lumbar vertebra, second lumbar vertebra, and so on
AP	anteroposterior	MG	myasthenia gravis
BE	below the elbow	ORTH, Ortho	orthopedics
BK	below the knee	RA	rheumatoid arthritis
C1, C2, to C7	first cervical vertebra, second cervical vertebra, and so on	S1, S2, to S5	first sacral vertebra, second sacral vertebra, and so on
CT	computed tomography	THR	total hip replacement
CTS	carpal tunnel syndrome	T1, T2, to T12	first thoracic vertebra, second thoracic vertebra, and so on
Fx	fracture	TKR	total knee replacement
HD	hemodialysis; hip disarticulation; hearing distance		

Additional Medical Terms

The following are additional terms related to the musculoskeletal system. Recognizing and learning these terms will help you understand the connection between a pathological condition, its diagnosis, and the rationale behind the method of treatment selected for a particular disorder.

Signs, Symptoms, and Diseases

Muscular Disorders

muscular dystrophy
MŬS-kū-lăr DĬS-trō-fē
muscul: muscle
  -ar: pertaining to
  dys-: bad; painful; difficult
  -trophy: development, nourishment
	Group of hereditary diseases characterized by gradual atrophy and weakness of muscle tissue
	There is no cure for muscular dystrophy, Duchenne dystrophy is the most common form with an average lifespan of 20 yrs.

myasthenia gravis (MG) mī-ăs-THĒ-nē-ă GRĂV-ĭs	Autoimmune neuromuscular disorder characterized by severe muscular weakness and progressive fatigue
rotator cuff injuries	Injuries to the capsule of the shoulder joint, which is reinforced by muscles and tendons; also called *musculotendinous rotator cuff injuries* *Rotator cuff injuries occur in sports in which there is a complete abduction of the shoulder, followed by a rapid and forceful rotation and flexion of the shoulder. (See Figure 10–2.) This type of injury occurs most commonly in baseball injuries when the player throws a baseball.*
sprain	Trauma to a joint that causes injury to the surrounding ligament, accompanied by pain and disability
strain	Trauma to a muscle from overuse or excessive forcible stretch
talipes equinovarus TĂL-ĭ-pēz ē-kwī-nō-VĀR-ŭs	Congenital deformity of the foot; also called *clubfoot* (See Figure 10–10.) *In talipes, the heel never rests on the ground. Treatment consists of applying casts to progressively straighten the foot and surgical correction for severe cases.*
tendinitis tĕn-dĭn-Ī-tĭs	Inflammation of a tendon, usually caused by injury or overuse; also called *tendonitis*
torticollis tōr-tĭ-KŎL-ĭs	Spasmodic contraction of the neck muscles, causing stiffness and twisting of the neck; also called *wryneck* *Torticollis may be congenital or acquired.*

Bones and Joints

carpal tunnel syndrome (CTS) KĂR-păl TŬN-ĕl SĬN-drōm	Pain or numbness resulting from compression of the median nerve within the carpal tunnel (wrist canal through which the flexor tendons and median nerve pass)

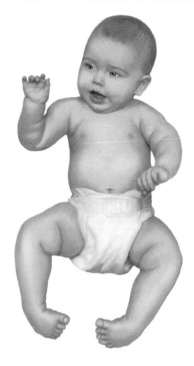

Figure 10-10   Talipes equinovarus.

contracture kŏn-TRĂK-chŭr	Fibrosis of connective tissue in the skin, fascia, muscle, or joint capsule that prevents normal mobility of the related tissue or joint
crepitation krĕp-ĭ-TĀ-shŭn	Grating sound made by movement of bone ends rubbing together, indicating a fracture or joint destruction
Ewing sarcoma Ū-ĭng săr-KŌ-mă	Malignant tumor that develops from bone marrow, usually in long bones or the pelvis *Ewing sarcoma occurs most commonly in adolescent boys.*
gout GOWT	Hereditary metabolic disease that is a form of acute arthritis, characterized by excessive uric acid in the blood and around the joints
herniated disk HĔR-nē-āt-ĕd	Herniation or rupture of the nucleus pulposus (center gelatinous material within an intervetebral disk) between two vertebrae; also called *prolapsed disk* (See Figure 10–11.) *A herniated disk places pressure on a spinal root nerve or the spinal cord. Displacement of the disk irritates the spinal nerves, causing muscle spasms and pain. It occurs most commonly in the lower spine.*

osteoporosis
ŏs-tē-ō-pōr-Ō-sĭs
  oste/o: bone
  -porosis: porous
	Decrease in bone density with an increase in porosity, causing bones to become brittle and increasing the risk of fractures

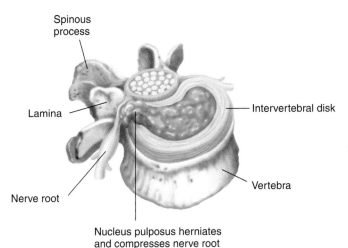

Figure 10-11 Herniated disk.

Paget disease PĂJ-ĕt dĭ-ZĒZ	Skeletal disease affecting elderly people that causes chronic inflammation of bones, resulting in thickening and softening of bones and bowing of long bones; also called *osteitis deformans*
rheumatoid arthritis (RA) ROO-mă-toyd ăr-THRĪ-tĭs *arthr:* joint *-itis:* inflammation	Chronic, systemic inflammatory disease affecting the synovial membranes of multiple joints, eventually resulting in crippling deformities (See Figure 10–12.) *As RA develops, there is congestion and edema of the synovial membrane and joint, causing formation of a thick layer of granulation tissue. This tissue invades cartilage, destroying the joint and bone. Eventually, a fibrous immobility of joints (ankylosis) occurs, causing visible derformities and total immobility.*
subluxation sŭb-lŭk-SĀ-shŭn	Partial or complete dislocation

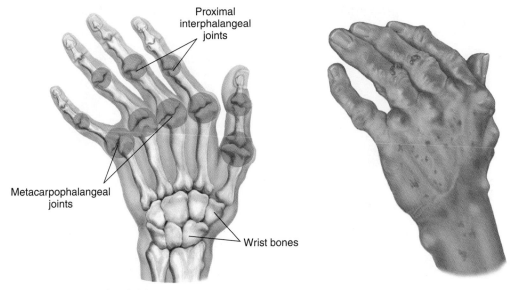

Figure 10-12 Rheumatoid arthritis.

sequestrum sē-KWĔS-trŭm	Fragment of a necrosed bone that has become separated from surrounding tissue

Spinal Disorders

ankylosing spondylitis ăng-kĭ-LŌS-ĭng spŏn-dĭl-Ī-tĭs *spondyl/o:* vertebra (backbone) *-itis:* inflammation	Chronic inflammatory disease of unknown origin that first affects the spine and is characterized by fusion and loss of mobility of two or more vertebrae; also called *rheumatoid spondylitis* *Treatment includes nonsteroidal anti-inflammatory drugs and, in advanced cases of a badly deformed spine, surgery.*
kyphosis kī-FŌ-sĭs *kyph:* humpback *-osis:* abnormal condition; increase (used primarily with blood cells)	Increased curvature of the thoracic region of the vertebral column, leading to a humpback posture; also called *hunchback* *Kyphosis may be caused by poor posture, arthritis, or osteomalacia. (See Figure 10–13.)*

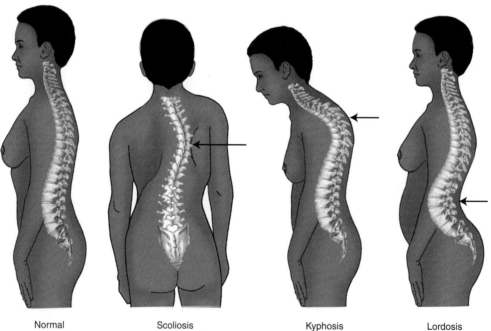

Normal   Scoliosis   Kyphosis   Lordosis

Figure 10-13 Spinal curvatures.

lordosis lōr-DŌ-sĭs *lord:* curve, swayback *-osis:* abnormal condition; increase (used primarily with blood cells)	Forward curvature of lumbar region of the vertebral column, leading to a swayback posture *Lordosis may be caused by increased weight in the abdomen, such as during pregnancy. (See Figure 10–13.)*
scoliosis skō-lē-Ō-sĭs *scoli:* crooked, bent *-osis:* abnormal condition; increase (used primarily with blood cells)	Abnormal sideward curvature of the spine to the left or right *Scoliosis eventually causes back pain, disk disease, or arthritis. It is commonly a congenital disease, but may result from poor posture. (See Figure 10–13.)*
spondylolisthesis spŏn-dĭ-lō-lĭs-THĒ-sĭs *spondyl/o:* vertebra (backbone) *-listhesis:* slipping	Partial forward dislocation of one vertebra over the one below it, most commonly the fifth lumbar vertebra over the first sacral vertebra; also called *spinal cord compression*

Diagnostic Procedures

arthrocentesis ăr-thrō-sĕn-TĒ-sĭs *arthr/o:* joint *-centesis:* surgical puncture	Puncture of a joint space with a needle to remove fluid *Arthrocentesis is performed to obtain samples of synovial fluid for diagnostic purposes. It may also be used to instill medications and remove accumulated fluid from joints to relieve pain.*
rheumatoid factor ROO-mă-toyd	Blood test to detect the presence of rheumatoid factor, a substance present in patients with rheumatoid arthritis

Medical and Surgical Procedures

arthroplasty ĂR-thrō-plăs-tē *arthr/o:* joint *-plasty:* surgical repair	Surgical reconstruction or replacement of a painful, degenerated joint to restore mobility in rheumatoid or osteoarthritis or to correct a congenital deformity (See Figure 10–6.)

sequestrectomy sē-kwĕs-TRĔK-tō-mē *sequestr:* separation *-ectomy:* excision, removal	Excision of a sequestrum (segment of necrosed bone)

Pharmacology

bone reabsorption inhibitors	Agents that reduce the reabsorption of bone in the treatment of weak and fragile bones as seen in osteoporosis and Paget disease
gold salts	Agents that treat rheumatoid arthritis by inhibiting activity within the immune system by preventing further disease progression
nonsteroidal anti-inflammatory drugs (NSAIDs) nŏn-STĔR-oyd-ăl ăn-tē-ĭn-FLĂM-ă-tō-rē	Drugs that relieve mild to moderate pain and reduce inflammation in treatment of musculoskeletal conditions, such as sprains and strains, and inflammatory disorders, including rheumatoid arthritis, osteoarthritis, bursitis, gout, and tendinitis

Additional Medical Terms Review

Match the medical term(s) below with the definitions in the numbered list.

ankylosis	Ewing sarcoma	myasthenia gravis	sequestrectomy	torticollis
arthroplasty	gout	osteoporosis	sequestrum	
arthroscopy	herniated disk	Paget disease	sprain	
contracture	kyphosis	RA	strain	
crepitation	lordosis	rheumatoid factor	talipes	
CTS	muscular dystrophy	scoliosis	tendinitis	

1. _____ means decrease in bone density and an increase in porosity, causing the risk of fractures.

2. _____ means inflammation of a tendon.

3. _____ refers to trauma to a joint, causing injury to the surrounding ligament.

4. _____ refers to trauma to a muscle that results from overuse or excessive, forcible stretch.

5. _____ means hunchback or humpback.

6. _____ is a malignant tumor that develops from bone marrow, usually in long bones or the pelvis, and occurs most commonly in adolescent boys.

7. _____ means wryneck.

8. _____ is a disease characterized by excessive uric acid in the blood and around the joints.

9. _____ is a disease characterized by inflammatory changes in joints and related structures that result in crippling deformities.

10. _____ is a skeletal disease of the elderly with chronic inflammation of bones, resulting in thickening and softening of bones and bowing of long bones; also called _osteitis deformans._

11. _____ is a fragment of necrosed bone that has become separated from surrounding tissue.

12. _____ means replacement of a joint.

13. _____ is a grating sound made by the ends of bone rubbing together.

14. _____ is a neuromuscular disorder characterized by muscular weakness and progressive fatigue.

15. _____ means forward curvature of the lumbar spine; also called _swayback._

16. _____ refers to a group of hereditary diseases characterized by gradual atrophy and weakness of muscle; the most common form is called _Duchenne._

17. _____ is connective tissue fibrosis that prevents normal mobility of the related tissue or joint.

18. _____ means immobility of a joint.

19. _____ refers to rupture of the nucleus pulposus between two vertebrae.

20. _____ is pain or numbness resulting from compression of the median nerve within the carpal tunnel.

21. _____ is excision of a necrosed piece of bone.

22. _____ is a blood test to detect a substance present in the blood of patients with rheumatoid arthritis.

23. _____ is a congenital foot deformity; also called _clubfoot._

24. _____ means visual examination of a joint.

25. _____ is abnormal sideward curvature of the spine to the left or right.

Competency Verification: Check your answers in Appendix B, Answer Key, page 579. If you are not satisfied with your level of comprehension, review the additional medical terms and retake the review.

Correct Answers _____ × 4 = _____ % Score

Medical Record Activities

Medical reports included in the following activities reflect common, real-life clinical scenarios using medical terminology to document patient care.

MEDICAL RECORD ACTIVITY 10-1

Degenerative, Intervertebral Disk Disease

Terminology

Terms listed in the table below come from the medical report *Degenerative, Intervertebral Disk Disease* that follows. Use a medical dictionary such as Taber's *Cyclopedic Medical Dictionary,* the appendices of this book, or other resources to define each term. Then practice reading the pronunciations aloud for each term.

Term	Definition
anteroposterior ăn-tĕr-ō-pŏs-TĒ-rē-ŏr	
bilateral bī-LĂT-ĕr-ăl	
degenerative dĕ-JĔN-ĕr-ă-tĭv	
hypertrophic hī-pĕr-TRŌF-ĭk	
intervertebral ĭn-tĕr-VĔRT-ĕ-brăl	
L5	
laminectomies lăm-ĭ-NĔK-tĕ-mēz	
lateral views LĂT-ĕr-ăl	
lipping LĬP-ĭng	
lumbar LŬM-băr	
lumbosacral lŭm-bō-SĀ-krăl	
S1	

Term	Definition
sacroiliac sā-krō-ĬL-ē-ăk	_____
sacrum SĀ-krŭm	_____

 Listen and Learn Online! will help you master pronunciations of selected medical words from this medical record activity. Visit _http://davisplus.fadavis.com/gylys/simplified_ to find instructions on completing the _Listen and Learn Online!_ exercise for this section and to practice pronunciations.

Reading

Practice pronunciation of medical terms by reading the following medical report aloud.

Degenerative, Intervertebral Disk Disease

Anteroposterior and lateral views of the lumbar spine and an AP view of the sacrum show a displacement of L5 on S1. The L5-S1 intervertebral disk space contains a slight shadow of decreased density. There is now slight narrowing of the L3-L4 and L4-L5. Bilateral laminectomies appear to have been done at L5-S1. Slight hypertrophic lipping of the upper lumbar vertebral bodies is now seen, as is slight lipping of the upper margin of the body of L4. The sacroiliac joint spaces are well preserved. Lateral views of the lumbosacral spine taken with the spine in flexion and extension show slight motion at all of the lumbar and lumbosacral levels.

IMPRESSION: 1. Degenerative, intervertebral disk disease at L5-S1, now also accompanied by slight narrowing of the L3-L4 and L4-L5.
2. Slight motion at all of the lumbar and lumbosacral levels.

Evaluation

Review the medical report above to answer the following questions. Use a medical dictionary such as _Taber's Cyclopedic Medical Dictionary_ and other resources if needed.

1. Why does the x-ray show a decreased density at L5-S1?

_____

_____

2. What is the most common cause of degenerative intervertebral disk disease?

_____

_____

3. What happens to the gelatinous material of the disk as aging occurs?

_____

_____

4. What is the probable cause of the narrowing of the L3-L4 and L4-L5?

_____

_____

Rotator Cuff Tear, Right Shoulder

Terminology

Terms listed in the table below come from the medical report *Rotator Cuff Tear, Right Shoulder* that follows. Use a medical dictionary such as *Taber's Cyclopedic Medical Dictionary,* the appendices of this book, or other resources to define each term. Then practice reading the pronunciations aloud for each term.

Term	Definition
AC joint	
acromial ăk-RŌ-mē-ăl	
acromioclavicular ă-krō-mē-ō-klă-VĬK-ū-lăr	
arthritis ăr-THRĪ-tĭs	
arthroscopy ăr-THRŎS-kō-pē	
biceps BĪ-sĕps	
bursectomy bŭr-SĔK-tō-mē	
calcification kăl-sĭ-fĭ-KĀ-shŭn	
degenerative dĕ-JĔN-ĕr-ă-tĭv	
glenohumeral glē-nō-HŪ-mĕr-ăl	
glenoid GLĒ-noyd	
gouty GOW-tē	
intra-articular ĭn-tră-ăr-TĬK-ū-lăr	
labra (singular, *labrum*) LĂ-bră	

Term	Definition
osteoarthritis ŏs-tē-ō-ăr-THRĪ-tĭs	_____
osteophyte ŎS-tē-ō-fīt	_____
spur spŭr	_____
subacromial sŭb-ă-KRŌ-mē-ăl	_____
tendinitis tĕn-dĭn-Ī-tĭs	_____
tuberosity tū-bĕr-ŎS-ĭ-tē	_____

Listen and Learn Online! will help you master pronunciations of selected medical words from this medical record activity. Visit *http://davisplus.fadavis.com/gylys/simplified* to find instructions on completing the *Listen and Learn Online!* exercise for this section and to practice pronunciations.

Reading

Practice pronunciation of medical terms by reading the following medical report aloud.

Rotator Cuff Tear, Right Shoulder

PREOPERATIVE DIAGNOSIS: Rotator cuff tear, right shoulder. Degenerative arthritis, right acromioclavicular joint. Calcific tendinitis at the level of the superior glenoid tuberosity, right shoulder. Early degenerative osteoarthritis of the right shoulder. History of gouty arthritis.

POSTOPERATIVE DIAGNOSIS: Rotator cuff tear, right shoulder. Degenerative arthritis, right acromioclavicular joint. Calcific tendinitis at the level of the superior glenoid tuberosity, right shoulder. Early degenerative osteoarthritis of the right shoulder. History of gouty arthritis.

OPERATION: Open repair of rotator cuff, open incision outer end of clavicle, anterior acromioplasty, glenohumeral and subacromial arthroscopy with arthroscopic bursectomy.

FINDINGS: A glenohumeral arthroscopy revealed the superior, anterior, inferior, and posterior glenoid labra were intact. There was some fraying of the anterior glenoid labrum. The long head of the biceps was intact. We were unable to visualize any intraarticular calcification. We observed the takeoff of the long head of the biceps from the posterior-superior edge of the glenoid labrum and the glenoid tuberosity. There was an osteophyte inferiorly on the humeral head. There was a deep surface tear of the rotator cuff at the posterior-superior corner of the greater tuberosity of the humerus at the infraspinatus insertion. There was an extremely dense subacromial bursal scar. There was prominence of the inferior edge of the AC joint, with inferior AC joint and anterior acromial spurs.

Evaluation

Review the medical report above to answer the following questions. Use a medical dictionary such as *Taber's Cyclopedic Medical Dictionary* and other resources if needed.

1. What type of arthritis did the patient have?

   _____

   _____

2. Did the patient have calcium deposits in the right shoulder?

   _____

   _____

3. What type of instrument did the physician use to visualize the glenoid labra?

   _____

   _____

4. What are labra?

   _____

   _____

5. Did the patient have any outgrowths of bone? If so, where?

   _____

   _____

6. Did they find any deposits of calcium salts within the shoulder joint?

   _____

   _____

Chapter Review

Word Elements Summary

The table below summarizes CFs, suffixes, and prefixes related to the musculoskeletal system.

Word Element	Meaning	Word Element	Meaning
Combining Forms			
arthr/o	joint	lumb/o	loin (lower back)
calc/o	calcium	metacarp/o	metacarpus (hand bones)
calcane/o	calcaneum (heel bone)	myel/o	bone marrow; spinal cord
carp/o	carpus (wrist bones)	my/o	muscle
cephal/o	head	oste/o	bone
cervic/o	neck; cervix uteri (neck of uterus)	patell/o	patella (kneecap)
chondr/o	cartilage	sacr/o	sacrum
cost/o	ribs	spin/o	spine
crani/o	cranium (skull)	spondyl/o, vertebr/o	vertebra (backbone)
encephal/o	brain	stern/o	sternum (breastbone)
femor/o	femur (thigh bone)	tend/o	tendon
fibul/o	fibula (smaller, outer bone of lower leg)	tibi/o	tibia (larger inner bone of lower leg)
humer/o	humerus (upper arm bone)		
OTHER COMBINING FORMS			
cyt/o	cell	proxim/o	near
cyst/o	bladder	radi/o	radiation, x-ray; radius (lower arm bone on thumb side)
dist/o	far, farthest	roentgen/o	x-rays
enter/o	intestine (usually small intestine)	scler/o	hardening; sclera (white of eye)
hepat/o	liver		

(continued)

Word Element	Meaning	Word Element	Meaning
Suffixes			
SURGICAL			
-centesis	surgical puncture	**-rrhaphy**	suture
-ectomy	excision, removal	**-tomy**	incision
-plasty	surgical repair		
DIAGNOSTIC, SYMPTOMATIC, AND RELATED			
-algia, -dynia	pain	**-logist**	specialist in study of
-cele	hernia, swelling	**-malacia**	softening
-cyte	cell	**-meter**	instrument for measuring
-emia	blood condition	**-oma**	tumor
-genesis	forming, producing, origin	**-osis**	abnormal condition
-gram	record, writing	**-pathy**	disease
-graphy	process of recording	**-plegia**	paralysis
-ist	specialist	**-rrhexis**	rupture
-itis	inflammation		
Prefixes			
en-	in, within	**inter-**	between
hemi-	one half	**peri-**	around
hypo-	under, below, deficient	**quadri-**	four

 Enhance your study and reinforcement of word elements with the power of *Davis Plus*. Visit *http://davisplus.fadavis.com/gylys/simplified* for this chapter's flash-card activity. We recommend you complete the flash-card activity before completing the word elements review below.

Word Elements Review

After you review the word elements summary, complete this activity by writing the meaning of each element in the space provided.

Word Element	Meaning	Word Element	Meaning
Combining Forms			
1. arthr/o	_____	14. lumb/o	_____
2. calc/o	_____	15. metacarp/o	_____
3. calcane/o	_____	16. myel/o	_____
4. carp/o	_____	17. my/o	_____
5. cephal/o	_____	18. oste/o	_____
6. cervic/o	_____	19. patell/o	_____
7. chondr/o	_____	20. sacr/o	_____
8. cost/o	_____	21. spin/o	_____
9. crani/o	_____	22. spondyl/o	_____
10. encephal/o	_____	23. vertebr/o	_____
11. femor/o	_____	24. stern/o	_____
12. fibul/o	_____	25. tend/o	_____
13. humer/o	_____	26. tibi/o	_____

OTHER COMBINING FORMS

27. proxim/o	_____	28. radi/o	_____

Suffixes

SURGICAL

29. -centesis	_____	31. -plasty	_____
30. -ectomy	_____		

DIAGNOSTIC, SYMPTOMATIC, AND RELATED

32. -cyte	_____	39. -malacia	_____
33. -genesis	_____	40. -meter	_____
34. -gram	_____	41. -oma	_____
35. -graphy	_____	42. -osis	_____
36. -ist	_____	43. -pathy	_____
37. -itis	_____	44. -plegia	_____
38. -logist	_____		

Prefixes

45. en-	_____	48. inter-	_____
46. hemi-	_____	49. peri-	_____
47. hypo-	_____	50. quadri-	_____

Competency Verification: Check your answers in Appendix A, Glossary of Medical Word Elements, page 538. If you are not satisfied with your level of comprehension, review the word elements and retake the review.

Correct Answers: _____ × 2 _____ % Score

Vocabulary Review

Match the medical terms below with the definitions in the numbered list.

AP	bone marrow	distal	proximal
arthrocentesis	cephalometer	intervertebral	quadriplegia
articulation	cervical vertebrae	myelogram	radiologist
atlas	closed fracture	myorrhexis	radiology
bilateral	diaphysis	open fracture	spondylomalacia

1. _____ is the study of x-rays and radioactive substances used for diagnosing and treating diseases.

2. _____ means shaft or main part of the bone.

3. _____ means passing from the front to the rear.

4. _____ is a fracture in which the bone is broken, but there is no external wound and surrounding tissue damage is minimal.

5. _____ means pertaining to or affecting two sides.

6. _____ means near the point of attachment to the trunk.

7. _____ is the place of union between two or more bones; a joint.

8. _____ is a fracture in which the broken end of a bone has moved so that it pierces the skin, with possibly extensive damage to surrounding blood vessels, nerves, and muscles.

9. _____ is the first cervical vertebra, which supports the skull.

10. _____ is a surgical puncture of a joint to remove fluid.

11. _____ is soft tissue that fills the medullary cavities of long bones.

12. _____ is an instrument used to measure the head.

13. _____ refers to a radiograph of the spinal canal after injection of a contrast medium.

14. _____ means rupture of a muscle.

15. _____ means softening of vertebrae.

16. _____ is a directional term that means farthest from the point of attachment to the trunk.

17. _____ is a physician who specializes in the use of x-rays for diagnosis and the treatment of disease.

18. _____ are bones that form the skeletal framework of the neck.

19. _____ is situated between two adjacent vertebrae.

20. _____ means paralysis of all four extremities.

Competency Verification: Check your answers in Appendix B, Answer Key, page 580. If you are not satisfied with your level of comprehension, review the chapter vocabulary and retake the review.

Correct Answers: _____ × 5 _____ % **Score**

11 Special Senses: Eyes and Ears

OBJECTIVES

Upon completion of this chapter, you will be able to:

- Describe the type of medical treatment the ophthalmologist and otolaryngologist provide.
- Identify the structures of the eye and ear by labeling them on the anatomical illustrations.
- Describe the primary functions of the eye and ear.
- Describe common diseases related to the eye and ear.
- Describe common diagnostic, medical, and surgical procedures related to the eye and ear.
- Apply your word-building skills by constructing various medical terms related to the eye and ear.
- Describe common abbreviations and symbols related to the eye and ear.
- Reinforce word elements by completing flash card activities.
- Recognize, define, pronounce, and spell terms correctly.
- Demonstrate your knowledge of this chapter by successfully completing the frames, reviews, and medical report evaluations.

Medical Specialties

Ophthalmology

Ophthalmology is the branch of medicine concerned with diagnosis and treatment of eye disorders. The medical specialist in ophthalmology is called an **ophthalmologist.**

Although ophthalmologists specialize in the treatment of the eyes only, it is important for them to be cognizant of other abnormalities that may be revealed during an eye examination. The importance of an eye examination cannot be underestimated because it commonly reveals the first signs of systemic illnesses (such as diabetes) that may be taking place in other parts of the body. The medical practice of ophthalmology includes prescribing corrective lenses and performing various types of corrective eye surgeries. Specialized surgeries involve techniques that are as delicate and precise as that of neurosurgery and are commonly performed using magnifying glasses and utilizing laser beams. Corrective eye surgeries include cornea transplantation, cataract removal, repair of ocular muscle dysfunction, glaucoma treatment, lens removal, and radial keratotomy.

Two other health care practitioners, the *optometrist* and *optician*, specialize in providing corrective lenses for the eyes. They are not medical doctors, but they are licensed to examine and test the eyes and treat visual defects by prescribing corrective lenses. The optician also specializes in filling prescriptions for corrective lenses.

Otolaryngology

Otolaryngology is the oldest medical specialty in the United States. Fifty years ago, otolaryngology was practiced along with **ophthalmology**. During that time, the medical practice consisted mainly of removing tonsils and adenoids and irrigating (cleansing a canal by flushing it with water or other fluids) the sinuses and ear canals.

Today, otolaryngology is greatly expanded to include medical and surgical management of patients with disorders of the ear, nose, and throat (ENT) and related structures of the head and neck. **Otolaryngologist**s, also known as *ENT physicians*, commonly treat disorders related to the sinuses, including allergies and disorders of the sense of smell. Their diagnostic techniques are used to detect the causes of such symptoms as hoarseness, hearing and breathing difficulty, and swelling around the head or neck. Another important part of the ENT physician's practice is treatment of sleep disorders, most commonly sleep apnea. Various types of procedures, including but not limited to surgery, may be performed to treat sleep apnea or snoring disorders. ENT physicians are also involved in introducing rehabilitative programs for children and adults who have suffered hearing loss. Such programs commonly include collaborations with community agencies to identify hearing-impaired individuals (through public screenings) and provide them with needed medical treatment. Another health care practitioner, the *audiologist* (not an MD), detects, evaluates, and treats hearing loss.

Anatomy and Physiology Overview

The major senses of the body are sight, hearing, smell, taste, touch, and balance. These sensations are identified with specific body organs. Senses of smell and taste were discussed in previous chapters. This chapter focuses on the eyes and ears, which include the senses of sight, hearing, and balance.

Eyes

The eyes and their accessory structures are receptor organs that provide vision. As one of the most important sense organs of the body, the eyes provide most of the information about what we see, but also of what we learn from printed material. Similar to other sensory organs, the eyes are constructed to detect stimuli in the environment and to transmit those observations to the brain for visual interpretation.

WORD ELEMENTS

This section introduces combining forms (CFs) related to the eye. Included are key suffixes; prefixes are defined in the right-hand column as needed. Review the following table, and pronounce each word in the word analysis column aloud before you begin to work the frames.

Word Element	Meaning	Word Analysis
Combining Forms		
blephar/o	eyelid	**blephar/o/spasm** (BLĔF-ă-rō-spăzm): involuntary contraction of eyelid muscles
		-spasm: involuntary contraction, twitching
		Blepharospasm may be due to eye strain or nervous irritability.
conjunctiv/o	conjuctiva	**conjunctiv/itis** (kŏn-jŭnk-tĭ-VĪ-tĭs): inflammation of the conjunctiva; also called *pinkeye*
		The conjunctiva has the ability to repair itself rapidly if it is scratched.

Word Element	Meaning	Word Analysis
choroid/o	choroid	**choroid**/o/pathy (kō-roy-DŎP-ă-thē): noninflammatory degeneration of the choroid *-pathy:* disease *The choroid is a thin, highly vascular layer of the eye between the retina and sclera.*
corne/o	cornea	**corne**/itis (kŏr-nē-Ī-tĭs): inflammation of the cornea; also called *keratitis* *-itis:* inflammation
cor/o	pupil	aniso/**cor**/ia (ăn-ĭ-sō-KŌ-rē-ă): inequality of pupil size *aniso:* unequal, dissimilar *-ia:* condition *Anisocoria may be congenital or associated with a neurological injury or disease.*
core/o		**core**/o/meter (kō-rē-ŎM-ĕ-tĕr): instrument for measuring the pupil *-meter:* instrument for measuring
pupill/o		**pupill**/ary (PŪ-pĭ-lĕr-ē): pertaining to the pupil *-ary:* pertaining to
dacry/o	tear; lacrimal apparatus (duct, sac, or gland)	**dacry**/o/rrhea (dăk-rē-ō-RĒ-ă): excessive secretion of tears *-rrhea:* discharge, flow
lacrim/o		**lacrim**/ation (lăk-rĭ-MĀ-shŭn): secretion and discharge of tears *-ation:* process (of)
dipl/o	double	**dipl**/opia (dĭp-LŌ-pē-ă): two images of an object seen at the same time; also called *double vision* *-opia:* vision
irid/o	iris	**irid**/o/plegia (ĭr-ĭd-ō-PLĒ-jē-ă): paralysis of the sphincter of the iris *-plegia:* paralysis
kerat/o	horny tissue; hard; cornea	**kerat**/o/plasty (KĔR-ă-tō-plăs-tē): replacement of a cloudy cornea with a transparent one, typically derived from an organ donor; also called *corneal transplant.* *-plasty:* surgical repair
ocul/o	eye	intra/**ocul**/ar (ĭn-tră-ŎK-ū-lăr): within the eyeball *intra-:* in, within *-ar:* pertaining to
ophthalm/o		**ophthalm**/o/scope (ŏf-THĂL-mō-skōp): instrument for examining the interior of the eye, especially the retina *-scope:* instrument for examining

(continued)

Word Element	Meaning	Word Analysis
opt/o	eye, vision	**opt**/ic (ŎP-tĭk): pertaining to the eye or to sight *-ic:* pertaining to
retin/o	retina	**retin**/o/pathy (rĕt-ĭn-ŎP-ă-thē): disease of the retina *-pathy:* disease
scler/o	hardening; sclera (white of eye)	**scler**/itis (sklĕ-RĪ-tĭs): inflammation of the sclera *-itis:* inflammation

Suffixes

-opia	vision	ambly/**opia** (ăm-blē-Ō-pē-ă): reduction or dimness of vision, usually in one eye, with no apparent pathological condition; also called *lazy eye* *ambly:* dull, dim
-opsia		heter/**opsia** (hĕt-ĕr-ŎP-sē-ă): inequality of vision in the two eyes *heter-:* different
-ptosis	prolapse, downward displacement	blephar/o/**ptosis** (blĕf-ă-rō-TŌ-sĭs): drooping of the upper eyelid *blephar/o:* eyelid
-tropia	turning	hyper/**tropia** (hī-pĕr-TRŌ-pē-ă): ocular deviation with one eye located higher than the other *hyper-:* excessive, above normal

Pronunciation Help	Long Sound Short Sound	ā in rāte ă in ălone	ē in rēbirth ĕ in ĕver	ī in īsle ĭ in ĭt	ō in ōver ŏ in nŏt	ū in ūnite ŭ in cŭt

Listen and Learn, the audio CD-ROM included in this book, will help you master pronunciation of selected medical words. Use it to practice pronunciations of the above-listed medical terms and for instructions to complete the *Listen and Learn* exercise for this section.

SECTION REVIEW 11-1

For the following medical terms, first write the suffix and its meaning. Then translate the meaning of the remaining elements starting with the first part of the word. The first word is completed for you.

Term	Meaning
1. aniso/cor/ia	*-ia: condition; unequal, dissimilar; pupil*
2. blephar/o/ptosis	
3. ambly/opia	
4. retin/o/pathy	
5. scler/itis	
6. ophthalm/o/scope	
7. intra/ocul/ar	
8. dacry/o/rrhea	
9. dipl/opia	
10. blephar/o/spasm	

Competency Verification: Check your answers in Appendix B, Answer Key, page 580. If you are not satisfied with your level of comprehension, review the vocabulary and retake the review.

Correct Answers _____ ×10= _____ % Score

11–1 The eye is a globe-shaped, hollow structure set within a bony cavity. The bony cavity, or *orbit,* houses the eyeball and associated structures, such as the eye muscles, nerves, and blood vessels. Most of the eyeball is protected from trauma by the orbit's bony cavity. The wall of the eyeball contains three layers: the (1) **sclera,** the white outer layer of the eyeball, is composed of fibrous connective tissue. On the most anterior portion of the eye, the sclera forms a transparent, domed structure called the (2) ***cornea.*** The cornea also protects the front part of the eye from injury and is the first structure of the eye that refracts light rays. In addition, the cornea is avascular (without blood vessels or capillaries), but is well supplied with nerve endings, most of which are pain fibers. For this reason, some people can never adjust to wearing contact lenses. Label the structures in Figure 11–1 as you observe the location and layers of the eyeball.

11–2 The (3) **choroid** layer lies below the sclera and contains blood vessels. It also contains a dark, pigmented tissue that prevents glare within the eyeball because of its ability to absorb light. The anterior portion of the choroid is modified and forms the (4) **ciliary body** (or muscle) and the (5) **iris,** the colored portion of the eye. Observe the location of the three structures discussed in this frame as you label them in Figure 11–1.

11-3   The (6) **retina** lines the posterior two-thirds of the eyeball. It contains rods and cones, the sensory receptors for vision and image formation. Rods perceive the presence of light only, whereas cones perceive different wavelengths of light as colors. Cones are concentrated in the depression near the center of the retina called the (7) **fovea,** which is the area of sharpest vision. Surrounding the fovea is the yellowish *macula,* which also has an abundance of cones. In addition, the retina is the only place in the body where blood vessels can be seen directly. Label Figure 11–1 as you observe the location of the structures responsible for image formation.

---

scler/itis
sklĕ-RĪ-tĭs

choroid/itis
kō-royd-Ī-tĭs

retin/itis
rĕt-ĭ-NĪ-tĭs

11-4   The CF **scler/o** refers to *hardening; sclera (white of eye);* **choroid/o** refers to the *choroid;* and **retin/o** refers to the *retina.*
Use these CFs to build medical terms that mean *inflammation of the*

sclera: _____ / _____

choroid: _____ / _____

retina: _____ / _____

---

choroid/o/pathy
kō-roy-DŎP-ă-thē

retin/o/pathy
rĕt-ĭn-ŎP-ă-thē

11-5   Practice building medical words that mean *disease of the*

choroid: _____ / _____ / _____

retina: _____ / _____ / _____

---

kerat/o/rrhexis
kĕr-ă-tō-RĔK-sĭs

irid/o/cele
ĭ-RĬD-ō-sēl

11-6   The CF **kerat/o** refers to *horny tissue; hard; cornea.* The CF **irid/o** refers to the *iris.*
Use these CFs to build medical terms that mean

rupture of the cornea: _____ / _____ / _____

herniation of the iris: _____ / _____ / _____

---

kerat/o

11-7   Kerat/itis, a vision-threatening infection, can occur if contact lenses are not cleaned and disinfected properly.
From *kerat/itis,* construct the CF for *cornea.*

_____ / _____

---

scler/itis
sklĕ-RĪ-tĭs

scler/o/malacia
sklĕ-rō-mă-LĀ-shē-ă

11-8   Form medical words that mean

inflammation of the sclera: _____ / _____

softening of the sclera: _____ / _____ / _____

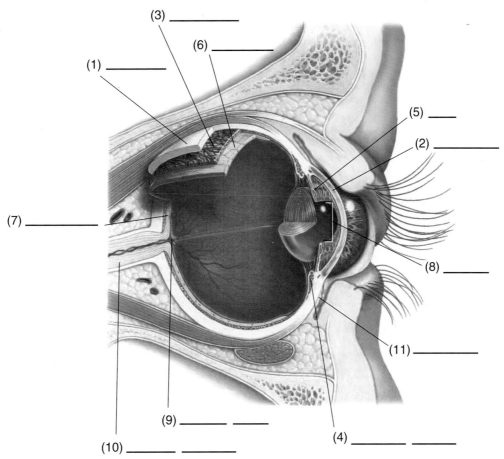

Figure 11-1 Eye structures.

<table>
<tr><td>**kerat/o/tomy**
kĕr-ă-TŎT-ō-mē</td><td>**11-9** In some cases, laser kerat/o/tomy can be used to correct vision. Doing so eliminates the need for contact lenses or glasses. Shallow, bloodless, hairline, radial incisions are made using a laser in the outer portion of the cornea, where they will not interfere with vision. This allows the cornea to flatten and helps to correct nearsightedness.
About two-thirds of patients are able to eliminate the use of glasses or contact lenses by undergoing the surgical procedure called *laser*

_____ / _____ / _____.</td></tr>
</table>

11-10 The opening in the center of the iris is called the (8) **pupil.** The amount of light entering the eye is controlled by contractions and dilations of the pupil. Constriction of the pupil permits a sharper near vision. It is also a reflex that protects the retina from intense light. Label the pupil in Figure 11–1.

11-11 Sensory receptors of vision, rods and cones, contain light-sensitive molecules *(photopigments)* that convert light energy into electrical impulses. Impulses generated by rods and cones are transmitted by retinal nerve fibers to the cortex of the brain. Retinal nerve fibers unite at the (9) **optic disc** and cut across through the wall of the eyeball as the (10) **optic nerve.** Because the optic disk has no rods or cones, it is known as the *blind spot.* Label the structures in Figure 11–1 as you learn about the location and role these structures play in providing vision.

ŏf-THĂL-mō

11-12 Words with *ophthalm/o (eye)* may be difficult to pronounce when you first encounter them. To avoid confusion, write the pronunciation *ŏf-THĂL-mō* and practice saying it aloud.

_____

---

instrument

11-13 An ophthalm/o/scope is an _____ for examining the interior of the eye.

---

ophthalm/o/scopy
ŏf-thăl-MŎS-kō-pē

11-14 The word that means *visual examination of the eye* is

_____ / _____ / _____.

---

ophthalm/algia
ŏf-thăl-MĂL-jē-ă

11-15 High blood pressure may cause ophthalm/o/dynia, or

_____ / _____.

---

eye(s)

11-16 An ophthalm/o/logist is a physician who specializes in disorders and treatment of the _____.

---

ophthalm/ectomy
ŏf-thăl-MĚK-tō-mē
ophthalm/o/malacia
ŏf-thăl-mō-mă-LĀ-shē-ă
ophthalm/o/plegia
ŏf-thăl-mō-PLĒ-jē-ă

11-17 Use *ophthalm/o* to build words that mean

surgical excision of the eye: _____ / _____

softening of the eye: _____ / _____ / _____

paralysis of the eye: _____ / _____ / _____

---

ophthalm/o/plegia
ŏf-thăl-mō-PLĒ-jē-ă

11-18 A stroke can prevent eye movement and cause paralysis of eye muscles. A person with paralysis of eye (muscles) has a condition called

_____ / _____ / _____.

---

conjuctiv/itis
kŏn-jŭnk-tĭ-VĪ-tĭs

11-19 The (11) **conjunctiva** is a thin mucous-secreting membrane that lines the interior surface of the eyelids and the exposed anterior surface of the eyeballs. Conjuctiv/itis is often caused by allergies and is manifested by itchy, watery, red eyes.

The medical term for inflammation of the conjunctiva is

_____ / _____.

Competency Verification: Check your labeling of Figure 11–1 with Appendix B, Answer Key, page 580.

blephar/o/plasty BLĔF-ă-rō-plăs-tē	**11-20** The surgical procedure to remove wrinkles from the eyelids is known as *blephar/o/plasty*. This procedure is performed for functional and cosmetic reasons. Surgical repair of the eyelid(s) is known as _____ / ____ / _____.
blephar/o/plasty BLĔF-ă-rō-plăs-tē	**11-21** Excessive skin around the upper eyelids may cause a decrease or lack of peripheral vision. To improve vision, the surgical procedure to remove the excessive skin is performed. This procedure is known as _____ / ____ / _____.
blephar/ectomy blĕf-ă-RĔK-tō-mē **blephar/o/tomy** blĕf-ă-RŎT-ō-mē **blephar/o/spasm** BLĔF-ă-rō-spăzm **blephar/o/plegia** blĕf-ă-rō-PLĒ-jē-ă	**11-22** Form medical words that mean *excision of part or all of the eyelid:* _____ / _____ *surgical incision of eyelid:* _____ / ____ / _____ *twitching or spasm of eyelid:* _____ / ____ / _____ *paralysis of an eyelid:* _____ / ____ / _____
red **yellow**	**11-23** The suffix *-opia* is used in words to mean *vision*. *Erythr/opia* is a condition in which objects that are not supposed to be red appear to be _____. *Xanth/opia* is a condition in which objects that are not yellow appear to be _____.
dipl/opia dĭp-LŌ-pē-ă	**11-24** Elements *dipl-* and ***dipl/o*** mean *double*. *Dipl/opia* occurs when both eyes are used but are not in focus. A person with double vision has a condition called _____ / _____.
dipl/opia dĭp-LŌ-pē-ă	**11-25** *Dipl/opia* can occur with brain tumors, strokes, head trauma, and migraine headaches. Write the word in this frame that means double vision. _____ / _____

hyper- **-opia** **my/o**	**11-26** Two common vision defects are *my/opia* (nearsightedness) and *hyper/opia* (farsightedness). See Figure 11–2 to compare a normal eye (emmetropia) with my/opia and hyper/opia. Write the element in this frame that means *excessive, above normal:* _____ *vision:* _____ *muscle:* _____ / _____
hyper/opia hī-pĕr-Ō-pē-ă	**11-27** In normal vision, the lens focuses the visual image on the retina. Hyper/opia occurs when the lens focuses the visual image beyond the retina (see Figure 11–2), causing difficulty in seeing objects that are close. This is a condition common in people over 40 years of age, but can be corrected with "reading" glasses. The medical term for *farsightedness* is _____ / _____.
close	**11-28** People with hyper/opia (farsightedness) have difficulty seeing objects that are _____.
my/opia mī-Ō-pē-ă	**11-29** If the eyeball is too long, the visual image falls in front of the retina (see Figure 11–2), causing difficulty seeing objects that are far away. The medical term for *nearsightedness* is _____ / _____.

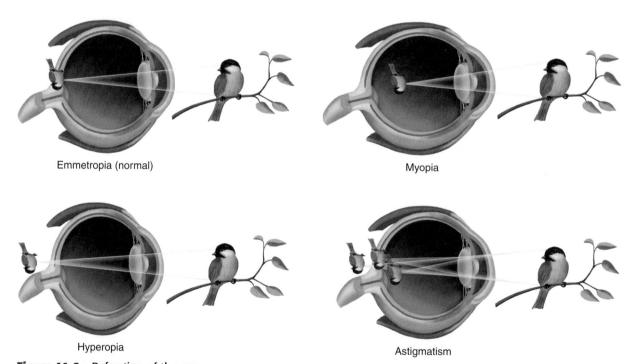

Emmetropia (normal)   Myopia

Hyperopia   Astigmatism

Figure 11-2   Refraction of the eye.

hyper/opia hī-pĕr-Ō-pē-ă	**11-30** The opposite of *my/opia* is _____ / _____.

11-31 Eyelids shade the eyes during sleep, protect them from excessive light and foreign objects, and spread lubricating secretions over the eyeballs.
Use ***blephar/o*** *(eyelid)* to construct medical words that mean

blephar/o/plasty BLĔF-ă-rō-plăs-tē	*surgical repair of eyelid:* _____ / ____ / _____
blephar/o/spasm BLĔF-ă-rō-spăzm	*twitching of an eyelid:* _____ / ____ / _____
blephar/o/ptosis blĕf-ă-rō-TŌ-sĭs	*prolapse of an eyelid:* _____ / ____ / _____

11-32 Blephar/o/ptosis is commonly seen after a stroke, because the muscles leading to the eyelids become paralyzed.
Indicate the elements in this frame that mean

blephar/o	*eyelid:* _____ / ____
-ptosis	*prolapse, downward displacement:* _____

11-33 The (1) **lacrimal gland** is located above the outer corner of each eye. These glands produce tears, which keep the eyeballs moist. The (2) **lacrimal sac** collects and drains tears into the (3) **nasolacrimal duct**. Label the lacrimal structures in Figure 11–3.

tears	**11-34** The CF ***dacry/o*** is used in words to mean *tear; lacrimal sac. Dacry/o/rrhea* is an excessive flow of _____.

(1) _____ _____

(2) _____ ____

(3) _____ ____

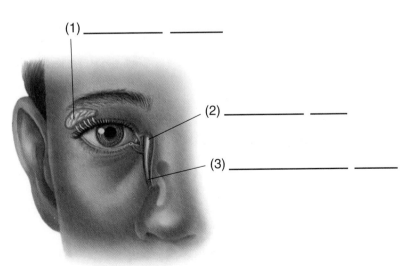

Figure 11-3 Lacrimal apparatus.

pain	**11-35** *Dacry/aden/algia* is _____ in a tear gland.

tear gland	**11-36** *Dacry/aden/itis* is an inflammation of a _____ _____.

Competency Verification: Check your labeling of Figure 11–3 with the answers in Appendix B, Answer Key, page 580.

Ears

The ears and their accessory structures are receptor organs that enable us to hear and maintain balance. Each ear consists of three divisions: the external ear, middle ear, and inner ear. The external and middle ear conduct sound waves through the ear. The inner ear contains auditory structures that receive sound waves and transmit them to the brain for interpretation. The inner ear also contains specialized receptors that maintain balance and equilibrium in response to fluctuations in body position and motion.

WORD ELEMENTS

This section introduces CFs related to the ear. Included are key suffixes; prefixes are defined in the right-hand column as needed. Review the following table and pronounce each word in the word analysis column aloud before you begin to work the frames.

Word Element	Meaning	Word Analysis
Combining Forms		
acous/o	hearing	**acous**/tic (ă-KOOS-tik): pertaining to sound or the sense of hearing *-tic:* pertaining to
audi/o		**audi**/o/meter (aw-dē-ŎM-ĕ-tĕr): instrument for testing hearing *-meter:* instrument for measuring
audit/o		**audit**/ory (AW-dĭ-tō-rē): pertaining to sense of hearing *-ory:* pertaining to

Word Element	Meaning	Word Analysis
myring/o	tympanic membrane (eardrum)	**myring/o/tomy** (mĭr-ĭn-GŎT-ō-mē): incision of the tympanic membrane *-tomy:* incision
tympan/o		**tympan/o/plasty** (tĭm-păn-ō-PLĂS-tē): surgical repair of the tympanic membrane *-plasty:* surgical repair *A tympanoplasty is any one of several surgical procedures designed to cure a chronic inflammatory process in the middle ear or restore function to the sound-transmitting mechanism of the middle ear.*
ot/o	ear	**ot/o/rrhea** (ō-tō-RĒ-ă): inflammation of the ear with purulent discharge *-rrhea:* discharge, flow
salping/o	tube (usually fallopian or eustachian [auditory] tubes)	**salping/o/pharyng/eal** (săl-pĭng-gō-fă-RĬN-jē-ăl): concerning the eustachian tube and pharynx *pharyng:* pharynx (throat) *-eal:* pertaining to

Suffixes

-acusis	hearing	**an/acusis** (ăn-ă-KŪ-sĭs): total deafness *an-:* without, not

Pronunciation Help						
	Long Sound	ā in rāte	ē in rēbirth	ī in īsle	ō in ōver	ū in ūnite
	Short Sound	ă in ălone	ĕ in ĕver	ĭ in ĭt	ŏ in nŏt	ŭ in cŭt

 Listen and Learn, the audio CD-ROM included in this book, will help you master pronunciation of selected medical words. Use it to practice pronunciations of the above-listed medical terms and for instructions to complete the *Listen and Learn* exercise for this section.

SECTION REVIEW 11-2

For the following medical terms, first write the suffix and its meaning. Then translate the meaning of the remaining elements starting with the first part of the word. The first word is completed for you.

Term	Meaning
1. tympan/o/centesis	*-centesis: surgical puncture; tympanic membrane (eardrum)*
2. acous/tic	
3. hyper/tropia	
4. ot/o/rrhea	
5. an/acusis	
6. myring/o/tomy	
7. tympan/o/plasty	
8. audi/o/meter	
9. ot/o/scope	
10. salping/o/pharyng/eal	

Competency Verification: Check your answers in Appendix B, Answer Key, page 581. If you are not satisfied with your level of comprehension, review the vocabulary and retake the review.

Correct Answers _____ × 10 = _____ % Score

11-37 The ear can be divided into three anatomical sections: external, middle, and inner. The external ear includes the (1) **auricle,** which directs sound waves to the (2) **ear canal.** Eventually, the sound waves hit the (3) **tympanic membrane** (eardrum) and make the eardrum vibrate. Transmission of sound waves ultimately generates impulses that are transmitted to and interpreted by the brain as sound. Label Figure 11–4 as you learn about the ear.

ot/algia
ō-TĂL-jē-ă

11-38 Swimmer's ear, resulting from an infection transmitted in the water of a swimming pool, may cause severe ot/o/dynia or _____ / _____.

eardrum

11-39 The CFs *tympan/o* and *myring/o* refer to the *tympanic membrane (eardrum). Tympan/itis* is an inflammation of the tympanic membrane, or _____.

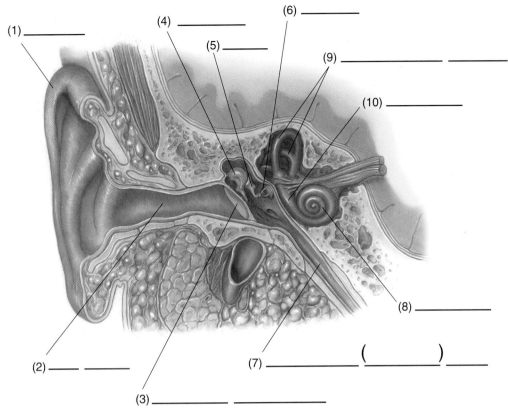

(1) _____

(4) _____

(5) _____

(6) _____

(9) _____ _____

(10) _____

(8) _____

(2) _____ _____

(3) _____ _____

(7) _____ (_____) _____

Figure 11-4 Ear structures.

	11–40 The tympan/ic membrane is stretched across the end of the ear canal and vibrates when sound waves strike it.
	The CFs for the tympanic membrane (eardrum) are
tympan/o, myring/o	_____ / _____ and _____ / _____.

	11–41 Vibrations of the tympanic membrane are transmitted to the three auditory bones in the middle ear: the (4) **malleus,** the (5) **incus,** and the (6) **stapes.** The (7) **eustachian (auditory) tube** leads from the middle ear to the nasopharynx and permits air to enter or leave the middle ear cavity. Label and review the position of the middle ear structures in Figure 11–4.

salping/itis	**11–42** The CF *salping/o* means *tube (usually fallopian or eustachian [auditory] tubes).* Inflammation of the eustachian tube would be diagnosed as
săl-pĭn-JĪ-tĭs	_____ / _____.

salping/o/scope
săl-PĬNG-gō-skōp

salping/o/scopy
săl-pĭng-GŎS-kō-pē

salping/o/stenosis
săl-pĭng-gō-stĕn-NŌ-sĭs

11-43 The eustachian tube equalizes air pressure in the middle ear with that of the outside atmosphere. Air pressure must be equalized for the eardrum to vibrate properly.
Build medical words that mean

instrument for examining the eustachian tube:

_____ / _____ / _____

visual examination of the eustachian tube:

_____ / _____ / _____

narrowing or stricture of the eustachian tube:

_____ / _____ / _____

11-44 Components of the inner ear include the (8) **cochlea** for hearing, the (9) **semicircular canals** for equilibrium, and the (10) **vestibule,** which is a chamber that joins the cochlea and semicircular canals. Label inner ear structures in Figure 11–4.

11-45 The inner ear, also called the *labyrinth,* consists of complicated, mazelike structures, all of which contain the functional organs for hearing and equilibrium. (See Figure 11–5.)
Use your medical dictionary to define *labyrinth* and list two types of inner ear labyrinths.

_____

_____

ot/o

11-46 The CF *ot/o* refers to the *ear.* From *ot/o/sclero/sis,* determine the CF for ear.

_____ / _____

ot/o/sclerosis
ō-tō-sklĕ-RŌ-sĭs

11-47 Ot/o/sclerosis is a hereditary condition of unknown cause in which irregular ossification occurs in the ossicles of the middle ear, especially of the stapes, causing hearing loss.
Chronic progressive deafness, especially for low tones, may be caused by a hereditary condition called _____ / _____ / _____.

staped/ectomy
stā-pē-DĔK-tō-mē

11-48 A patient diagnosed with ot/o/scler/osis may have hearing restored with a surgical procedure called *staped/ectomy.*
To improve hearing, especially in cases of ot/o/scler/osis, the surgeon may excise the stapes using a surgical procedure called

_____ / _____.

staped/ectomy
stā-pē-DĔK-tō-mē

11-49 Staped/ectomy involves removal of the stapes and replacement by a prosthesis to restore hearing loss.
When the surgeon excises the stapes, the surgery performed is called

_____ / _____.

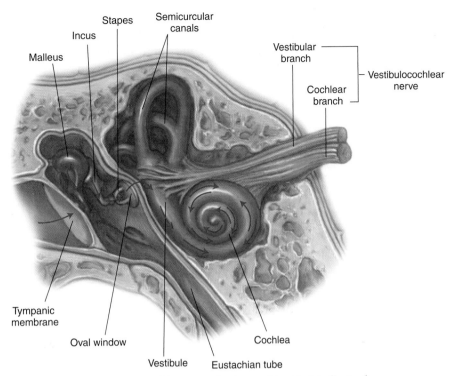

Figure 11-5 The labyrinths of the inner ear with arrows in the cochlea that indicate the path of vibrations.

pain, ear	**11–50** The inner ear contains the receptors for two senses: hearing and equilibrium. Ot/o/dynia is _____ in the _____.
ot/algia ō-TĂL-jē-ă	**11–51** Ot/o/dynia is also known as an *earache*. Can you think of another term for pain in the ear? _____ / _____
ot/o/scopy ō-TŎS-kŏ-pē	**11–52** Ear infections can be diagnosed with an ot/o/scope. Visual examination of the ear is known as _____ / ____ / _____.
URI	**11–53** Ot/itis media, infection of the middle ear, usually occurs following upper respiratory infection (URI). Upon ot/o/scopy, redness and stiffness of the tympanic membrane is observed, indicating inflammation. The abbreviation for *upper respiratory infection* is _____.

11–54 Ot/itis media caused by bacteria is commonly treated with antibiotics. When the condition persists and becomes chronic, a myring/o/tomy may be required. During this surgical procedure, a pressure-equalizing (PE) tube is inserted into the eardrum to relieve pressure and promote drainage. (See Figure 11–6.)

Build the medical word that means *incision into the eardrum*.

myring/o/tomy

_____ / ____ / _____

ot/o/plasty
Ō-tō-plăs-tē

11–55 Plastic surgery of the ear (to correct defects and deformities) is called _____ / ____ / _____.

Competency Verification: Check your labeling of Figure 11–4 with the answers in Appendix B, Answer Key, page 581.

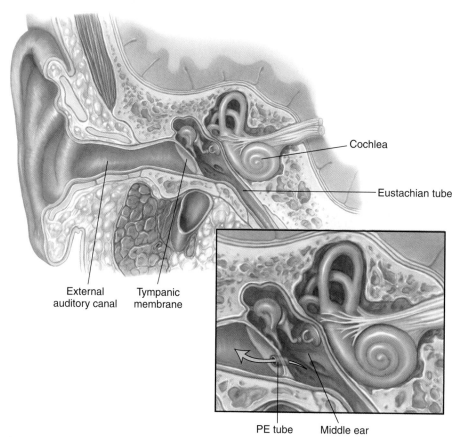

Figure 11-6   Placement of pressure-equalizing (PE) tubes.

SECTION REVIEW 11-3

Using the following table, write the CF, suffix, or prefix that matches its definition in the space provided to the left of the definition. There may be more than one word element that matches a definition.

Combining Forms		Suffixes		Prefixes
aden/o	myring/o	-acusis	-spasm	dipl-
audi/o	ophthalm/o	-edema	-stenosis	hyper-
blephar/o	ot/o	-logist		
choroid/o	retin/o	-malacia		
corne/o	salping/o	-opia		
dacry/o	scler/o	-opsia		
dipl/o	tympan/o	-ptosis		
irid/o	xanth/o	-rrhexis		
kerat/o		-salpinx		

1. _____ excessive, above normal

2. _____ choroid

3. _____ horny tissue; hard; cornea

4. _____ double

5. _____ ear

6. _____ tube (usually fallopian or eustachian [auditory] tube)

7. _____ eye

8. _____ eyelid

9. _____ gland

10. _____ hardening; sclera (white of eye)

11. _____ involuntary contraction, twitching

12. _____ iris

13. _____ prolapse, downward displacement

14. _____ specialist in study of

15. _____ retina

16. _____ rupture

17. _____ softening

18. _____ hearing

19. _____ narrowing, stricture

20. _____ swelling

21. _____ tear; lacrimal apparatus (duct, sac, or gland)

22. _____ tympanic membrane (eardrum)

23. _____ cornea

24. _____ vision

25. _____ yellow

Competency Verification: Check your answers in Appendix B, Answer Key, page 581. If you are not satisfied with your level of comprehension, go back to Frame 11–1 and rework the frames.

Correct Answers _____ × 4 = _____ % Score

Abbreviations

This section introduces abbreviations related to the eyes and ears and their meanings. Included are abbreviations contained in the medical record activities that follow.

Abbreviation	Meaning	Abbreviation	Meaning
Eyes			
ARMD	age-related macular degeneration	**Myop**	myopia
Ast	astigmatism	**OD**	right eye
D	diopter (lens strength)	**O.D.**	Doctor of Optometry
ECCE	extracapsular cataract extraction	**OS**	left eye
Em	emmetropia	**OU**	both eyes
EOM	extraocular movement	**REM**	rapid eye movement
IOL	intraocular lens	**SICS**	small incision cataract surgery
IOP	intraocular pressure	**ST**	esotropia
mix astig	mixed astigmatism	**VA**	visual acuity
MVR	mitral valve replacement; massive vitreous retraction (blade)	**VF**	visual field
		XT	exotropia
Ears			
AC	air conduction	**ENT**	ear, nose, and throat
AD	right ear	**NIHL**	noise-induced hearing loss
AS	left ear	**OM**	otitis media
AU	both ears	**PE**	physical examination; pulmonary embolism; pressure-equalizing (tube)
BC	bone conduction		

Additional Medical Terms

The following are additional terms related to the eyes and ears. Recognizing and learning these terms will help you understand the connection between a pathological condition, its diagnosis, and the rationale behind the method of treatment selected for a particular disorder.

Signs, Symptoms, and Diseases

Eye

achromatopsia ă-krō-mă-TŎP-sē-ă *a-:* without, not *chromat:* color *-opsia:* vision	Congenital deficiency in color perception; also called *color blindness* *Achromatopsia is more common in men.*
astigmatism ă-STĬG-mă-tĭzm *a-:* without, not *stigmat:* point, mark *-ism:* condition	Defective curvature of the cornea and lens, which causes light rays to focus unevenly over the retina rather than being focused on a single point, resulting in a distorted image (See Figure 11–2.)
cataract KĂT-ă-răkt	Degenerative disease in which the lens of the eye becomes progressively cloudy, causing decreased vision *Cataracts are usually a result of the aging process, caused by protein deposits on the surface of the lens that slowly build up until vision is lost. Treatment includes surgical intervention to remove the cataract.*
conjunctivitis kŏn-jŭnk-tĭ-VĪ-tĭs *conjunctiv:* conjunctiva *-itis:* inflammation	Inflammation of the conjunctiva that can be caused by bacteria, allergy, irritation, or a foreign body; also called *pinkeye*
diabetic retinopathy dī-ă-BĔT-ĭk rĕt-ĭn-ŎP-ă-thē *retin/o:* retina *-pathy:* disease	Retinal damage marked by aneurysmal dilation and bleeding of blood vessels or the formation of new blood vessels, causing visual changes *Diabetic retinopathy occurs in people with diabetes, manifested by small hemorrhages, edema, and formation of new vessels leading to scarring and eventual loss of vision.*

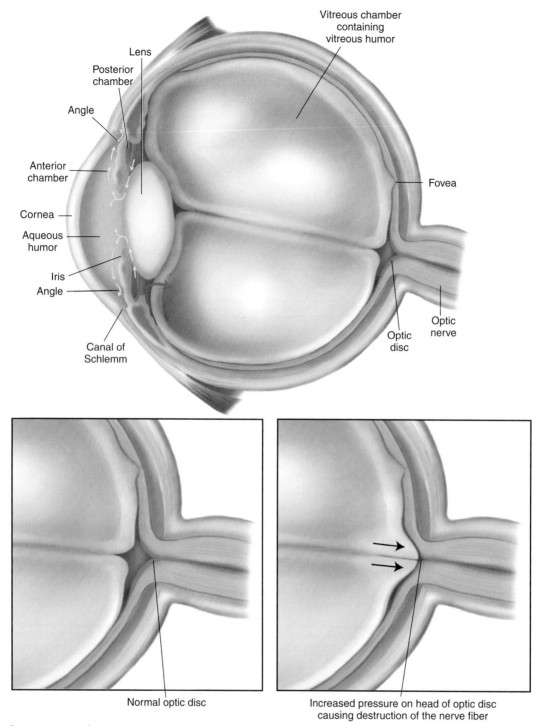

Figure 11-7 Glaucoma.

glaucoma glaw-KŌ-mă *glauc:* gray *-oma:* tumor	Condition in which aqueous humor fails to drain properly and accumulates in the anterior chamber of the eye, causing elevated intraocular pressure (IOP) (See Figure 11–7.) *Glaucoma eventually leads to loss of vision and, commonly, blindness. Treatment for glaucoma includes miotics (eyedrops) that cause the pupils to constrict, permitting aqueous humor to escape from the eye, thereby relieving pressure. If miotics are ineffective, surgery may be necessary.*
open-angle	Most common form of glaucoma that results from degenerative changes that cause congestion and reduce flow of aqueous humor through the *canal of Schlemm* *Open-angle glaucoma is painless but destroys peripheral vision, causing tunnel vision.*
closed-angle	Type of glaucoma caused by an anatomically narrow angle between the iris and the cornea, which prevents outflow of aqueous humor from the eye into the lymphatic system, causing a sudden increase in IOP *Closed-angle glaucoma constitutes an emergency situation. Symptoms include severe pain, blurred vision, and photophobia.*
hordeolum hor-DĒ-ō-lŭm	Small, purulent inflammatory infection of a sebaceous gland of the eyelid; also called *sty* (See Figure 11–8.)
macular degeneration MĂK-ū-lăr	Breakdown of the tissues in the macula, resulting in loss of central vision *Macular degeneration is the most common cause of visual impairment in persons over age 50. (See Figure 11–9.)*
photophobia fō-tō-FŌ-bē-ă *phot/o:* light *-phobia:* fear	Unusual intolerance and sensitivity to light *Photophobia occurs in such disorders as meningitis, eye inflammation, measles, and rubella.*
retinal detachment RĔT-ĭ-năl *retin:* retina *-al:* pertaining to	Separation of the retina from the choroid, which disrupts vision and results in blindness if not repaired *Retinal detachment may follow trauma, choroidal hemorrhages, or tumors and may be associated with diabetes mellitus.*

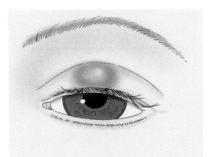

Figure 11-8   Hordeolum.

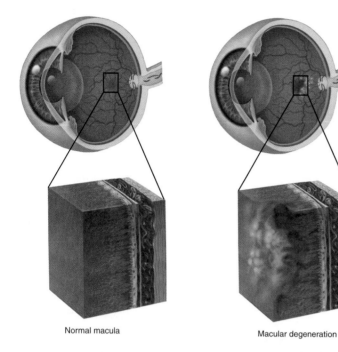

Normal macula

Macular degeneration

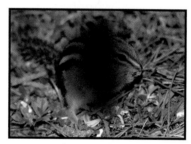

Normal vision

Central vision loss

Figure 11-9 Macular degeneration.

strabismus stră-BĬZ-mŭs	Muscular eye disorder in which the eyes turn from the normal position so that they deviate in different directions *Various forms of strabismus are referred to as tropias, their direction being indicated by the appropriate prefix, such as esotropia and exotropia. (See Figure 11–10.)*
esotropia ĕs-ō-TRŌ-pē-ă *eso-:* inward *-tropia:* turning	Strabismus in which there is deviation of the visual axis of one eye toward that of the other eye, resulting in diplopia; also called *cross-eye* and *convergent strabismus* (See Figure 11–10.)
exotropia ĕks-ō-TRŌ-pē-ă *exo-:* outside, outward *-tropia:* turning	Strabismus in which there is deviation of the visual axis of one eye away from that of the other eye, resulting in diplopia; also called *wall-eye* and *divergent strabismus* (See Figure 11–10.)

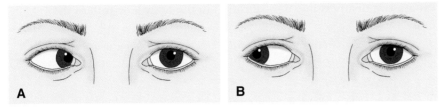

Figure 11-10 Types of strabismus. (A) Esotropia. (B) Exotropia.

Ear

acoustic neuroma a-KOOS-tĭk nū-RŌ-mă *acous:* hearing *-tic:* pertaining to *neur:* nerve *-oma:* tumor	Benign tumor that develops from the eighth cranial (vestibulocochlear) nerve and grows within the auditory canal *Depending on the location and size of the tumor, progressive hearing loss, headache, facial numbness, dizziness, and an unsteady gait may result.*
hearing loss	Decreased ability to perceive sounds compared to what the individual or examiner would regards as normal
anacusis ăn-ă-KŪ-sĭs *an-:* without, not *-acusis:* hearing	Total deafness (complete hearing loss)
conductive kŏn-dŭk-TĬV	Hearing loss due to an impairment in the transmission of sound waves because of an obstruction of the ear canal, or damage to the eardrum, or ossicles (tiny bones)
Ménière disease mĕn-ē-ĀR	Rare disorder of unknown etiology within the labyrinth of the inner ear that can lead to a progressive loss of hearing *Symptoms of Ménière disease include vertigo, hearing loss, tinnitus, and a sensation of pressure in the ear.*
otitis media (OM) ō-TĪ-tĭs MĒ-dē-ă *ot:* ear *-itis:* inflammation *med:* middle *-ia:* condition	Inflammation of the middle ear, which is commonly the result of an upper respiratory infection (URI)
serous	Noninfectious inflammation of the middle ear with accumulation of serum (clear fluid) *Treatment for serous OM may include myringotomy to aspirate fluid and the surgical insertion of pressure equalizing (PE) tubes. (See Figure 11–6.)*
suppurative	Inflammation of the middle ear with pus formation *Suppurative OM is a common affliction in infants and young children, due to the horizontal orientation and small diameter of the eustachian tube in such patients, which predisposes them to infection. If left untreated, complications include ruptured tympanic membrane, mastoiditis, labyrinthitis, hearing loss, and meningitis.*

otosclerosis ō-tō-sklĕ-RŌ-sĭs *ot/o:* ear *scler:* hardening; sclera (white of eye) *-osis:* abnormal condition; increase (used primarily with blood cells)	Progressive deafness due to ossification in the bony labyrinth of the inner ear *Treatment for otosclerosis includes stapedectomy or stapedotomy, which is usually successful in restoring hearing.*
presbycusis prĕz-bĭ-KŪ-sĭs *presby:* old age *-cusis:* hearing	Impairment of hearing that results from the aging process
tinnitus tĭn-Ī-tĭs	Ringing or tinkling noise heard constantly or intermittently in one or both ears, even in a quiet environment *Tinnitus may be a sign of injury to the ear, some disease process, or toxic levels of some medications (such as aspirin).*
vertigo VĔR-tĭ-gō	Sensation of moving around in space or a feeling of spinning or dizziness *Vertigo usually results from inner ear structure damage associated with balance and equilibrium.*

Diagnostic Procedures

Eye

tonometry tōn-ŎM-ĕ-trē *ton/o:* tension *-metry:* act of measuring	Screening test to detect glaucoma that measures intraocular pressure (IOP) by determining the resistance of the eyeball to pressure indentation by an applied force (See Figure 11–11.) *IOP pressure is measured by pressing the small, flat disk of the tonometer against the corner to record IOP.*
visual acuity test ă-KŪ-ĭ-tē	Standard eye examination to determine the smallest letters a person can read on a Snellen chart, or *E chart*, at a distance of 20 feet *Visual acuity is expressed as a ratio. The first number is the distance at which a person reads the chart, the second is the distance at which a person with normal vision can read the same chart. For example 20/20 indicates that the person correctly read letters at 20 feet that could be read by a person with normal vision at 20 feet. Normal vision is 20/20.*

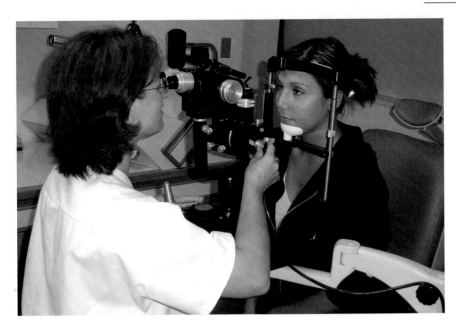

Figure 11-11   Tonometry.

Ear

audiometry ăw-dē-ŎM-ĕ-trē *audi/o:* hearing *-metry:* act of measuring	Test that measures hearing acuity at various sound frequencies *In audiometry, an instrument called an audiometer delivers acoustic stimuli at different frequencies, and results are plotted on a graph called an audiogram.*
otoscopy ō-TŎS-kŏ-pē *ot/o:* ear *-scopy:* visual examination	Visual examination of the external auditory canal and the tympanic membrane using an otoscope
pneumatic	Otoscopic procedure that assesses the ability of the tympanic membrane to move in response to a change in air pressure *In pneumatic otoscopy, the increase and decrease in pressure causes the healthy tympanic membrane to move in and out. Lack of movement indicates increased impedance or eardrum perforation.*
Rinne test RĬN-nē	Hearing acuity test performed with a vibrating tuning fork that is first placed on the mastoid process and then in front of the external auditory canal to test bone and air conduction *The Rinne test is useful for differentiating between conductive and sensorineural hearing loss.*

Medical and Surgical Procedures

Eye

cataract surgery KĂT-ă-răkt	Excision of a lens affected by a cataract *Extracapsular cataract extraction(ECCE) and phacoemulsification and are the two primary ways to remove a cataract. In both surgeries, the central part of the lens is removed and replaced with an artificial introcular lens (IOL) implant.*
extracapsular cataract extraction (ECCE) ĕks-tră-KĂP-sū-lăr KĂT-ă-răkt	Excision of the the anterior segment of the lens capsule along with the lens, allowing for the insertion of an intraocular lens implant
phacoemulsification FĂK-ō-ē-mŭl-sĭ-fĭ-kā-shŭn	Excision of the lens by ultrasonic vibrations that break the lens into tiny particles, which are suctioned out of the eye; also called *small incision cataract surgery (SICS)* (See Figure 11–12.)
corneal transplant KŎR-nē-ăl *corne:* cornea *-al:* pertaining to, relating to	Surgical transplantation of a donor cornea (from a cadaver) into the eye of a recipient; also called *keratoplasty*
iridectomy ĭr-ĭ-DĔK-tŏ-mē *irid:* iris *-ectomy:* excision, removal	Excision of a portion of the iris used to relieve intraocular pressure in patients with glaucoma *Iridectomy is usually performed to create an opening through which aqueous humor can drain.*

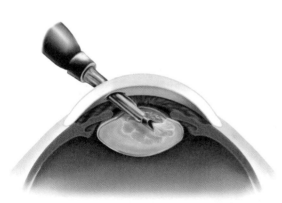
Cataract removal

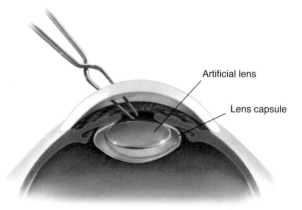
Artificial lens

Lens capsule

Artificial lens insertion

Figure 11-12 Phacoemulsification.

Ear

cochlear implant KŎK-lē-ăr *cochle:* cochlea *-ar:* pertaining to	Electronic transmitter surgically implanted into the cochlea of a deaf person to restore hearing
myringoplasty mĭr-ĬN-gō-plăst-ē *myring/o:* tympanic membrane (eardrum) *-plasty:* surgical repair	Surgical repair of a perforated eardrum with a tissue graft; also called *tympanoplasty* *Myringoplasty is performed to correct hearing loss.*
myringotomy mĭr-ĭn-GŎT-ō-mē *myring/o:* tympanic membrane (eardrum) *-tomy:* incision	Incision of the eardrum to relieve pressure and release pus or serous fluid from the middle ear or to insert PE tubes (tympanostomy tubes) in the eardrum via surgery (See Figure 11–6.) *Tympanostomy tubes provide ventilation and drainage of the middle ear when repeated ear infections do not respond to antibiotic treatment. They are used when persistent, severely negative middle ear pressure is present.*

Pharmacology

antiglaucoma drugs ăn-tĭ-glaw-KŌ-mă	Drugs that reduce intraocular pressure by lowering the amount of aqueous humor in the eyeball, reducing its production, or increasing its outflow
miotics mī-ŎT-ĭks	Agents that cause the pupil to constrict
mydriatics mĭd-rē-ĂT-ĭks	Agents that cause the pupil to dilate and prepare the eye for an internal examination
vertigo and motion sickness drugs VĔR-tĭ-gō	Drugs that decrease sensitivity of the inner ear to motion and prevent nerve impulses from the inner ear from reaching the vomiting center of the brain
wax emulsifiers ē-MŬL-sĭ-fī-ĕrs	Agents that loosen and help remove impacted ceruman (ear wax)

Additional Medical Terms Review

Match the medical term(s) below with the definitions in the numbered list.

achromatopsia	conjunctivitis	myringotomy	presbycusis
acoustic neuroma	diabetic retinopathy	otitis media	retinal detachment
anacusis	glaucoma	otosclerosis	Rinne test
astigmatism	hordeolum	phacoemulsification	strabismus
cataract	iridectomy	tinnitus	tonometry
conductive hearing loss	macular degeneration	photophobia	vertigo
	Ménière disease		

1. _____ means ringing in the ears.

2. _____ is progressive deafness due to ossification in the bony labyrinth of the inner ear.

3. _____ means color blindness.

4. _____ is a rare disorder characterized by progressive deafness, vertigo, and tinnitus, possibly caused by swelling of membranous structures within the labyrinth.

5. _____ is a disorder in which both eyes cannot focus on the same point, resulting in looking in different directions at the same time.

6. _____ means total deafness.

7. _____ refers to middle ear infection that is most commonly seen in young children.

8. _____ refers to *pinkeye*.

9. _____ means intolerance or unusual sensitivity to light.

10. _____ is hearing loss due to old age.

11. _____ refers to increased intraocular pressure caused by the failure of the aqueous humor to drain.

12. _____ refers to a feeling of spinning or dizziness.

13. _____ refers to separation of the retina from the choroid.

14. _____ is another term for *sty*.

15. _____ is abnormal curvature of the cornea, which causes light rays to focus unevenly over the retina, resulting in a distorted image.

16. _____ is a benign tumor of the eighth cranial nerve that may or may not produce symptomatic changes.

17. _____ measures intraocular pressure and is used to diagnose glaucoma.

18. _____ refers to excision of a portion of the iris.

19. _____ is hearing loss caused by an impairment in sound transmission because of damage to the eardrum, ossicles, or ear canal obstruction.

20. _____ refers to opacity (cloudiness) of the lens as a result of protein deposits on its surface.

21. _____ is a type of cataract surgery.

22. _____ is a hearing acuity test that is performed with a vibrating tuning fork.

23. _____ refers to retinal damage marked by aneurysmal dilation of blood vessels.

24. _____ loss of central vision that is the most common cause of visual impairment in persons older than age 50.

25. _____ is an incision of the eardrum to relieve pressure and release pus or serous fluid from the middle ear.

Competency Verification: Check your answers in Appendix B, Answer Key, page 581. If you are not satisfied with your level of comprehension, review the additional medical terms and retake the review.

Correct Answers: _____ × 4 _____ % Score

Medical Record Activities

Medical reports included in the following activities reflect common, real-life clinical scenarios using medical terminology to document patient care.

MEDICAL RECORD ACTIVITY 11-1

Retinal Detachment

Terminology

Terms listed in the table below come from the medical report *Retinal Detachment* that follows. Use a medical dictionary such as *Taber's Cyclopedic Medical Dictionary,* the appendices of this book, or other resources to define each term. Then practice reading the pronunciations aloud for each term.

Term	Definition
akinesia ă-kĭ-NĒ-zē-ă	
anesthesia ăn-ĕs-THĒ-zē-ă	
anteriorly ăn-TĒR-ē-or-lē	
cannula KĂN-ū-lă	
conjunctival kŏn-jŭnk-TĪ-văl	
EKG	
hemorrhage HĔM-ĕ-rĭj	
IV	
limbus LĬM-bŭs	
mm	
MVR	
retinal detachment RĔT-ĭ-năl	
retinitis rĕt-ĭ-NĪ-tĭs	

Term	Definition
retrobulbar rĕt-rō-BŬL-băr	
sclerotomy sklĕ-RŎT-ō-mē	
vitrectomy vĭ-TRĔK-tō-mē	

 Listen and Learn Online! will help you master pronunciations of selected medical words from this medical record activity. Visit *http://davisplus.fadavis.com/gylys/simplified* to find instructions on completing the *Listen and Learn Online!* exercise for this section and to practice pronunciations.

Reading

Practice pronunciation of medical terms by reading the following medical report aloud.

Retinal Detachment

DIAGNOSIS: Total retinal detachment, left eye, secondary to complications of retinitis.

PROCEDURE: Patient was taken to the operating room, placed on the operating table, IV infusion begun, EKG lead monitor attached, and retrobulbar anesthetic given, achieving good anesthesia and akinesia. The patient was scrubbed, prepped, and draped in a standard sterile fashion for retinal surgery. A 360-degree conjunctival opening was made and 2-0 silk sutures were placed around each rectus muscle. Four millimeters from the limbus, a mark in the sclera was made and preplaced 5-0 Mersiline suture was passed; MVR stab incision made, and 4-mm infusion cannula was slipped into position and visualized inside the eye. Similar sclerotomy sites were made superior nasally and superior temporally. Trans pars plana vitrectomy was undertaken. Dense vitreous hemorrhage and debris were found, which were removed. There was incomplete posterior vitreous attachment. The retina was almost totally detached, and a small amount of nasal retina was still attached. A linear retinal break was seen just above the disk along a vessel. Gradually, all peripheral vitreous was removed.

Air-fluid exchange was performed with some difficulty because some sort of vitreous was found anteriorly, which loculated the bubble. It gave me a peculiar view, but slowly the retina became totally flat, and we treated the retinal break with the diode laser. A 240 band was wrapped around the eye and fixed with the Watke's sleeve superior temporally. The sclerotomies were all sewn closed. Before the last sclerotomy was closed, the air was exchanged for silicone. The eye was left soft because the patient had poor perfusion.

Evaluation

Review the medical report above to answer the following questions. Use a medical dictionary such as *Taber's Cyclopedic Medical Dictionary* and other resources if needed.

1. Where is the retina located?

2. Was the anesthetic administered behind or in front of the eyeball?

_____

_____

3. How much movement remained in the eye following anesthesia?

_____

_____

4. Where was the hemorrhage located?

_____

_____

5. What type of vitrectomy was undertaken?

_____

_____

6. Why was the eye left soft?

_____

_____

MEDICAL RECORD ACTIVITY 11-2

Otitis Media

Terminology

Terms listed in the table below come from the medical report *Otitis Media* that follows. Use a medical dictionary such as *Taber's Cyclopedic Medical Dictionary,* the appendices of this book, or other resources to define each term. Then practice reading the pronunciations aloud for each term.

Term	Definition
cholesteatoma kō-lē-stē-ă-TŌ-mă	_____
ENT	_____
general anesthesia ăn-ĕs-THĒ-zē-ă	_____
mucoserous mū-kō-SĒR-ŭs	_____
otitis media ō-TĪ-tĭs MĒ-dē-ă	_____
postoperatively pōst-ŎP-ĕr-ă-tĭv-lē	_____
tympanoplasty tĭm-păn-ō-PLĂS-tē	_____

Listen and Learn Online! will help you master pronunciations of selected medical words from this medical record activity. Visit *http://davisplus.fadavis.com/gylys/simplified* to find instructions on completing the *Listen and Learn Online!* exercise for this section and to practice pronunciations.

Reading

Practice pronunciation of medical terms by reading the following medical report aloud.

Otitis Media

A 25-year-old white woman with a diagnosis of mucoserous otitis media in the right ear was seen by the ENT specialist. The patient was admitted to the hospital and developed cholesteatoma. A tube was inserted for the chronic adhesive otitis media with secondary cholesteatoma. The patient progressed favorably postoperatively, but the cholesteatoma continued to enlarge in size. Currently, she has been admitted to the hospital for a right tympanoplasty performed under general anesthesia.

Evaluation

Review the medical record above to answer the following questions. Use a medical dictionary such as *Taber's Cyclopedic Medical Dictionary* and other resources if needed.

1. Where was the patient's infection located?

_____

_____

2. What complication developed while the patient was hospitalized?

_____

_____

3. What is the purpose of the tube placement?

_____

_____

4. What surgery is being performed to resolve the cholesteatoma?

_____

_____

5. Will the patient be asleep during the surgery?

_____

_____

Chapter Review

Word Elements Summary

The table below summarizes combining forms, suffixes, and prefixes related to the special senses.

Word Element	Meaning	Word Element	Meaning
Combining Forms			
acous/o, audi/o, audit/o	hearing	**irid/o**	iris
aden/o	gland	**kerat/o**	horny tissue; hard; cornea
blephar/o	eyelid	**myring/o, tympan/o**	tympanic membrane (eardrum)
choroid/o	choroid	**ocul/o, ophthalm/o**	eye
chromat/o	color	**ot/o**	ear
cochle/o	cochlea	**retin/o**	retina
corne/o	cornea	**salping/o**	tube (usually fallopian or eustachian [auditory] tubes)
dacry/o, lacrim/o	tear; lacrimal apparatus (duct, sac, or gland)	**scler/o**	hardening; sclera (white of eye)
dipl/o	double		
OTHER COMBINING FORMS			
erythr/o	red	**presby/o**	old age
my/o	muscle	**ton/o**	tension
neur/o	nerve	**xanth/o**	yellow
Suffixes			
SURGICAL			
-ectomy	excision, removal	**-tomy**	incision
-plasty	surgical repair		
DIAGNOSTIC, SYMPTOMATIC, AND RELATED			
-acusis	hearing	**-pathy**	disease
-algia, -dynia	pain	**-ptosis**	prolapse, downward displacement
-edema	swelling	**-rrhexis**	rupture

Word Element	Meaning	Word Element	Meaning
-itis	inflammation	-salpinx	tube (usually fallopian or eustachian [auditory] tubes)
-logist	specialist in study of	-scope	instrument for examining
-logy	study of	-scopy	visual examination
-malacia	softening	-spasm	involuntary contraction, twitching
-metry	act of measuring	-stenosis	narrowing, stricture
-oma	tumor	-tomy	incision
-opia, -opsia	vision	-tropia	turning
-osis	abnormal condition; increase (used primarily with blood cells)		

Prefixes			
a-	without, not	eso-	inward
ana-	against; up; back	exo-	outside, outward
dipl-	double	hyper-	excessive, above normal

Enhance your study and reinforcement of word elements with the power of *Davis Plus.* Visit *http://davisplus.fadavis.com/gylys/simplified* for this chapter's flash-card activity. We recommend you complete the flash-card activity before completing the word elements review below.

Word Elements Review

After you review the word elements summary, complete this activity by writing the meaning of each element in the space provided.

Word Element	Meaning	Word Element	Meaning
Combining Forms			
1. acous/o, audi/o, audit/o	_____	8. myring/o, tympan/o	_____
2. aden/o	_____	9. ocul/o, ophthalm/o	_____
3. blephar/o	_____	10. ot/o	_____
4. choroid/o	_____	11. retin/o	_____
5. corne/o, kerat/o	_____	12. salping/o	_____
6. dacry/o, lacrim/o	_____	13. scler/o	_____
7. irid/o	_____		
Suffixes			
DIAGNOSTIC, SYMPTOMATIC, AND RELATED			
14. -acusis	_____	18. -ptosis	_____
15. -edema	_____	19. -rrhexis	_____
16. -opia	_____	20. -salpinx	_____
17. -pathy	_____	21. -stenosis	_____
Prefixes			
22. ana-	_____	24. exo-	_____
23. dipl-	_____	25. hyper-	_____

Competency Verification: Check your answers in Appendix A, Glossary of Medical Word Elements, page 538. If you are not satisfied with your level of comprehension, review the word elements and retake the review.

Correct Answers: _____ × 4 = _____ % Score

Vocabulary Review

Match the medical word(s) below with the definitions in the numbered list.

blepharoptosis	diplopia	labyrinth	otitis media
cholesteatoma	eustachian tube	mastoid surgery	postoperatively
chronic	general anesthetic	mucoserous	salpingostenosis
dacryorrhea	hyperopia	myopia	sclera
diagnosis	keratitis	ophthalmologist	tympanic membrane

1. _____ means double vision.

2. _____ refers to white of eye.

3. _____ is the eardrum; it vibrates when sound waves strike it.

4. _____ means excessive flow of tears.

5. _____ equalizes the air pressure in the middle ear with that of the outside atmosphere.

6. _____ refers to inflammation of the cornea due to a vision-threatening infection; sometimes occurs when contact lenses are not disinfected properly.

7. _____ is a process of determining the cause and nature of a pathological condition.

8. _____ means composed of mucus and serum.

9. _____ is inflammation of the middle ear.

10. _____ is a tumorlike sac filled with keratin debris most commonly found in the middle ear.

11. _____ is an operation on the mastoid process of the temporal bone.

12. _____ is anesthesia that affects the entire body with loss of consciousness.

13. _____ is a physician who specializes in the treatment of eye disorders.

14. _____ means *of long duration*, designating a disease showing little change or slow progression

15. _____ means farsightedness.

16. _____ means occurring after surgery.

17. _____ is a system of intercommunicating canals, especially of the inner ear.

18. _____ is prolapse of an eyelid.

19. _____ is a narrowing or stricture of the eustachian tube.

20. _____ means nearsightedness.

Competency Verification: Check your answers in Appendix B, Answer Key, page 582. If you are not satisfied with your level of comprehension, review the chapter vocabulary and retake the review.

Correct Answers: _____ × 5 = _____ % Score

A Glossary of Medical Word Elements

Medical Word Element	Meaning	Medical Word Element	Meaning
A		**ambly/o**	dull, dim
a-	without, not	**amni/o**	amnion (amniotic sac)
ab-	from, away from	**an-**	without, not
abdomin/o	abdomen	**an/o**	anus
abort/o	to miscarry	**ana-**	against; up; back
-ac	pertaining to	**andr/o**	male
acid/o	acid	**aneurysm/o**	widened blood vessel
acous/o	hearing	**angi/o**	vessel (usually blood or lymph)
acr/o	extremity		
acromi/o	acromion (projection of scapula)	**aniso-**	unequal, dissimilar
		ankyl/o	stiffness; bent, crooked
-acusis	hearing	**ante-**	before, in front of
-ad	toward	**anter/o**	anterior, front
ad-	toward	**anthrac/o**	coal, coal dust
aden/o	gland	**anti-**	against
adenoid/o	adenoids	**aort/o**	aorta
adip/o	fat	**append/o**	appendix
adren/o	adrenal glands	**appendic/o**	appendix
adrenal/o	adrenal glands	**aque/o**	water
aer/o	air	**-ar**	pertaining to
af-	toward	**-arche**	beginning
agglutin/o	clumping, sticking together	**arteri/o**	artery
		arteriol/o	arteriole
agora-	marketplace	**arthr/o**	joint
-al	pertaining to	**-ary**	pertaining to
albin/o	white	**asbest/o**	asbestos
albumin/o	albumin (protein)	**-asthenia**	weakness, debility
-algesia	pain	**astr/o**	star
-algia	pain	**-ate**	having the form of, possessing
allo-	other		
alveol/o	alveolus; air sac	**atel/o**	incomplete; imperfect

Medical Word Element	Meaning	Medical Word Element	Meaning
ather/o	fatty plaque	-cele	hernia, swelling
-ation	process (of)	-centesis	surgical puncture
atri/o	atrium	cephal/o	head
audi/o	hearing	-ceps	head
audit/o	hearing	-ception	conceiving
aur/o	ear	cerebell/o	cerebellumnt
auricul/o	ear	cerebr/o	cerebrum
auto-	self, own	cervic/o	neck; cervix uteri (neck of uterus)
ax/o	axis, axon		
azot/o	nitrogenous compounds	chalic/o	limestone
B		cheil/o	lip
bacteri/o	bacteria (singular, bacterium)	chem/o	chemical; drug
		chlor/o	green
balan/o	glans penis	chol/e	bile, gall
bas/o	base (alkaline, opposite of acid)	cholangi/o	bile vessel
		cholecyst/o	gallbladder
bi-	two	choledoch/o	bile duct
bi/o	life	chondr/o	cartilage
bil/i	bile, gall	chori/o	chorion
-blast	embryonic cell	choroid/o	choroid
blast/o	embryonic cell	chrom/o	color
blephar/o	eyelid	chromat/o	color
brachi/o	arm	-cide	killing
brachy-	short	cine-	movement
brady-	slow	circum-	around
bronch/o	bronchus (plural, bronchi)	cirrh/o	yellow
bronchi/o	bronchus (plural, bronchi)	-cision	a cutting
bronchiol/o	bronchiole	-clasia	to break; surgical fracture
bucc/o	cheek	-clasis	to break; surgical fracture
C		-clast	to break
calc/o	calcium	clavicul/o	clavicle (collar bone)
calcane/o	calcaneum (heel bone)	-cleisis	closure
-capnia	carbon dioxide (CO_2)	clon/o	clonus (turmoil)
carcin/o	cancer	-clysis	irrigation, washing
cardi/o	heart	coccyg/o	coccyx (tailbone)
-cardia	heart condition	cochle/o	cochlea
carp/o	carpus (wrist bones)	col/o	colon
cata-	down	colon/o	colon
caud/o	tail	colp/o	vagina
cauter/o	heat, burn	condyl/o	condyle
cec/o	cecum	coni/o	dust
		conjunctiv/o	conjunctiva

(continued)

Medical Word Element	Meaning	Medical Word Element	Meaning
-continence	to hold back	dipl/o	double
contra-	against, opposite	dips/o	thirst
cor/o	pupil	-dipsia	thirst
core/o	pupil	dist/o	far, farthest
corne/o	cornea	dors/o	back (of body)
coron/o	heart	duct/o	to lead; carry
corp/o	body	-duction	act of leading, bringing, conducting
corpor/o	body		
cortic/o	cortex	duoden/o	duodenum (first part of small intestine)
cost/o	ribs		
crani/o	cranium (skull)	dur/o	dura mater; hard
crin/o	secrete	-dynia	pain
-crine	secrete	dys-	bad; painful; difficult
cruci/o	cross	**E**	
cry/o	cold	-eal	pertaining to
crypt/o	hidden	ec-	out, out from
culd/o	cul-de-sac	echo-	a repeated sound
-cusia	hearing	-ectasis	dilation, expansion
-cusis	hearing	ecto-	outside, outward
cutane/o	skin	-ectomy	excision, removal
cyan/o	blue	-edema	swelling
cycl/o	ciliary body of eye; circular; cycle	ef-	away from
		electr/o	electricity
-cyesis	pregnancy	-ema	state of; condition
cyst/o	bladder	embol/o	embolus (plug)
cyt/o	cell	-emesis	vomiting
-cyte	cell	-emia	blood condition
D		emphys/o	to inflate
dacry/o	tear; lacrimal apparatus (duct, sac, or gland)	en-	in, within
		encephal/o	brain
dacryocyst/o	lacrimal sac	end-	in, within
dactyl/o	fingers; toes	endo-	in, within
de-	cessation	enter/o	intestine (usually small intestine)
dendr/o	tree		
dent/o	teeth	eosin/o	dawn (rose-colored)
derm/o	skin	epi-	above, upon
-derma	skin	epididym/o	epididymis
dermat/o	skin	epiglott/o	epiglottis
-desis	binding, fixation (of a bone or joint)	episi/o	vulva
		erythem/o	red
di-	double	erythemat/o	red
dia-	through, across	erythr/o	red
dipl-	double	eschar/o	scab

Medical Word Element	Meaning
-esis	condition
eso-	inward
esophag/o	esophagus
esthes/o	feeling
-esthesia	feeling
eti/o	cause
eu-	good, normal
ex-	out, out from
exo-	outside, outward
extra-	outside
F	
faci/o	face
fasci/o	band, fascia (fibrous membrane supporting and separating muscles)
femor/o	femur (thigh bone)
-ferent	to carry
fibr/o	fiber, fibrous tissue
fibul/o	fibula (smaller bone of lower leg)
fluor/o	luminous, fluorescence
G	
galact/o	milk
gangli/o	ganglion (knot or knotlike mass)
gastr/o	stomach
-gen	forming, producing, origin
gen/o	forming, producing, origin
-genesis	forming, producing, origin
genit/o	genitalia
gest/o	pregnancy
gingiv/o	gum(s)
glauc/o	gray
gli/o	glue; neuroglial tissue
-glia	glue; neuroglial tissue
-globin	protein
glomerul/o	glomerulus
gloss/o	tongue
glott/o	glottis
gluc/o	sugar, sweetness

Medical Word Element	Meaning
glucos/o	sugar, sweetness
glyc/o	sugar, sweetness
glycos/o	sugar, sweetness
gnos/o	knowing
-gnosis	knowing
gon/o	seed (ovum or spermatozoon)
gonad/o	gonads, sex glands
-grade	to go
-graft	transplantation
-gram	record, writing
granul/o	granule
-graph	instrument for recording
-graphy	process of recording
-gravida	pregnant woman
gyn/o	woman, female
gynec/o	woman, female
H	
hallucin/o	hallucination
hedon/o	pleasure
hem/o	blood
hemangi/o	blood vessel
hemat/o	blood
hemi-	one half
hepat/o	liver
hetero-	different
hidr/o	sweat
hist/o	tissue
histi/o	tissue
home/o	same, alike
homeo-	same, alike
homo-	same
humer/o	humerus (upper arm bone)
hydr/o	water
hyp-	under, below, deficient
hyp/o	under, below, deficient
hyper-	excessive, above normal
hypn/o	sleep
hypo-	under, below, deficient
hyster/o	uterus (womb)
I	
-ia	condition
-iac	pertaining to

(continued)

Medical Word Element	Meaning	Medical Word Element	Meaning
-iasis	abnormal condition (produced by something specified)	-itis	inflammation
		-ive	pertaining to
		-ization	process (of)
iatr/o	physician; medicine; treatment	**J**	
-iatry	medicine; treatment	jaund/o	yellow
-ic	pertaining to	jejun/o	jejunum (second part of small intestine)
-ical	pertaining to		
-ice	noun ending	**K**	
ichthy/o	dry, scaly	kal/i	potassium (an electrolyte)
-ician	specialist	kary/o	nucleus
-icle	small, minute	kerat/o	horny tissue; hard; cornea
-icterus	jaundice	ket/o	ketone bodies (acids and acetones)
idi/o	unknown, peculiar		
-ile	pertaining to	keton/o	ketone bodies (acids and acetones)
ile/o	ileum (third part of small intestine)		
		kinesi/o	movement
ili/o	ilium (lateral, flaring portion of hip bone)	-kinesia	movement
		kinet/o	movement
im-	not	kyph/o	humpback
immun/o	immune, immunity, safe	**L**	
in-	in; not	labi/o	lip
-ine	pertaining to	labyrinth/o	labyrinth (inner ear)
infer/o	lower, below	lacrim/o	tear; lacrimal apparatus (duct, sac, or gland)
infra-	below, under		
inguin/o	groin	lact/o	milk
insulin/o	insulin	-lalia	speech, babble
inter-	between	lamin/o	lamina (part of vertebral arch)
intra-	in, within		
-ion	the act of	lapar/o	abdomen
-ior	pertaining to	laryng/o	larynx (voice box)
irid/o	iris	later/o	side, to one side
-is	noun ending	lei/o	smooth
isch/o	to hold back; block	leiomy/o	smooth muscle (visceral)
ischi/o	ischium (lower portion of hip bone)	-lepsy	seizure
		lept/o	thin, slender
-ism	condition	leuk/o	white
iso-	same, equal	lingu/o	tongue
-ist	specialist	lip/o	fat
-isy	state of; condition	lipid/o	fat
-itic	pertaining to		

Medical Word Element	Meaning	Medical Word Element	Meaning
-listhesis	slipping	ment/o	mind
-lith	stone, calculus	meso-	middle
lith/o	stone, calculus	meta-	change, beyond
lob/o	lobe	metacarp/o	metacarpus (hand bones)
log/o	study of	metatars/o	metatarsus (foot bones)
-logist	specialist in the study of	-meter	instrument for measuring
-logy	study of	metr/o	uterus (womb); measure
lord/o	curve, swayback	metri/o	uterus (womb)
-lucent	to shine; clear	-metry	act of measuring
lumb/o	loins (lower back)	mi/o	smaller, less
lymph/o	lymph	micr/o	small
lymphaden/o	lymph gland (node)	micro-	small
lymphangi/o	lymph vessel	mono-	one
-lysis	separation; destruction; loosening	morph/o	form, shape, structure
		muc/o	mucus
M		multi-	many, much
		muscul/o	muscle
macro-	large	mut/a	genetic change
mal-	bad	my/o	muscle
-malacia	softening	myc/o	fungus (plural, fungi)
mamm/o	breast	mydr/o	widen, enlarge
-mania	state of mental disorder, frenzy	myel/o	bone marrow; spinal cord
		myos/o	muscle
mast/o	breast	myring/o	tympanic membrane (eardrum)
mastoid/o	mastoid process		
maxill/o	maxilla (upper jaw bone)	myx/o	mucus
meat/o	opening, meatus	**N**	
medi-	middle		
medi/o	middle	narc/o	stupor; numbness; sleep
mediastin/o	mediastinum	nas/o	nose
medull/o	medulla	nat/o	birth
mega-	enlargement	natr/o	sodium (an electrolyte)
megal/o	enlargement	necr/o	death, necrosis
-megaly	enlargement	neo-	new
melan/o	black	nephr/o	kidney
men/o	menses, menstruation	neur/o	nerve
mening/o	meninges (membranes covering brain and spinal cord)	neutr/o	neutral; neither
		nid/o	nest
		noct/o	night
		nucle/o	nucleus
meningi/o	meninges (membranes covering brain and spinal cord)	nulli-	none
		nyctal/o	night

(continued)

Medical Word Element	Meaning	Medical Word Element	Meaning
O		**-para**	to bear (offspring)
obstetr/o	midwife	**parathyroid/o**	parathyroid glands
ocul/o	eye	**-paresis**	partial paralysis
odont/o	teeth	**patell/o**	patella (kneecap)
-oid	resembling	**path/o**	disease
-ole	small, minute	**-pathy**	disease
olig/o	scanty	**pector/o**	chest
-oma	tumor	**ped/i**	foot; child
omphal/o	navel (umbilicus)	**ped/o**	foot; child
onc/o	tumor	**pedicul/o**	lice
onych/o	nail	**pelv/i**	pelvis
oophor/o	ovary	**pelv/o**	pelvis
-opaque	obscure	**pen/o**	penis
ophthalm/o	eye	**-penia**	decrease, deficiency
-opia	vision	**-pepsia**	digestion
-opsia	vision	**per-**	through
-opsy	view of	**peri-**	around
opt/o	eye, vision	**perine/o**	perineum (area between scrotum [or vulva in the female] and anus)
optic/o	eye, vision		
or/o	mouth		
orch/o	testis (plural, testes)	**peritone/o**	peritoneum
orchi/o	testis (plural, testes)	**-pexy**	fixation (of an organ)
orchid/o	testis (plural, testes)	**phac/o**	lens
-orexia	appetite	**phag/o**	swallowing, eating
orth/o	straight	**-phage**	swallowing, eating
-ory	pertaining to	**-phagia**	swallowing, eating
-ose	pertaining to; sugar	**phalang/o**	phalanges (bones of fingers and toes)
-osis	abnormal condition; increase (used primarily with blood cells)	**pharmaceutic/o**	drug, medicine
		pharyng/o	pharynx (throat)
-osmia	smell	**-phasia**	speech
oste/o	bone	**-phil**	attraction for
ot/o	ear	**phil/o**	attraction for
-ous	pertaining to	**-philia**	attraction for
ovari/o	ovary	**phleb/o**	vein
ox/i	oxygen	**-phobia**	fear
ox/o	oxygen	**-phonia**	voice
-oxia	oxygen	**-phoresis**	carrying, transmission
P		**-phoria**	feeling (mental state)
		phot/o	light
palat/o	palate (roof of mouth)	**phren/o**	diaphragm; mind
pan-	all	**-phylaxis**	protection
pancreat/o	pancreas	**-physis**	growth
para-	near, beside; beyond		

Medical Word Element	Meaning	Medical Word Element	Meaning
pil/o	hair	pupill/o	pupil
pituitar/o	pituitary gland	py/o	pus
-plakia	plaque	pyel/o	renal pelvis
plas/o	formation, growth	pylor/o	pylorus
-plasia	formation, growth	pyr/o	fire
-plasm	formation, growth	**Q, R**	
-plasty	surgical repair	quadri-	four
-plegia	paralysis	rachi/o	spine
pleur/o	pleura	radi/o	radiation, x-ray; radius (lower arm bone on thumb side)
-plexy	stroke		
-pnea	breathing		
pneum/o	air; lung	radicul/o	nerve root
pneumon/o	air; lung	rect/o	rectum
pod/o	foot	ren/o	kidney
-poiesis	formation, production	reticul/o	net, mesh
poikil/o	varied, irregular	retin/o	retina
poli/o	gray; gray matter (of brain or spinal cord)	retro-	backward, behind
		rhabd/o	rod-shaped (striated)
poly-	many, much	rhabdomy/o	rod-shaped (striated) muscle
polyp/o	small growth		
-porosis	porous	rhin/o	nose
post-	after, behind	rhytid/o	wrinkle
poster/o	back (of body), behind, posterior	roentgen/o	x-rays
		-rrhage	bursting forth (of)
-potence	power	-rrhagia	bursting forth (of)
-prandial	meal	-rrhaphy	suture
pre-	before, in front of	-rrhea	discharge, flow
presby/o	old age	-rrhexis	rupture
primi-	first	-rrhythm/o	rhythm
pro-	before, in front of	rube/o	red
proct/o	anus, rectum	**S**	
prostat/o	prostate gland	sacr/o	sacrum
proxim/o	near, nearest	salping/o	tube (usually fallopian or eustachian [auditory] tubes)
pseudo-	false		
psych/o	mind		
-ptosis	prolapse, downward displacement	-salpinx	tube (usually fallopian or eustachian [auditory] tubes)
ptyal/o	saliva		
-ptysis	spitting		
pub/o	pelvis bone (anterior part of pelvic bone)	sarc/o	flesh (connective tissue)
		-sarcoma	malignant tumor of connective tissue
pulmon/o	lung		

(continued)

Medical Word Element	Meaning	Medical Word Element	Meaning
scapul/o	scapula (shoulder blade)	steth/o	chest
-schisis	a splitting	sthen/o	strength
schiz/o	split	stigmat/o	point, mark
scler/o	hardening; sclera (white of eye)	stomat/o	mouth
scoli/o	crooked, bent	-stomy	forming an opening (mouth)
-scope	instrument for examining	sub-	under, below
-scopy	visual examination	sudor/o	sweat
scot/o	darkness	super-	upper, above
seb/o	sebum, sebaceous	super/o	upper, above
semi-	one half	supra-	above; excessive; superior
semin/i	semen; seed	sym-	union, together, joined
semin/o	semen; seed	syn-	union, together, joined
sept/o	septum	synapt/o	synapsis, point of contact
sequestr/o	separation	synov/o	synovial membrane, synovial fluid
ser/o	serum		
sial/o	saliva, salivary gland	**T**	
sider/o	iron		
sigmoid/o	sigmoid colon	tachy-	rapid
sin/o	sinus, cavity	tax/o	order, coordination
sinus/o	sinus, cavity	-taxia	order, coordination
-sis	state of; condition	ten/o	tendon
somat/o	body	tend/o	tendon
somn/o	sleep	tendin/o	tendon
son/o	sound	-tension	to stretch
-spadias	slit, fissure	test/o	testis (plural, *testes*)
-spasm	involuntary contraction, twitching	thalam/o	thalamus
sperm/i	spermatozoa, sperm cells	thalass/o	sea
sperm/o	spermatozoa, sperm cells	thec/o	sheath (usually refers to meninges)
spermat/o	spermatozoa, sperm cells	thel/o	nipple
sphygm/o	pulse	therapeut/o	treatment
-sphyxia	pulse	-therapy	treatment
spin/o	spine	therm/o	heat
spir/o	breathe	thorac/o	chest
splen/o	spleen	-thorax	chest
spondyl/o	vertebra (backbone)	thromb/o	blood clot
squam/o	scale	thym/o	thymus gland
staped/o	stapes	-thymia	mind; emotion
-stasis	standing still	thyr/o	thyroid gland
steat/o	fat	thyroid/o	thyroid gland
sten/o	narrowing, stricture	tibi/o	tibia (larger bone of lower leg)
-stenosis	narrowing, stricture	-tic	pertaining tong
stern/o	sternum (breastbone)		

Medical Word Element	Meaning	Medical Word Element	Meaning
-tocia	childbirth, labor	**ureter/o**	ureter
tom/o	to cut	**urethr/o**	urethra
-tome	instrument to cut	**-uria**	urine
-tomy	incision	**urin/o**	urine, urinary tract
ton/o	tension	**-us**	condition; structure
tonsill/o	tonsils	**uter/o**	uterus (womb)
tox/o	poison	**uvul/o**	uvula
-toxic	poison	**V**	
toxic/o	poison	**vagin/o**	vagina
trabecul/o	trabecula (supporting bundles of fibers)	**valv/o**	valve
		varic/o	dilated vein
trache/o	trachea (windpipe)	**vas/o**	vessel; vas deferens; duct
trans-	across, through	**vascul/o**	vessel (usually blood or lymph)
tri-	three		
trich/o	hair	**ven/o**	vein
trigon/o	trigone (triangular region at base of bladder)	**ventr/o**	belly, belly side
		ventricul/o	ventricle (of heart or brain)
-tripsy	crushing	**-version**	turning
-trophy	development, nourishment	**vertebr/o**	vertebra (backbone)
-tropia	turning	**vesic/o**	bladder
-tropin	stimulate	**vesicul/o**	seminal vesicle
tubercul/o	a little swelling	**vest/o**	clothes
tympan/o	tympanic membrane (eardrum)	**viscer/o**	internal organs
		vitr/o	vitreous body (of eye)
U		**vitre/o**	glassy
-ula	small, minute	**vol/o**	volume
-ule	small, minute	**vulv/o**	vulva
uln/o	ulna (lower arm bone on opposite side of thumb)	**X, Y, Z**	
		xanth/o	yellow
ultra-	excess, beyond	**xen/o**	foreign, strange
-um	structure, thing	**xer/o**	dry
umbilic/o	umbilicus, navel	**xiph/o**	sword
ungu/o	nail	**-y**	condition; process
uni-	one		
ur/o	urine, urinary tract		

Chapter 1: Introduction to Programmed Learning and Medical Word Building

Frame 1–51

Medical Term	Combining Form (Root + *o*)	Word Root	Suffix
arthr/o/scop/ic ăr-thrōs-KŎP-ĭk	*arthr/o*	*scop*	*-ic*
erythr/o/cyt/osis ĕ-rĭth-rō-sī-TŌ-sĭs	erythr/o	cyt	-osis
append/ix ă-PĔN-dĭks		append	-ix
dermat/itis dĕr-mă-TĪ-tĭs		dermat	-itis
gastr/o/enter/itis găs-trō-ĕn-tĕr-Ī-tĭs	gastr/o	enter	-itis
orth/o/ped/ic or-thō-PĒ-dĭk	orth/o	ped	-ic
oste/o/arthr/itis ŏs-tē-ō-ăr-THRĪ-tĭs	oste/o	arthr	-itis
vagin/itis văj-ĭn-Ī-tĭs		vagin	-itis

Section Review 1–1

1. breve
2. macron
3. long
4. short
5. pn
6. hard
7. n
8. eye
9. second
10. separate

Surgical Suffixes

Term	Meaning
arthr/o/**centesis** ăr-thrō-sĕn-TĒ-sĭs *arthr/o:* joint	*surgical puncture of a joint*
oste/o/**clast** ŎS-tē-ō-klăst *oste/o:* bone	Area of broken-down bone
arthr/o/**desis** ăr-thrō-DĒ-sĭs *arthr/o:* joint	binding or fixation of a joint
append/**ectomy** ăp-ĕn-DĔK-tō-mē *append:* appendix	excision or removal of the appendix
thromb/o/**lysis** thrŏm-BŎL-ĭ-sĭs *thromb/o:* blood clot	separation, destruction, or loosening of a blood clot
mast/o/**pexy** MĂS-tō-pĕks-ē *mast/o:* breast	fixation of the breast(s)
rhin/o/**plasty** RĪ-nō-plăs-tē *rhin/o:* nose	surgical repair of the nose (to change shape or size)
my/o/**rrhaphy** mī-OR-ă-fē *my/o:* muscle	suture of a muscle
trache/o/**stomy** trā-kē-ŎS-tō-mē *trache/o:* trachea (windpipe)	forming an opening (mouth) into the trachea
oste/o/**tome** ŎS-tē-ō-tōm *oste/o:* bone	instrument to cut bone
trache/o/**tomy** trā-kē-ŎT-ō-mē *trache/o:* trachea (windpipe)	incision into the trachea
lith/o/**tripsy** LĬTH-ō-trĭp-sē *lith/o:* stone, calculus	crushing a stone or calculus

Diagnostic Suffixes

Term	Meaning
electr/o/cardi/o/**gram** ē-lĕk-trō-KĂR-dē-ō-grăm *electr/o:* electricity *cardi/o:* heart	record of electrical activity of the heart
cardi/o/**graph** KĂR-dē-ō-grăf *cardi/o:* heart	instrument to record electrical activity of the heart
angi/o/**graphy** ăn-jē-ŎG-ră-fē *angi/o:* vessel (usually blood or lymph)	process of recording images of blood vessels (recording images of blood vessels after injection of a contrast medium)
pelv/i/**meter** pĕl-VĬM-ĕ-tĕr *pelv/i:* pelvis	instrument for measuring the pelvis
pelv/i/**metry** pĕl-VĬM-ĕ-trē *pelv/i:* pelvis	act of measuring the pelvis
endo/**scope** ĔN-dō-skōp *endo-:* in, within	instrument for examining within (or inside a hollow organ or cavity)
endo/**scopy** ĕn-DŎS-kō-pē *endo-:* in, within	visual examination within (a cavity or canal using a specialized lighted instrument called an endoscope)

Pathologic Suffixes

Term	Meaning
neur/**algia** nū-RĂL-jē-ă *neur:* nerve	pain of a nerve (or pain along the path of a nerve)
ot/o/**dynia** ō-tō-DĬN-ē-ă *ot/o:* ear	pain in the ear (earache)
hepat/o/**cele** hĕ-PĂT-ō-sēl *hepat/o:* liver	hernia or swelling of the liver

Term	Meaning
bronchi/**ectasis** brŏng-kē-ĔK-tă-sĭs *bronchi:* bronchus (plural, bronchi)	abnormal dilation or expansion of a bronchus or bronchi
lymph/**edema** lĭmf-ĕ-DĒ-mă *lymph:* lymph	swelling of lymph tissue (swelling resulting from accumulation of tissue fluid)
hyper/**emesis** hī-pĕr-ĔM-ĕ-sĭs *hyper-:* excessive, above normal	excessive or above normal vomiting
an/**emia** ă-NĒ-mē-ă *an-:* without, not	literally means without blood (blood condition caused by iron deficiency or decrease in red blood cells)

chol/e/lith/**iasis**
kō-lē-lĭ-THĪ-ă-sĭs
  chol/e: bile, gall
    lith: stone, calculus
	presence or formation of gallstones (in the gallbladder or common bile duct)

gastr/**itis** găs-TRĪ-tĭs *gastr:* stomach	inflammation of the stomach
chol/e/**lith** KŌ-lē-lĭth *chol/e:* bile, gall	gallstone
chondr/o/**malacia** kŏn-drō-mă-LĀ-shē-ă *chondr/o:* cartilage	softening of cartilage
cardi/o/**megaly** kăr-dē-ō-MĔG-ă-lē *cardi/o:* heart	enlargement of the heart
neur/**oma** nū-RŌ-mă *neur:* nerve	tumor composed of nerve cells
cyan/**osis** sī-ă-NŌ-sĭs *cyan:* blue	abnormal condition of dark blue (bluish or purple discoloration of the skin and mucous membrane)
my/o/**pathy** mī-ŎP-ă-thē *my/o:* muscle	any disease of muscle

(continued)

Term	Meaning
erythr/o/**penia** ĕ-rĭth-rō-PĒ-nē-ă *erythr/o:* red	abnormal decrease or deficiency in red (blood cells)
hem/o/**phobia** hē-mō-FŌ-bē-ă *hem/o:* blood	fear of blood
hemi/**plegia** hĕm-ē-PLĒ-jē-ă *hemi-:* one half	paralysis of one half (paralysis of one side of the body)
hem/o/**rrhage** HĔM-ĕ-rĭj *hem/o:* blood	bursting forth of blood (loss of large amounts of blood within a short period, externally or internally)
men/o/**rrhagia** mĕn-ō-RĀ-jē-ă *men/o:* menses, menstruation	bursting forth of menses (profuse discharge of blood during menstruation)
dia/**rrhea** dī-ă-RĒ-ă *dia-:* through, across	discharge or flow through (abnormally frequent discharge or flow of fluid fecal matter from the bowel)
arteri/o/**rrhexis** ăr-tē-rē-ō-RĔK-sĭs *arteri/o:* artery	rupture of an artery
arteri/o/**stenosis** ăr-tē-rē-ō-stĕ-NŌ-sĭs *arteri/o:* artery	narrowing or stricture of an artery
hepat/o/**toxic** HĔP-ă-tō-tŏk-sĭk *hepat/o:* liver	potentially destructive to the liver
dys/**trophy** DĬS-trō-fē *dys-:* bad; painful; difficult	bad development or nourishment (abnormal condition caused by defective nutrition or metabolism)

Section Review 1–2

Singular	Plural	Rule
1. sarcoma	*sarcomata*	*Retain the* ma *and add* ta.
2. thrombus	thrombi	Drop *us* and add *i*.
3. appendix	appendices	Drop *ix* and add *ices*.
4. diverticulum	diverticula	Drop *um* and add *a*.
5. ovary	ovaries	Drop *y* and add *ies*.
6. diagnosis	diagnoses	Drop *is* and add *es*.
7. lumen	lumina	Drop *en* and add *ina*.
8. vertebra	vertebrae	Retain the *a* and add *e*.
9. thorax	thoraces	Drop the *x* and add *ces*.
10. spermatozoon	spermatozoa	Drop *on* and add *a*.

Common Prefixes

Term	Meaning
a/mast/ia ă-MĂS-tē-ă 　*mast:* breast 　　*-ia:* condition	without a breast
an/esthesia ăn-ĕs-THĒ-zē-ă 　*-esthesia:* feeling	without feeling (partial or complete loss of sensation with or without loss of consciousness)
circum/duction sĕr-kŭm-DŬK-shŭn 　*-duction:* act of leading, 　　　　bringing, 　　　　conducting	act of leading around (movement of a part, such as an extremity, in a circular direction)
peri/odont/al pĕr-ē-ō-DŎN-tăl 　*odont:* teeth 　　*-al:* pertaining to	pertaining to around a tooth
dia/rrhea dī-ă-RĒ-ă 　*-rrhea:* discharge, flow	flow through
trans/vagin/al trăns-VĂJ-ĭn-ăl 　*vagin:* vagina 　　*-al:* pertaining to	pertaining to across the vagina

(continued)

Term	Meaning
dipl/opia dĭp-LŌ-pē-ă *-opia:* vision	double vision

diplo/bacteri/al
dĭp-lō-băk-TĒR-ē-ăl
  bacteri: bacteria
    -al: pertaining to
	pertaining to bacteria linked together in pairs

endo/crine ĔN-dō-krĭn *-crine:* secrete	secrete within

intra/muscul/ar
ĭn-tră-MŬS-kū-lăr
  muscul: muscle
    -ar: pertaining to
	pertaining to within the muscle

homo/graft HŌ-mō-grăft *-graft:* transplantation	literally means transplantation of same (transplantion of tissue between the same species)
homeo/plasia hō-mē-ō-PLĀ-zē-ă *-plasia:* formation, growth	formation or growth of new tissue similar to that already existing in a part

hypo/derm/ic
hī-pō-DĔR-mĭk
  derm: skin
    -ic: pertaining to
	pertaining to under the skin (under or inserted under the skin, as in a hypodermic injection)

macro/cyte MĂK-rō-sīt *-cyte:* cell	abnormally large cell (usually erythrocyte), such as those found in pernicious anemia
micro/scope MĬ-krō-skōp *-scope:* instrument for examining	instrument for examining minute objects
mono/cyte MŎN-ō-sīt *-cyte:* cell	large mononuclear leukocyte

uni/nucle/ar
ū-nĭ-NŪ-klē-ăr
  nucle: nucleus
    -ar: pertaining to
	pertaining to one nucleus

post/nat/al
pōst-NĀ-tăl
  nat: birth
    -al: pertaining to
	pertaining to (the period) after birth

Term	Meaning

pre/nat/al
prē-NĀ-tăl
  nat: birth
   -al: pertaining to
	pertaining to (the period) before birth

pro/gnosis prŏg-NŌ-sĭs *-gnosis:* knowing	before knowing; knowing beforehand (prediction of the course and end of a disease, and the estimated chance of recovery)
primi/gravida prī-mĭ-GRĂV-ĭ-dă *-gravida:* pregnant woman	woman during her first pregnancy
retro/version rĕt-rō-VĔR-shŭn *-version:* turning	literally means turning backward (tipping backward of an organ (such as the uterus) from its normal position)
super/ior soo-PĒ-rē-or *-ior:* pertaining to	pertaining to upper or above (toward the head or upper portion of a structure)

Chapter 2: Body Structure

Section Review 2–1

Term	Meaning
1. dist/al	*-al: pertaining to; far, farthest*
2. poster/ior	-ior: pertaining to; back (of body), behind, posterior
3. hist/o/logist	-logist: specialist in study of; tissue
4. dors/al	-al: pertaining to; back (of body)
5. anter/ior	-ior: pertaining to; anterior, front
6. later/al	-al: pertaining to; side, to one side
7. medi/ad	-ad: toward; middle
8. cyt/o/toxic	-toxic: poison; cell
9. proxim/al	-al: pertaining to; near, nearest
10. ventr/al	-al: pertaining to; belly, belly side

Section Review 2–2

1. hist/o	**4.** proxim/o	**7.** ventr/o	**10.** caud/o	**13.** infer/o
2. -al, -ior	**5.** -logy	**8.** -toxic	**11.** -logist	**14.** -lysis
3. medi/o	**6.** cyt/o	**9.** -ad	**12.** dist/o	**15.** later/o

Section Review 2–3

Term	Meaning
1. ili/ac	*-ac: pertaining to; ilium (lateral, flaring portion of hip bone)*
2. abdomin/al	-al: pertaining to; abdomen
3. inguin/al	-al: pertaining to; groin
4. spin/al	-al: pertaining to; spine
5. peri/umbilic/al	-al: pertaining to; around; umbilicus, navel
6. cephal/ad	-ad: toward; head
7. gastr/ic	-ic: pertaining to; stomach
8. thorac/ic	-ic: pertaining to; chest
9. cervic/al	-al: pertaining to; neck, cervix uteri (neck of uterus)
10. lumb/ar	-ar: pertaining to; loins (lower back)

Section Review 2–4

1. -ad	4. pelv/o	7. -ac, -al, -ic, -ior	10. hypo-	13. umbilic/o
2. inguin/o	5. chondr/o	8. lumb/o	11. crani/o	14. poster/o
3. gastr/o	6. epi-	9. thorac/o	12. spin/o	15. abdomin/o

Additional Medical Terms Review

1. CT	4. MRI	7. anastomosis	10. radiopharmaceutical	13. adhesion
2. fluoroscopy	5. PET	8. SPECT	11. endoscopy	14. radiography
3. US	6. endoscope	9. tomography	12. cauterize	15. sepsis

Chapter 3: Integumentary System

Section Review 3–1

Term	Meaning
1. hypo/derm/ic	*-ic: pertaining to; under, below, deficient; skin*
2. melan/oma	-oma: tumor; black
3. kerat/osis	-osis: abnormal condition, increase (used primarily with blood cells); horny tissue; hard; cornea
4. cutane/ous	-ous: pertaining to; skin
5. lip/o/cyte	-cyte: cell; fat
6. onych/o/malacia	-malacia: softening; nail

Term	Meaning
7. scler/o/derma	-derma: skin; hardening; sclera (white of eye)
8. dia/phoresis	-phoresis: carrying, transmission; through, across
9. dermat/o/myc/osis	-osis: abnormal condition, increase (used primarily with blood cells); skin; fungus
10. cry/o/therapy	-therapy: treatment; cold

Competency Verification, Figure 3–2

Identifying Integumentary Structures, Page 69

1. epidermis   **3.** stratum corneum   **5.** hair follicle   **7.** sudoriferous (sweat) gland
2. dermis   **4.** basal layer   **6.** sebaceous (oil) gland   **8.** subcutaneous tissue

Competency Verification, Figure 3–3

Structure of a Fingernail, Page 77

1. nail root   **3.** cuticle   **5.** nail body
2. matrix   **4.** nail bed   **6.** lunula

Section Review 3–2

1. -pathy   **5.** trich/o, pil/o   **9.** derm/o, dermat/o, cutane/o, -derma   **12.** epi-
2. xer/o   **6.** scler/o   **13.** -osis
3. lip/o, adip/o, steat/o   **7.** -cele   **10.** -malacia   **14.** hidr/o
4. -rrhea   **8.** onych/o   **11.** -logist   **15.** hypo-

Section Review 3–3

1. melan/o   **4.** cyt/o, -cyte   **7.** -rrhea   **10.** -derma   **13.** xanth/o
2. cyan/o   **5.** -penia   **8.** erythr/o   **11.** -oma   **14.** necr/o
3. -emia   **6.** -pathy   **9.** auto-   **12.** leuk/o   **15.** -osis

Additional Medical Terms Review

1. verruca   **4.** furuncle   **7.** biopsy   **10.** cryosurgery   **13.** alopecia
2. vitiligo   **5.** eczema   **8.** dermabrasion   **11.** debridement   **14.** comedo
3. tinea   **6.** urticaria   **9.** electrodesiccation   **12.** scabies   **15.** petechia

Medical Record Activity 3–1: Compound Nevus

Evaluation

1. What is a nevus?

   A mole; a type of skin tumor

2. Locate the vermilion border on your lip. Where is it located?

   It is the edge of the red portion of the upper or lower lip.

3. Was the lesion limited to a certain area?

   Yes, the right side of the lower lip

4. In the impression, the pathologist has ruled out melanoma. What does this mean?

   The nevus is not cancerous.

5. Is melanoma a dangerous condition? If so, explain why.

   Yes, it metastasizes rapidly.

Medical Record Activity 3–2: Psoriasis

Evaluation

1. What causes psoriasis?

   The etiology is unknown, but heredity is a significant determining factor

2. On what parts of the body does psoriasis typically occur?

   Scalp, elbows, knees, sacrum, and around the nails, arms, legs, and abdomen.

3. How is psoriasis treated?

   Mild to moderate psoriasis is treated with corticosteroids and phototherapy.

4. What is a histiocytoma?

   A tumor containing histiocytes, macrophages present in all loose connective tissue

Vocabulary Review

1. subcutaneous	6. suction lipectomy	11. onychoma	16. xeroderma
2. diaphoresis	7. onychomycosis	12. hirsutism	17. melanoma
3. trichopathy	8. pressure ulcers	13. pustule	18. lipocele
4. autograft	9. leukemia	14. papules	19. xanthoma
5. Kaposi sarcoma	10. ecchymosis	15. erythrocyte	20. onychomalacia

Chapter 4: Respiratory System

Section Review 4–1

Term	Meaning
1. laryng/o/scope	-scope: instrument for examining; larynx (voice box)
2. py/o/thorax	-thorax: chest; pus
3. hyp/oxia	-oxia: oxygen; under, below, deficient
4. trache/o/stomy	-stomy: forming an opening (mouth); trachea (windpipe)
5. a/pnea	-pnea: breathing; without, not
6. pulmon/o/logist	-logist: specialist in study of; lung
7. pneumon/ia	-ia: condition; air, lung
8. rhin/o/rrhea	-rrhea: discharge, flow; nose
9. an/osmia	-osmia: smell; without, not
10. pneum/ectomy	-ectomy: excision, removal; air, lung

Section Review 4–2

1. aer/o
2. para-
3. myc/o
4. -ectasis
5. -stomy
6. -tomy
7. -tome
8. laryng/o
9. -cele
10. neo-
11. nas/o, rhin/o
12. -plegia
13. pharyng/o
14. -stenosis
15. -phagia
16. trache/o
17. -therapy
18. a-, an-
19. -scopy
20. hydr/o

Competency Verification, Figure 4–2

Identifying Upper and Lower Respiratory Tracts, Page 111

1. nasal cavity
2. pharynx (throat)
3. larynx (voice box)
4. epiglottis
5. trachea (windpipe)
6. right and left primary bronchi
7. bronchioles
8. left lung
9. alveoli
10. pulmonary capillaries
11. pleura
12. diaphragm

Section Review 4–3

1. -osis
2. brady-
3. dys-
4. melan/o
5. -pnea
6. bronch/o, bronchi/o
7. hem/o
8. thorac/o
9. -ectasis
10. -phobia
11. myc/o
12. eu-
13. -cele
14. -scope
15. -spasm
16. macro-
17. tachy-
18. pneum/o, pneumon/o
19. pleur/o
20. micro-
21. orth/o
22. -stenosis
23. -centesis
24. a-
25. chondr/o

Additional Medical Terms Review

1. stridor   **6.** cystic fibrosis   **10.** crackle   **14.** atelectasis   **18.** SIDS

2. epistaxis   **7.** lung cancer   **11.** bronchodilators   **15.** epiglottitis   **19.** hypoxia

3. influenza   **8.** pleural effusion   **12.** ARDS   **16.** pertussis   **20.** rhonchi

4. acidosis   **9.** pneumothorax   **13.** MRI   **17.** consolidation

5. coryza

Medical Record Activity 4–1: Upper Airway Obstruction

Evaluation

1. What types of patients are at risk for nasal polyps?

Patients with chronic inflammation of the nasal cavity and sinus mucosa that is usually due to allergies

2. When is a polypectomy indicated?

When the patient fails to respond to medical treatment or if there is severe nasal obstruction

3. Were the patient's nasal polyps cancerous?

No, polyps are benign

4. What contributed to the patient's death?

Papillary carcinoma that metastasized to the lymph node

5. Why was a biopsy of the liver performed?

Enlarged liver nodes; to check for metastasis

6. What does "patient expired at home" mean?

Patient died at home

Medical Record Activity 4–2: Bronchoscopy

Evaluation

1. What does "bronchoscope was inserted transnasally" mean?

It was inserted through the nose

2. What was seen in the left lower bronchus?

Endobronchial friable mucosal lesion, partially occluding the entire left lower lobe bronchus

3. What kinds of biopsies were obtained during the bronchoscopy?

Transbronchial biopsies of the left lower lung area, transbronchial needle aspiration, bronchial brush biopsies, and bronchial brush washings

4. What type of radiographic procedure was used to enhance visualization to obtain biopsies for cytology evaluation?

Fluoroscopic

5. What condition results from the bacterium *Legionella?*

Legionnaire disease

Vocabulary Review

1. pyothorax	**5.** tracheostomy	**9.** aspirate	**13.** pharyngoplegia	**17.** rhinoplasty
2. thoracentesis	**6.** diagnosis	**10.** chondroma	**14.** pleurisy	**18.** TB
3. asthma	**7.** apnea	**11.** atelectasis	**15.** *Pneumocystis*	**19.** COPD
4. croup	**8.** aerophagia	**12.** anosmia	**16.** catheter	**20.** pneumothorax

Chapter 5: Cardiovascular and Lymphatic

Section Review 5–1

Term	Meaning
1. endo/cardi/um	-um: structure, thing; in, within; heart
2. cardi/o/megaly	-megaly: enlargement; heart
3. aort/o/stenosis	-stenosis: narrowing, stricture; aorta
4. tachy/cardia	-cardia: heart condition; rapid
5. phleb/itis	-itis: inflammation; vein
6. thromb/o/lysis	-lysis: separation, destruction, loosening; blood clot
7. vas/o/spasm	-spasm: involuntary contraction, twitching; vessel; vas deferens; duct
8. ather/oma	-oma: tumor; fatty plaque
9. electr/o/cardi/o/graphy	-graphy: process of recording; electricity; heart
10. atri/o/ventricul/ar	-ar: pertaining to; atrium; ventricle (of heart or brain)

Competency Verification, Figure 5–2

Heart Structures, Page 157

1. endocardium	**5.** right atrium	**8.** pulmonary trunk	**11.** left atrium
2. myocardium	**6.** superior vena cava	**9.** right lung	**12.** right pulmonary veins
3. pericardium	**7.** inferior vena cava	**10.** left lung	**13.** left pulmonary veins
4. aorta			

Competency Verification, Figure 5–3

Internal Structures of the Heart, Page 161

1. right atrium (RA)
2. left atrium (LA)
3. right ventricle (RV)
4. left ventricle (LV)
5. interventricular septum (IVS)
6. superior vena cava (SVC)
7. inferior vena cava (IVC)
8. tricuspid valve
9. pulmonary valve
10. right pulmonary artery
11. left pulmonary artery
12. right pulmonary veins
13. left pulmonary veins
14. mitral valve
15. aortic valve
16. aorta
17. branches of the aorta
18. descending aorta

Competency Verification, Figure 5–5

Heart Structures Depicting Valves and Cusps, Page 170

1. tricuspid valve
2. mitral valve
3. chordae tendineae
4. pulmonary valve
5. aortic valve
6. three cusps
7. two cusps

Section Review 5–2

1. -osis
2. epi-
3. aort/o
4. peri-
5. arteri/o
6. atri/o
7. hem/o, hemat/o
8. -pnea
9. -pathy
10. -ectasis
11. scler/o
12. cardi/o
13. -spasm
14. my/o
15. tachy-
16. -rrhexis
17. brady-
18. -ole, -ule
19. -rrhaphy
20. -stenosis
21. -phagia
22. tri-
23. bi-
24. phleb/o, ven/o
25. ventricul/o

Competency Verification, Figure 5–6

Conduction Pathway of the Heart, Page 173

1. sinoatrial (SA) node
2. right atrium (RA)
3. atrioventricular (AV) node
4. bundle of His
5. bundle branches
6. Purkinje fibers

Section Review 5–3

Term	Meaning
1. agglutin/ation	*-ation: process (of); clumping, gluing*
2. thym/oma	-oma: tumor; thymus gland
3. phag/o/cyte	-cyte: cell; swallowing, eating
4. lymphaden/itis	-itis: inflammation; lymph gland (node)

Term	Meaning
5. splen/o/megaly	-megaly: enlargement; spleen
6. aden/o/pathy	-pathy: disease; gland
7. ana/phylaxis	-phylaxis: protection; against, up, back
8. lymphangi/oma	-oma: tumor; lymph vessel
9. lymph/o/poiesis	-poiesis: formation, production; lymph
10. immun/o/gen	-gen: forming, producing, origin; immune, immunity, safe

Competency Verification, Figure 5–9

Lymphatic System, Page 183

1. lymph capillaries

2. lymph vessels

3. thoracic duct

4. right lymphatic duct

5. cervical nodes

6. axillary nodes

7. inguinal nodes

8. tonsil

9. spleen

10. thymus

Section Review 5–4

1. aort/o

2. hem/o

3. thromb/o

4. -cyte

5. cerebr/o

6. necr/o

7. -pathy

8. electr/o

9. -megaly

10. cardi/o

11. lymph/o

12. my/o

13. -graphy

14. -gram

15. -al, -ic

16. -rrhexis

17. -lysis

18. -stenosis

19. -plasty

20. angi/o

Additional Medical Terms Review

1. varicose veins

2. mononucleosis

3. thrombolytic therapy

4. embolus

5. lymphadenitis

6. DVT

7. hypertension

8. arrhythmia

9. TIA

10. bruit

11. stroke

12. rheumatic heart disease

13. atherosclerosis

14. Holter monitor

15. Raynaud phenomenon

16. ischemia

17. Hodgkin disease

18. AIDS

19. HF

20. fibrillation

21. valvuloplasty

22. lymphangiography

23. tissue typing

24. troponin I

25. CABG

Medical Record Activity 5–1: Myocardial Infarction

Evaluation

1. What symptoms did the patient experience before admission to the hospital?

Generalized malaise, increased shortness of breath (SOB) while at rest, and dyspnea followed by periods of apnea and syncope

2. What was found during clinical examination?

Irregular radial pulse, uncontrolled atrial fibrillation with evidence of a recent myocardial infarction (MI)

3. What is the danger of atrial fibrillation?

A decrease in cardiac output and promotion of thrombus formation in the upper chambers, syncope, angina, palpitations, and HF

4. Did the patient have prior history of heart problems? If so, describe them.

Yes, sinus tachycardia attributed to preoperative anxiety and thyroiditis

5. Was the patient's prior heart problem related to her current one?

No.

Medical Record Activity 5–2: Cardiac Catheterization

Evaluation

1. What coronary arteries were under examination?

The left and right coronary arteries

2. Which surgical procedure was used to clear the stenosis?

Balloon angioplasty

3. What symptoms did the patient exhibit before balloon inflation?

The patient had significant ST elevations in the inferior leads and severe throat tightness and shortness of breath.

4. Why was the patient put on heparin?

To prevent postsurgical clots from forming.

Vocabulary Review

1. myocardium	**5.** systole	**9.** desiccated	**13.** MI	**17.** capillaries
2. tachypnea	**6.** diastole	**10.** cardiomegaly	**14.** agglutination	**18.** hemangioma
3. arteriosclerosis	**7.** ECG	**11.** aneurysm	**15.** tachyphagia	**19.** arterioles
4. phagocyte	**8.** malaise	**12.** angina pectoris	**16.** anaphylaxis	**20.** pacemaker

Chapter 6: Digestive System

Section Review 6–1

Term	Meaning
1. gingiv/itis	*-itis:* inflammation; gum(s)
2. dys/pepsia	-pepsia: digestion; bad, painful, difficult
3. pylor/o/tomy	-tomy: incision; pylorus
4. dent/ist	-ist: specialist; teeth
5. esophag/o/scope	-scope: instrument for examining; esophagus
6. gastr/o/scopy	-scopy: visual examination; stomach

Term	Meaning
7. dia/rrhea	-rrhea: discharge, flow; through, across
8. hyper/emesis	-emesis: vomiting; excessive, above normal
9. an/orexia	-orexia: appetite; without, not
10. sub/lingu/al	-al: pertaining to; under, below; tongue

Competency Verification, Figure 6–2

Oral Cavity, Esophagus, Pharynx, and Stomach, Page 215

1. oral cavity **3.** submandibular gland **5.** bolus **7.** esophagus

2. sublingual gland **4.** parotid gland **6.** pharynx (throat) **8.** stomach

Section Review 6–2

1. -oma **6.** myc/o **11.** sial/o **16.** dia- **21.** stomat/o, or/o

2. -al, -ary, -ic **7.** gingiv/o **12.** gastr/o **17.** lingu/o, gloss/o **22.** -algia, -dynia

3. peri- **8.** pylor/o **13.** -ist **18.** -scope **23.** -phagia

4. hypo- **9.** dys- **14.** orth/o **19.** -tomy **24.** an-

5. -rrhea **10.** hyper- **15.** dent/o, odont/o **20.** -orexia **25.** -pepsia

Section Review 6–3

Term	Meaning
1. duoden/o/scopy	*-scopy: visual examination; duodenum (first part of small intestine)*
2. appendic/itis	-itis: inflammation; appendix
3. enter/o/pathy	-pathy: disease; intestine (usually small intestine)
4. col/o/stomy	-stomy: forming an opening (mouth); colon
5. rect/o/cele	-cele: hernia, swelling; rectum
6. sigmoid/o/tomy	-tomy: incision; sigmoid colon
7. proct/o/logist	-logist: specialist in study of; anus, rectum
8. jejun/o/rrhaphy	-rrhaphy: suture; jejunum (second part of small intestine)
9. append/ectomy	-ectomy: excision, removal; appendix
10. ile/o/stomy	-stomy: forming an opening (mouth); ileum (third part of small intestine)

Competency Verification, Figure 6–3

Small Intestine and Colon, Page 231

1. duodenum

2. jejunum

3. ileum

4. ascending colon

5. transverse colon

6. descending colon

7. sigmoid colon

8. rectum

9. anus

Section Review 6–4

1. enter/o

2. -tome

3. rect/o

4. -spasm

5. ile/o

6. -scopy

7. jejun/o

8. col/o, colon/o

9. duoden/o

10. -stomy

11. proct/o

12. -stenosis

13. -rrhaphy

14. -tomy

15. sigmoid/o

Section Review 6–5

Term	Meaning
1. hepat/itis	*-itis: inflammation; liver*
2. hepat/o/megaly	-megaly: enlargement; liver
3. chol/e/lith	-lith: stone, calculus; bile, gall
4. cholangi/ole	-ole: small, minute; bile vessel
5. cholecyst/ectomy	-ectomy: excision, removal; gallbladder
6. post/prandial	-prandial: meal; after, behind
7. chol/e/lith/iasis	-iasis: abnormal condition (produced by something specified); bile, gall; stone, calculus
8. choledoch/o/tomy	-tomy: incision; bile duct
9. pancreat/o/lith	-lith: stone, calculus; pancreas
10. pancreat/o/lysis	-lysis: separation; destruction; loosening; pancreas

Competency Verification, Figure 6–6

Liver, Gallbladder, Pancreas, and Duodenum with Associated Ducts and Blood Vessels, Page 243

1. liver

2. gallbladder

3. pancreas

4. duodenum

5. common bile duct

6. right hepatic duct

7. left hepatic duct

8. hepatic duct

9. cystic duct

10. pancreatic duct

Section Review 6–6

1. -osis	**6.** -megaly	**11.** hepat/o	**16.** -gram
2. -iasis	**7.** -ectomy	**12.** -algia, -dynia	**17.** -lith
3. choledoch/o	**8.** -stomy	**13.** pancreat/o	**18.** -plasty
4. chol/e	**9.** cholecyst/o	**14.** toxic/o, tox/o, -toxic	**19.** -rrhaphy
5. cyst/o	**10.** therm/o	**15.** -graphy	**20.** -emesis

Additional Medical Terms Review

1. hemoccult	**6.** lithotripsy	**11.** hematochezia
2. nasogastric intubation	**7.** fistula	**12.** volvulus
3. polyp	**8.** jaundice	**13.** cirrhosis
4. ascites	**9.** barium enema	**14.** barium swallow
5. Crohn disease	**10.** IBD	**15.** IBS

Medical Record Activity 6–1: Rectal Bleeding

Evaluation

1. What is the patient's symptom that made him seek medical help?

   Weight loss of 40 pounds since his last examination

2. What surgical procedures were performed on the patient for regional enteritis?

   Ileostomy and appendectomy

3. What abnormality was found with the sigmoidoscopy?

   Dark blood and rectal bleeding

4. What is causing the rectal bleeding?

   It could be due to a polyp, bleeding, diverticulum, or rectal carcinoma.

5. Write the plural form of diverticulum.

   Diverticula

Medical Record Activity 6–2: Carcinosarcoma of the Esophagus

Evaluation

1. What surgery was performed on this patient?

   Resection of the esophagus with anastomosis of the stomach; mediastinal lymph node excision

2. What diagnostic testing confirmed malignancy?

   Pathology tests on the biopsy specimen from esophagoscopy

3. Where was the carcinosarcoma located?

   Middle third of the esophagus

4. Why was the adjacent lymph node excised?

   Metastasis was suspected.

Vocabulary Review

1. gastroscopy
2. dyspepsia
3. hematemesis
4. ultrasound
5. salivary glands
6. alimentary canal
7. stomatalgia
8. duodenotomy
9. hepatomegaly
10. dysphagia
11. cholecystectomy
12. anastomosis
13. sigmoidotomy
14. rectoplasty
15. GERD
16. ileostomy
17. cholelithiasis
18. friable
19. choledochal
20. bariatric

Chapter 7: Urinary System

Section Review 7–1

Term	Meaning
1. glomerul/o/scler/osis	-osis: abnormal condition, increase (used primarily with blood cells); glomerulus; hardening, sclera (white of eye)
2. cyst/o/scopy	-scopy: visual examination; bladder
3. poly/uria	-uria: urine; many, much
4. lith/o/tripsy	-tripsy: crushing; stone, calculus
5. dia/lysis	-lysis: separation; destruction; loosening; through, across
6. ureter/o/stenosis	-stenosis: narrowing, stricture; ureter
7. meat/us	-us: condition, structure; opening, meatus
8. ur/emia	-emia: blood condition; urine
9. nephr/oma	-oma: tumor; kidney
10. ureter/o/cele	-cele: hernia; swelling; ureter

Section Review 7–2

1. -osis
2. -iasis
3. supra-
4. -pathy
5. -megaly
6. dia-
7. -pexy
8. scler/o
9. -tome
10. -tomy
11. nephr/o, ren/o
12. -ptosis
13. lith/o
14. -rrhaphy
15. poly-

Competency Verification, Figure 7–2

Urinary System, page 277

1. right kidney
2. renal cortex
3. renal medulla
4. renal artery
5. renal vein
6. nephron
7. ureters
8. urinary bladder
9. urethra
10. urinary meatus

Section Review 7–3

1. -iasis
2. cyst/o, vesic/o
3. carcin/o
4. -pathy

5. -megaly
6. -ectomy
7. -ectasis
8. aden/o

9. -tomy
10. -itis
11. -scope
12. enter/o

13. pyel/o
14. rect/o
15. -lith
16. -plasty

17. -rrhaphy
18. -oma
19. ureter/o
20. urethr/o

Competency Verification, Figure 7–6

Structure of a Nephron, Page 294

1. renal cortex
2. renal medulla

3. glomerulus
4. collecting tubule

5. Bowman capsule

Section Review 7–4

1. cyst/o, vesic/o
2. hemat/o
3. cyt/o, -cyte
4. glomerul/o
5. scler/o

6. -ist
7. nephr/o, ren/o
8. py/o
9. erythr/o
10. pyel/o

11. olig/o
12. ureter/o
13. urethr/o
14. ur/o
15. leuk/o

16. -cele
17. poly-
18. -ptosis
19. intra-
20. a-, an-

Additional Medical Terms Review

1. urinalysis
2. Wilms tumor
3. azoturia
4. dysuria

5. diuresis
6. retrograde pyelography
7. hypospadias
8. interstitial nephritis

9. BUN
10. enuresis
11. catheterization
12. VCUG

13. uremia
14. renal hypertension
15. dialysis

Medical Record Activity 7–1: Cystitis

Evaluation

1. What was found when the patient had a cystoscopy?

   Cystitis

2. What are the symptoms of cystitis?

   Nocturia, urinary frequency, pelvic pain, and hematuria, in this case

3. What is the patient's past surgical history?

   Cholecystectomy, choledocholithotomy, and incidental appendectomy

4. What is the treatment for cystitis?

   Antibiotics and consumption of a lot of fluids

5. What are the dangers of untreated cystitis?

The spreading of infection to the kidneys or to the bloodstream (sepsis)

6. What instrument is used to perform a cystoscopy?

A cystoscope

Medical Record Activity 7–2: Dysuria with Benign Prostatic Hypertrophy

Evaluation

1. What prompted the consultation with the urologist, Dr. Moriarty?

Preoperative catheterization was not possible

2. What abnormality did the urologist discover?

Mild to moderate benign prostatic hypertrophy

3. Did the patient have any previous surgery on his prostate?

No

4. Where was the patient's hernia?

In the groin and scrotum (hydrocele)

5. What in the patient's past medical history contributed to his present urological problem?

Nothing in his past history contributed to his benign prostatic hypertrophy; he had a previous colon resection for carcinoma of the colon

Vocabulary Review

1. malignant	**6.** diuretics	**11.** nephroptosis	**16.** hematuria
2. nephrons	**7.** edema	**12.** ureteropyeloplasty	**17.** polyuria
3. cholelithiasis	**8.** benign	**13.** bilateral	**18.** oliguria
4. renal pelvis	**9.** nephrolithotomy	**14.** nocturia	**19.** anuria
5. IVP	**10.** acute renal failure	**15.** urinary incontinence	**20.** cystocele

Chapter 8: Reproductive System

Section Review 8–1

Term	Definition
1. primi/gravida	-gravida: pregnant woman; first
2. colp/o/scopy	-scopy: visual examination; vagina
3. gynec/o/logist	-logist: specialist in study of; woman, female
4. perine/o/rrhaphy	-rrhaphy: suture; perineum
5. hyster/ectomy	-ectomy: excision, removal; uterus (womb)

Term	Definition
6. oophor/oma	-oma: tumor; ovary
7. dys/tocia	-tocia: childbirth, labor; bad, painful, difficult
8. endo/metr/itis	-itis: inflammation; in, within; uterus (womb); measure
9. mamm/o/gram	-gram: record, writing; breast
10. amni/o/centesis	-centesis: surgical puncture; amnion (amniotic sac)

Section Review 8–2

1. cyst/o

2. hemat/o, hem/o

3. -rrhage, -rrhagia

4. hyster/o, uter/o, metr/o

5. -cele

6. -tomy

7. -tome

8. -scope

9. salping/o, -salpinx

10. -pexy

11. muc/o

12. oophor/o, ovari/o

13. -arche

14. metr/o

15. -ptosis

16. -oid

17. -logist

18. -logy

19. -plasty

20. colp/o, vagin/o

Competency Verification, Figures 8–2 and 8–3

Lateral View of the Female Reproductive System, Page 331

Anterior View of the Female Reproductive System, Page 331

1. ovary (singular)

2. fallopian tube (singular)

3. uterus

4. vagina

5. labia majora

6. labia minora

7. clitoris

8. Bartholin gland

9. cervix

Competency Verification, Figure 8–7

Structure of Mammary Glands, Page 345

1. adipose tissue

2. glandular tissue

3. lobe

4. lactiferous duct

5. nipple

6. areola

Section Review 8–3

1. post-

2. gynec/o

3. pre-

4. mamm/o, mast/o

5. -pathy

6. -ectomy

7. -rrhea

8. -itis

9. -tome

10. -scope

11. -scopy

12. men/o

13. cervic/o

14. -algia, -dynia

15. -ary, -ous

16. -logist

17. salping/o

18. colp/o, vagin/o

19. vulv/o, episi/o

20. dys-

Section Review 8–4

Term	Meaning
1. vas/ectomy	-ectomy: excision, removal; vessel, vas deferens, duct
2. balan/itis	-itis: inflammation; glans penis
3. spermat/i/cide	-cide: killing; spermatozoa, sperm cells
4. gonad/o/tropin	-tropin: stimulate; gonads, sex glands
5. orchi/o/pexy	-pexy: fixation (of an organ); testis (plural, *testes*)
6. a/sperm/ia	-ia: condition; without, not; spermatozoa, sperm cells
7. vesicul/itis	-itis: inflammation; seminal vesicle
8. orchid/ectomy	-ectomy: excision, removal; testis (plural, *testes*)
9. andr/o/gen	-gen: forming, producing, origin; male
10. crypt/orch/ism	-ism: condition; hidden; testis (plural, *testes*)

Competency Verification, Figure 8–10

Lateral View of the Male Reproductive System, Page 355

1. testis (singular) or testicle (singular)
2. scrotum
3. epididymis
4. vas deferens
5. seminal vesicle
6. prostate gland
7. bulbourethral gland
8. penis
9. glans penis
10. foreskin

Section Review 8–5

1. -rrhaphy
2. dys-
3. cyst/o
4. carcin/o
5. -cyte
6. -pathy
7. -megaly
8. -cele
9. -itis
10. -tome
11. vas/o
12. muc/o
13. neo-
14. -genesis
15. prostat/o
16. test/o, orchi/o, orchid/o
17. olig/o
18. spermat/o, sperm/o
19. -pexy
20. hyper-

Additional Medical Terms Review

1. cryptorchidism
2. pyosalpinx
3. sterility
4. anorchism
5. candidiasis
6. chlamydia
7. circumcision
8. cerclage
9. leukorrhea
10. endometriosis
11. mammography
12. gonorrhea
13. syphilis
14. toxic shock
15. trichomoniasis
16. D&C
17. phimosis
18. impotence
19. oligomenorrhea
20. gonadotropins

Medical Record Activity 8–1: Postmenopausal Bleeding

Evaluation

1. How many times has the patient been pregnant? How many children has the patient given birth to?

Four; four

2. Why is the patient being admitted to the hospital?

To have a gynecological laparoscopy and diagnostic D&C to rule out the neoplastic process

3. What is a D&C?

Dilatation and curettage; a surgical procedure that expands the cervical canal of the uterus so that the surface lining of the uterine wall can be scraped

4. What is the patient's past surgical history?

Simple mastectomy a year ago

5. At what sites did the patient have malignant growth?

Left breast with metastases to the axilla, liver, and bone

Medical Record Activity 8–2: Bilateral Vasectomy

Evaluation

1. What is the end result of a bilateral vasectomy?

Sterilization

2. Was the patient awake during the surgery? What type of anesthesia was used?

Yes; 1% Xylocaine

3. What was used to prevent bleeding?

Hemostats, cautery, and sutures

4. What type of suture material was used to close the incision?

2–0 chromic

5. What was the patient given for pain relief at home?

Darvocet-N 100

6. Why is it important for the patient to go for a follow-up visit?

To analyze his semen and confirm sterilization

Vocabulary Review

1. prostatomegaly

2. testopathy

3. testosterone

4. amenorrhea

5. estrogen, progesterone

6. oophoritis

7. aspermatism

8. gravida 4

9. uterus

10. prostatic cancer

11. epididymis

12. hydrocele

13. vas deferens

14. para 4

15. cervix uteri

16. dysmenorrhea

17. postmenopausal

18. aplasia

19. vasectomy

20. PID

Chapter 9: Endocrine and Nervous Systems

Section Review 9–1

Term	Definition
1. toxic/o/logist	-logist: specialist in study of; poison
2. pancreat/itis	-itis: inflammation; pancreas
3. thyr/o/megaly	-megaly: enlargement; thyroid gland
4. hyper/trophy	-trophy: development, nourishment; excessive, above normal
5. gluc/o/genesis	-genesis: forming, producing, origin; sugar, sweetness
6. hypo/calc/emia	-emia: blood condition; under, below, deficient; calcium
7. adrenal/ectomy	-ectomy: excision, removal; adrenal glands
8. poly/dipsia	-dipsia: thirst; many, much
9. aden/oma	-oma: tumor; gland
10. thyroid/ectomy	-ectomy: excision, removal; thyroid gland

Section Review 9–2

1. -osis	5. -emia	9. acr/o	13. -tome	17. -logist
2. hyper-	6. calc/o	10. anter/o	14. neur/o	18. poly-
3. poster/o	7. -pathy	11. aden/o	15. toxic/o	19. thyroid/o, thyr/o
4. dys-	8. -megaly	12. -tomy	16. radi/o	20. hypo

Competency Verification, Figure 9–3

Locations of Major Endocrine Glands, Page 395

1. pituitary gland	4. adrenal glands	7. thymus gland
2. thyroid gland	5. pancreas	8. ovaries
3. parathyroid glands	6. pineal gland	9. testes

Section Review 9–3

1. -iasis	6. -rrhea	11. -lysis	16. -dipsia
2. supra-	7. poly-	12. -lith	17. thym/o
3. adrenal/o, adren/o	8. para-	13. gluc/o, glyc/o	18. hypo-
4. -pathy	9. pancreat/o	14. -phagia	19. -uria
5. -pexy	10. -gen, -genesis	15. orch/o, orchi/o, orchid/o	20. toxic/o

Section Review 9–4

Term	Meaning
1. meningi/oma	*-oma: tumor; meninges*
2. neur/o/lysis	-lysis: separation, destruction, loosening; nerve
3. hemi/paresis	-paresis: partial paralysis; one half
4. myel/algia	-algia: pain; bone marrow, spinal cord
5. cerebr/o/spin/al	-al: pertaining to; cerebrum; spine
6. a/phasia	-phasia: speech; without, not
7. mening/o/cele	-cele: hernia, swelling; meninges
8. encephal/itis	-itis: inflammation; brain
9. gli/oma	-oma: tumor; glue; neuroglial tissue
10. quadri/plegia	-plegia: paralysis; four

Competency Verification, Figure 9–8

1. cervical nerves
2. thoracic nerves
3. lumbar nerves
4. sacral nerves
5. coccygeal nerve

Section Review 9–5

1. -osis
2. dys-
3. thromb/o
4. vascul/o
5. encephal/o
6. -rhage, -rrhagia
7. gli/o, -glia
8. scler/o
9. mening/o, meningi/o
10. neur/o
11. cerebr/o
12. -malacia
13. -phasia
14. myel/o
15. a-

Additional Medical Terms Review

1. Bell palsy
2. stroke
3. epilepsy
4. exophthalmos
5. Graves disease
6. insulinoma
7. myxedema
8. pheochromocytoma
9. Parkinson disease
10. poliomyelitis
11. sciatica
12. spina bifida
13. hydrocephalus
14. neuroblastoma
15. Alzheimer disease
16. MRI
17. type 1 diabetes
18. shingles
19. pituitarism
20. panhypopituitarism
21. Huntington chorea
22. lumbar puncture
23. CT
24. thalamotomy
25. PET

Medical Record Activity 9–1: Diabetes Mellitus

Evaluation

1. What symptoms of DM did the patient experience before his office visit?

   Glycosuria, elevated blood glucose of 400, polydipsia, and increased appetite

2. What confirmed the patient's new diagnosis of DM?

   Elevated blood glucose and glycosuria

3. What conditions had to be met before the patient could be discharged from the hospital?

   He had to be able to draw up and give his own insulin and perform fingersticks.

4. How many times a day does the patient have to take insulin?

   Two times, once in the morning and once in the afternoon

5. Why does the patient have to perform fingersticks four times a day?

   To monitor his blood glucose levels closely and ensure they are within the normal range

6. What is an ADA 2,000-calorie diet? Why is it important?

   A 2000-calorie diet designed by American Diabetic Association, which is important for maintaining the same number of calories each day to help control blood glucose levels

Medical Record Activity 9–2: Stroke

Evaluation

1. Did the patient have a history of cardiovascular problems before her stroke?

   No

2. What symptoms did the patient experience just before her stroke?

   Paralysis of the right arm and left leg, aphasia, and diplopia

3. What is the primary site of this patient's cancer?

   Head of the pancreas

4. What is cerebrovascular disease?

   A disorder resulting from a change within the blood vessel(s) of the brain

5. What is the probable cause of the patient's stroke?

   Metastatic lesion of the brain or cerebrovascular disease

Vocabulary Review

1. acromegaly	8. pancreatopathy	15. adrenalectomy	22. vertigo
2. pancreatolysis	9. polyphagia	16. adrenaline	23. jaundice
3. adenohypophysis	10. diabetes mellitus	17. glycogenesis	24. metastasis
4. cerebral palsy	11. hyperglycemia	18. meningocele	25. hormone
5. hypercalcemia	12. pancreatolith	19. neuromalacia	
6. insulin	13. polydipsia	20. pruritus	
7. neurohypophysis	14. thyrotoxicosis	21. deglutition	

Chapter 10: Musculoskeletal System

Section Review 10–1

Term	Meaning
1. my/o/sarcoma	-sarcoma: malignant tumor of connective tissue; muscle
2. my/o/rrhaphy	-rrhaphy: suture; muscle
3. hemi/plegia	-plegia: paralysis; one half
4. ten/o/tomy	-tomy: incision; tendon
5. cost/o/chondr/itis	-itis: inflammation; ribs; cartilage
6. tend/o/lysis	-lysis: separation, destruction, loosening; tendon
7. my/o/pathy	-pathy: disease; muscle
8. lumb/o/cost/al	-al: pertaining to; loins (lower back); ribs
9. tendin/itis	-itis: inflammation; tendon
10. my/algia	-algia: pain; muscle

Section Review 10–2

1. -osis	5. hemi-	9. hepat/o	13. -rrhexis	17. -tome
2. cyst/o	6. scler/o	10. my/o	14. -plasty	18. chondr/o
3. -cyte	7. -tomy	11. -plegia	15. -rrhaphy	19. -sarcoma
4. quadri-	8. enter/o	12. -genesis	16. ten/o, tendin/o, tend/o	20. -lysis

Section Review 10–3

Term	Meaning
1. dia/physis	-physis: growth; through, across
2. sub/cost/al	-al: pertaining to; under, below; ribs
3. oste/o/malacia	-malacia: softening; bone
4. lamin/ectomy	-ectomy: excision, removal; lamina (part of vertebral arch)
5. pelv/i/metry	-metry: act of measuring; pelvis
6. myel/o/cele	-cele: hernia, swelling; bone marrow, spinal cord
7. oste/o/porosis	-porosis: porous; bone
8. ankyl/osis	-osis: abnormal condition, increase (used primarily with blood cells); stiffness; bent, crooked
9. carp/o/ptosis	-ptosis: prolapse, downward displacement; carpus (wrist bones)
10. crani/o/tomy	-tomy: incision; cranium (skull)

Competency Verification, Figure 10–4

Longitudinal Section of a Long Bone (femur) and Interior Bone Structure, Page 463

1. diaphysis
2. periosteum
3. compact bone
4. medullary cavity
5. distal epiphysis
6. proximal epiphysis
7. spongy bone

Section Review 10–4

1. hyper-
2. peri-
3. -emia
4. oste/o
5. chondr/o
6. calc/o
7. -cyte
8. dist/o
9. scler/o
10. -cele
11. -tomy
12. -itis
13. proxim/o
14. my/o
15. -algia, -dynia
16. -graphy
17. -genesis
18. -gram
19. -malacia
20. -logist
21. myel/o
22. -rrhaphy
23. -oma
24. hypo-
25. radi/o

Competency Verification, Figure 10–7

Anterior View of the Skeleton, Page 473

1. crani/o
2. stern/o
3. cost/o
4. vertebr/o
5. humer/o
6. carp/o
7. metacarp/o
8. phalang/o
9. pelv/i, pelv/o
10. femor/o
11. patell/o
12. tibi/o
13. fibul/o
14. calcane/o

Competency Verification, Figure 10–8

Types of Fractures, Pages 475

1. closed fracture
2. open fracture
3. greenstick fracture
4. comminuted fracture
5. impacted fracture
6. complicated fracture
7. Colles fracture
8. incomplete fracture

Competency Verification, Figure 10–9

Vertebral Column, Lateral View, Page 477

1. intervertebral disks
2. cervical vertebrae
3. atlas
4. axis
5. thoracic vertebrae
6. lumbar vertebrae
7. sacrum
8. coccyx

Section Review 10–5

1. -osis
2. oste/o
3. encephal/o
4. thorac/o
5. -pathy
6. -ectomy
7. cephal/o
8. arthr/o
9. lumb/o
10. cervic/o
11. -um
12. cost/o
13. sacr/o
14. -centesis
15. spondyl/o, vertebr/o

Additional Medical Terms Review

1. osteoporosis
2. tendinitis
3. sprain
4. strain
5. kyphosis
6. Ewing sarcoma

7. torticollis
8. gout
9. RA
10. Paget disease
11. sequestrum
12. arthroplasty

13. crepitation
14. myasthenia gravis
15. lordosis
16. muscular dystrophy
17. contracture
18. ankylosis

19. herniated disk
20. CTS
21. sequestrectomy
22. rheumatoid factor
23. talipes
24. arthroscopy

25. scoliosis

Medical Record Activity 10–1: Degenerative, Intervertebral Disk Disease

Evaluation

1. Why does the x-ray show a decreased density at L5–S1?

    Appears that a bilateral laminectomy had been done

2. What is the most common cause of degenerative intervertebral disk disease?

    Aging; this is a common finding in individuals 50 years old and older

3. What happens to the gelatinous material of the disk as aging occurs?

    The gelatinous material is replaced by harder fibrocartilage

4. What is the probable cause of the narrowing of the L3–L4 and L4–L5?

    Narrowing commonly occurs as a result of degenerative intervertebral disk disease

Medical Record Activity 10–2: Rotator Cuff Tear, Right Shoulder

Evaluation

1. What type of arthritis did the patient have?

    Degenerative

2. Did the patient have calcium deposits in the right shoulder?

    No

3. What type of instrument did the physician use to visualize the glenoid labra?

    Arthroscope

4. What are labra?

    Liplike structures; in this case, edges or rims of bones

5. Did the patient have any outgrowths of bone? If so, where?

    Yes, spurs were found at the inferior and anterior acromioclavicular joint

6. Did they find any deposits of calcium salts within the shoulder joint?

    They were unable to visualize an intra-articular calcification.

Vocabulary Review

1. radiology
2. diaphysis
3. AP
4. closed fracture
5. bilateral

6. proximal
7. articulation
8. open fracture
9. atlas
10. arthrocentesis

11. bone marrow
12. cephalometer
13. myelogram
14. myorrhexis
15. spondylomalacia

16. distal
17. radiologist
18. cervical vertebrae
19. intervertebral
20. quadriplegia

Chapter 11 Special Senses: The Eyes and Ears

Section Review 11–1

Term	Meaning
1. aniso/cor/ia	*-ia: condition; unequal, dissimilar; pupil*
2. blephar/o/ptosis	-ptosis: prolapse, downward displacement; eyelid
3. ambly/opia	-opia: vision; dull, dim
4. retin/o/pathy	-pathy: disease; retina
5. scler/itis	-itis: inflammation; hardening, sclera (white of eye)
6. ophthalm/o/scope	-scope: instrument for examining; eye
7. intra/ocul/ar	-ar: pertaining to; within, in; eye
8. dacry/o/rrhea	-rrhea: discharge, flow; tear; lacrimal apparatus (duct, sac, or gland)
9. dipl/opia	-opia: vision; double
10. blephar/o/spasm	-spasm: involuntary contraction, twitching; eyelid

Competency Verification, Figure 11–1

Eye Structures, Page 505

1. sclera
2. cornea
3. choroid

4. ciliary body
5. iris
6. retina

7. fovea
8. pupil
9. optic disc

10. optic nerve
11. conjunctiva

Competency Verification, Figure 11–3

Lacrimal Apparatus, Page 509

1. lacrimal gland
2. lacrimal sac
3. nasolacrimal duct

Section Review 11–2

Term	Meaning
1. tympan/o/centesis	*-centesis: surgical puncture; tympanic membrane (eardrum)*
2. acous/tic	-tic: pertaining to; hearing
3. hyper/tropia	-tropia: turning; excessive, above normal
4. ot/o/rrhea	-rrhea: discharge, flow; ear
5. an/acusis	-acusis: hearing; without, not
6. myring/o/tomy	-tomy: incision; tympanic membrane (eardrum)
7. tympan/o/plasty	-plasty: surgical repair; tympanic membrane (eardrum)
8. audi/o/meter	-meter: instrument for measuring; hearing
9. ot/o/scope	-scope: instrument for examining; ear
10. salping/o/pharyng/eal	-eal: pertaining to; tube (usually fallopian or eustachian [auditory] tubes); pharynx (throat)

Figure 11–4 - Ear structures

1. auricle   **4.** malleus   **7.** eustachian (auditory) tube   **10.** vestibule

2. ear canal   **5.** incus   **8.** cochlea

3. tympanic membrane   **6.** stapes   **9.** semicircular canals

Section Review 11–3

1. hyper-   **6.** salping/o, -salpinx   **11.** -spasm   **16.** -rrhexis   **21.** dacry/o

2. choroid/o   **7.** ophthalm/o   **12.** irid/o   **17.** -malacia   **22.** tympan/o, myring/o

3. kerat/o   **8.** blephar/o   **13.** -ptosis   **18.** audi/o, -acusis   **23.** corne/o

4. dipl/o, dipl-   **9.** aden/o   **14.** -logist   **19.** -stenosis   **24.** -opia, -opsia

5. ot/o   **10.** scler/o   **15.** retin/o   **20.** -edema   **25.** xanth/o

Additional Medical Terms Review

1. tinnitus   **8.** conjunctivitis   **15.** astigmatism   **21.** phacoemulsification

2. otosclerosis   **9.** photophobia   **16.** acoustic neuroma   **22.** Rinne test

3. achromatopsia   **10.** presbycusis   **17.** tonometry   **23.** diabetic retinopathy

4. Ménière disease   **11.** glaucoma   **18.** iridectomy   **24.** macular degeneration

5. strabismus   **12.** vertigo   **19.** conductive hearing loss   **25.** myringotomy

6. anacusis   **13.** retinal detachment

7. otitis media   **14.** hordeolum   **20.** cataract

Medical Record Activity 11–1: Retinal Detachment

Evaluation

1. Where is the retina located?

The retina is the innermost layer of the eye

2. Was the anesthetic administered behind or in front of the eyeball?

Behind the eyeball (retrobulbar)

3. How much movement remained in the eye following anesthesia?

None; akinesia

4. Where was the hemorrhage located?

In the orbit of the eye behind the lens, where the vitreous humor is located

5. What type of vitrectomy was undertaken?

Trans pars plana vitrectomy

6. Why was the eye left soft?

Because it had poor perfusion

Medical Record Activity 11–2: Otitis Media

Evaluation

1. Where was the patient's infection located?

Right ear

2. What complication developed while the patient was hospitalized?

Cholesteatoma

3. What is the purpose of the tube placement?

It reduces the accumulation of fluid within the middle ear

4. What surgery is being performed to resolve the cholesteatoma?

Tympanoplasty, right ear

5. Will the patient be asleep during the surgery?

Yes, under general anesthesia

Vocabulary Review

1. diplopia
2. sclera
3. tympanic membrane
4. dacryorrhea
5. eustachian tube

6. keratitis
7. diagnosis
8. mucoserous
9. otitis media
10. cholesteatoma

11. mastoid surgery
12. general anesthetic
13. ophthalmologist
14. chronic
15. hyperopia

16. postoperatively
17. labyrinth
18. blepharoptosis
19. salpingostenosis
20. myopia

C Index of Diagnostic, Medical, and Surgical Procedures

This section provides a list of the diagnostic, medical, and surgical procedures covered in the textbook along with page numbers. Diagnostic procedures help the physician determine a patient's health status, evaluate the factors influencing that status, and determine a method of treatment. Medical and surgical procedures are performed to treat a specific disorder that is diagnosed by the physician.

Diagnostic Procedures

Medical and Surgical Procedures

D Drug Classifications

This section provides a quick reference of common drug categories. They include prescription and over-the-counter drugs that are used to treat symptoms, signs, and diseases of the various body systems.

Drug Classification	Description
alkylates	Treat certain types of malignancies *Alkylates break deoxyribonucleic acid (DNA) strands in the cancerous cell by substituting an alkyl group for a hydrogen molecule in the DNA.*
analgesics	Relieve minor to severe pain *Analgesics include nonprescription drugs, such as aspirin and other nonsteroidal anti-inflammatory agents, and those classified as controlled substances and available only by prescription.*
angiotensin-converting enzyme inhibitors	Lower blood pressure by inhibiting conversion of angiotensin I (an inactive enzyme) to angiotensin II (a potent vasoconstrictor)
androgens	Increase testosterone levels *Hyposecretion of testosterone may be due to surgical removal of testes, or decreased levels of luteinizing hormone (LH) from the anterior pituitary gland.*
anesthetics	Produce partial or complete loss of sensation, with or without loss of consciousness *General anesthetics act upon the brain to produce complete loss of feeling with loss of consciousness. Local anesthetics act upon nerves or nerve tracts to affect a local area only.*
antacids	Neutralize excess acid in the stomach and help relieve gastritis and ulcer pain *Antacids also are used to relieve indigestion and reflux esophagitis (heartburn).*
antianginals	Relieve angina pectoris by vasodilation
antianxiety drugs	Reduce anxiety and neurosis *Antianxiety drugs are classified as minor tranquilizers and anxiolytics.*
antiarrhythmics	Treat cardiac arrhythmias by stabilizing the electrical conduction of the heart

Drug Classification	Description
antibiotics	Inhibit growth of or destroy microorganisms *Antibiotics are used extensively in treatment of infectious diseases.*
anticoagulants	Prevent or delay blood coagulation *Anticoagulants prevent deep vein thrombosis (DVT) and postoperative clot formation and decrease the risk of stroke.*
anticonvulsants	Prevent or reduce the severity of epileptic or other convulsive seizures; also called *antiepileptics*
antidepressants	Regulate mood and reduce symptoms of depression by affecting the amount of neurotransmitters in the brain
antidiabetics	Stimulate the pancreas to produce more insulin and decrease peripheral resistance to insulin *Antidiabetics are taken orally to treat type 2 diabetes mellitus.*
antidiarrheals	Control loose stools and relieve diarrhea by absorbing excess water in the bowel or slowing peristalsis in the intestinal tract
antidiuretics	Reduce the production of urine
antiemetics	Prevent or suppress vomiting *Antiemetics are also used in the treatment of vertigo, motion sickness, and nausea.*
antifungals	Alter the cell wall of fungi or disrupt enzyme activity, resulting in cellular death
antihistamines	Counteract the effects of a histamine *Antihistamines inhibit allergic reactions of inflammation, redness, and itching, especially hay fever and other allergic disorders of the nasal passages.*
antihyperlipidemics	Lower lipid levels in the bloodstream *Antihyperlipidemics reduce the risk of heart attack by lowering lipid levels.*
antihypertensives	Lower blood pressure
anti-impotence	Treat erectile dysfunction (impotence) by increasing blood flow to the penis, resulting in an erection
anti-infectives, antibacterials, antifungals	Eliminate or inhibit bacterial or fungal infections *Anti-infectives, antibacterials, and antifungals can be administered either topically or systemically.*

(continued)

Drug Classification	Description
anti-inflammatories	Relieve the swelling, tenderness, redness, and pain of inflammation *Anti-inflammatories may be classified as steroidal (corticosteroids) or nonsteroidal.*
corticosteroids (glucocorticoids)	Relieve inflammation and replace hormones for adrenal insufficiency (Addison disease) *Corticosteroids are widely used to suppress the immune system's inflammatory response to tissue damage, controlling allergic reactions, reducing the rejection process in tissue and organ transplantation, and treating some cancers.*
nonsteroidals (NSAIDs)	Relieve inflammation associated with arthritis and related disorders
antimetabolites	Interfere with the use of enzymes required for cell division *Antimetabolites block folic acid, a B vitamin required for synthesis of some amino acids in the DNA of cancerous cells.*
antimicrobials	Destroy or inhibit the growth of bacteria, fungi, and protozoa, depending on the particular drug, generally by interfering with the functions of their cell membrane or their reproductive cycle
antiparkinsonians	Control tremors and muscle rigidity associated with Parkinson disease by increasing dopamine levels in the brain
antipruritics	Prevent or relieve itching
antipsychotics	Treat psychosis, paranoia, and schizophrenia by altering chemicals in the brain, including the limbic system (group of brain structures), which controls emotions
antiseptics	Topically applied agent that destroys or inhibits the growth of bacteria, preventing infection in cuts, scratches, and surgical incisions
antispasmodics	Act on the autonomic nervous system to reduce spasms in the bladder or GI tract
antithyroids	Treat hyperthyroidism by impeding the formation of T_3 and T_4 hormone
antituberculars	Used in the treatment of tuberculosis *Several of these drugs are used in combination to produce effective treatment.*
antitussives	Relieve or suppress coughing by blocking the cough reflex in the medulla of the brain
antivirals	Prevent replication of viruses within host cells *Antivirals are used in treatment of HIV infection and AIDS.*
astringents	Shrink the blood vessels locally, dry up secretions from seeping lesions, and lessen skin sensitivity

Drug Classification	Description
beta-adrenergic blockers	Treat cardiac arrhythmias, angina pectoris, and hypertension and improve outcomes after myocardial infarction; also called *beta blockers* *Beta-adrenergic blocking agents block the effect of epinephrine on beta receptors, slowing the nerve pulses that pass through the heart, thereby causing a decrease in heart rate and contractility. Some beta-adrenergic blockers are also used to treat glaucoma.*
bone resorption inhibitors	Inhibit breakdown of bone *Bone resorption inhibitors are used to treat osteoporosis.*
bronchodilators	Stimulate bronchial muscles to relax, thereby expanding air passages and resulting in increased air flow to the lungs
calcium channel blockers	Selectively block movement of calcium (required for blood vessel contraction) into myocardial cells and arterial walls, causing heart rate and blood pressure to decrease *Calcium channel blockers are used to treat angina pectoris, arrhythmias, heart failure, and hypertension.*
chrysotherapy	Treat certain diseases with gold compounds; also called *gold therapy* *Chrysotherapy is used to treat rheumatoid arthritis.*
contraceptives **birth control patch**	Prevent conception or ovulation; also called *birth control* Delivers two synthetic hormones, progestin and estrogen, through a transdermal patch, impeding pregnancy by preventing the ovaries from releasing eggs (ovulation) and thickening the cervical mucus *The patch is applied directly to the skin (buttocks, abdomen, upper torso, or upper outer arm) and has an effectiveness rate of 95%.*
injectable	Delivers a synthetic drug similar to progesterone (medroxyprogesterone acetate) through an injection administered four times per year that prevents the ovaries from releasing eggs (ovulation) and thickens the cervical mucus *When used as directed, an injectable contraceptive (Depo-Provera) may prevent pregnancy more than 99% of the time.*
oral	Inhibits ovulation and pituitary secretion of luteinizing hormone (LH), causing changes in cervical mucus that render it unfavorable to penetration by sperm and altering the nature of the endometrium; also called *birth control pills* *Oral contraceptives (OCs) contain mixtures of estrogen and progestin in various levels of strength. When used as directed, oral contraceptives (OCs) are nearly 100% effective.*
cycloplegics	Paralyze the ciliary muscles, resulting in pupil dilation *Cycloplegics are used to dilate the pupils to facilitate certain eye examinations and surgical procedures.*

(continued)

Drug Classification	Description
cytotoxics	Disrupt nucleic acid and protein synthesis, causing immunosuppression and cancer cell death *Cytotoxics are used to treat cancer and autoimmune diseases, such as inflammatory bowel disease and systemic vasculitis. They are also used to prevent rejection in transplant recipients.*
decongestants	Decrease congestion of mucous membranes of sinuses and nose *Decongestants are used for temporary relief of nasal congestion associated with the common cold, hay fever, other upper respiratory allergies, and sinusitis.*
diuretics	Act on the kidney to promote the excretion of sodium and water *Diuretics are used to treat edema and hypertension.*
emetics	Used to induce vomiting, especially in cases of poisoning
estrogen hormone	Used in estrogen replacement therapy (ERT) during menopause to correct estrogen deficiency and as chemotherapy for some types of cancer, including tumors of the prostate
expectorants	Liquefy respiratory secretions so that they are more easily dislodged during coughing episodes
fibrinolytics	Trigger the body to produce plasmin, an enzyme that dissolves clots *Fibrinolytics are used to treat acute pulmonary embolism and, occasionally, deep vein thrombosis.*
gonadotropins	Raise sperm count in infertility cases
growth hormone replacements	Increase skeletal growth in children and growth hormone deficiencies in adults
H_2 blockers	Block histamine-2 (H_2) receptors in the stomach to decrease the release of hydrochloric acid *H_2 blockers are used to treat peptic ulcers.*
hemostatics	Prevent or control bleeding *Hemostatics are used to treat blood disorders and certain bleeding problems associated with surgery.*
hypnotics	Depress the central nervous system (CNS) to induce or maintain sleep
inotropics, cardiotonics	Increase the efficiency of contractions of the heart muscle *Inotropics are used to treat cardiac arrhythmias and cardiac failure.*
insulins	Synthetic form of insulin hormone for diabetes administered by injection to lower the glucose (sugar) level in the blood

Drug Classification	Description
keratolytics	Destroy and soften the outer layer of skin so that it is sloughed off or shed. *Strong keratolytics are effective for removing warts and corns. Milder preparations are used to promote the shedding of scales and crusts in eczema, psoriasis, and seborrheic dermatitis. Weak keratolytics irritate inflamed skin, acting as tonics that speed up the healing process.*
laxatives (cathartic, purgative)	Induce bowel movements or loosen stool *When used in smaller doses, laxatives relieve constipation. When used in larger doses, they evacuate the entire gastrointestinal tract; for example, as preparation for surgery or intestinal radiologic examinations.*
miotics	Constrict the pupil of the eye *Miotics are used in the treatment of glaucoma.*
mucolytics	Liquefy sputum or reduce its viscosity so that it can be coughed up more easily
mydriatics	Dilate the pupil and paralyze the muscles of accommodation of the iris *Mydriatics are used to prepare the eye for internal examination and to treat inflammatory conditions of the iris.*
nitrates	Treat angina pectoris by dilating arteries and increasing blood flow to the myocardium
opiates	Relieve pain *Opiates contain opium or its derivative. They are commonly prescribed on a short-term basis due to their strong addictive property.*
parasiticides	Destroy systemic parasites, such as pinworm or tapeworm, in oral form, or insect parasites, such as mites and lice, in topical form
potassium supplements	Increase the potassium level of the blood *Potassium can be administered orally or intravenously (IV) when dangerously low levels occur. It is used as a replacement for potassium loss due to diuretics.*
prostaglandins	Used to induce labor, terminate pregnancy, or treat erectile dysfunction, patent ductus arteriosis, or pulmonary hypertension
protectives	Function by covering, cooling, drying, or soothing inflamed skin *Protectives do not penetrate or soften the skin but form a long-lasting film that protects the skin from air, water, and clothing during the natural healing process.*
proton pump inhibitors	Block the final stage of hydrochloric acid production in the stomach *Proton pump inhibitors are used to treat peptic ulcers and gastroesophageal reflux disease (GERD).*

(continued)

Drug Classification	Description
psychotropics	Alter chemical balance in the brain, causing changes in perception, mood, and behavior *Psychotropics are commonly employed in the management of psychiatric disorders.*
relaxants	Reduce tension, causing relaxation of muscles or bowel
salicylates	Relieve mild to moderate pain and reduce inflammation
sedatives	Exert a calming or tranquilizing effect
skeletal muscle relaxants	Relieve muscle spasms and stiffness
spermicides	Chemically destroy sperm *Spermicidals consist of jellies, creams, and foams and do not require a prescription. They are commonly used within the woman's vagina for contraceptive purposes.*
statins	Lower cholesterol in the blood and reduce its production in the liver by blocking the enzyme that produces it
thrombolytics	Dissolve blood clots by destroying their fibrin strands *Thrombolytics are used to break apart, or lyse, thrombi.*
thyroid supplements	Replace or supplement thyroid hormones
topical anesthetics	Block sensation of pain by numbing the skin layers and mucous membranes *Topical anesthetics are applied directly in sprays, creams, gargles, suppositories, and other preparations. They are also used to numb the skin to make the injection of medication more comfortable.*
tranquilizers	Calm anxiousness or agitation without decreasing consciousness
uricosurics	Increase urinary excretion of uric acid, reducing the concentration of uric acid in the blood *Uricosurics are used in treatment of gout.*
uterine stimulants	Induce labor at term, control postpartum hemorrhage, and induce therapeutic abortion; also called *oxytocic agents* *Oxytocin is a pharmaceutically prepared chemical that is similar to the pituitary hormone oxytocin. Uterine stimulants are also used to treat infertility in females.*
vasoconstrictors	Narrow or constrict the diameter of blood vessels *Vasoconstrictors are used to decrease blood flow and increase blood pressure.*
vasodilators	Dilate the diameter of blood vessels *Vasodilators are used in treatment of angina pectoris and hypertension.*
vitamin B$_{12}$	Treats pernicious anemia *Vitamin B$_{12}$ is delivered by nasal spray or intramuscular (IM) injection.*

Abbreviations

The table below lists common abbreviations used in health care and related fields along with their meanings.

Abbreviations	Meaning	Abbreviations	Meaning
A		**AI**	artificial insemination
A&P	anatomy and physiology; auscultation and percussion	**AICD**	automatic implantable cardioverter defibrillator
A, B, AB, O	blood types in ABO blood group	**AIDS**	acquired immune deficiency syndrome
AAA	abdominal aortic aneurysm	**AK**	above the knee
AB, Ab, ab	antibody; abortion	**ALL**	acute lymphocytic leukemia
ABC	aspiration biopsy cytology	**ALS**	amyotrophic lateral sclerosis (also called *Lou Gehrig disease*)
ABG	arterial blood gas(es)		
a.c.*	Before meals	**ALT**	alanine aminotransferase
ACL	anterior cruciate ligament	**AM, a.m.**	in the morning, or before noon
ACTH	adrenocorticotropic hormone	**AML**	acute myelogenous leukemia
AD*	Right ear		
ad lib.	as desired	**ANS**	autonomic nervous system
AD*	right ear	**ant**	anterior
ADH	antidiuretic hormone (vasopressin)	**AOM**	acute otitis media
		AP	anteroposterior
ADHD	attention-deficit hyperactivity disorder	**ARDS**	acute respiratory distress syndrome
ADLs	activities of daily living	**ARF**	acute renal failure
AE	above the elbow	**ARMD, AMD**	age-related macular degeneration
AED	automatic external defibrillator	**AS**	aortic stenosis
AF	atrial fibrillation	**AS***	left ear
AFB	acid-fast bacillus (TB organism)	**ASD**	atrial septal defect
		ASHD	arteriosclerotic heart disease
AGN	acute glomerulonephritis	**AST**	angiotensin sensitivity test

(continued)

Abbreviations	Meaning	Abbreviations	Meaning
Ast	astigmatism	CAH	chronic active hepatitis; congenital adrenal hyperplasia
AU*	both ears		
AV	atrioventricular; arteriovenous	CAT	computed axial tomography
		Cath	catheterization; catheter
B		CBC	complete blood count
Ba	barium	CC	cardiac catheterization; chief complaint
baso	basophil (type of white blood cell)	cc*	cubic centimeters; same as milliliters (1/1000 of a liter)
BBB	bundle branch block		
BC	bone conduction		
BCC	basal cell carcinoma	CCU	coronary care unit
BE	barium enema; below the elbow	CDH	congenital dislocation of the hip
BG	blood glucose	CF	cystic fibrosis
b.i.d.*	twice a day	CHD	coronary heart disease
BK	below the knee	chemo	chemotherapy
BKA	below-knee amputation	CHF	congestive heart failure
BM	bowel movement	Chol	cholesterol
BMI	body mass index	CLL	chronic lymphocytic leukemia
BMR	basal metabolic rate		
BNO	bladder neck obstruction	CK	creatine kinase (cardiac enzyme); conductive keratoplasty
BP, B/P	blood pressure		
BPH	benign prostatic hyperplasia; benign prostatic hypertrophy		
		cm	centimeter (1/100 of a meter)
BS	blood sugar	CML	chronic myelogenous leukemia
BSE	breasrt self-examination		
BSO	bilateral salpingo-oophorectomy	CNS	central nervous system
		c/o	complains of, complaints
BUN	blood urea nitrogen	CO	cardiac output
Bx, bx	biopsy	CO₂	carbon dioxide
C		COPD	chronic obstructive pulmonary disease
C1, C2, and so on	first cervical vertebra, second cervical vertebra, and so on	CP	cerebral palsy
		CPAP	continuous positive airway pressure
CA	cancer; chronological age; cardiac arrest	CPD	cephalopelvic disproportion
Ca	calcium; cancer	CPK	creatine phosphokinase (enzyme released into the bloodstream after a heart attack)
CABG	coronary artery bypass graft		
CAD	coronary artery disease		

Abbreviations	Meaning	Abbreviations	Meaning
CPR	cardiopulmonary resuscitation	D.P.M.	Doctor of Podiatric Medicine
CRF	chronic renal failure	DPT	diphtheria, pertussis, tetanus
CRRT	continuous renal replacement therapy	DRE	digital rectal examination
C&S	culture and sensitivity	DSA	digital subtraction angiography
CS, C-section	cesarean section	DUB	dysfunctional uterine bleeding
CSF	cerebrospinal fluid	DVT	deep vein thrombosis; deep venous thrombosis
CT	computed tomography		
CTS	carpal tunnel syndrome	Dx	diagnosis
CV	cardiovascular	**E**	
CVA	cerebrovascular accident; costovertebral angle	EBV	Epstein-Barr virus
CVD	cardiovascular disease	ECCE	extracapsular cataract extraction
CVS	chorionic villus sampling	ECG, EKG	electrocardiogram; electrocardiography
CWP	childbirth without pain		
CXR	chest x-ray, chest radiograph	ECHO	echocardiogram; echocardiography; echoencephalogram; echoencephalography
cysto	cystoscopy		
D			
D	diopter (lens strength)	ED	erectile dysfunction; emergency department
dc, DC, D/C*	discharge; discontinue		
D&C	dilatation (dilation) and curettage	EEG	electroencephalography; electroencephalogram
Decub.	decubitus (lying down)	EENT	eyes, ears, nose, and throat
derm	dermatology	EF	ejection fraction
DES	diffuse esophageal spasm; drug-eluting stent	EGD	esophagogastroduodenoscopy
		ELT	endovenous laser ablation; endoluminal laser ablation
DEXA, DXA	dual energy x-ray absorptiometry		
DI	diabetes insipidus; diagnostic imaging	Em	emmetropia
		EMG	electromyography
diff	differential count (white blood cells)	ENT	ears, nose, and throat
		EOM	extraocular movement
DJD	degenerative joint disease	eos	eosinophil (type of white blood cell)
DKA	diabetic ketoacidosis		
DMARDs	disease modifying antirheumatic drugs	ERCP	endoscopic retrograde cholangiopancreatography
DM	diabetes mellitus	ESR	erythrocyte sedimentation rate
DNA	deoxyribonucleic acid		
D.O., DO	Doctor of Osteopathy	ESRD	end-stage renal disease
DOE	dyspnea on exertion	ESWL	extracorporeal shock-wave lithotripsy
DPI	dry powder inhaler	ETT	exercise tolerance test

(continued)

Abbreviations	Meaning	Abbreviations	Meaning
F		**HDL**	high-density lipoprotein
FBS	fasting blood sugar	**HDN**	hemolytic disease of the newborn
FECG, FEKG	fetal electrocardiogram	**HDV**	hepatitis D virus
FH	family history	**HEV**	hepatitis E virus
FHR	fetal heart rate	**HF**	heart failure
FHT	fetal heart tone	**HIV**	human immunodeficiency virus
FS	frozen section		
FSH	follicle-stimulating hormone	**HMD**	hyaline membrane disease
FTND	full-term normal delivery	**HNP**	herniated nucleus pulposus (herniated disk)
FVC	forced vital capacity	**H₂O** H_2O	water
Fx	fracture	**HP**	hemipelvectomy
G		**HPV**	human papillomavirus
G	gravida (pregnant)	**HRT**	hormone replacement therapy
g, gm	gram		
GB	gallbladder	**h.s.***	at bedtime
GBS	gallbladder series (x-ray studies)	**hs***	half strength
		HSG	hysterosalpingography
GC	gonococcus (*Neisseria gonorrhoeae*)	**HSV**	herpes simplex virus
		HTN	hypertension
G-CSF	granulocyte colony-stimulating factor	**Hx**	history
		I, J	
GER	gastroesophageal reflux	**IAS**	interatrial septum
GERD	gastroesophageal reflux disease	**I&D**	incision and drainage; irrigation and debridement
GH	growth hormone		
GI	gastrointestinal	**IBD**	irritable bowel disease
GTT	glucose tolerance test	**IBS**	irritable bowel syndrome
GU	genitourinary	**ICD**	implantable cardioverter-defibrillator
GVHD	graft-versus-host disease		
GVHR	graft-versus-host reaction	**ICP**	intracranial pressure
GYN	gynecology	**ICU**	intensive care unit
		ID	intradermal
H		**IDDM**	insulin-dependent diabetes mellitus
HAV	hepatitis A virus		
Hb, Hgb, hgb	hemoglobin	**Ig**	immunoglobulin
HBV	hepatitis B virus	**IM**	intramuscular; infectious mononucleosis
HCG	human chorionic gonadotropin		
HCl	hydrochloric acid	**IMP**	impression (synonymous with diagnosis)
HCT, Hct	hematocrit		
HCV	hepatitis C virus	**IOL**	intraocular lens
HD	hemodialysis; hip disarticulation; hearing distance	**IT**	intensive therapy
		IVP	intravenous pyelogram; intravenous pyelography

Abbreviations	Meaning	Abbreviations	Meaning
IOP	intraocular pressure	LPR	laryngopharyngeal reflux
IPPB	intermittent positive-pressure breathing	LS	lumbosacral spine
		LSO	left salpingo-oophorectomy
IRDS	infant respiratory distress syndrome	lt	left
		LUQ	left upper quadrant
IT	intensive therapy	LV	left ventricle
IUD	intrauterine device	lymphos	lymphocytes
IUGR	intrauterine growth rate; intrauterine growth retardation	**M**	
		MCH	mean cell hemoglobin (average amount of hemoglobin per red cell)
IV	intravenous		
IVC	intravenous cholangiogram; intravenous cholangiography	MCHC	mean cell hemoglobin concentration (average concentration of hemoglobin per red cell)
IVF	in vitro fertilization		
IVF-ET	in vitro fertilization and embryo transfer	MCV	mean cell volume (average volume or size per red cell)
IVP	intravenous pyelography	MDI	metered-dose inhaler
K		MEG	magnetoencephalography
K	potassium (an electrolyte)	MG	myasthenia gravis
KD	knee disarticulation	mg	milligram (1/1000 of a gram)
KUB	kidney, ureter, bladder		
L		mg/dl, mg/dL	milligram per deciliter
L	liter	MI	myocardial infarction
L1, L2, and so on	first lumbar vertebra, second lumbar vertebra, and so on	mix astig	mixed astigmatism
		ml, mL	milliliter (1/1000 of a liter)
		mm	millimeter (1/1000 of a meter)
LA	left atrium		
LASIK	laser-assisted in situ keratomileusis	mm Hg	millimeters of mercury
		MR	mitral regurgitation
LAT, lat	lateral	MRA	magnetic resonance angiogram; magnetic resonance angiography
LBBB	left bundle branch block		
LD	lactate dehydrogenase; lactic acid dehydrogenase (cardiac enzyme)		
		MRI	magnetic resonance imaging
		MS	mitral stenosis; musculoskeletal; multiple sclerosis; mental status; magnesium sulfate
LDL	low-density lipoprotein		
LES	lower esophageal sphincter		
LFT	liver function test		
LH	luteinizing hormone	MSH	melanocyte-stimulating hormone
LLQ	left lower quadrant		
LMP	last menstrual period	MUGA	multiple-gated acquisition (scan)
LOC	loss of consciousness		
LP	lumbar puncture	MVP	mitral valve prolapse

(continued)

Abbreviations	Meaning	Abbreviations	Meaning
MVR	mitral valve replacement; massive vitreous retraction (blade); microvitreoretinal	PAC	premature atrial contraction
		Pap	Papanicolaou (test)
Myop	myopia (nearsightedness)	para 1, 2, 3 and so on	unipara, bipara, tripara and so on (number of viable births)
N		PAT	paroxysmal atrial tachycardia
Na	sodium (an electrolyte)	PBI	protein-bound iodine
NB	newborn	pc, p.c.*	after meals
NCV	nerve conduction velocity	PCL	posterior cruciate ligament
NG	nasogastric	PCNL	percutaneous nephrolithotomy
NIDDM	non–insulin-dependent diabetes mellitus	Pco_2	partial pressure of carbon dioxide
NIHL	noise-induced hearing loss	PCP	*Pneumocystis* pneumonia; primary care physician; phencyclidine (hallucinogen)
NK	natural killer cell		
NMT	nebulized mist treatment		
NPO, n.p.o.*	nothing by mouth	PE	physical examination; pulmonary embolism; pressure-equalizing (tube)
NSAID	nonsteroidal anti-inflammatory drug		
NSR	normal sinus rhythm		
O		PERRLA	pupils equal, round, and reactive to light and accommodation
O_2	oxygen		
OB	obstetrics		
OCP	oral contraceptive pill	PET	positron emission tomography
O.D.	Doctor of Optometry	PFT	pulmonary function test
OD	overdose	PGH	pituitary growth hormone
OD*	right eye	pH	symbol for degree of acidity or alkalinity
OM	otitis media		
OP	outpatient; operative procedure	PID	pelvic inflammatory disease
OR	operating room	PIH	pregnancy-induced hypertension
ORTH, ortho	orthopedics		
OS*	left eye; by mouth (pharmacology)	PKD	polycystic kidney disease
		PMH	past medical history
OSA	obstructive sleep apnea	PMI	point of maximum impulse
OU*	both eyes	PMN, PMNL	polymorphonuclear leukocyte
P			
P	phosphorus; pulse	PMP	previous menstrual period
PA	posteroanterior; pernicious anemia; pulmonary artery; physician assistant	PMS	premenstrual syndrome
		PND	paroxysmal nocturnal dyspnea
		PNS	peripheral nervous system

Abbreviations	Meaning	Abbreviations	Meaning
p.o.*	by mouth	RGB	Roux-en-Y gastric bypass
Po$_2$	partial pressure of oxygen	RK	radial keratotomy
poly	polymorphonuclear leukocyte	RLQ	right lower quadrant
		R/O	rule out
post	posterior	ROM	range of motion
p.r.n.*	as required	RP	retrograde pyelogram; retrograde pyelography
PSA	prostate-specific antigen		
pt	patient	RSO	right salpingo-oophorectomy
PT	prothrombin time; physical therapy	rt	right
		RUQ	right upper quadrant
PTCA	percutaneous transluminal coronary angioplasty	RV	residual volume; right ventricle
PTH	parathyroid hormone (also called *parathormone*)	**S**	
		S1, S2, and so on	first sacral vertebra, second sacral vertebra, and so on
PTHC	percutaneous transhepatic cholangeography	SA, S-A	sinoatrial
		Sao$_2$	arterial oxygen saturation
PTT	partial thromboplastin time	SD	shoulder disarticulation
PUD	peptic ulcer disease	SIADH	syndrome of inappropriate antidiuretic hormone
PVC	premature ventricular contraction	SICS	small incision cataract surgery
Q		SIDS	sudden infant death syndrome
q.2h.*	every 2 hours	SLE	systemic lupus erythematosus; slit-lamp examination
qAM*	every morning		
q.d.*	every day		
q.h.*	every hour		
q.i.d.*	four times a day	SMAS	superficial musculoaponeurotic system (flap)
q.o.d.*	every other day		
qPM*	every evening	SNS	sympathetic nervous system
R		SOB	shortness of breath
RA	right atrium; rheumatoid arthritis	sono	sonogram
		SPECT	single photon emission computed tomography
RAI	radioactive iodine		
RAIU	radioactive iodine uptake	sp. gr.	specific gravity
RBC, rbc	red blood cell	ST	esotropia
RD	respiratory distress	stat., STAT	immediately
RDS	respiratory distress syndrome	STD	sexually transmitted disease
		subcu, Sub-Q, subQ*	subcutaneous (injection)
RF	rheumatoid factor; radio frequency	Sx	symptom

(continued)

Abbreviations	Meaning	Abbreviations	Meaning
T		**TVH-BSO**	total vaginal hysterectomy–bilateral salpingo-oophorectomy
T1, T2, and so on	first thoracic vertebra, second thoracic vertebra, and so on	**Tx**	treatment
T₃	triiodothyronine (thyroid hormone)	**U**	
T₄	thyroxine (thyroid hormone)	**UA**	urinalysis
T&A	tonsillectomy and adenoidectomy	**UC**	uterine contractions
TAH	total abdominal hysterectomy	**UGI**	upper gastrointestinal
TB	tuberculosis	**UGIS**	upper gastrointestinal series
TFT	thyroid function test	**U&L, U/L**	upper and lower
THA	total hip arthroplasty	**ung**	ointment
ther	therapy	**UPP**	uvulopalatopharyngoplasty
THR	total hip replacement	**URI**	upper respiratory infection
TIA	transient ischemic attack	**US**	ultrasound; ultrasonography
t.i.d.*	three times a day	**UTI**	urinary tract infection
TKA	total knee arthroplasty	**V**	
TKR	total knee replacement	**VA**	visual acuity
TPPV	trans pars plana vitrectomy	**VC**	vital capacity
TPR	temperature, pulse, and respiration	**VCUG**	voiding cystourethrography
TRAM	transverse rectus abdominis muscle	**VD**	venereal disease
TSE	testicular self-examination	**VF**	visual field
TSH	thyroid-stimulating hormone	**VSD**	ventricular septal defect
TSS	toxic shock syndrome	**VT**	ventricular tachycardia
TURP	transurethral resection of the prostate	**VUR**	vesicoureteral reflux
TVH	total vaginal hysterectomy	**W**	
		WBC, wbc	white blood cell
		WD	well-developed
		WN	well-nourished
		WNL	within normal limits
		X, Y, Z	
		XP, XDP	xeroderma pigmentosum
		XT	exotropia

*Although these abbreviations are currently found in medical records and clinical notes, they are easily misinterpreted. Thus, the Joint Commission (formerly JCAHO) requires their discontinuance. Instead, they recommend to write out their meanings. For a summary of these abbreviations, see the table below.

Summary of Discontinued Abbreviations

As noted above, the Joint Commission has recommended the discontinuance of certain abbreviations that are easily misinterpreted in medical records. The table below lists these abbreviations along with their meanings.

Abbreviation	Meaning
Medication and Therapy Time Schedule	
a.c.	before meals
b.i.d.	twice a day
hs	half strength
h.s.	at bedtime
NPO, n.p.o.	nothing by mouth
p.c.	after meals
p.o.	by mouth (orally)
p.r.n.	as required
qAM	every morning
q.d.	every day
q.h.	every hour
q.2h.	every 2 hours
q.i.d.	four times a day
q.o.d.	every other day
qPM	every evening
t.i.d.	three times a day
Other Related Abbreviations	
AD	right ear
AS	left ear
AU	both ears
cc	cubic centimeters; same as ml (1/1000 of a liter) *Use ml for milliliters or write out the meaning.*
dc, DC, D/C	discharge; discontinue
OD	right eye
OS	left eye
OU	both eyes
subcu, Sub-Q, subQ	subcutaneous (injection)
U	unit

Common Symbols

The table below lists some common symbols used in health care and related fields.

Symbol	Meaning	Symbol	Meaning
@	at	−	minus, negative
āā	of each	±	plus or minus; either positive or negative; indefinite
′	foot	∅	no
″	inch	#	number; following a number; pounds
c̄	with	÷	divided by
Δ	change; heat	/	divided by
p̄	after	×	multiplied by; magnification
pH	degree of acidity or alkalinity	=	equals
℞	prescription, treatment, therapy	≈	approximately equal
s̄	without	°	degree
→	to, in the direction of	%	percent
↑	increase(d), up	♀	female
↓	decrease(d), down	♂	male
+	plus, positive		

F Medical Specialties

Medical Specialty	Medical Specialist	Description of Medical Specialty
Allergy	Allergist	Diagnosis and treatment of allergic disorders caused by hypersensitivity to foods, pollens, dusts, and medicines
Anesthesiology	Anesthesiologist	Administration of agents capable of bringing about loss of sensation with or without loss of consciousness
Cardiology	Cardiologist	Diagnosis and treatment of heart and vascular disorders
General practice (GP)	General Practitioner (GP)	Coordination of total health care delivery to all members of the family, regardless of sex, including counseling; also known as *family medicine* *The GP encompasses several branches of medicine, including internal medicine, preventive medicine, pediatrics, surgery, obstetrics, and gynecology.*
Geriatrics	Geriatrician	Understanding of the physiologic characteristics of aging and the diagnosis and treatment of diseases affecting elderly patients; also known as *gerontology*
Gynecology	Gynecologist	Diagnosis and treatment of diseases of the female reproductive organs
Hematology	Hematologist	Diagnosis and treatment of diseases of the blood and blood-forming tissues
Immunology	Immunologist	Study of various elements of the immune system and their functions *Immunology includes treatment of immunodeficiency diseases such as AIDS; autoimmune diseases such as lupus erythematosus, allergies, and various cancer types related to the immune system.*

(continued)

Medical Specialty	Medical Specialist	Description of Medical Specialty
Internal medicine	Internist	Study of the physiological and pathological characteristcs of internal organs and the diagnosis and treatment of these organs
Neonatology	Neonatologist	Care and treatment of neonates
Nephrology	Nephrologist	Diagnosis and management of kidney disease, kidney transplantation, and dialysis therapies
Neurosurgery	Neurosurgeon	Surgery of the brain, spinal cord, and peripheral nerves
Obstetrics	Obstetrician	Care of women during pregnancy, childbirth, and postnatal care
Oncology	Oncologist	Diagnosis, treatment, and prevention of cancer *Oncologists are internal medicine physicians who specialize in the treatment of solid tumors (such as carcinomas and sarcomas) and liquid tumors (including hematologic malignancies such as leukemias).*
Ophthalmology	Ophthalmologist	Diagnosis and treatment of eye diseases, including prescribing corrective lenses
Optometry	Optometrist	Primary eye care, including testing the eyes for visual acuity, diagnosing and managing eye health, prescribing corrective lenses, and recommending eye exercises *An optometrist, licensed by the state, is not a medical doctor but is known as a Doctor of Optometry (OD).*
Orthopedics	Orthopedist	Prevention, diagnosis, care, and treatment of musculoskeletal disorders *Musculoskeletal disorders include injury to or disease of bones, joints, ligaments, muscles, and tendons.*
Otolaryngology	Otolaryngologist	Medical and surgical management of disorders of the ear, nose, and throat (ENT) and related structures of the head and neck
Pathology	Pathologist	Study and cause of disease *A pathologist usually specializes in autopsy or in clinical or surgical pathology.*
Pediatrics	Pediatrician	Diagnosis and treatment of disease in infants, children, and adolescents
Plastic surgery	Plastic surgeon	Surgery to alter, replace, and restore a body structure due to a defect or for cosmetic reasons

Medical Specialty	Medical Specialist	Description of Medical Specialty
Physiatry	Physiatrist	Prevention, diagnosis, and treatment of disease or injury and the rehabilitation from resultant impairment and disability; also called *physical medicine* *Physiatrists are physicians who use physical agents such as light, heat, cold water, therapeutic exercise, mechanical apparatus and, sometimes, pharmaceutical agents.*
Pulmonology	Pulmonologist	Diagnosis and treatment of diseases involving the lungs, its airways and blood vessels, and the chest wall (thoracic cage); also called *pulmonary medicine*
Psychiatry	Psychiatrist	Diagnosis, treatment, and prevention of disorders of the mind *Psychiatry is different from others discussed in this book because it deals with pathological conditions of the mind, an entity that is not considered a body system.*
Radiology	Radiologist	Diagnosis using x-ray and other diagnostic procedures, such as ultrasound (US), computed tomography (CT), and magnetic resonance imaging (MRI) *Radiology also employs various radiation techniques to treat disease through other subspecialties of radiology, such as interventional radiology and nuclear medicine.*
Rheumatology	Rheumatologist	Diagnosis and treatment of inflammatory and degenerative diseases of the joints
Surgery	Surgeon	Use of operative procedures to treat deformity, injury, and disease
Thoracic surgery	Thoracic surgeon	Use of operative procedures to treat disease or injury of the thoracic area
Urology	Urologist	Diagnosis and treatment of the male urinary and reproductive systems and the female urinary system

G Glossary of English-to-Spanish Translations

This appendix provides guidelines to help health care practitioners communicate with their Spanish-speaking patients. The following list includes selected terms commonly used in various medical specialties.

Spanish Sounds

Although the spelling of some Spanish terms resembles English terms, the terms are still pronounced with a Spanish accent. Because of these similarities, the practitioner should learn the meaning and pronunciations of certain Spanish words. The first step in communicating with Spanish-speaking patients is to learn the Spanish sound system. This section provides Spanish pronunciations of vowels and consonants. The table below lists vowels and their Spanish pronunciations. Practice the pronunciations before continuing with the other information in this appendix.

Letter	Spanish Pronunciation Sounds Like
Vowels	
a	*ah* as in father
e	*eh* as in net
i	*ee* as in keep
o	*oh* as in no
u	*oo* as in spoon; silent following q or g
y	*ee* as in bee
Consonants	
c	*k* as in kitten (before *a*, *o*, *u*, and any consonant except *h*); *s* as in sit (before *e* or *i*); *k* after *e* or *i*
g	*h* as in hit (when followed by *e* or *i*); otherwise, like *g* as in gold

Letter	Spanish Pronunciation Sounds Like
h	silent; never pronounced unless preceded by *c*
j	*h* as in hot
ll	*y* as in yellow
ñ	*ni* as in onion
qu*	*k* as in kite
r	trilled *r*
rr*	strongly trilled *r*
v	*v* as in void
z	*s* as in sun

*Note: *qu* and *rr* are not consonants but rather sounds. As such they are not part of the Spanish alphabet. We include them here purely as an aid in pronunciation for non–Spanish speaking health care providers.

Emphasis in Spanish

In the table below, capitalization is used to indicate primary emphasis of Spanish words. The capital letters in the Spanish pronunciation column indicate that emphasis is placed on the capitalized syllable. You will note that some Spanish terms, such as *perspiración* and *úlcera*, have a diacritical mark above a vowel. This mark indicates emphasis that falls on a syllable other than the one predicted by the rules of Spanish pronunciation.

Although there are some exceptions to these rules, the suggested guidelines here will help you learn Spanish terms and pronunciations of selected key terms in each chapter. Start by reviewing English and Spanish terms, and then practice Spanish pronunciations by applying the English system of phonetics.

Adjective Endings

Many Spanish adjectives change the last letter of the word to denote the gender of the noun being modified. If the noun is feminine, the letter will be *a;* for a masculine noun, the letter used is *o*. For example, the adjective *lenta* (slow) modifies a feminine noun. The same adjective when modifying a masculine noun ends with the letter *o*, so it would be *lento*. To change the gender of an adjective to correspond with the noun it modifies, change the ending vowel. For example, if the noun is masculine, change the ending vowel to *o*. The table below clearly identifies Spanish adjectives that should receive a specific gender.

English-to-Spanish Translations

The following selected terms are used in the medical environment to denote anatomical structures and their functions; signs, symptoms, and diseases; as well as other related terms.

English	Spanish	Spanish Pronunciation
abdomen	abdomen	**ab-DOH-men**
adrenal gland	glándula adrenal	**GLAN-doo-lah ah-dreh-NAHL**
adrenaline	adrenalina	**ah-dreh-nah-LEE-nah**
allergy	alergia	**ah-LEHR-hee-ah**
alveolus	alvéolo	**ahl-VEH-oh-loh**
aneurysm	aneurisma	**a-neh-oo-REES-mah**
ankle	tobillo	**toh-BEE-yoh**
antacid	antiácido	**ahn-tee-AH-see-doh**
appendix	apéndice	**ah-PEHN-dee-seh**
appetite	apetito	**ah-peh-TEE-toh**
arm	brazo	**BRAH-soh**
artery	arteria	**ahr-TEH-ree-ah**
arthritis	artritis	**ahr-TREE-tees**
asphyxia	asfixia	**ahs-FEEK-see-ah**
asthma	asma	**AHS-mah**
belch	eructar	**eh-rook-TAHR**
belly	barriga	**bahr-REE-gah**
benign	benigno	**beh-NEEG-noh**
birth	nacimiento	**nah-see-mee-ENH-toh**
black	negra (feminine)	**NEH-grah**
	negro (masculine)	**NEH-groh**
bladder	vejiga	**beh-HEE-gah**
blepharospasm	blefaroespasmo	**bleh-fah-roh-ehs-PAHS-moh**
blister	ampolla	**am-PO-yah**
blood	sangre	**SAHN-greh**
blood clot	coágulo de sangre	**koh-AH-goo-loh deh SAHN-greh**
blood pressure	presión sanguínea	**preh-see-OHN san-GEE-nee-ah**
blue	azul	**ah-SOOL**
bones	huesos	**oo-EH-sohs**
brain	cerebro	**seh-REH-broh**
breast	pecho	**PEH-cho**

English	Spanish	Spanish Pronunciation
breathe	respirar	**rehs-pee-RAHR**
breathing	respiración	**rehs-pee-rah-see-OHN**
bronchus	bronquios	**BROHN-kee-ohs**
brown	marrón	**mahr-ROHN**
	or	
	café	**cah-FAY**
burn	quemar	**keh-MAHR**
calcium	calcio	**KAHL-see-oh**
calculus	cálculo	**KAHL-coo-loh**
capillary	capilar	**kah-pee-LAHR**
cartilage	cartílago	**kahr-TEE-lah-goh**
catheter	catéter	**kah-TEH-tehr**
catheterization	cateterización	**kah-teh-teh-ree-sah-see-OHN**
cerumen	cera de los oídos	**CEH-rah deh lohs oh-EE-dohs**
cervix	cervix	**SERH-beex**
cesarean section	cesárea	**seh-SAH-reh-ah**
chew	masticar	**mahs-tee-KAHR**
choroidopathy	coroidopatía	**coh-roh-ee-doh-pah-TEE-ah**
circumcision	circuncisión	**seer-koon-see-see-OHN**
clear	clara (feminine)	**KLAH-rah**
	claro (masculine)	**KLAH-roh**
cloudy	nublado	**noo-BLAH-doh**
collarbone	clavícula	**klah-BEE-coo-lah**
colon	colon	**KOH-lohn**
colonoscopy	colonoscopia	**koh-loh-nohs-koh-PEE-ah**
conception	concepción	**khon-sehp-see-OHN**
concussion	concusión	**kohn-koo-see-OHN**
condom	condón	**kohn-DOHN**
conscious	consciente	**kohns-see-EHN-teh**
constipation	estreñimiento	**ehs-treh-nyee-mee-EHN-toh**
cough	toser	**toh-SEHR**
cystoscopy	cistoscopia	**sees-toh-scoh-PEE-ah**

(continued)

English	Spanish	Spanish Pronunciation
dark	obscuro	obs-COO-roh
deafness	sordera	sohr-DEH-rah
defecate	defecar	deh-feh-KAHR
dermatology	dermatologia	der-mah-to-lo-HEE-ah
diabetes	diabetes	dee-ah-BEH-tehs
dialysis	diálisis	dee-AH-lee-sees
diaphragm	diafragma	de-ah-FRAHG-mah
diarrhea	diarrea	dee-ah-RREH-ah
digestion	digestión	dee-hes-tee-OHN
diplopia	diplopia	dee-ploh-PEE-ah
diuretic	diurético	dee-oo-REH-tee-coh
dizzy	mareado	mah-reh-AH-doh
dyspepsia	dispepsia	dees-PEHP-see-ah
dysphagia	disfagia	dees-FAH-hee-ah
dysuria	disuria	dee-SOO-ree-ah
eardrum	tímpano del oído	TEEM-pah-noh dehl oh-EE-doh
ears	oídos	oh-EE-dohs
encephalopathy	encefalopatía	ehn-ceh-fah-loh-pah-TEE-ah
endometriosis	endometriosis	ehn-doh-meh-tree-OH-sees
epiglottis	epiglotis	eh-pee-GLOH-tees
epilepsy	epilepsia	eh-pee-LEHP-see-ah
erection	erección	eh-rek-see-OHN
esophagus	esófago	eh-SOH-fah-goh
excretion	excreción	ex-kreh-see-OHN
eyelid	párpado	PAHR-pah-doh
eyes	ojos	OH-hohs
fainting	desmayo	dehs-MAH-yoh
fracture	fractura	frahk-TOO-rah
gallbladder	vesícula biliar	beh-SEE-koo-lah bee-lee-AHR
gallstone	cálculo biliar	KAHL-koo-loh bee-lee-AHR

English	Spanish	Spanish Pronunciation
genitalia	genitalia	**heh-nee-TAH-lee-ah**
glucose	glucosa	**gloo-KO-sah**
goiter	bocio	**BOH-see-oh**
gums	encia	**ehn-SEE-ah**
hair	pelo	**PEH-loh**
hardening	endurecimiento	**en-doo-reh-see-mee-EHN-toh**
heart	corazón	**koh-rah-SOHN**
heart attack	ataque al corazón *or* ataque cardíaco	**ah-TAH-keh ahl koh-rah-SOHN** **ah-TAH-keh kar-DEE-ah-koh**
heart rate	ritmo cardíaco	**REET-moh kar-DEE-ah-koh**
hematuria	hematuria	**eh-mah-TOO-ree-ah**
hernia	hernia	**EHR-nee-ah**
herniated disk	disco herniado	**DEES-coh ehr-nee-AH-doh**
hip	cadera	**kah-DEH-rah**
hormone replacement	reemplazo de hormonas	**reh-ehm-PLAH-soh deh or-MOH-nahs**
hyperopia	hiperopía	**ee-pehr-oh-PEE-ah**
hysterectomy	histerectomía	**ees-teh-rek-toh-MEE-ah**
impotency	impotencia	**eem-poh-TEHN-see-ah**
influenza	influenza	**een-floo-EHN-sah**
inner ear	oído interior	**oh-EE-doh een-teh-ree-OHR**
insulin	insulina	**in-soo-LEE-nah**
intestine	intestino	**een-tehs-TEE-noh**
iodine	yodo	**YOH-doh**
iris	iris	**EE-rees**
jaundice	ictericia	**eek-teh-REE-see-ah**
joint	coyunturas	**ko-yoon-TOO-rahs**
kidney	riñón	**ree-NYOHN**
knee	rodilla	**roh-DEE-yah**
kneecap	rótula	**ROH-too-lah**
laparoscopy	laparoscopía	**lah-pah-rohs-KOH-pee-ah**

(continued)

English	Spanish	Spanish Pronunciation
larynx	laringe	lah-REEN-heh
leukorrhea	leucorrea	leh-oo-koh-RREH-ah
ligament	ligamento	lee-gah-MEHN-toh
light	luz	loos
liver	hígado	EE-gah-doh
lobe	lóbulo	LOH-boo-loh
lungs	pulmones	pool-MOH-nehs
lymph	linfa	LEEN-fah
lymph node	nódulo linfatico	NOH-doo-loh leen-FAH-tee-coh
lymphatic	linfático	leen-FAH-tee-coh
macular degeneration	degeneración macular	deh-heh-neh-rah-see-OHN mah-coo-LAHR
malignant	maligno	mah-LEEG-noh
mammogram	mamografía	mah-moh-grah-FEE-ah
masculine	masculino	mahs-koo-LEE-noh
menopause	menopausia	meh-noh-PAH-oo-see-ah
menstruation	menstruación	mehns-troo-ah-see-OHN
mouth	boca	BOH-kah
movement	movimiento	moh-bee-mee-EHN-toh
muscle	músculo	MOOS-koo-loh
myopia	miopía	mee-o-PEE-ah
nails	sarpullidos	sar-pooh-YEE-dohs
nerve	nervio	NER-bee-oh
newborn	recién nacida (feminine)	re-see-EHN nah-SEE-dah
	recién nacido (masculine)	re-see-EHN nah-SEE-doh
nocturia	nocturia	nok-TOO-ree-ah
nose	nariz	nah-REES
nostril	orificio de la nariz	o-ree-FEE-see-oh deh lah nah-REES
obstruction	obstrucción	obs-trook-see-OHN
oliguria	oliguria	oh-lee-GOO-ree-ah

English	Spanish	Spanish Pronunciation
ophthalmoscopy	oftalmoscopía	ohf-tahl-mohs-coh-PEE-ah
otalgia	otalgía	oh-tahl-HEE-ah
otitis media	otitis media	oh-TEE-tees MEH-dee-ah
otoscope	otoscopio	oh-tohs-COH-pee-oh
otoscopy	otoscopía	oh-tohs-coh-PEE-ah
ovary	ovario	oh-BAH-ree-oh
pain	dolor	doh-LOHR
pancreas	páncreas	PAHN-kreh-ahs
paralysis	parálisis	pah-RAH-lee-sees
penis	pene	PEH-neh
perspiration	perspiración	pehr-spee-rah-see-OHN
pink	rosada (female)	roh-SAH-dah
	rosado (male)	roh-SAH-doh
pituitary	pituitaria	pee-too-ee-TAH-ree-ah
pneumonia	pulmonía	pool-moh-NEE-ah
pregnant	embarazada	ehm-bah-rah-SAH-dah
prostate	próstata	PROHS-tah-tah
protein	proteína	proh-teh-EE-nah
pulse	pulso	POOL-soh
rapid	rápida (feminine)	RAH-pee-dah
	rápido (masculine)	RAH-pee-doh
rectum	recto	REHK-toh
reduction	reducción	reh-dook-see-OHN
renal pelvis	pelvis renal	PEHL-bees reh-NAHL
retina	retina	reh-TEE-nah
retinitis	retinitis	reh-tee-NEE-tees
rhythm	ritmo	REET-moh
rib	costilla	coh-STEE-yah
sacrum	sacro	SAH-croh
sclera	esclera	es-KLEH-rah

(continued)

English	Spanish	Spanish Pronunciation
seizure	convulsion	con-vuhl-see-OHN
	or	
	ataque de apoplejía	ah-TAH-keh deh ah-pohp-leh-HEE-uh
sensation	sensación	sen-sah-see-OHN
sexual intercourse	coito	KOH-ee-toh
shoulder	hombro	OHM-broh
sigmoidoscopy	sigmoidoscopia	seeg-moh-ee-doh-SKOH-pee-ah
sinus	seno	SEH-noh
skin	piel	pee-EHL
slow	lenta (feminine)	LEHN-tah
	lento (masculine)	LEHN-toh
sore	llaga	YAH-gah
	or	
	úlcera	OOL-seh-rah
spinal column	espina dorsal	ehs-PEE-nah dohr-SAHL
sprain	torcer	tohr-SEHR
sputum	esputo	ehs-POO-toh
sternum	esternón	ehs-tehr-NOHN
stiff	dura (feminine)	DOO-rah
	duro (masculine)	DOO-roh
stomach	estómago	es-TOH-mah-goh
stroke	ataque	ah-TAH-keh
stroke	ataque cerebral	ah-TAH-keh seh-reh-BRAHL
support	soporte	soh-POHR-teh
swallow	tragar	trah-GAHR
symptom	síntoma	SEEN-toh-mah
syncope	síncope	SEEN-coh-peh
teeth	diente	dee-EHN-teh
tendon	tendón	tehn-DOHN
testicle	testículo	tehs-TEE-koo-loh
thigh	muslo	MOOS-loh
thyroid	tiroides	tee-ROH-ee-dehs
tinnitus	tinitus	tee-NEE-toos

English	Spanish	Spanish Pronunciation
tissue	tejido	**teh-HEE-doh**
toe, finger	dedo	**DEH-doh**
tonsil	amígdala	**ah-MEEG-dah-lah**
trachea	tráquea	**TRAH-keh-ah**
ulcer	úlcera	**OOL-seh-rah**
ultrasonography	ultrasonografía	**ool-trah-soh-noh-grah-FEE-ah**
unconscious	inconsciente	**een-kons-see-EHN-teh**
ureter	uréter	**oo-REH-tehr**
urethra	uretra	**oo-REH-trah**
urinalysis	urinalisis	**oo-reh-NAH-lee-sees**
urinary	urinario	**oo-ree-NAH-ree-oh**
urinary tract infection	infección del tracto urinario	**een-fek-see-OHN dehl TRAK-toh oo-ree-NAH-ree-oh**
urinate	orinar	**oh-ree-NAHR**
urine	orina	**oh-REE-nah**
urology	urología	**ooh-roh-loh-HEE-ah**
uterus	útero	**OO-teh-roh**
vagina	vagina	**vah-HEE-NAH**
valve	válvula	**BAHL-boo-lah**
varicose vein	vena varicosa	**BEH-nah bah-ree-KOH-sah**
vein	vena	**BEH-nah**
ventricle	ventrículo	**behn-TREE-koo-loh**
vertebrae	vértebra	**BEHR-teh-brah**
vision	visión	**bee-see-OHN**
voice	voz	**bohs**
vomit	vómito	**BOH-mee-toh**
wound	herida	**eh-REE-dah**
wrist	muñeca	**moo-NYEH-kah**
x-ray	rayos equis *or* radiografía	**RAH-yohs EH-kees** **rah-dee-oh-grah-FEE-yah**
yellow	amarilla (feminine) amarillo (masculine)	**ah-mah-REE-yah** **ah-mah-REE-yoh**

Index